Bacterial Wilt Disease
and the
Ralstonia solanacearum
Species Complex

Edited by

Caitilyn Allen
University of Wisconsin-Madison
U.S.A.

Philippe Prior
INRA Centre de Avignon
Montfavet, France

A. C. Hayward
The University of Queensland
Brisbane, Australia

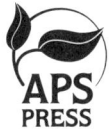

APS
PRESS

The American Phytopathological Society
St. Paul, Minnesota U.S.A.

Financial Sponsor
Australian Centre for International Agricultural Research

Cover photographs: Kenyan farmers planting potatoes by the seed-plot technique (courtesy Julian Smith, CAB International); see chapter by Kinyua et al. *Ralstonia solanacearum* cells expressing green fluorescent protein (GFP) colonizing tomato roots (courtesy Jian Yao, University of Wisconsin, and Jacques Vasse, INRA-Toulouse); see chapter by Vasse et al. Background, GFP-expressing *R. solanacearum* cells in a cross section of a tomato stem (courtesy Tim Denny, University of Georgia); see chapter by Denny.

This book has been reproduced directly from computer-generated copy submitted in final form to APS Press by the editors of the volume. No editing or proofreading has been done by the Press.

Reference in this publication to a trademark, proprietary product, or company name by personnel of the U.S. Department of Agriculture or anyone else is intended for explicit description only and does not imply approval or recommendation to the exclusion of others that may be suitable.

Library of Congress Control Number: 2005921793
International Standard Book Number: 0-89054-329-1

Printed in the United States of America on acid-free paper

The American Phytopathological Society
3340 Pilot Knob Road
St. Paul, Minnesota 55121, U.S.A.

Table of Contents

Preface

The bacterial wilt diseases caused by members of the *Ralstonia solanacearum* species complex have never been more important. The research presented in this volume reveals a pathogen on the move, with a growing global profile. While these diseases inflict ongoing and increasing crop losses on subsistence farmers, the pathogen now has significant political and economic impact in the developed world. The presence of the brown rot pathogen, *R. solanacearum* race 3 biovar 2, in European potato fields and waterways makes *R. solanacearum* a contentious topic in agricultural trade negotiations in the European Union. Since the Third International Bacterial Wilt Symposium (3rd IBWS), race 3 biovar 2 has been listed as a Select Agent in the U.S. Agroterrorism Protection Act of 2002, making it subject to strict new quarantine and eradication regulations. When geranium cuttings infected with race 3 biovar 2 were accidentally imported into the U.S. in 2003, the problem came full circle. This legislation had unforeseen economic impacts on laborers in Kenya and Guatemala, where race 3 biovar 2 is endemic and millions of ornamental plant cuttings are produced for the North American and European markets. More than ever, scientists who work with this pathogen must recognize that although bacterial wilt certainly can cause severe crop losses on a local scale, it also plays a complex and significant role in the worldwide agricultural matrix.

This volume is divided into seven subsections on topics ranging from the basic biology of the host-pathogen interaction to very applied research designed to immediately address disease losses in the field. With the intention of making this book a useful reference with a longer shelf life than a simple meeting proceedings, the organizers of the 3rd IBWS asked experts in various aspects of our subject to write brief overviews focusing on the pressing research needs in each area. These overview chapters open each subsection and are intended to give the reader our best current understanding of the topic and to suggest promising directions for future research.

The 3rd IBWS featured several substantial sessions on special topics of particular interest or controversy. To transmit the contents of these sessions, Dick Van Elsas and co-authors here summarize our current understanding (and lack thereof) concerning the viable-but-non-culturable (VBNC) form of *R. solanacearum*. Maria Lopez and Elena Biosca describe the significant challenges for understanding and controlling brown rot of potato. Reports at the 3rd IBWS indicated that the most rapid and alarming increases in bacterial wilt disease incidence around the world are on potatoes and on banana and plantain.

In addition, the book opens with two key general reviews. Chris Hayward presents a thoughtful analysis of international collaborations on bacterial wilt research in the context of a review of the literature published on this topic. He makes a compelling case that bacterial wilt researchers in the developing world have a critical need for access to published information and effective collaborations with colleagues in more developed nations. John Elphinstone accepted the Herculean task of compiling a global assessment of the current impact of bacterial wilt. Although there are still significant gaps and many estimates are of necessity based on incomplete data, thanks to his hard work and the many respondents to his inquiries we have for the first time a general idea of the real impact and extent of these diseases around the world.

The 3rd IBWS and this volume would not have been possible without the generous support of the Rockefeller Foundation, the U.S. National Science Foundation, CSIRO in Australia, the South African Agricultural Research Council, and all the authors who present their research here.

Caitilyn Allen
Madison, Wisconsin

Bacterial Wilt Disease
and the
Ralstonia solanacearum
Species Complex

Research on Bacterial Wilt: A Perspective on International Linkages and Access to the Literature

A.C. Hayward

Department of Microbiology and Parasitology,The University
of Queensland, St. Lucia 4072 Qld Australia

Bacterial wilt caused by *Ralstonia solanacearum* affects a wide range of crop plants and has a distribution extending throughout much of the wet tropics, sub-tropics and some warm temperate regions of the world (J. Elphinstone, this volume; 4,7,8). In recent decades a specific strain of the pathogen causing brown rot of potato has been found in many cool temperate regions of the northern and southern hemisphere where previously it was unknown or not recognized. Recent European and African experience has shown that there is potential for gross contamination of the environment – for example, of waterways as a result of infection of weed hosts (eg. *Solanum dulcamara*) growing at river margins. In potato and other susceptible host species the density of biomass generated in the vascular tissue probably far exceeds that of any other bacterial plant pathogen. There have been four reviews in the *Annual Review of Phytopathology* in the past three decades (3,4,6,15), an indication of the global impact and scientific interest of the disease.

The purpose of this chapter is to describe the development of international collaboration in bacterial wilt research and the benefits of networking and communication. Although in the age of the internet communication potentially occurs with greater ease and rapidity than ever before, the reality is that the benefits of information technology are denied to many in the developing world where bacterial wilt has greatest impact. Communication within the developing world and to and from the developing world is often slow and erratic. The *International Bacterial Wilt Symposia* provide opportunities for personal interaction and are one potent means of overcoming this difference in access to information on bacterial wilt.

1

International Linkages

Three of the international agriculture centers, the International Potato Center (CIP), the International Crops Research Institute for the Semi-Arid Tropics (ICRISAT) and the Asian Vegetable Research and Development Center (AVRDC) have pioneered collaborative research on bacterial wilt in the tropics and sub-tropics; they continue to promote research on the control of the disease on the crops for which they have a mandate: potato (CIP), peanut (ICRISAT), and tomato, eggplant, and pepper (AVRDC). Their major contributions have been in integrated disease management, collection, conservation and distribution of new sources of disease-resistant germplasm, plant breeding, and the evaluation of new lines and cultivars in multilocational field trials. The first phase of more broadly based collaborative linkages was marked by the *Planning Conference and Workshop on the Ecology and Control of Bacterial Wilt caused by Pseudomonas solanacearum* held in Raleigh, North Carolina in July, 1976, which was supported by grants from the US Agency for International Development, the University of California/AID Pest Management and Related Environmental Project, and CIP (16). Later meetings sponsored by the international centers addressed bacterial wilt on potato (1) and peanut (9,10,11). The *International Workshop on Bacterial Wilt* held at Los Banos, Philippines in October 1985, sponsored by the Australian Centre for International Agricultural Research (ACIAR) among other agencies, had a regional rather than a single crop focus (13). *The International Bacterial Wilt Symposia* (IBWS) began in Kaohsiung, Taiwan, in October 1992. This first meeting, sponsored by AVRDC, ACIAR, ICRISAT, CIP, and ODA (now DFID), led to two major publications on bacterial wilt (5,7). The second IBWS, sponsored by the French agencies INRA, CIRAD, and ORSTOM, held in Guadeloupe, French West Indies, in June 1997, also resulted in a substantial publication (14). The third, sponsored by the South African Agricultural Research Council, was held at White River, RSA, in February, 2002. The 4th IBWS will be held in the United Kingdom in 2007, continuing the five-year periodicity which experience has shown is a sufficient interval to enable new work to be produced, and for collaborative linkages established at earlier meetings to bear fruit.

There has long been recognition that research effort on bacterial wilt was widely scattered throughout the tropics and subtropics and lacked coordination. In general research on the fundamental questions of the genetic basis of virulence, pathogenicity, and regulation of gene expression has been carried out in the developed countries of Europe and North America (3,15), whereas research on disease resistance, disease management, and many aspects of epidemiology and disease biology has been carried out in the countries of the developing world. As will be shown there is a marked disparity in the ease of interchange of information within and between the developed and developing world. In an attempt to improve communication and information exchange, the *ACIAR Bacterial Wilt Newsletter* was started in 1986; the last print issue (No. 16) appeared in May 1999. The Newsletter is likely to be revived as both an on-line and a print version following the establishment by Prior and Fegan of the Bacterial Wilt Consortium and the *Web of Bacterial Wilt* (http://ibws.nexenservices.com/). This website is proving to be a major resource for networking and information exchange, including linkage with the *Groundnut Bacterial Wilt Working Group* with its own Newsletter started by Liao Boshou of the Oil Crops Research Institute of the Chinese Academy of Agricultural Sciences, on behalf of ICRISAT.

The Literature on Bacterial Wilt

In spite of all the positive developments in international collaboration, the marked disparity continues in the dissemination of research findings between developed and developing world.

In the developed world the trend has been towards publication in on-line journals with high impact factors; at the same time library budgets have either been cut or have not kept pace with inflation or currency fluctuations, leading to a general reduction in holdings of many regional and national publications from the developing world. For example in North America between 1986-99, journal unit costs rose by 207% and journal expenditure by 170%, whereas journals and monographs purchased decreased by 6% and 26%, respectively. Similarly in Australia from 1986-99, journal unit costs rose by 474% and serials expenditure by 263%, at the same time that titles purchased decreased by 37% (2). These global trends in library acquisitions affect the dissemination of publications on bacterial wilt research as they do the results of any scholarly endeavour, but the effect will be proportionately greater in institutions lacking the infrastructure for on-line library services.

In this context it is illuminating to compare publications on bacterial wilt research shown in the single major monograph on bacterial wilt with the trends of the past five decades. For anyone wishing to read the early literature on bacterial wilt, the review by Kelman (8) provides masterly coverage for the period 1881 to 1952. There are 876 references in the bibliography of which 294 were in languages other than English. Many were in Dutch, reflecting the large contribution of Dutch plant pathologists between the last decade of the 19th and the first four decades of the 20th century in the former Dutch East Indies. In the past five decades the number of papers has increased to about 4500 and the profile of journals in which the literature appears has undergone a profound change; some journals have ceased

Table 1. List of Journals in which Research on Bacterial Wilt Was Published, 1998-2001[a]

Acta Phytopathologica Sinica	Journal of Immunological Methods
African Crop Science Journal	*Journal of Magnetic Resonance*
Annals of the Phytopathological Society of Japan	Journal of Phytopathology (Phytopathologische Zeitschrift)
Annual Review of Phytopathology	Journal of the Faculty of Agriculture
Applied and Environmental Microbiology	Kyushu University
	Journal of the Japanese Society for
Applied Engineering in Agriculture	Horticultural Science
Biological Control	Journal of Tropical Agriculture
Biometrics	Malaysian Applied Biology
Botanical Bulletin of Academic Sinica Taipei	*Microbiology (UK)*
	Molecular Genetics and Genomics
Breeding Science	*Molecular Microbiology*
Bulletin OEPP-EPPO Bulletin	*Molecular Plant Pathology*
Canadian Journal of Microbiology	*Molecular Plant-Microbe Interactions*
Canadian Journal of Plant Pathology	*Nemotropica*
Crop Protection	Philippine Agricultural Scientist
Crop Science	*Physiological and Molecular Plant*
Current Science (India)	*Pathology*
EMBO Journal	*Phytochemical Analysis*
Environmental Microbiology	*Phytopathology*
European Journal of Plant Pathology	*Plant Disease*
Forest Pathology	*Plant Journal*
Genetics	*Plant Pathology (UK)*
Indian Phytopathology	*Plant Physiology and Biochemistry*
Infomusa	Plant Protection Bulletin – Taichung
International Journal of Pest Management	*Plant Science*
	Planta
Japan Agricultural Research Quarterly	Potato Research
Journal of Agricultural and Food Chemistry	Seed Science and Technology
	Soil Science and Plant Nutrition
Journal of Bacteriology	Summa Phytopathologica
Journal of Bacteriological Control	*Systematic and Applied Microbiology*
Journal of Chemical Ecology	*Theoretical and Applied Microbiology*
Journal of General Plant Pathology (Japan)	*World Journal of Microbiology and Biotechnology*

[a] Journals for which the table of contents, abstracts and full text are available on-line from a website are shown in italics; for all of other journals listed tables of contents and abstracts only are available on-line or on CD-ROM from Biological Abstracts, the Commonwealth Agricultural Bureau, or Web of Science (*Current Contents*).

publication or changed their name, and there has been a dramatic increase in the range and diversity of journals being published. Table 1 lists the principal journals, including all of those which are available on-line and have high impact factors, in which bacterial wilt research was published between 1998 and 2001.

All of the journals listed have published one or more papers devoted to either some aspect of disease biology or management or some specialized property of the pathogen. In addition to the 61 periodicals listed in Table 1 there are several others of high impact or wide circulation that published occasional papers on bacterial wilt prior to 1998 but not in the specified four year period; these include *American Potato Journal, Australasian Plant Pathology, Euphytica, Journal of the American Society for Horticultural Science, Plant and Soil, Soil Biology and Biochemistry*, and *Tropical Agriculture (Trinidad)*. Early in 2002 there were papers in *Journal of Microbiological Methods, Nature* (London), *Proceedings of the National Academy of Sciences USA*, and *Synthetic Metals*. When the total of 72 periodicals is compared with those covered by Kelman's review there are just nine in common: *American Potato Journal, Annals of the Phytopathological Society of Japan, Current Science (India), Indian Phytopathology, Nature (London), Phytopathology, Plant Disease Reporter* (now *Plant Disease*) and *Tropical Agriculture (Trinidad)*. Many of the papers published between 1998 and 2001 dealt with the genetic basis of virulence, the regulation of expression of genes involved in pathogenesis, with diagnosis using DNA-based methods or molecular phylogeny; all of these papers were published in journals of relatively recent origin and none of the journals were in print at the time Kelman's review was completed.

There are many other publications containing significant information on bacterial wilt, mainly from the developing world, of lesser impact and distribution than those listed in Table 1. They include national and institutional publications, annual reports, seminar proceedings, extension bulletins, and abstracts of papers presented at national congresses. Many of these publications are abstracted by the Commonwealth Agricultural Bureau (CAB) and appear in the *Review of Plant Pathology*, and tables of contents and abstracts are available to subscribers either on-line or on CD-ROM; many others appear in *Biological Abstracts*. However, these publications are delayed in access to the scientific community and the coverage is not universal. One significant and inexplicable anomaly in coverage concerns two papers on the fruit rot of cooking banana (Saba and Cardaba ABB/BBB genotype) in the Philippines caused by insect transmitted strains of *Ralstonia solanacearum* race 2. The first comprehensive description of disease biology was published in *Philippine Phytopathology* in 1994 (17) and the same authors provided brief summary descriptions soon after in two other publications which are available on-line; unfortunately neither of the summary accounts made reference to the full description (18,19). A second significant paper on disease control by debudding of the male inflorescence was published in *Philippine Phytopathology* in 1996 (12). A recent authoritative review of bacterial diseases of the banana published in 2000 makes no reference to either publication (20). A search of library databases showed that 1990 was the last year in which *Philippine Phytopathology* could be found in a bibliographic database and this was in Microbiology Abstracts A and B in the Cambridge Scientific Abstracts service. The CAB database only had three records for *Philippine Phytopathology*, added in 1995; it does not index the journal. Two major alerting services, *Ingenta* (previously *unCover Reveal*) and *Swetsnet,* which send tables of contents to recpients via e-mail, do not have *Philippine Phytopathology* included in the journals they cover, although each index has approximately 20,000 journal titles.

Conclusion

In the age of the internet there is the potential for rapid transfer of information on a global basis but the dissemination of information to the developing world and, in particular, from the developing world to the developed world remains slow and erratic. This disparity is greater now than it was before the advent of the internet. In contrast information exchange among scientists of whatever provenance goes on all the time through a multiplicity of informal networks or more formally through aid agencies or the international centers. The most powerful catalyst is personal contact and interaction as made possible through the *International Bacterial Wilt Symposia*; they serve to identify gaps in knowledge needed for better disease management and they enable groups of people to decide on focal points for collaboration and set goals for the future. The first two symposia provide ample evidence of fruitful outcomes in the cause of better basic understanding of bacterial wilt and all aspects of management and control.

Acknowledgements

I wish to thank Sue Curlewis, Librarian, Biological Sciences Library, University of Queensland, for her expert advice on access to databases, and the AusAID International Seminar Support Scheme for financial assistance that enabled my attendance at the 3rd IBWS.

Literature Cited

1. Anon. 1988. Bacterial Diseases of the Potato, Report of the Planning Conference on Bacterial Diseases of the Potato 1987. International Potato Center (CIP), Lima, Peru.
2. Blixrud, J. 2001. Igniting change in the scholarly communication system. Scholarly Publishing and Academic Resources Coalition (SPARC). Seminar, University of Queensland, December 2001. (Website: www.arl.org/sparc).
3. Boucher, C.A., Gough, C., and Arlat, M.F. 1992. Molecular genetics of pathogenicity determinants of *Pseudomonas solanacearum* with special emphasis on *hrp* genes. Annu. Rev. Phytopathol. 30: 443-461.
4. Buddenhagen, I.W., and Kelman, A. 1964. Biological and physiological aspects of bacterial wilt caused by *Pseudomonas solanacearum*. Annu. Rev. Phytopathol. 2: 203-230.
5. Hartman, G.L., and Hayward, A.C., eds. 1992. Bacterial Wilt: Proceedings of an international conference held at Kaohsiung, Taiwan, 28-31 October. ACIAR Press, Canberra.
6. Hayward, A.C. 1991. Biology and epidemiology of bacterial wilt caused by *Pseudomonas solanacearum*. Annu. Rev. Phytopathol. 29: 65-87.
7. Hayward, A.C., and Hartman, G.L., eds. 1994. Bacterial Wilt: the Disease and its Causative Agent *Pseudomonas solanacearum*. CAB International in association with AVRDC, Wallingford, UK.
8. Kelman, A. 1953. The bacterial wilt caused by *Pseudomonas solanacearum*. N.C. Agr. Res. Sta. Tech. Bull.: 99.
9. Mehan, V.K., and Hayward, A.C., eds. 1993. Groundnut bacterial wilt: proceedings of the Second Working Group meeting, 2 November 1992. Asian Vegetable Research and Development Center, Tainan, Taiwan. India: International Crops Research Institute for the Semi-Arid Tropics.
10. Mehan, V.K., and McDonald, D., eds. 1994. Groundnut bacterial wilt in Asia: proceedings of the Third Working Group meeting, 4-5 July 1994, Oil Crops Research Institute, Wuhan,China. India: International Crops Research Institute for the Semi-Arid Tropics.
11. Middleton, K.J., and Hayward, A.C., eds. 1990. Bacterial wilt of groundnut: An ACIAR/ICRISAT collaborative research planning meeting, Malaysia, 18-19 March, 1990. ACIAR Press, Canberra.
12. Molina, G.C. 1996. Integrated management of 'Tibaglon' a bacterial fruit rot disease of cooking bananas under farmer's field. Philippine Phytopath. 32: 83-91.
13. Persley, G.J., ed. 1986. Bacterial Wilt Disease in Asia and the South Pacific: proceedings of an international workshop held at PCARRD, Los Banos, Philippines, 8-10 October 1985. ACIAR Press, Canberra.

14. Prior, P., Allen, C., and Elphinstone, J. 1998. Bacterial Wilt Disease: Molecular and Ecological Aspects. Report of the Second International Bacterial Wilt Symposium, Guadeloupe, France, 22-27 June 1997. Springer Verlag, Heidelburg, and INRA, Paris.
15. Schell, M.A. 2000. Control of virulence and pathogenicity genes of *Ralstonia solanacearum* by an elaborate sensory network. Annu. Rev. Phytopathol. 38: 263-292.
16. Sequeira, L., and Kelman, A., eds. Proceedings of the First International Planning Conference and Workshop on the Ecology and Control of Bacterial Wilt caused by *Pseudomonas solanacearum*. Raleigh, North Carolina State University.
17. Soguilon, C.E., Magnaye, L.V., and Natural, M.P. 1994. Bugtok disease of cooking bananas: 1. Etiology and diagnostic symptoms. Philippine Phytopath. 30: 26-34.
18. Soguilon, C.E., Magnaye, L.V., and Natural, M.P. 1994. Bugtok disease of cooking bananas in the Philippines. InfoMusa 3: 21-22..
19. Soguilon, C.E., Magnaye, L.V., and Natural, M.P. 1995. Bugtok disease of banana. Musa Disease Fact Sheet No. 6. INIBAP, Montpellier, France.
20. Thwaites, R., Eden-Green, S.J., and Black, R. 2000. Diseases caused by bacteria. pp. 213-239 in: Diseases of Banana, Abaca and Enset. D.R. Jones ed. CAB International, Wallingford, UK.

The Current Bacterial Wilt Situation: A Global Overview

J.G. Elphinstone
Plant Health Group, Central Science Laboratory
Sand Hutton, York, YO41 1LZ, UK.

There have been over 450 publications on *Ralstonia solanacearum* since the 2nd International Bacterial Wilt Symposium, held in Guadeloupe in 1997 (49). Broadly classifying the topics that have been reported, 24% concern breeding and selection for resistance, while the others address pathogen diversity, distribution, and host range (22%), disease management and control (18%), pathogenicity and host-pathogen interactions (17%), biological control (10%), detection and diagnosis (4%), and epidemiology and ecology (3%). Among the host crops studied were tomato (35%), potato (24%), eggplant (11%), tobacco (9%), *Capsicum* (7%), groundnut (3%), banana (3%), and ginger (2%). The remainder (5%) described work on newly or less studied crop hosts including *Anthurium*, artichoke, *Eucalyptus*, jute, loofah, *Moringa oleifera*, mulberry, *Pelargonium*, *Piper hispidinervium*, *Pogostemon patchouli*, pumpkin, sesame, and turmeric.

The worldwide distribution of *R. solanacearum* was recently summarized by CAB International (CABI) and the European and Mediterranean Plant Protection Organisation (EPPO) in their updated series of distribution maps of plant diseases (6). Three maps indicate the distribution of race 1 on a range of economically important hosts (Map 783), race 2 on banana and other Musaceae (Map 784), and race 3 on potato and other Solanaceae (Map 785). Revised maps are published every two years and on-line data (which are revised annually) are also now commercially available via the internet (http://www.cabi.org/compendia) or on CD-ROM. The data are mostly taken from published articles held on EPPO and CABI databases and there are inevitably time lags between occurrences of the pathogen in new areas and appearance of the data on the distribution maps. Furthermore, there are still many areas where distribution data have not been published, where old findings have not been updated, where suspect findings have not been confirmed, or where surveys have not been carried out at all.

This overview highlights current information on the global situation of bacterial wilt through review of the recent literature and over 100 additional reports submitted for presentation at the 3rd International Bacterial Wilt Symposium, South Africa, 2002. In order to obtain a more detailed impression of the current situation in some areas, a questionnaire was distributed to 56 experts in 25 countries and the opinions obtained are reported below. Currently-used diagnostic methods and their role in surveying pathogen distribution and preventing further spread are also discussed.

Geographical Distribution and Current Status on Major Crops

NORTH AMERICA

The predominant strains found in North America all fall within Phylotype II (Fegan, this volume), show the biovar 1 phenotype, and mainly affect tobacco and tomato in the southeastern USA. In North and South Carolina, occurrences of Granville wilt on tobacco have increased dramatically as a result of increased mechanisation (Fortnum and Kluepfel, this volume). The pathogen is now considered widespread in southeastern North Carolina and eastern South Carolina, where it is currently one of the top two pathogens affecting tobacco and the single most important in seasons which favour bacterial wilt development (B. Fortnum and A. Robertson, pers. comm.). The same strains are also regarded among the top five pathogens of tomato in isolated locations of the southeastern USA where they frequently occur in North and South Carolina, southern Georgia and Florida (B. Fortnum, A. Robertson, T. Momol, pers. comm.). CABI/ EPPO (6) also report the occurrence of race 1 in Alabama, Arkansas, and Hawaii. There have also been occasional references to findings of biovar 1 strains on sunflower and certain ornamentals (including *Dahlia*, *Hibiscus*, *Pothos*, *Verbena,* and *Zinnia*) although these are not currently considered economically important (T. Momol, pers. comm.). A suspected occurrence of biovar 1 (race 2) on banana reported in Florida (6) requires substantiation. Declining yields of ginger due to bacterial wilt caused by biovar 3 strains, have been recently reported in Hawaii (Alvarez *et al*, this volume). A recent report of the occurrence of biovar 2 (race 3) on greenhouse-grown geraniums (*Pelargonium* x *hortorum*) in Wisconsin and South Dakota (67) represents the first report of disease caused by biovar 2 in North America. *R. solanacearum* is not established in Canada.

Phylotype II of *R. solanacearum* is reported to be present in several countries of Central America and the Caribbean (6, Fegan, this volume). Race 1 strains are quoted as widespread in Belize, restricted in Mexico, and of unknown distribution in at least seven other countries. Race 2 (biovar 1) strains are currently known to be distributed in at least 11 countries within this region (6) where it has become established in wild *Heliconia* spp. (54). Moko disease has been declared widespread in Grenada, of restricted distribution in Belize, and of unknown distribution in the other countries. Expert opinion from Mexico (L. Fujikovsky, pers. comm.) indicates that moko is the most important disease of banana in the state of Chiapas where it is widespread and there are also unconfirmed reports of spread to ornamental *Heliconia* plantations. Biovar 1 (race 1) has occurred in the past on tobacco in the state of Oaxaca but is not currently of economic importance. Biovar 2 (race 3) has occurred sporadically in several Mexican states (including Sinaloa, Chihuahua, Coahuila, Queretaro, Morelos, and Michoacan) but is currently of minor economic importance and is thought to have been eradicated completely from the state of Tlaxcala. Elsewhere in Central America, biovar 2 strains are also currently reported only in Costa Rica and Guadeloupe (6) where their distribution is unknown.

SOUTH AMERICA

Phylotype II strains also predominate in South America (Fegan, this volume). CABI/EPPO (11) report *R. solanacearum* race 1 strains as present but of unknown distribution in at least four countries (Brazil, Colombia, Guyana and Peru) but as eradicated from Uruguay. Biovar 2 (race 3) strains are reported as present in seven South American countries (Argentina, Bolivia, Brazil, Chile, Colombia, Peru, and Uruguay). Race 3 is declared widespread in Chile, and is present in six of the 12 regions (17).

Expert opinion clarifies the current status in Peru and Bolivia (S. Priou, pers. comm.) and in Colombia (G.A. Granada, pers. comm.). *R. solanacearum* has been detected in 12 of the 24 departments of Peru. Race 3 (biovar 2A) may be considered widespread on potato (in 10 departments), whereas the distribution of race 1 (biovar 1) and biovar 2T is more restricted to six and two departments respectively. Recent surveys have shown that approximately eight to 10,000 Ha, among a total of 57,200 Ha of potato notably in the Cajamarca and Huánuco regions, are affected by bacterial wilt (53). In Bolivia, the distribution of biovar 2A is currently restricted to some 15,000 Ha of potato in four departments in which the disease occurs frequently (18). In both Peru and Bolivia, bacterial wilt is considered the second most important disease of potato after late blight (*Phytophthora infestans*). In Colombia, race 1 strains are among the five most damaging pathogens of tobacco in Santander region and can also significantly affect tomato production, whereas race 3 occurs frequently on potato and infrequently on tree tomato in isolated regions (e.g. Antioquia).

Survey results (37) and expert opinion from Brazil (C.A. Lopes, pers. comm.) clarifies the current status there. In both the tropical north, which is hot and humid, and the northeast, which is the driest region, bacterial wilt (caused by *R. solanacearum* biovars 1 and 3) is the most serious disease affecting tomato production. Surveys from 1998 – 2000 in 20 municipalities of Amazonas region found bacterial wilt to be present in all tomato fields visited (9). In the northern region, bacterial wilt is also among the five most important diseases of sweet pepper, which is also significantly affected in all other regions. In the main potato producing areas in the temperate, sub-tropical south and southeastern regions, biovar 2 and occasionally biovar 1 are among the top five pathogens and the main cause of rejection of seed potato crops during certification. Bacterial wilt is also seriously limiting in winter-irrigated tomato and potato production in central Brazil where predominantly biovar 1 is isolated but biovar 2 has also been imported, probably on infected seed from the south.

Moko disease (caused by strains of biovar 1, race 2) is reported as present but of unknown distribution in seven South American countries (Brazil, Colombia, Guyana, Paraguay, Peru, Suriname, and Venezuela) and as reported but not confirmed in Argentina and Ecuador (6). New reports clarify the current status in Brazil and Colombia. In Brazil the disease is the most limiting constraint to banana production in the Amazonia region (Coelho-Netto and Nutter, this volume) and it has been reported for the first time on *Heliconia* spp. in the state of Pernambuco where it is seriously damaging ornamental plantation production (Assis et al, this volume). In Colombia, moko is currently considered the most important disease affecting banana and plantain and, as a result of trade in contaminated planting material and insufficient attention to control measures, is now widespread wherever *Musa* spp. are grown (G. Grenada, pers. comm.).

EUROPE

The status of *R. solanacearum* in European and Mediterranean countries of the EPPO region was reviewed at a workshop in 1997 (22). As discussed previously (13,26,31), sporadic outbreaks of potato brown rot caused by biovar 2A (race 3) have been reported since 1989 in restricted areas of nine of the 15 member states of the European Community (Belgium, France, Germany, Greece, Italy, the Netherlands, Portugal, Spain and the UK). Isolated potato brown rot outbreaks have also recently been reported in Hungary (6). New information from Turkey (M. Ozakman, pers. comm.)

also confirms recent infrequent outbreaks of biovar 2 on potato in isolated areas.

In all EC countries where potato brown rot has recently occurred, strict control measures have been imposed through an official EC Control Directive (1), which aims to determine the extent of pathogen distribution in outbreak areas and to contain and eventually eradicate it. Eradication has been complicated by the fact that the pathogen has been found in some countries to persist on wild *Solanum dulcamara* inhabiting river banks and has been dispersed in river water used for irrigation (13,31). Systematic detection surveys on potato stocks and surface water, as well as official demarcation and prohibition of the use of infested land and waterways, have significantly reduced the risk of spread of the organism to potato crops. As a result, infections in potato crops have been reduced almost to zero, although it is generally too early to claim successful eradication of the pathogen. In the Netherlands, where brown rot outbreaks were most extensive in 1995, testing of some 60,000 potato samples per year and 14,000 water and *S. dulcamara* samples (31) have reduced findings to less than 0.01% of tested lots (J. D. Janse, pers. comm.). Recent surveys in Sweden (47) indicated that eradication of the pathogen was successfully achieved by removal of infected *S. dulcamara* over a 5-year period from 30 km of a contaminated watercourse following isolated potato brown rot outbreaks in the 1970s (40).

As in the USA, *R. solanacearum* biovar 2A has recently been detected on imported *Pelargonium* cuttings (Janse *et al.*, this volume). Although there have also been occasional interceptions of *R. solanacearum* race 1 strains on ornamentals imported into Europe from Asia (31), it is generally understood that none of these strains have become established. Reports of suspected findings of race 1 in Georgia, Moldovia, the Ukraine, and in restricted areas of Russia (6) require substantiation.

ASIA AND THE MIDDLE EAST

R. solanacearum Phylotype I strains (biovars 3 or 4) have been reported from at least 20 Asian and Middle Eastern countries (6, Fegan, this volume). In China, the distribution is reported as restricted with presence in at least 15 provinces (Anhui, Fujian, Guandong, Guangxi, Hebei, Henan, Hong Kong, Hubei, Hunan, Jiangsu, Jiangxi, Shandong, Sichuan,Yunnan, and Zhejiang) but without further published details. Distribution of strains with biovar 3, 4 and 2T phenotype is also reported in several regions of Japan (29). In India, race 1 is reported as widespread and present in 11 states (Andhra Pradesh, Assam, Himachal Pradesh, Indian Punjab, Karnataka, Kerala, Maharashtra, Nagaland, Orissa, Uttar Pradesh, and West Bengal). For other countries there is little published information on current status or distribution.

Phylotype 1 strains (biovars 3 and 4) are widespread and affect a very wide range of economically important crops across Asia. The most important crop affected is tomato; experts consistently rated bacterial wilt as either the most important or at least among the top five diseases of this crop in the major production areas of all affected countries. In areas where off-season tomato production is increasing (e.g. along the Mekong River in north-east Thailand), high temperatures at the time of transplanting are increasing losses due to this disease even further (J.F. Wang, pers. comm.). Bacterial wilt is also widely ranked among the top five diseases of other solanaceous crops, including eggplant, sweet pepper, and chili.

Bacterial wilt of ginger has become very destructive in many parts of Asia in the last decade (A.C. Hayward, pers. comm.). The disease occurs frequently in the traditional Indian ginger producing areas of Kerala state (Wyanad) and in the north-eastern states of Sikkim and Assam where it is among the five most important diseases of the crop. The disease has similar current status on ginger in the Philippines (M. Natural, pers. comm.). Bacterial wilt is regarded as the most important disease of ginger and the related *Curcuma alismatifolia* (patumma) in the production areas of northern Thailand (N. Thaveechai and V. Dittapongpitch, pers. comm.) where *R. solanacearum* biovar 4 is widespread. It is also regarded as the most important disease of ginger in Indonesia (Supriadi, pers comm.). In the Kochi Prefecture of Japan, strains of biovar 4 have spread in epidemic scale from *Curcuma* to ginger and the related mioga (*Zingiber mioga*) in recent years (62).

Bacterial wilt is currently considered the most damaging disease of groundnut in Indonesia (Supriadi, pers comm.) and among the top five diseases on this host in Vietnam (N. X. Hong, pers comm.), especially in areas where dry-land cropping systems are employed. Groundnut is also currently significantly affected in the Philippines and Thailand (M. Natural and N. Thaveechai, pers comm.) although there are at least five pathogens which cause higher losses. The disease has also occurred in isolated areas of India, including Kerala state, but is currently considered of minor economic importance.

R. solanacearum has been reported on banana in several Asian countries, although further investigation is required to substantiate suspected cases reported from India (Maharashtra, Tamil Nadu, and West Bengal), Malaysia (Sabah), Sri Lanka, Taiwan, Thailand and Vietnam (6). Current information from the Philippines (M. Natural, pers. comm.) confirms that *R. solanacearum* is still widespread throughout the country and is currently among the top five pathogens affecting banana and plantain. Moko disease is highly damaging in commercial banana plantations (54) and bugtok (also known as tapurok or tibaglon) disease is commonly found on cooking banana cultivars (BBB and ABB) grown by small-scale producers throughout the country. Although the symptoms differ, both diseases are caused by Phylotype II (biovar 1, race 2) strains which are indistinguishable genetically (Raymundo et al., this volume). In Indonesia, the banana blood disease bacterium is spreading and, in addition to being widespread in Sulawesi, outbreaks have now been reported on several other islands including West Java, Sumatra, West Kalimantan (Supriadi, this volume) and most recently on Irian Jaya, but not yet in the most Western province of neighbouring Papua New Guinea (11). According to Supriadi (pers. comm.) it is in the top five most important diseases of cooking and dessert bananas and is the most important disease of some susceptible (ABB) cooking banana cultivars in some areas of Indonesia. The blood disease bacterium belongs to Phylotype IV (Fegan, this volume) and is genetically distinct from the other banana strains of *R. solanacearum*. Its continued spread at up to 200 km per year (probably involving insect transmission) is an important threat to both cooking and dessert banana production in South East Asia.

CABI/EPPO (6) report the occurrence of race 3 (biovar 2) in nine Asian (Bangladesh, China, India, Indonesia, Japan, Nepal, Pakistan, Philippines, and Sri Lanka) and two Middle Eastern (Lebanon and Iran) countries, in which the distribution is either given as restricted or unknown). It is known to have occurred in at least six provinces of China (Fujian, Guandong, Guangxi, Hebei, Jiangsu, and Hejiang) and nine Indian states (Himachal Pradesh, Madhya Pradesh, Maharashtra, Manipur, Meghalaya, Tamil Nadu, Tripura, Uttar Pradesh, and West Bengal). In Nepal, it is now widespread in potato growing areas (P.M.P. Pradhanang, pers. comm.). Bacterial wilt is one of the five most important potato diseases in the highland production areas of Thailand where biovar 2 strains are present (N. Thaveechai, pers comm.). Bacterial wilt is also one of the five most important potato diseases in Indonesia. The relative importance of race 3 and race 1 strains is unclear and both may be isolated from the same affected crop. Strains with the biovar 2T phenotype, also isolated from potato in West Java, belong to Phylotype IV and thus differ genetically from those found in South America and Africa (Fegan, this volume). In the Philippines, bacterial wilt of potato occurs frequently in isolated areas of the country. Crops are affected by both races 1 and 3 although current opinion suggests that biovar 2 is less frequently isolated than biovar 3, particularly in lower elevation production areas (M. Natural, pers. comm.).

AFRICA

R. solanacearum race 1 strains have been reported in at least 21 countries in Africa. Biovar 2 (race 3) has been reported on potato in at least 10 countries (Burundi, Egypt, Ethiopia, Kenya, Libya, Reunion, Rwanda, South Africa, Tanzania, and Uganda) (6, 20, Fortnum and

Kleupfel, this volume; M. Osiru, pers. comm.). In addition, potato isolates collected in Kenya, Nigeria and Cameroon, were found to have the biovar 2T phenotype (57). Furthermore, biovar 1 strains isolated in southern Africa (including Angola, Madagascar, Reunion Island and Zimbabwe) have been shown to form a new subdivision within *R. solanacearum* (48), now designated Phylotype III (Fegan, this volume). There are therefore three of the four known phyloytpes (I, II and III) of *R. solanacearum* present on the African continent.

In almost all cases, there is little or no published information on distribution or importance. There are also references (6) to suspect findings of *R. solanacearum* on Musaceae in some African countries (including Ethiopia, Libya, Nigeria, Senegal and Sierra Leone) although further substantiation is required.

Current information from South Africa (J. Terblanche, pers. comm.) indicates that biovar 3 occurs frequently on tobacco only in sub-tropical regions and also affects *Capsicum*. In addition, biovar 2 is widespread throughout the country on potato and tomato. Bacterial wilt is regarded as one of the five most important diseases on all of these crops in S. Africa. In Zimbabwe, bacterial wilt is currently considered of minor importance on tobacco, potato, and tomato (A. Robertson, pers. comm.). Biovar 3 occurs frequently on tobacco in the Mvurwi/Concession tobacco-growing area, whereas biovar 2 occurs infrequently and only in isolated parts of the country. A recent survey indicated that biovar 3 was probably among the five most important pathogens of tobacco in Malawi (J. Terblanche, pers. comm.), and of potato, tomato, *Anthurium,* and tobacco in Mauritius (A. Dookun, pers. comm.), where it is also of minor economic importance on bean (*Phaseolus vulgaris*) and groundnut. In Uganda, biovar 2 (race 3) is currently considered widespread in highland potato-growing areas whereas strains of biovar 3 are widespread in the lowlands (M. Osiru, pers. comm.). Bacterial wilt is considered one of the five most important diseases of tomato, potato, and tobacco in Uganda and also significantly affects groundnut production and has minor importance on bean (*Phaseolus vulgaris*). In Egypt, recent extensive testing of potatoes for export to Europe has indicated that biovar 2 occurs frequently in restricted areas within the country (Janse, pers. comm.), permitting the mapping of pathogen-free areas over several seasons from which potatoes with significantly lower risk of infection have been exported.

OCEANIA

Biovars 1, 2, 3, and 4 have all previously been reported in Australia. Biovar 1 (race 2) isolated from imported Heliconia plants at a nursery in

North Queensland in 1989 did not spread and is believed to have been totally eradicated (30).

Biovar 2 (race 3) has previously been reported in almost all potato-growing areas, situated in isolated parts of Queensland (including Lockyer Valley, Darling Downs, and other areas around Brisbane as well as many records for the Atherton Tableland), Victoria (parts of East Gippsland, particularly the Koo Wee Rup swamp area) and New South Wales (Ebor-Dorrigo area of Northern NSW, other coastal regions, and several outbreaks in irrigated areas near Deniliquin). Sporadic outbreaks have occurred previously in South Australia (south-east of Adelaide) and in Western Australia (south and south-east of Perth) but are believed to have been eradicated (T. Wicks, pers. comm.). Sporadic outbreaks have been associated with crops grown from infected seed tubers originating from Victoria.

Biovar 3 strains of race 1 are endemic and widespread in the tropical, high rainfall areas of Northern Queensland (east of the continental divide from Brisbane to Cape York peninsula) and in the Northern Territory (S. Akiew, M. Fegan, A.C. Hayward, pers. comm.). In these areas, *R. solanacearum* is probably the most important bacterial pathogen of a wide range of solanaceous crops (including tomato, potato, eggplant, *Capsicum*, and tobacco) and ornamentals (including palms, *Lesianthus*, *Anthurium*, *Heliconia*, *Strelitzia*, *Lilium*, and *Tagetes*). In addition, it has a significant but less important effect on fruit trees (including custard apple, black sapote and neem) and *Eucalyptus*. Bacterial wilt is considered among the top five diseases in tomato-growing areas of central and southern Queensland. Biovar 4 is uncommon and is believed to have been eradicated from ginger in southern Queensland as a result of quarantine measures imposed following outbreaks of severe and rapid wilt in the past (25, 46). Outside of Australia, biovars 3 and 4 (race 1) strains together with biovar 2 (race 3) have been previously reported in Papua New Guinea (61). Race 1 has also been reported in Fiji (6).

STATUS ON NEW AND LESS-STUDIED HOSTS

There are many crop plants affected by race 1, although their economic importance and current status have been less studied. Bacterial wilt of sesame has been reported in Assam, India, is currently rated as significantly important in Thailand and Vietnam (N. Thaveechai and N.X. Hong, pers. comm.), and may be caused by the same biovar 4 strains that affect ginger and *Curcuma* (59). In the Indian state of Kerala, race 1 strains are also causing significant losses on cucurbits where it frequently occurs in isolated areas (K.V. Peter, pers. comm.). Race 1 strains also have minor economic importance in cowpea, hyacinth beans (*Dolichos lablab*), and patchouli (*Pogostemon patchouli*), and have little or no current importance on nutmeg, moringa (*Moringa olerifera*), or mulberry. In Thailand, bacterial wilt is currently considered one of the five most important diseases of marigold (*Tagetes* spp.). Bacterial wilt of *Eucalyptus* was recently found to be common on trees less than two years old in the Republic of Congo, South Africa, and Uganda (Coutinho *et al.,* this volume). Minor economic damage on *Eucalyptus* trees is also currently reported from Thailand (Thaveechai, pers. comm.), Australia (Hayward, pers. comm.) and Brazil (C.A. Lopes, pers. comm.). Significant economic losses due to race 1 are occurring in cowpea and winged bean in the Philippines while infections on abaca and *Heliconia* spp. are considered of minor or no current economic importance (M. Natural, pers. comm). Bacterial wilt of mulberry, caused by *R. solanacearum* biovar 5 was previously thought to occur only in China although new information suggests that it has also been isolated on rare occasions in Vietnam (N.X. Hong, pers. comm.).

In Taiwan, several more unusual host crops are currently affected by race 1 strains (J-F Wang, pers. comm.). Bacterial wilt is now considered among the five most important pathogens of water spinach or kankong (*Ipomoea reptans*) and of strawberry. On Kankong, it is widespread across the country, particularly occurring in wetland and in mechanically-harvested crops. On strawberry, it occurs frequently in isolated areas of the country where it is spreading through movement of non-certified latently infected runners. Race 1 is also frequently and significantly affecting production of custard apple (*Annona squamosa*), *Anthurium,* and jute (*Corchorus* spp.) in isolated areas of the country, although in each case there are at least five other more important pathogens. Strains of race 1 have infrequently caused minor economic damage in isolated areas on wax apple (*Syzygium samarangese*). Dye and condiment production from *Perilla crispa* is now very minor due to the high losses which resulted from infection by biovar 3 strains which spread during mechanical clipping (28). Bacterial wilt of radish has been reported previously in Taiwan but is now believed to have been eradicated.

Economic Importance

There is little general information on the economic impact of *R. solanacearum* worldwide. Direct yield losses vary widely according to host, cultivar, climate, soil type, cropping practices and pathogen strain. In areas where the organism has quarantine status, considerable economic losses can result from the destruction of entire infected crops, additional eradication measures and restriction on further production on contaminated land. Association of *R. solanacearum* with root knot nematodes can apparently change plant physiology, thus causing increased bacterial wilt severity in several hosts including tobacco (8), banana (45), and eggplant (63). The following recent examples illustrate current economic damage levels as experienced on some major host crops:

Tomato. In Taiwan, bacterial wilt incidence in field-grown tomato was 15-26% in improved hybrids as opposed to 55% in other hybrids (24). In India, a yield loss study with one cultivar showed 10-100% mortality of plants and 0-91% yield loss, with maximum losses occurring in crops infected before 60 days and during the summer season (33). A survey of 17 dis-tricts of Uganda in 1998 showed that 88% of tomato farms visited were af-fected by bacterial wilt caused by biovar 3 (Katafiire, this volume). Average yield losses in tomato and eggplant in Australia have been estimated at 5-15% although extreme cases may reach 70% (M. Fegan and A.C. Hayward, pers. comm.). Disease incidence in South Carolina, USA, has been estimated at 15% of fields affected per year, leading to yield losses of 1-5% (T. Keinath, pers. comm.).

Potato. Bacterial wilt of potato has been estimated to affect some three million farm families (about 1.5 million Ha) in around 80 countries with global damage estimates currently exceeding $950 million annually (64). China, Bangladesh, Bolivia and Uganda were thought to be among the most seriously affected countries. In Bolivia, yield loss estimates at harvest ranged from 30-90% and losses during storage were as high as 98% (35, Coelho-Netto and Nutter, this volume). In recent surveys in Venezuela, *R. solanacearum* had spread to 24 of 38 localities in the main potato production zones between 1167 and 3000 m above sea level (20). Bacterial wilt disease incidence was found to have increased from 22% in 1992 to 37% in 1996 with the infested area per farm ranging from 5 to 75%. Current reports from Bangladesh quote some regions as having more than 30% of potato crops affected by bacterial wilt in the last two seasons with over 14% reduction in yield (T. Dey, pers. comm.). In Nepal, tuber rotting occurred in an average of 10% of stored potatoes with a maximum of 50% in some cases (56). Crop losses in small farms in the Nepalese hills were up to 100%, mainly due to poor cultural practices and keeping seed from infected crops (23). Significant losses have been recorded in litigation cases involving sale of allegedly infected seed stocks. For example, a recent case in South Australia led to costs of 70 million Australian dollars (T. Wicks, pers. comm.). In comparison, insurance claims in the Netherlands in 1998 and 1999 as a result of potato brown rot outbreaks have been estimated at US $2.7 million (36).

Tobacco. Good economic loss data exists for tobacco production in the southeast USA where the importance of bacterial wilt has significantly increased in recent years (19, 21, 38, Fortnum and Kluepfel, this volume). In some counties of South Carolina, some 95% of farm fields were found to be affected in 1998 with 7% of the total crop affected. In the same year, economic losses in North and South Carolina were estimated at $40 million. Average tobacco yield losses were estimated to be less than 5% in Zimbabwe (50) and 10-30% in Australia (M. Fegan and A.C. Hayward, pers. comm.).

Banana. Over the years, moko disease has affected susceptible bananas and plantains over thousands of square miles in central and south America (54). It remains potentially the most damaging disease of banana and plantain in most areas where it occurs, particularly for small subsistence farmers. Resistance is lacking, transmission (especially by insects) can be rapid, and expensive control measures are only effectively managed by large plantation companies. Recent surveys in Colombia (5) showed that losses in plantain crops over the period 1998-2000 exceeded $570,000 in only six municipalities of one region (Quindío). In the Philippines, a survey of 163 farmers fields on Negros Oriental showed a 60-92% incidence of *R. solanacearum* race 2 causing bugtok (or tibaglon) disease on cooking bananas (39). With 80-100% of fingers left unfit for consumption, this major source of livelihood for many farmers was devastated by the disease. Similarly, the rapid spread of banana blood disease in Indonesia is seriously threatening banana and plantain production there and potentially in the neighbouring countries. In other areas race 2 has caused serious economic loss due to severe quarantine measures, as for example, following findings on *Heliconia* in Australia (30).

Groundnut. In Vietnam, bacterial wilt incidence on groundnut was found to range from 0.2% in paddy rice:groundnut rotations to 16.9% in dryland cropping systems on sandy soils along riverbanks and in upland areas (27). Groundnut varieties latently infected by the bacterium (so-called tolerant varieties) showed no apparent yield reduction (34). Groundnut infected by biovars 3 and 4 has been reported from 16 provinces in China with the infested area estimated at >200,000 Ha (58, 69). Annual incidence ranged from 4 to 8% on resistant cultivars and the annual loss in pod yield was estimated at 36,000 t. Yield losses of up to 20% were found, and were most serious in southern provinces. Losses of up to 10% have also been recorded in Uganda (42).

Ginger. Bacterial wilt of ginger was present in 80% of 310 fields surveyed in Himachal Pradesh, India (55) and severe losses were also reported from Thailand (60). Bacterial wilt is also common in wild and cultivated turmeric (*Curcuma* spp.) in Thailand and Indonesia (59). *R. solanacearum* intercepted from rhizomes exported for cut flower production in Europe caused serious economic problems when severe quarantine measures had to be taken in greenhouses (62).

Disease Diagnosis and Quarantine Control

Rapid and reliable diagnostic capabilities are essential for accurate determination of pathogen distribution, to understand its ability to establish and persist in the environment and to identify and eliminate the risks of spread to new areas. Despite extensive research on diagnostic methods, much reliance at the practical level is still placed on isolation of the organism using modifications of the tetrazolium medium described by Kelman (32). Variations on the SMSA medium developed in South Africa (12, 15) have been widely used in recent years for semi-selective isolation as well as for enrichment purposes to amplify serological and DNA-based assays (66, Biosca et al.,this volume).

In Europe, official testing schemes have been standardized and validated in ring tests among 20 plant health diagnostic laboratories (14). These are mainly based on the recommended EPPO procedure (16) which involves immunofluorescence microscopy and bioassay in tomato seedlings, but with complimentary selective isolation and optional confirmatory testing using various PCR (4, 41, 43, 44, 52), ELISA (7, 51) and fluorescent in situ hybridization (68) protocols. Adoption of similar testing schemes in other countries is having a positive effect on bacterial wilt control. For example, in Cuba (J. Garcia, pers. comm) the introduction of the immunofluorescence test has apparently coincided with the elimination of bacterial wilt from potato production there. Similarly in Egypt, systematic testing of potato lots using this test has permitted the identification of R. solanacearum-free areas for production of potatoes for export to Europe with significantly reduced risk of infection (J.D. Janse, pers. comm.).

On-site serological tests, such as the NCM ELISA kit produced by the International Potato Center (Priou et al., this volume) and a new "Pocket Diagnostic" lateral flow device (10) offer particularly practical means to monitor and control R. solanacearum directly in the field. The NCM ELISA kits have already been applied in relatively inexpensive survey work to monitor pathogen distribution on potato in Bolivia (O. Antezana, pers. comm), Peru (Priou et al., this volume), Kenya (Kinuya et al., this volume), Burundi (A. Ntahimpera, pers. comm.), Thailand (T. Boonsuebsakul, pers. comm.), Bangladesh (T. Dey, pers. comm.) and to test imported seed potatoes in the Philippines (A. Bacho, pers. comm.). Further practical applications for these test kits include testing ginger rhizomes (Kumar et al., this volume), banana suckers and Pelargonium cuttings (Janse et al., this volume).

The adoption of PCR into routine testing schemes, with potential advantages of increased sensitivity and specificity, has been largely inhibited by the tendency for false negative test results due to inhibitors of DNA polymerases in plant and soil material. Positive advances for the future include multiplex assays with internal PCR controls as well as assays which amplify species- and strain-specific DNA targets for rapid and accurate pathogen identification (44, 65, Prior and Fegan, this volume). In addition, quantitative PCR methods offer gel-free, automated detection and can indicate pathogen viability during enrichment (66).

Conclusions

The information presented above is intended to depict the current global status of R. solanacearum, as far as it is known at the time of writing. It is also intended as a reminder of the importance of accurate and timely reporting of reliable data on current distribution and economic importance of this pathogen wherever it occurs. This information is vital for continued assessment of the risks of spread at national and international levels and for appropriate decision making and policy formulation on control measures and future research strategy. It is therefore the duty of all bacterial wilt researchers to continuously check the validity of published information on disease distribution and economic importance in their respective regions and to stress the importance of continued survey work as an essential component of bacterial wilt control.

Acknowledgements

All participants in the expert opinion questionnaire (indicated in the text as personal communications) are gratefully acknowledged. The participation of J.G. Elphinstone in the 3rd IBWS was supported by the UK Department for Environment, Food and Rural Affairs (DEFRA) and the British Society for Plant Pathology (BSPP).

Literature Cited

1. Anon. 1998. Council Directive 98/57/EC of 20 July 1998 on the control of *Ralstonia solanacearum* (Smith) Yabuuchi *et al.* Official J. Eur. Commun. L235: 1-39.
2. Barea, O., Michel, W., and Fernandez-Northcote, E.N. 1996. Incidencia y distribución de la marchitez bacteriana en la provincia Tomina del departamento de Chuquisaca. In: IBTA. Cuarta reunión nacional de papa: Compendio de exposiciones. Cochabamba (Bolivia). 8-11 Oct 1996. Cochabamba (Bolivia).

3. Black, R., Seal, S., Abubakar, Z., Nono-Womdim, R., and Swai, I.
    1999. Wilt pathogens of Solanaceae in Tanzania: *Clavibacter
    michiganensis* subsp. *michiganensis, Pseudomonas corrugata* and
    Ralstonia solanacearum. Plant Dis. 83: 1070.
4. Boudazin, G., Le Roux, A.C., Josi, K., Labarre, P., and Jouan, B.
    1999. Design of division specific primers of *Ralstonia solanacearum*
    and application to the identification of European isolates. Eur. J. Plant
    Pathol. 105: 373-380.
5. Buitrago Gallego, E. 2001. Impacto socio-económico de la
    enfermedad del moko en plantaciones de plátano y banano en seis
    municipios del departamento del Quindío, Julio 1998-Diciembre 2000.
    In: Seminario Taller "Manejo integrado de sigatokas, moko y picudo
    negro del plátano en el eje cafetero". Armenia 24-25 Mayo, 2001.
6. CABI/EPPO. 1999. Distribution maps of plant diseases. CAB
    International, Wallingford, UK.
7. Caruso, P., Gorris, M.T., Cambra, M., Palomo, J.L., Collar, J., and
    Lopez, M.M. 2002. Enrichment Double-Antibody Sandwich Indirect
    Enzyme-Linked Immunosorbent Assay that uses a specific monoclonal
    antibody for sensitive detection of *Ralstonia solanacearum* in
    asymptomatic potato tubers. Appl Environ. Microbiol. 68: 3634-3638.
8. Chen, W.Y. 1984. Influence of the root-knot nematode on wilt
    resistance of flue-cured tobacco infested by *Pseudomonas
    solanacearum*. Bulletin of the Tobacco Research Institute 21: 44-48.
9. Coelho Netto, R.A., Pereira, B.G., Noda, H., and Boher, B. 2004.
    Bacterial wilt in Amazonas state. Fitopatologia Brasileira 29: 17-23.
10. Danks, C., and Barker, I. 2000. On-site detection of plant pathogens
    using lateral flow devices. EPPO Bulletin 30: 421-426.
11. Davis, R.I., Fegan, M., Tjahjono, B., and Rahamma, S. 2000. An
    outbreak of blood disease of banana in Irian Jaya, Indonesia. Austral.
    Plant Pathol. 29: 152.
12. Elphinstone, J. G., Hennessy, J., Wilson, J. K., and Stead, D. E. 1996.
    Sensitivity of detection of *Ralstonia solanacearum* in potato tuber
    extracts. EPPO Bulletin 26: 663-678
13. Elphinstone, J.G., Stanford, H., and Stead, D.E. 1998. Detection of
    Ralstonia solanacearum in potato tubers, *Solanum dulcamara* and
    associated irrigation water. Pages 133-139 in: Bacterial Wilt Disease:
    Molecular and Ecological Aspects. P. Prior, C. Allen, and J.G.
    Elphinstone, eds. Springer-Verlag Berlin.
14. Elphinstone, J.G., Stead, D.E., *et al.* 2000. Standardization of methods
    for detection of *Ralstonia solanacearum* in potato. EPPO Bulletin 30:
    391-396.
15. Englebrecht, M. C. 1994. Modification of a semi-selective medium for
    the isolation and quantification of *Pseudomonas solanacearum*. Pages

3-5 in: Bacterial Wilt Newsletter 10. A. C. Hayward, ed. Australian Centre for International Agricultural Research, Canberra, Australia.

16. EPPO. 1990. Quarantine procedures no. 26. *Pseudomonas solanacearum*. OEPP/EPPO Bulletin 20: 255-262.

17. EPPO. 2000. New records or new detailed records on quarantine pests in Argentina, Brazil and Chile. EPPO Reporting Service 2000, No. 01: 2000/006.

18. Fernández-Northcote, E.N. 1996. Marchitez bacteriana de la papa en Bolivia. Pages 19-25 in: Memoria IV Reunión Nacional de la Papa. October 8-11, 1996. Cochabamba, Bolivia.

19. Fortnum, B.A. 2001. Disease management. Pages 38-59 in: South Carolina tobacco growers guide 2001. D.T. Gooden, ed. Co-operative Extension Service, Clemson University, Clemson, SC, USA.

20. Garcia, R., Garcia, A., and Delgado, L. 1999. Distribucion, incidencia y variabilidad de *Ralstonia solanacearum*, agente causal de la marchitez bacteriana de la papa en el estado Merida, Venezuela. Bioagro 11:12-23.

21. Gooden, D.T., Christenbury, G.D., Fortnum, B.A., Manley, D.G., Murdock, E.C., and Sutton, R.W. 2000. In: South Carolina tobacco growers guide 2001. Cooperative Extension Service. Clemson University, Clemson SC, USA.

22. Grousset, F., Roy, A.S., and Smith, I.M. 1998. Situation of *Ralstonia solanacearum* in the EPPO region in 1997. EPPO Bulletin 28:53-63.

23. Gurung, T.B., and Vaidya, A.K. 1997. Baseline study report of a community participatory bacterial wilt management programme in Ulleri and Jhilibarang villages of western Nepal. Working-Paper No. 97. Lumle Regional Agricultural Research Centre, Nepal.

24. Hartman, G.L., Hong, W.F., and Wang, T.C. 1991. Survey of bacterial wilt on fresh market hybrid tomatoes in Taiwan. Plant Protection Bulletin, Taiwan 33: 197-203.

25. Hayward, A.C., Moffett, M.L., and Pegg, K.G. 1967. Bacterial wilt of ginger in Queensland. Queensland Journal of Agricultural and Animal Science 24: 1-5.

26. Hayward, A.C., Elphinstone, J.G., Caffier, D., Janse, J., Stefani, E., French, E.R., and Wright, A.J. 1998. Round table on bacterial wilt (brown rot) of potato. Pages 420-430 in: Bacterial Wilt Disease: Molecular and Ecological Aspects. P. Prior, C. Allen, and J.G. Elphinstone, eds. Springer-Verlag Berlin/Heidelberg.

27. Hong, N.X., Mehan, V.K., Ly, N.T., and Vinh, M.T. 1994. Status of groundnut bacterial wilt research in Vietnam. Groundnut bacterial wilt in Asia. Pages 135-141 in: Proceedings of the third groundnut wilt working group meeting 4-5 July 1994, Oil Crops Research Institute, Wuhan, China.

28. Hong, W.F., Hsu, S.T., and Tzeng, K.C. 1993. Bacterial wilt of *Perilla crispa*: New host and new transmission method. Pages 373-376 in: Bacterial Wilt. Proceedings of an International Conference held at Kaohsiung, Taiwan, 28-31 October 1992. G.L. Hartman and A.C. Hayward, eds. ACIAR Proceedings No. 45, Canberra, Australia.

29. Horita, M., and Tsuchiya, K. 2001. Genetic diversity of Japanese strains of *Ralstonia solanacearum*. Phytopathology 91: 399-407.

30. Hyde, K.D., McCulloch, B., Akiew, E., Peterson, R.A., and Diatloff, A. 1992. Strategies used to eradicate bacterial wilt of *Heliconia* (race 2) in Cairns, Australia, following introduction of the disease from Hawaii. Australasian Plant Pathology 21: 29-31.

31. Janse, J.D., Araluppan, F.A.X., Schans, J., Wenneker, M., and Westerhuis, W. 1998. Experiences with bacterial brown rot, *Ralstonia solanacearum* biovar 2 race 3, in the Netherlands. Pages 146-154 in: Bacterial Wilt Disease: Molecular and Ecological Aspects. P. Prior, C. Allen, and J.G. Elphinstone, eds. Springer-Verlag Berlin/Heidelberg.

32. Kelman, A. 1954. The relationship of pathogenicity of *Pseudomonas solanacearum* to colony appearance on a tetrazolium medium. Phytopathology 44: 693-695.

33. Kishun, R. 1987. Loss in yield of tomato due to bacterial wilt caused by *Pseudomonas solanacearum*. Indian Phytopath. 40: 152 - 155.

34. Liao, B.S., Shan, Z.H., Lei, Y., Tan, Y.J., Li, D., and Duan, N.X. 1998. Reaction of groundnut (*Arachis hypogaea*) to latent infection by bacterial wilt (*Ralstonia solanacearum*). Chinese J. Oil Crop Sci. 20: 66-70.

35. López, O., Cardoso, H., and Fernandez-Northcote, E.N. 1999. Incidencia y distribución de la marchitez bacteriana de la papa en el Departamento de Tarija. Es. Cochabamba (Bolivia). Fundación Proyecto Manejo Integrado de la Marchitez Bacteriana de la Papa (PROINPA).

36. Meiners, U. 2000. Bacterial ring rot: possibilities and limits of insurance coverage. Kartoffelbau 51:536-539.

37. Melo, M.S., de Furuya, N., Iiyama, K., Khan, A.A., and Matsuyama, N. 1999. Geographical distribution of biovars of *Ralstonia solanacearum* in Brazil. J. Facul. Agricul. Kyushu University, 44: 9-15.

38. Melton, T.A., and Broadwell, A. 2001. Disease Management. Pages 94-118 in: Flue-cured Tobacco Information. Cooperative Extension Service, North Carolina State University, Raleigh, NC, USA.

39. Molina, G.C. 1996. Integrated management of 'tibaglon' a bacterial fruit rot disease of cooking banana under farmers field. Philippine Phytopathol. 32: 83-91.

40. Olsson, K. 1976. Experience of brown rot caused by *Pseudomonas solanacearum* in Sweden. EPPO Bulletin 6:199-207.

41. Opina, N., Tavner, F., Holloway, G., Wang, J.-F., Li, T.-H., Maghirang, R., Fegan, M., Hayward, A.C., Krishnapillai, V., Hong, W.F., Holloway, B.W., and Timmis, J.N. 1997. A novel method for development of species and strain-specific DNA probes and PCR primers for identifying *Burkholderia solanacearum* (formerly *Pseudomonas solanacearum*). Asian-Pac. J. Mol. Biol. Biotechnol. 5: 19-33.

42. Opio, A.F., and Busolo-Bulafu, C.M. 1990. Status of bacterial wilt on groundnut in Uganda. Pages 54-55 in: Proceedings of an ACIAR/ICRISAT collaborative research planning meeting, 18-19 March 1990. K.J. Middleton and A.C. Hayward, eds. ACIAR Proceedings No. 31. Canberra , Australia.

43. Pastrik, K.H., and Maiss, E. 2000. Detection of *Ralstonia solanacearum* in potato tubers by polymerase chain reaction. J. Phytopathol. 148:619-626.

44. Pastrik, K. H., Elphinstone, J.G., and Pukall, R. 2002. Differentiation and identification of *Ralstonia solanacearum* biovars by RAPD-PCR and analysis of amplified 16S-23S ribosomal intergenic spacer region. Eur. J. Plant Pathol. 108: 831-842.

45. Pathak, K.N., Roy, S., Ojha, K.L., and Jha, M.M., 1999. Influence of *Meloidogyne incognita* on the fungal and bacterial wilt complex of banana. Indian J. Nem. 29: 39-43.

46. Pegg, K.G., and Moffett, M.L. 1971. Host range of the ginger strain of *Pseudomonas solanacearum* in Queensland.. Australian J. Expt. Agricul. Animal Husb. 11: 696-698.

47. Persson, P. Successful eradication of *Ralstonia solanacearum* from Sweden. 1998. EPPO Bulletin 28: 113-119.

48. Poussier, S., Trigalet-Demery, D., Vanderwalle, P., Goffinet, B., Luisetti, J., and Trigalet, A. 2000. Genetic diversity of *Ralstonia solanacearum* as assessed by PCR-RFLP of the hrp gene region, AFLP and 16S rRNA sequence analysis, and identification of an African subdivision. Microbiology 146: 1679-1692.

49. Prior, P., Allen, C., and Elphinstone, J.G. eds. 1998. Bacterial Wilt Disease: Molecular and Ecological Aspects. Springer-Verlag Berlin/Heidelberg.

50. Robertson, A.E. 1999. Characterisation, epidemiology and management of bacterial wilt of tobacco, caused by *Ralstonia solanacearum* in Zimbabwe. M. Phil Thesis. University of Zimbabwe.

51. Robinson-Smith, A., Jones, P., Elphinstone, J.G., and Forde, S.M.D. 1995. Production of antibodies to *Pseudomonas solanacearum*, the causative agent of bacterial wilt. Food Agricul. Immunol. 7:67-79.

52. Seal, S.E., Jackson, L.A. Young, J.P.W., and Daniels, M.J. 1993. Detection of *Pseudomonas solanacearum*, *Pseudomonas syzygii*, *Pseudomonas pickettii* and Blood Disease Bacterium by partial 16S rRNA sequencing: construction of oligonucleotide primers for sensitive detection by polymerase chain reaction. J. Gen. Microbiol. 139: 1587-1594.

53. SENASA. 1999. Results of a survey on potato diseases in Peru in 1998-1999. International Potato Center, Lima Peru.

54. Sequeira, L. 1998. Bacterial wilt: the missing element in international banana improvement programs. Pages 6-16 in: Bacterial Wilt Disease: Molecular and Ecological Aspects. P. Prior, C. Allen, and J.G. Elphinstone, eds. Springer-Verlag Berlin.

55. Sharma, B.K., and Rana, K.S. 1999. Bacterial wilt: A threat to ginger cultivation in Himachal Pradesh. Plant Dis. Res. 14:216-217.

56. Shrestha, S.K. 1996. Bacterial wilt of potato in Nepal: spread, losses and magnitude of disease. Pages 11-18 in: Integrated management of bacterial wilt of potato: Lessons from the hills of Nepal. P.M. Pradhanang and J.G. Elphinstone, eds. Proceedings of a national workshop held at Lumle Agricultural Research Centre, Pokhara, Nepal, 4-5 November 1996.

57. Smith, J.J., Offord, L.C., Holderness, M., and Saddler, G.S. 1995. Genetic diversity of *Burkholderia solanacearum* (syn. *Pseudomonas solanacearum*) race 3 in Kenya. Appl. Environ. Microbiol. 61: 4263-68.

58. Tan, Y.J., Duan, N.X., Liao, B.S., Xu, Z.Y., He, L.Y., and Zheng, G.R. 1994. Status of groundnut bacterial wilt research in China. Pages 107-113 in: Groundnut bacterial wilt in Asia. Proceedings of the third working group meeting 4-5 July 1994, Oil Crops Research Institute, Wuhan, China.

59. Thammakijjawat, P., Thaveechai, N., Paradhonuwat, A., Wannakairoj, S., and Suthirawut, S. 1999. Bacterial rhizome rot of patumma and detection of seed-borne rhizome. [Thai]. Pages 295-302 in: The 37th Kasetsart University Annual Conference, 3-5 February, 1999. Text and Journal Publication Co, Ltd, Bangkok, Thailand.

60. Titatarn, V. 1986. Bacterial wilt in Thailand. Pages 65-67 in: Bacterial wilt disease in Asia and the South Pacific. Proceedings of an international workshop held at PCARRD, Los Baños, Philippines, 8-10 October 1885. Persley, G.J. ed. ACIAR Proceedings No. 13, Canberra, Australia.

61. Tomlinson, D.L., and Gunther, M.T. 1986. Bacterial wilt in Papua New Guinea. Pages 35-39 in: Bacterial wilt diseases in Asia and the South Pacific. Proceedings of an international workshop held at

PCARRD, Los Baños, Philippines, 8-10 October 1885. G.J. Persley, ed. ACIAR Proceedings No. 13, Canberra, Australia.

62. van der Tuin, W.R., Nahumury, E.T., Spit, B.E., and Janse, J.D. 1996. *Pseudomonas (Ralstonia) solanacearum* race 1, biovar 4 in *Curcuma longa*. Verslagen en Meded. Plantenziektenk. Dienst 186, 1997, Annual Report 1996: 17.

63. Verma, S.K., Gupta, N.N., and Phogat, K.P.S. 1997. Studies on the interaction between root-knot nematodes, *Meloidogyne* spp.; fungi, *Fusarium oxysporum* and *F. solani* and bacterium, *Pseudomonas solanacearum* (*Ralstonia solanacearum*) on brinjal, *Solanum melongena L.* under valley condition of Garhwal hills. Progres. Hort. 29: 188-193.

64. Walker, T., and Collion, M-H. 1998. Priority setting at CIP for the 1998-2000 Medium Term Plan. International Potato Center, Lima, Peru.

65. Weller, S.A., Elphinstone, J.G., Smith, N., Stead, D.E., and Boonham, N. 1999. Detection of *Ralstonia solanacearum* strains using an automated and quantitative fluorogenic 5' nuclease TaqMan assay. Appl. & Environ. Microbiol. 66: 2853-2858.

66. Weller S.A., Elphinstone J.G., Smith N., and Stead D.E. 2000. Detection of *Ralstonia solanacearum* from potato tissue by post enriched TaqMan™ PCR. EPPO Bulletin 30: 381-384.

67. Williamson, L., Nakaho, K., Hudelson, B., and Allen, C. 2002. *Ralstonia solanacearum* race 3, biovar 2 stains isolated from Geranium are pathogenic on potato. Plant Disease 86: 987-991.

68. Wullings, B.A., van Beuningen, A.R., Janse, J.D., and Akkermans, A.D.L. 1998. Detection of *Ralstonia solanacearum*, which causes brown rot of potato, by fluorescent in situ hybridization with 23s rRNA-targeted probes. Appl. Environ. Microbiol. 64:4546-4554.

69. Yeh, W.L. 1990. A review of bacterial wilt on groundnut in Guangdong Province, Peoples' Republic of China. ACIAR Proceedings 31: 48-51.

Introduction and Prospectus
on the Survival of *R. solanacearum*

Teresa A. Coutinho

Department of Microbiology and Plant Pathology
Forestry and Agricultural Biotechnology Institute (FABI)
University of Pretoria, Pretoria 0002, Republic of South Africa

Bacterial wilt, caused by *Ralstonia solanacearum*, is a major constraint to the production of a number of economically important agricultural crops. The disease is widely distributed, occurring in tropical, subtropical and temperate regions of the world (12). Timms-Wilson *et al.* (39) speculated that the recent occurrence of bacterial wilt on potato crops in Northern Europe was due to the selection and proliferation of a novel variant of the pathogen adapted to cooler environments. [Editor's note: This seems unlikely, given that the race 3 potato-infecting strains are successful at cool temperatures at their origin in the High Andes. Moreover, phylogenetic data indicate that this group of strains is highly genetically uniform worldwide, with no indication that European strains are in any way different from others. A more probable explanation is simply that race 3 strains were introduced into Europe and have become established there.] The epidemiology of bacterial wilt is considered to be complicated, involving many interacting factors (2,14,19). This review will focus on recent developments in our understanding of *R. solanacearum* survival, including both the means of pathogen dispersal and sources of inoculum.

Some aspects of *R. solanacearum* dispersal, such as the dissemination of the pathogen on farm implements (Fortnum, this volume, 24) and root-to-root transmission (21) are well understood. Other aspects are less well understood, such as occurrence of the bacterium in seed, soil, and water, and latent infections in both hosts and alternative weed hosts. Several sensitive detection methods have been described over the past decade (31,33,37,41, 46). Development of methods for detecting the bacterium in these environmental samples has been delayed because *R. solanacearum* constitutes a complex, phenotypically heterogeneous species complex.

Strains of *R. solanacearum* have been divided into five host-specific races and five biovars based on biochemical properties (3,11). Further

29

studies, based on phenotypic and genotypic analysis of different strains from all over the world, have found two distinct groups within the complex species (4,38,39,46). In this volume, Fegan and Prior proposed a new phylogenetic scheme for classifying *R. solanacearum* based on genetic diversity. In this scheme, strains are also epidemiologically grouped into clusters that relate to pathogenicity, host range and/or geographic origin.

The reliable, sensitive methods for detecting *R. solanacearum* that are now available have provided information on the source and virulence of isolates (Fegan and Prior, this volume, 39). Low densities of the pathogen in watercourses, soils and plant materials can also now be detected (42,43). As will be illustrated below, these detection methods have provided a greater understanding of the survival strategies used by this pathogen and the extent of its distribution and persistence in plant material, irrigation water and soils.

Survival in Plant Material

Both short- and long-distance dispersal of *R. solanacearum* on vegetatively propagation material has been known for many years (2). Dispersal in propagation material is especially important for banana, ginger, and potato (22). Recently, the detection of the pathogen in geranium cuttings imported into Belgium, Germany, the Netherlands, and the United States from Kenya (Janse, this volume) has highlighted the importance of enforcing strict quarantine regulations related to the movement of plant material over international borders.

The discovery that both solanaceous and non-solanaceous plants can be infected by *R. solanacearum* without showing any symptoms has had a great impact on quarantine and breeding strategies. The movement of latently-infected seed potatoes in Northern and Southern Europe has resulted in outbreaks of the disease where it had not previously occurred (40). The occurrence of *R. solanacearum* as latent infections in plants not exhibiting wilt symptoms, and thus regarded as resistant, has highlighted the importance of selecting planting stock under conditions conducive for disease expression (14). If plants are selected at low temperatures and the material is then planted at temperatures favorable for the disease, the consequences can be devastating.

A number of methods have been developed to detect *R. solanacearum* where it exists as a latent pathogen, particularly in potato. These include indirect immunofluorescence (IIF) microscopy (46), followed by isolations on semi-selective media (6), fatty acid analysis (16), and pathogenicity tests on indicator plants such as tomato. A PCR detection method has been used as an alternative to IIF (34) but has been found to be unreliable (17).

Recently, fluorescent *in situ* hybridization (FISH) with 23s rRNA-targeted probes has rapidly and reliably detected latent infections (46). These methods also detected the pathogen in soil, water and root tissue of a weed host, *Solanum dulcamara* (bittersweet) in contaminated areas [Editor's note: For further information on detection methods, see also Diversity and Diagnosis section of this volume, especially references from Priou *et al.*).

There are few reports on the survival of *R. solanacearum* on or in true seed from infected plants, but the evidence is conflicting. Seed transmission has been demonstrated in groundnut (23) and artificially contaminated seeds of tomato and capsicum were also reported to transmit the disease (26). However, seed from naturally-infected tomato plants appears to be pathogen-free (Martins *et al.*, this volume). Survival of the pathogen in groundnut seed was found to be closely linked to the water content, that is, when the water content of the seed was below 10% the pathogen could not be detected (47). Although seed transmission of *R. solanacearum* is not prevalent, it may have epidemiological significance in some situations.

The range and variety of weed hosts of *R. solanacearum* is extensive (14,19). Some of these hosts are susceptible, others tolerant, while still others may act as latent or symptomless carriers (11,25). Weed hosts can increase bacterial populations in the soil and may also serve as alternate hosts whenever non-host plants are cultivated (15). A few studies have also considered the rhizosphere of weeds as a protected survival site (1,11).

Survival in Irrigation Water

Irrigation water contaminated with *R. solanacearum* has been responsible for outbreaks of bacterial wilt on a number of crops (7). In the case of potato, contaminated surface water was associated with effluent from the potato processing industry and municipal water purification plants that handled diseased potatoes (5,17). In Egypt, the bacterium was found in both irrigation and drainage canals near infected potato fields (8) while in Kenya, infection of geranium cuttings was apparently due to the use of contaminated irrigation water (Janse, this volume).

Ralstonia solanacearum can survive for considerable periods of time in water (19), and this has important implications for agricultural practices (29). Prolonged survival and even growth has been shown to take place in sterile water under appropriate environmental conditions (20,43,44). Temperature, pH, salt level, surfaces provided by particulate matter, and the presence of competing, antagonistic or parasitic organisms are the key factors influencing the bacterium's ability to survive in aquatic habitats (43). The survival of *R. solanacearum* was strongly dependent on temperature irrespective of inoculum density and physiological state, with maximum survival occurring at 12°, 20° and 28° C. The water biota can have a marked effect on survival of the bacterium at these temperatures, since the persistence of the strain studied was significantly enhanced in sterilized drainage water (43). Furthermore, both incident light and seawater salts were detrimental to strain survival. *R. solanacearum* persisted in canal sediment saturated with drainage water but died out when the sediment was dried (43).

The viable but nonculturable state (VBNC) of *R. solanacearum* may be involved in the long-term survival of this bacterium in water and soil and at different stages in plant infection (12,43). The strain studied by van Elsas *et al.* (43) converted to this state in water microcosms kept at 4°C but not those at 20° C. The potential occurrence of VBNC cells in natural water poses a problem for the detection of *R. solanacearum* by cultivation-based methods. A more detailed discussion of the VBNC state in *R. solanacearum* is presented by van Elsas *et al.* (this volume).

Weed hosts of *R. solanacearum* commonly inhabit the edges of watercourses in Europe (43). The semi-aquatic weed *S. dulcamara* (bittersweet nightshade) has been found to act as a reservoir of this pathogen, accumulating and continuously releasing the bacterium into the water (5,18). Other weeds growing in watercourses such as *Urtica dioica* (stinging nettle) may play a similar role (43). An enhanced liberation of cells from bittersweet has been postulated to explain the increase in numbers of *R. solanacearum* in the period following winter, when water temperatures rise and exceed 15° C (45). Alternatively, van Elsas *et al.* hypothesize that the resuscitation of VBNC cells present in low temperatures would increase with the gradual warming of the water (43). Further studies on the survival mechanisms of this pathogen in natural water systems are needed.

Survival in Soil

There are conflicting reports on the ability of *R. solanacearum* to survive in soils. Most of the available evidence suggests that this pathogen does not survive in bulk soil away from plant material except for short periods of time (9). In a study of soil survival in temperate soils by van Elsas *et al.* (42), the population density of *R. solanacearum* biovar 2 declined progressively over time. In two of the three fields studied, the bacterium persisted in the soil for periods of 12 months or longer. Indications were also found in this study that the bacterium can exist in the VBNC state in some of these soil types.

Long-term survival of *R. solanacearum* in the soil is believed by many researchers to reflect the ability of the organism to infect the roots of susceptible or latent plant hosts, or to colonize the rhizosphere of non-hosts

(1,10,11). Plant debris provides temporary sheltered sites for the bacterium (1). Graham (10) showed that plant debris could harbor *R. solanacearum* for 33 weeks after the potato crop was harvested. Van Elsas (42) suggested the presence of potato volunteer plants, weeds and plant debris in the fields may have contributed to the pathogen's survival, although they could not exclude the survival of the bacterium directly in the soil or in soil-associated water, possibly in deeper layers, as an important factor determining the fate of this pathogen.

Soil moisture content, temperature and soil type can all play a critical role in the survival of *R. solanacearum* in this habitat (27,28,36,42). The extent to which these factors affect survival can vary and the ultimate effect depends on the physiological and physical requirements of *R. solanacearum* as well as the interactions between these factors. This was evident in the study by van Elsas *et al.* (42), where *R. solanacearum* persistence in soil microcosms depended on abiotic conditions, temperature and moisture content.

It is clear from the above that the survival mechanisms as well as strategies for persistence of *R. solanacearum* in soil are complicated and remain poorly understood. One of the reasons for this is that pathogenic populations in soils decline over time to an undetectable level. The use of selective media can only provide reliable information above a concentration of 10^2 CFU/g soil (11). Other methods such as serological and immunological procedures have similar or lesser sensitivity (35). Recently, a nested PCR technique was described by Pradhanang (31), which was used to detect *R. solanacearum* at very low concentrations in soils. Also, Poussier (this volume) reported reliable PCR detection of *R. solanacearum* in the environment after using different strategies for DNA capture and extraction. The means are thus now available to allow us to investigate strategies and mechanisms deployed by this pathogen in soil habitats.

Prospectus

In the epilogue of the book "Bacterial Wilt: The Disease and its Causative Agent, *Pseudomonas solanacearum*", Sequeira (35) states that there is little mention in the literature on the great potential of modern detection methods for ecological studies. Over the past decade, a number of techniques have been developed for this purpose and these have also found an application in quarantine procedures. These techniques are typically molecular because of their advantageous increased specificity and sensitivity. With the development of *R. solanacearum*-specific PCR methods, Seal *et al.* (34) were able to detect 16S rDNA sequences from a single cell grown in culture. Although highly sensitive *in vitro*, the routine application of

PCR for pathogen detection is currently limited because of the presence of PCR-inhibitory compounds in soil and plant extracts (30,32). It is possible to remove these compounds but the procedures are time-consuming, hazardous or expensive and, therefore, not suited to routine diagnostics. Other methods that have proved reliable include IF, SMSA media and PCR, fatty acid profiles, rep-PCR and sample dilution and enrichment in SMSA broth followed by a two-stage nested PCR protocol. Sequeira (35) stated that a primary need in our studies on *R. solanacearum* is to improve our understanding of survival of this organism. More specifically he states that "Survival is an issue that is fundamental not only to our knowledge of the biology of this organism but to the implementation of rational methods of control". We have made some progress in this regard. *R. solanacearum* can now be detected, even in low concentrations, in plant material, water and soil. Over the next decade, the application of recently described detection methods and those still to be developed will provide additional insight to how this bacterium survives in the absence of its host.

Literature Cited

1. Akiew, E., and Trevorrow, P.R. 1994. Management of bacterial wilt of tobacco. Pages 179-198 in: Bacterial Wilt: The Disease and its Causative Agent, *Pseudomonas solanacearum*. A.C. Hayward and G.L. Hartman eds. CAB International, United Kingdom.
2. Buddenhagen, I., and Kelman, A. 1964. Biological and physiological aspects of bacterial wilt caused by *Pseudomonas solanacearum*. Ann. Rev. Phytopathol. 2:203-230.
3. Buddenhagen, I.W., Sequeira, L., and Kelman, A. 1962. Designation of races of *Pseudomonas solanacearum*. Phytopathology 52:726.
4. Cook, D., Barlow, E., and Sequeira, L. 1989. Genetic diversity of *Pseudomonas solanacearum*: detection of restriction fragment length polymorphisms with DNA that specify virulence and the hypersensitive response. Mol. Plant-Microbe Inter. 2:113-121.
5. Elphinstone, J.G. 1996. Survival and possible extinction of *Pseudomonas solanacearum* (Smith) Smith in cool climates. Potato Res. 39:403-410.
6. Elphinstone, J.G., Hennessy, J., Wilson, J.K., and Stead, D.E. 1996. Sensitivity of different methods for the detection methods for *Ralstonia solanacearum* in potato tuber extracts. Bull. OEPP/EPPO Bull. 26:663-678.
7. Elphinstone, J.G., Stanford, H., and Stead, D.E. 1998. Detection of *Ralstonia solanacearum* in potato tubers, *Solanum dulcamara* and associated irrigation water. Pages 133-139 in: Bacterial Wilt Disease:

Molecular and Ecological Aspects. P. Prior, C. Allen, and J. Elphinstone, eds. Springer-Verlag, Heidelberg, Germany.

8. Faraq, N., Stead, D. E., and Janse, J. D. 1999. *Ralstonia* (*Pseudomonas*) *solanacearum* race 3, biovar 2, detected in surface (irrigation) water in Egypt. J. Phytopathol. 147:485-487.

9. Graham, J., and Lloyd, A.B. 1979. Survival of potato strain (race 3) of *Pseudomonas solanacearum* in the deeper soil layers. Aust. J. Agri. Res. 30:489-496.

10. Graham, J., Jones, D.A., and Lloyd, A.B. 1979. Survival of *Pseudomonas solanacearum* race 3 in plant debris and in latently infected potato tubers. Phytopathology 69:1100-1103.

11. Granada, G.A., and Sequeira, L. 1983. Survival of *Pseudomonas solanacearum* in soil, rhizosphere and plant roots. Can. J. Microbiol. 29:433-440.

12. Grey, B.E., and Steck, T.R. 2001. The viable but nonculturable state of *Ralstonia solanacearum* may be involved in long-term survival and plant infection. Appl. Environ. Microbiol. 67:3866-3872.

13. Hayward, A.C. 1964. Characteristics of *Pseudomonas solanacearum*. J. Appl. Bacteriol. 27:265-277.

14. Hayward, A.C. 1991. Biology and epidemiology of bacterial wilt caused by *Pseudomonas solanacearum*. Ann. Rev. Phytopathol. 29:65-87.

15. Hayward, A.C. 1994. The hosts of *Pseudomonas solanacearum*. Pages 9-24 in: Bacterial Wilt: The Disease and its Causative Agent, *Pseudomonas solanacearum*. A.C. Hayward and G.L. Hartman, eds. CABI International, United Kingdom.

16. Janse, J.D. 1991. Infra- and intraspecific classification of *Pseudomonas solanacearum* strains, using whole cell fatty acid analysis. Syst. Appl. Microbiol. 12:335-345.

17. Janse, J.D. 1996. Potato brown rot in Western Europe: history, present occurrence and some remarks on possible origin, epidemiology and control strategies. Bull. OEPP/EPPO Bull. 26:679-665.

18. Janse, J.D., Araluppen, F.A.X., Schans, J., Wenneker, M., and Westerhuis, W. 1998. Experiences with bacterial brown rot *Ralstonia solanacearum* biovar 2, race 3 in the Netherlands. Pages 146-152 in: Bacterial Wilt Disease. Molecular and Ecological Aspects. P. Prior, C. Allen, and J. Elphinstone, eds. Springer-Verlag, Heidelberg, Germany.

19. Kelman, A. 1953. The bacterial wilt caused by *Pseudomonas solanacearum*. A literature review and bibliography. N.C. Agri. Exp. Stat. Tech. Bull. 99, Raleigh, North Carolina State University.

20. Kelman, A. 1956. Survival of *Pseudomonas solanacearum* in water. Phytopathology 46:16-17.

21. Kelman, A., and Sequeira, L. 1965. Root-root spread of *Pseudomonas solanacearum*. Phytopathology 60:833-838.
22. Kelman, A., Hartman, G.L., and Hayward, A.C. 1994. Introduction. Pages 1-8 in: Bacterial Wilt: The Disease and its Causative Agent, *Pseudomonas solanacearum*. A.C. Hayward and G.L. Hartman, eds. CAB International, United Kingdom.
23. Machmund, M., and Middleton, K.J. 1991. Transmission of *Pseudomonas solanacearum* through groundnut seed. ACIAR Bact. Wilt News. 7:4-5.
24. McCarter, S.M., and Jaworski, C.A. 1968. Greenhouse studies on the spread of *Pseudomonas solanacearum* in tomato plants by clipping. Plant Dis. 52:330-334.
25. Moffett, M.L., and Hayward, A.C. 1980. The role of weed species in the survival of *Pseudomonas solanacearum* in tomato cropping land. Aust. Plant Pathol. Soc. News. 9:6-8.
26. Moffett, M.L., Wood, B.A., and Hayward, A.C. 1981. Seed and soil: sources of inoculum for the colonization of the foliage of solanaceous hosts by *Pseudomonas solanacearum*. Annals App. Biol. 98:403-411.
27. Nesmith, W.C., and Jenkins, S.F., Jr. 1983. Survival of *Pseudomonas solanacearum* in selected North Carolina soils. Phytopathology 73:1300-1304.
28. Nesmith, W.C., and Jenkins, S.F., Jr. 1985. Influence of antagonists and controlled matrix potential on the survival of *Pseudomonas solanacearum* in four North Carolina soils. Phytopathology 75:1182-1187.
29. Olsson, K. 1976. Experience of brown rot caused by *Pseudomonas solanacearum* (Smith) Smith in Sweden. Bull. OEPP/EPPO Bull. 6:199-207.
30. Picard, C., Ponsonnet, C., Paget, E., Nesme, X., and Simonet, P. 1992. Detection and enumeration of bacteria in soil by direct DNA extraction and polymerase chain reaction. Appl. Envir. Microbiol. 58:2717-2722.
31. Pradhanang, P.M., Elphinstone, J.G., and Fox, R.T.V. 2000. Sensitive detection of *Ralstonia solanacearum* in soil: a comparison of different detection techniques. Plant Pathol. 49:414-422.
32. Seal, S. 1995. PCR-based detection and characterization of *Pseudomonas solanacearum* for use in less developed countries. Bull. OEPP/EPPO Bull. 25:227-231.
33. Seal, S.E., Jackson, L.A., and Daniels, M.J. 1992. Use of tRNA consensus primers to indicate subgroups of *Pseudomonas solanacearum* by PCR amplification. Appl. Envir. Microbiol. 58:3759-3761.
34. Seal, S.E., Jackson, L.A., Young, J.P.W., and Daniels, M.J. 1993. Differentiation of *Pseudomonas solanacearum, Pseudomonas syzygii,*

Pseudomonas picketti and blood disease bacterium by partial 16S rRNA sequencing: construction of oligonucleotide primers for sensitive detection by polymerase chain reaction. J. Gen. Microbiol. 139:1587-1594.

35. Sequeira, L. 1994. Epilogue: life with a "mutable and treacherous tribe". Pages 235-248 in: Bacterial Wilt: The Disease and its Causative Agent, *Pseudomonas solanacearum*. A.C. Hayward and G.L. Hartman, eds. CAB International, United Kingdom.

36. Shekhawat, G.S., and Perombelon, M.C.M. 1991. Factors affecting survival in soil and virulence of *Pseudomonas solanacearum*. Z. Pflanzenk. u. Pflanzenschutz. 98:258-267.

37. Smith, J.J., Offord, L.C., Holderness, M., and Saddler, G.S. 1995. Pulse field gel electrophoresis analysis of *Pseudomonas solanacearum*. Bull. OEPP/EPPO Bull. 25:163-167.

38. Taghavi, M., Hayward, C., Sly, I., and Fegan, M. 1996. Analysis of the phylogenetic relationships of strains of *Burkholderia solanacearum*, *Pseudomonas syzygi*, and the blood disease bacterium of banana based on 16S rRNA gene sequences. International J. Syst. Bacteriol. 46:10-15.

39. Timms-Wilson, T.M., Bryant, T., and Bailey, M.J. 2001. Strain characterization and 16S-23S probe development for differentiating geographically dispersed isolates of the phytopathogen *Ralstonia solanacearum*. Environ. Microbiol. 3:785-797.

40. Turco, P., Saccardi, A., Piazzi, E., Martini, G., Melegatti, A., Xodo, E., and Gambin, E. 1998. Monitoring of *Ralstonia solanacearum* in the Veneto region (Italy). Bull. OEPP/EPPO Bull. 28:85-92.

41. Van der Wolf, J.M., Vriend, S.G.C., and van Vuurde, J.W.L. 2000. Immunofluorescence colony-staining (IFC) for detection and quantification of *Ralstonia* (*Pseudomonas*) *solanacearum* biovar 2 (race 3) in soil and verification of positive results by PCR and dilution plating. Eur. J. Plant Pathol. 106:123-133.

42. Van Elsas, J.D., Kastelein, P., van Bekkum, P., van der Wolf, J.M., de Vries, P.M., and van Overbeek, L.S. 2000. Survival of *Ralstonia solanacearum* biovar 2, the causative agent of potato brown rot, in field and microcosm soils in temperate climates. Phytopathology 90:1338-1366.

43. Van Elsas, J.D., Kastelein, P., de Vries, P.M., and van Overbeek, L.S. 2001. Effects of ecological factors on the survival and physiology of *Ralstonia solanacearum* bv. 2 in irrigation water. Can. J. Microbiol. 47:842-854.

44. Wakimoto Utatsu, I., Matsuo, N., and Hayashi, I. 1982. Multiplication of *Pseudomonas solanacearum* in pure water. Ann. Rev. Phytopathol., Soc. Jap. 48: 620-627.

45. Wenneker, M., Verdel, M.S.W., Groenewald, R.M.W., Kempenaar, C., Van Beuningen, A.R., and Janse, J.D. 1999. *Ralstonia (Pseudomonas) solanacearum* race 3 (biovar 2) in surface water and natural weed hosts: first report on stinging nettle (*Urtica dioica*). Eur. J. Plant Pathol. 106:123-133.
46. Wullings, B.A., Van Beuningen, A.R., Janse, J.D., and Akkermans, A.D.L. 1998. Detection of *Ralstonia solanacearum*, which causes brown rot of potato, by fluorescent *in situ* hybridization with 23S rRNA-targeted probes. Appl. Environ. Microbiol. 64:4546-4554.
47. Zhang, Y.X., Hua, J.Y., and He, L.Y. 1993. Effect of groundnut seeds on transmission of *Pseudomonas solanacearum*. Bact. Wilt News. 9:9-10.

Fate of *Ralstonia solanacearum* Biovar 2 as Affected by Conditions and Soil Treatments in Temperate Climate Zones

J.D. Van Elsas[1], L.S. Van Overbeek[1], M.J. Bailey[2], J. Schönfeld[3], and K. Smalla[3]

[1] Plant Research International, Wageningen, The Netherlands; [2] Institute of Virology and Environmental Microbiology (IVEM-NERC), Oxford; [3] Federal Biological Research Centre for Agriculture and Forestry, Braunschweig, Germany

In the past decade, bacterial wilt of potato, caused by *Ralstonia solanacearum* biovar 2 (race 3) has appeared in Northwest Europe. A considerable amount of farmland has been found to be infested by this pathogen, which has resulted in large economic losses (26,31). In addition, a range of water-ways in the infested regions has been shown to be persistently infested. As *R. solanacearum* biovar 2 may thus have become established in European ecosystems, it is urgent that tactics for efficient management of the pathogen are developed. Soil management methods, which ideally result in an enhanced suppression of the pathogen, can either involve soil treatments using simple farmer's measures, or an educated choice of the most suitable follow up crop. As postulated by van Bruggen and Semenov (24), the key effects brought about by soil management methods relate to the composition and/or activity of the soil microbiota. Thus, to be effective, measures should impact the soil microbial community in such a way that the disease suppressive activity of that community – the natural biological control capacity – is enhanced. Alternative strategies can be based upon the actual application of microorganisms that perform well in the ecosystem, taking advantage of their natural inclination to antagonize *R. solanacearum*. One such strategy was based on the potential offered by non-pathogenic (*hrp* gene mutant) forms of the pathogen (23,21).

A European Research Consortium with participation of partners from five member states as its main aims wants to enhance the understanding of the fate and physiology of *R. solanacearum* biovar 2 in temperate climate habitats, and to develop strategies that can lead to measures that stimulate the pathogen-suppressive activity of the natural microflora in soils. The current chapter will review the state-of-the-art in these two important areas.

Fate and Physiology of *R. solanacearum* Biovar 2 in Soil and Water

METHODS

For the specific detection of *R. solanacearum* biovar 2 cells in natural habitats, we have relied on immunofluorescence colony staining (IFC) based on the use of a highly specific antibody raised against *R. solanacearum* strain 1609 (29,25,26). The method has been validated as an adequate method for ecological monitoring, as it specifically identified and enumerated IFC-culturable cells of *R. solanacearum*. The method was complemented by the application of division II-specific PCR with the primer set recommended by Boudazin and colleagues (2) or by targeting unique 23S rRNA sequences that further distinguish European isolates (22). These characterization methods were supported by checking isolates for their capacity to cause wilting of susceptible tomato plants.

For detection at the total cell level, we used direct immunofluorescence (IF) (16,14,5) using the same antiserum mentioned above. These methods were complemented with methods that assess the viability of cells, i.e. the direct viable count (DVC) method recommended by Kogure (15) and CTC membrane activity measurements (11); see chapter on VBNC cells in this volume.

Molecular approaches were also developed to identify novel transcripts in *R. solanacearum* following exposure to stress and inability to be isolated on selective media. The method described by Dellagi and colleagues (3) was adapted to monitor differential gene expression in *R. solanacearum*. Subtractive hybridization and cDNA–AFLP analysis of differentially expressed mRNA (Bryant and Bailey, unpublished) identified novel transcripts, when compared with genome sequence data (17). Following the incubation of bacterial cells in filter-sterilized water, *de novo* synthesis of mRNA was monitored and compared to the rate of cellular activity, measured by 23S ribosomal RNA levels.

Recent studies performed in microcosms and in the field assessed the survival of *R. solanacearum* biovar 2 (strain 1609) in soil and water from infested regions in the Netherlands (26,27). In general, the pathogen revealed the capacity to survive for considerable periods of time in several soil and aquatic habitats. Survival in soil extended as long as one year after outbreak, even including a winter period; a key role for potato volunteers (9) was indicated in this survival. Temperature was shown to strongly affect the survival of *R. solanacearum* in both soil and water systems. Maximal survival, in particular in the water systems, was demonstrated at physiologically favorable temperatures, whereas progressive reductions in the sizes of the *R. solanacearum* culturable populations were observed at low temperatures. We obtained evidence for the progressive appearance of viable-but-non-culturable (VBNC) cells of the pathogen (26,27). The characterization of these VBNC cells will be further discussed below as well as in a separate chapter. Other key factors that regulated the population size of *R. solanacearum* biovar 2 were (soil) moisture content, the presence of indigenous organisms and the presence of sediment (in water). Rapid drying of soil resulted in an irreversible loss of culturability of *R. solanacearum* cells. The presence of sediment in water systems led to a greatly enhanced survival rate, but drying of this sediment resulted in quick eradication. Most importantly, *R. solanacearum* biovar 2 showed great capacity to grow when present in low numbers in sterile ultrapure water (27). Even upon several serial transfers to new ultrapure water, this growth was still observed. The substrates upon which this growth took place are so far unknown. However, the capability of *R. solanacearum* to actively grow at very low substrate concentrations is revealing in that it points to a possible life strategy of this organism in oligotrophic environments.

PHYSIOLOGY

Physiological responses of *R. solanacearum* biovar 2 that might affect its survival in natural habitats have been poorly studied so far. On the one hand, it is known that this pathogen, much like other plant pathogens, possesses a very sophisticated machinery that enables it to interact with a potential host plant, leading to infection and pathogenesis (18). In the invasive process, there is molecular signaling involving quorum sensing, and it is likely that a highly concerted sequence of events takes place, in which periods of motility are alternated with periods of non-motility and high enzymatic activity. The invasive process almost certainly involves groups of cells rather then single cells. However, we are far from understanding the intricacies of all events that take place during the invasive process. On the other hand, the physiological status of *R. solanacearum* in the environment in the absence of host plants is less well understood. As outlined above, *R. solanacearum* biovar 2 multiplies at the expense of very minute amounts of substrate, suggesting that the organism is an avid scavenger of scarce nutrients in the environment (27,30). In sterilized oligotrophic water systems, *R. solanacearum* biovar 2 was shown to survive for over 2 years, and the surviving forms were still able to cause wilting disease in susceptible tomato plants. The majority of these forms were not in a VBNC state, as evidenced by direct comparison of IF and IFC counts. Rather, *R. solanacearum* biovar 2 was shown to produce cells with enhanced resistance to secondary stresses upon exposure to oligotrophic conditions, as evidenced by challenging the starved cells with hydrogen peroxide (Van Overbeek, unpublished).

As outlined in the foregoing, the decline noted at low temperature (4°C) in soil and water systems could consistently be linked to the appearance of VBNC cells, that is, cells that do not form colonies on plates or multiply otherwise, yet are metabolically active and, thus, alive. As described above, incubating *R. solanacearum* strain 1609 inocula in river water at 4°C or 18°C reduced culturability from 5×10^6 CFU to at or below detection limits (5 CFU per ml) after 10 and 30 days, respectively. However, direct detection methods like immunofluorescence and FISH targeting 23S rRNA (22) showed no loss in total cell numbers in the same samples. That these cells show activities other than those shown by DVC and CTC methods became apparent in recent work performed at IVEM-NERC, Oxford. An RT-PCR assay was developed to monitor transcription of mRNA produced in response to stress. We used cDNA-AFLP to compare cellular mRNA profiles from bacteria after prolonged incubation in water to those from bacteria incubated in broth. Several novel transcripts were identified in the water-stressed populations, including the *de novo* expression of the *aphC* gene (alkyl hydroperoxide reductase); moreover 23S rRNA levels declined more than 100-fold. These data demonstrate the continuing transcriptional activity of cells that appear to have entered a phase where they are recalcitrant to culture on agar. Despite the promise of these observations that uniquely indicate sustained metabolic activity in these populations, there is a caveat. The limits of detection for plate isolation were 5-10 cells per ml, so it is possible, though unlikely when compared to the controls, that the RT-PCR assay detects these few potentially culturable bacteria. Clearly, the occurrence of VBNC *R. solanacearum* cells presents an enormous challenge to research and agricultural practice alike (26,10). We need a greater understanding of the ecology of these types of cells and their importance for plant health and disease.

Strategies for Management of *R. solanacearum* Biovar 2 by Soil Treatments and Effects on the Soil Microbiota

METHODS

As many, if not most, of the available soil management methods have an impact on the soil microbiota, and often these effects can be causal, it is important to assess the structures of soil microbial communities. To achieve this aim, a range of molecular community fingerprinting methods based on soil DNA have been developed (1). The advantage of these direct methods is that they take into account the as-yet-uncultured fraction of soil microbial communities, which form the majority of the soil microbiota in most, if not all, soil habitats on earth. A very powerful method, PCR-denaturing gradient gel electrophoresis (DGGE) based on 16S or 18S ribosomal RNA genes, allows such fingerprints to be made of microbial communities in bulk soil (7), rhizosphere soil (4,12,20) and in plant tissue (6). The method can be geared to detect either broad bacterial or fungal groups or narrower groupings such as the beta-Proteobacteria (8). It enables an assessment of shifts in relative abundance of specific microbial groups in complex systems, which might pinpoint organisms involved in suppression of plant pathogens, or might otherwise just reveal the abundance of indicator organisms. On the other hand, it is key to our understanding of the antagonistic interactions in complex systems like soil, that the players "behind" the community fingerprints and their activities become known, in other words, that isolates from the systems are matched to the fingerprints obtained. A direct method on plates, in which dilutions of soil suspensions are tested for effects on *R. solanacearum*, has been successfully developed and applied in our laboratories (28). Isolates with consistent antagonistic action against the pathogen are being tested in soil/plant microcosms for their *in situ* activity.

SOIL SUPPRESSIVENESS TOWARDS *R. SOLANACEARUM*

Effects of management. Key strategies feasible for application in common farming systems should be simple, cheap, easy to execute and should ideally be non-chemical. Such strategies could either directly limit the survival of *R. solanacearum*, or, indirectly, affect this pathogen by virtue of effects on the indigenous antagonistic microflora. Strategies can range from additions of organic matter such as compost, manure or other commonly-available substrates, to solarization or liming. For instance, the addition of compost, with or without solarization, can enhance the suppressiveness of soils towards a range of mainly fungal plant pathogens (13). The suppressiveness of the system - defined as the capacity of soils to restrict the survival and activity of plant pathogens (24) - might be enhanced as a result of

43

the increased abundance and activity of antagonistic microbial populations induced by these measures. In addition, abiotic factors such as soil texture, soil organic matter content and pH are also important in determining the fate of suppressive and pathogenic organisms alike.

Recently, we investigated the effects of compost addition and simulated solarization treatments of soil on the survival of *R. solanacearum* biovar 2, as well as on the structure of indigenous bacterial communities, in soil microcosms (19). In addition, we assessed the effects of these treatments on the invasion of tomato test plants by the pathogen. In untreated soil, *R. solanacearum* strain 1609 showed a slow progressive decline, from about 10^7 to 10^5 CFU/g of dry soil over a period of 54 days. Moreover, all six test plants growing in this soil developed symptoms of wilting and revealed the presence of the pathogen in their lower stem parts, as evidenced by IFC and PCR. Solarization of unamended soil also did not affect *R. solanacearum* strain 1609 survival or plant invasiveness. However, both the addition of household compost and the combination of compost addition with solarization resulted in significantly enhanced population decline rates, as well as a reduction of the numbers of diseased plants in the suppressiveness test. Surprisingly, some healthy-looking plants, primarily from the soils treated with compost only, contained strain 1609 in their lower stem parts, as evidenced by IFC supported by PCR. Bacteria with antagonistic activity towards *R. solanacearum* were isolated from all soils independent from the previous treatment, indicating that potential *R. solanacearum* antagonists are amongst the numerically dominant culturable bacteria. The majority of the potential antagonists were streptomycetes. The increased suppressiveness of the soils amended with compost could thus result from an enhanced metabolic activity of potential antagonists present.

Analysis of the composition of the total bacterial as well as the β-subgroup proteobacterial communities revealed that compost amendment led to changes in the composition of the eubacterial and β-proteobacterial communities of the soil, which were detectable until the end of the experiment. The relative abundance of *R. solanacearum* clearly decreased in soils amended with compost, as evidenced by DGGE analysis of the β-proteobacterial communities. Two bands, identified as related to *Variovorax paradoxus* and *Aquaspirillum psychrophylum*, were consistently amplified from the compost treatment, and are proposed as putative bio-indicators for this treatment. Whether or not these bio-indicators have a causal relationship with the antagonism is at present unknown.

Concluding Remarks

It is clear that novel tools developed for the study of *R. solanacearum* in its natural habitat have been very helpful in describing and elucidating the events taking place with this organism at the population level. However, as is apparent from the above results, we are only beginning to understand the ecological behavior of *R. solanacearum* biovar 2 in soil and water habitats. Although the organism can survive in culturable forms for considerable periods of time, its behavior in relation to other organisms, to several key habitat conditions, and to the initial stages of host plant invasion are barely known. The discovery of a VBNC state in *R. solanacearum* is also intriguing and, for the time being, raises more questions than it answers. For instance, there is no knowledge so far with respect to the possible reversion of VBNC *R. solanacearum* cells to culturable or even fully aggressive forms, and their putative relationship to phenotype conversion (PC) mutants is still unexplored. It is of utmost importance that these questions are answered in the near future. A better understanding of the ecological behavior of *R. solanacearum* in its natural habitat would also be helpful for predicting suppression of this organism as a result of the application of simple agronomical measures. For instance, the finding of a strong effect on *R. solanacearum* strain 1609 by compost amendment and, in particular, the combined compost amendment and simulated solarization hinted at potential use for these, and possibly other, simple soil treatments in pathogen management. However, we are still far from establishing the scientific basis for the enhanced suppressiveness, even though it is likely that specific suppressive organisms play a role in it. Only on the basis of a thorough understanding of all factors that play a role in pathogen suppression can future soil management strategies be designed and guided. It is a challenge for future research to close this gap, i.e. to connect the observed microbial community changes to changes in pathogen suppressiveness.

From all studies performed so far, *R. solanacearum* biovar 2 appears to be an organism with a remarkable genetic and physiological versatility. In addition to its sophisticated machinery for invasion of plant tissue, it also possesses a surprising capacity to grow at very low substrate concentrations, as well as to convert to a VBNC form at low temperature. It is likely that these very divergent behavioral patterns evolved in response to the biphasic life strategy that the organism had to develop in order to successfully compete in highly divergent habitats. We are looking forward to ecological studies with this organism using gene arrays to exploit the enormous information from the complete genomic sequence (17).

45

Acknowledgements

This work was supported by the EU-FAIR program (acronym FATE, PL97-3632) as well as funds supplied by the Dutch Ministry for Agriculture. We thank partners of the FATE Consortium for providing some of their data and for helpful discussions.

Literature Cited

1. Akkermans, A.D.L., Van Elsas J.D., and de Bruijn, F.J., eds. 1995. Molecular Microbial Ecology Manual, Kluwer Academic Publishers, Dordrecht/Boston/London.
2. Boudazin, G., Le Roux, A.C., Josi, K., Labarre, P., and Jouan, B., 1999. Design of division specific primers of *Ralstonia solanacearum* and application to the identification of European isolates. Eur. J. Plant Pathol. 105: 373-380.
3. Dellagi, A., Birch, P.R.J., Heilbronn, J., Lyon, G.D., and Toth, I.K. 2000. cDNA-AFLP analysis of differential gene expression in the prokaryotic plant pathogen *Erwinia carotovora*. Microbiol. 146: 165-171.
4. Duineveld, B.M., Rosado, A.S., Van Elsas, J.D., and Van Veen, J.A. 1998. Analysis of the dynamics of bacterial communities in the rhizosphere of the chrysanthemum via denaturing gradient gel electrophoresis and substrate utilization patterns. Appl. Environ. Microbiol. 64: 4950-4957.
5. Elphinstone, J.G., Hennessy, J., Wilson, J.K., and Stead, D.K. 1996. Sensitivity of different methods for the detection of *Pseudomonas solanacearum* (Smith) Smith in potato tuber extracts. Bull. OEPP/EPPO Bull. 26: 663-678.
6. Garbeva, P., Van Overbook, L.S., Van Vuurde, J.W.L., and Van Elsas, J.D. 2001. Analysis of endophytic bacterial communities of potato by plating and denaturing gradient gel electrophoresis (DGGE) of 16S rDNA based PCR fragments. Microb. Ecol. 41: 369-383.
7. Gelsomino, A., Keijzer-Wolters, A.C., Cacco, G., and Van Elsas, J.D. 1999. Assessment of bacterial community structure in soil by polymerase chain reaction and denaturing gradient gel electrophoresis. J. Microbiol. Meth. 38: 1-15.
8. Gomes, N.C.M., Heuer, H., Schönfeld, J., Costa, R., Hagler-Mendonca, L., and Smalla, K. 2001. Bacterial diversity of the rhizosphere of maize (*Zea mays*) grown in tropical soil studied by temperature gradient gel electrophoresis. Plant and Soil 232: 167-180.

9. Graham, J., Jones, D.A., and Lloyd, A.B. 1979. Survival of *Pseudomonas solanacearum* race 3 in plant debris and in latently infected potato tubers. Phytopathology 69: 1100-1103.

10. Grey, B.E., and Steck, T.R. 2001. The viable but nonculturable state of *Ralstonia solanacearum* may be involved in long-term survival and plant infection. Appl. Environ. Microbiol. 67: 3866-3872.

11. Heijnen, C E., Page, S., and van Elsas, J.D. 1995. Metabolic activity of *Flavobacterium* strain P25 during starvation and after introduction into bulk soil and the rhizosphere of wheat. FEMS Microbiol. Ecol. 18: 129-138.

12. Heuer, H., and Smalla, K. 1997. Application of denaturing gradient gel electrophoresis (DGGE) and temperature gradient gel electrophoresis (TGGE) for studying soil microbial communities. Pages 353-373 in: Modern Soil Microbiology. J.D. Van Elsas, E.M.H. Wellington, and J.T. Trevors, eds. Marcel Dekker, Inc., New York, NY.

13. Hoitink, H.A.J., and Fahy, P.C. 1986. Basis for the control of soilborne plant pathogens with compost. Ann Rev. Phytopathol. 24: 93-114.

14. Janse, J.D. 1988. A detection method for *Ralstonia solanacearum* in symptomless potato tubers and some data on its sensitivity and specificity. Bull. OEPP/EPPO Bull. 18: 343-351.

15. Kogure, K., Simidu, U., and Taga, N. 1979. A tentative direct microscopic method for counting living marine bacteria. Can. J. Microbiol. 25: 415-420.

16. Postma, J., Van Elsas, J.D., Govaert, J.M., and Van Veen, J.A. 1988. The dynamics of *Rhizobium leguminosarum* biovar *trifolii* introduced into soil as determined by immunofluorescence and selective plating techniques. FEMS Microbiol. Ecol. 53: 251-260.

17. Salanoubat, M., Genin, S., Artiguenave, F., Gouzy, J., Mangenot, S., Arlat, M., Billault, A., Brottier, P., Camus, J.C., Cattolico, L., Chandler, M., Choisne, N., Claudel-Renard, C., Cunnac, S., Demange, N., Gaspin, C., Lavle, M., Moisan, A., Robert, C., Saurin, W., Schiex, T., Sguier, P., Thëbault, P., Whalen, M., Wincker, P., Levy, M., Weissenbach, J., and Boucher, C.A. 2002. Genome sequence of the plant pathogen *Ralstonia solanacearum*. Nature 415: 497-502.

18. Schell, M. 2000. Control of virulence and pathogenicity genes of *Ralstonia solanacearum* by an elaborate sensory network. Ann. Rev. Phytopathol. 38: 263-292.

19. Schönfeld, J., Gelsomino, A., Van Overbeek, L.S., and Van Elsas, J.D. 2003. Effects of compost addition and simulated solarisation on the fate of *Ralstonia solanacearum* biovar 2 and indigenous bacteria in soil. FEMS Microbiol. Ecol. 43:63-74.

20. Smalla, K., Wieland, G., Buchner, A., Zick, A., Parzy, J., Kaiser, S., Roskot, N., Heuer, H., and Berg, G. 2001. Bulk and rhizosphere soil

bacterial communities studied by denaturing gradient gel electrophoresis: plant-dependent enrichment and seasonal shifts revealed. Appl. Environ. Microbiol. 67: 4742-4751.
21. Smith, J.J., Offord, L.C., Kibata, G.N., Murimi, Z.K., Trigalet, A., Saddler, G.S., 1998, The development of a biological control agent against *Ralstonia solanacearum* Race 3 in Kenya. Pages 337-342 in: Bacterial Wilt Disease. P. Prior, C. Allen, and J. Elphinstone, eds. Bacterial Wilt Disease, Springer-Verlag, Berlin.
22. Timms-Wilson, T.M., Bryant, K., and Bailey, M.J. 2002. Strain characterisation and 16S-23S probe development for differentiating geographically dispersed isolates of the phytopathogen *Ralstonia solanacearum*. Environmental Microbiology 3: 785-797.
23. Trigalet, A., Trigalet-Demery, D., and Prior, P. 1998. Elements of biocontrol of tomato bacterial wilt. Pages 332-336 in: Bacterial Wilt Disease. P. Prior, C. Allen, and J. Elphinstone, eds. Springer-Verlag, Berlin.
24. Van Bruggen, A.H.C. and A.M. Semenov. 2000. In search of biological indicators for soil health and disease suppression. Appl. Soil Ecol. 15: 13-24.
25. Van der Wolf, J.M., Van Bekkum, P.J., Van Elsas, J.D., Nijhuis, E.H., Vriend, S.G.C., and Ruissen, M.A. 1998. Immunofluorescence colony staining and selective enrichment in liquid medium for studying the population dynamics of *Ralstonia solanacearum* (race 3) in soil. Bull. OEPP/EPPO Bull. 28, 71-79.
26. Van Elsas, J.D., Kastelein, P., Van Bekkum, P., Van der Wolf, J.M., de Vries, P.M., and Van Overbeek, L.S. 2000. Survival of *Ralstonia solanacearum* biovar 2, the causative agent of potato brown rot, in field and microcosm soils in temperate climates. Phytopathology 90: 1358-1366.
27. Van Elsas, J.D., Kastelein, P., de Vries, P.M., and Van Overbeek, L.S. 2001. Effects of ecological factors on the survival and physiology of *Ralstonia solanacearum* biovar 2 in agricultural drainage water. Can. J. Microbiol. 47: 842-854.
28. Van Overbeek, L.S., Cassidy, M., Kozdroj, J., Trevors. J.T., and van Elsas, J.D. 2001. A polyphasic approach for studying the interaction between *Ralstonia solanacearum* and potential control agents in the tomato rhizosphere. J. Microbiol. Meths. 48: 69-86.
29. Van Vuurde, J.W.L., and Van der Wolf, J.M. 1995. Immuno-fluorescence colony-staining (IFC). Pages 1-19 in: Molecular Microbiology Ecology Manual. A.D.L. Akkermans, J.D. Van Elsas, and F.J. de Bruijn, eds. Kluwer Academic Publishers, Dordrecht.

30. Wakimoto, Utatsu, I., Matsuo, N., and Hayashi, I. 1982. Multiplication of *Pseudomonas solanacearum* in pure water. Ann. Rev. Phytopathol. Soc. Japan 48: 620-627.

31. Wenneker, M, Verdel, M.S.W., Groeneveld, R.M.W., Kempenaar, C., van Beuningen, A.R., and Janse, J.D., 1999. *Ralstonia (Pseudomonas) solanacearum* race 3 (biovar 2) in surface water and natural weed hosts: First report on stinging nettle (*Urtica dioica*). Eur. J. Plant Pathol.105: 307-315.

Mechanization Has Contributed to the Spread of Bacterial Wilt on Flue-Cured Tobacco in the Southeastern USA

Bruce A. Fortnum[1] and Dan Kluepfel[2]

[1] Department of Plant Pathology and Physiology, Clemson University, Pee Dee Research and Education Center, 2200 Pocket Rd., Florence 29506-9706; [2] Department of Plant Pathology and Physiology, Clemson University, Clemson, SC

Bacterial wilt, caused by *Ralstonia solanacearum*, is an extremely damaging disease of flue cured tobacco. Bacterial wilt losses in South Carolina, expressed as the percentage of total crop production, have increased from 0.2% in 1981 to 7.2% in 1998. Consolidation of tobacco allotments from 24,000 in 1981 to < 5000 in 1998 has resulted in larger farming units, and increased mechanization in flower (topping) and leaf removal (mechanical leaf harvesters).

The role of mechanical topping in the spread of bacterial wilt was evaluated in randomized complete block factorial experiments on the Pee Dee Research and Education Center and in large-scale on-farm trials. Main blocks were method of flower removal (hand vs. mechanical) and subplots were tobacco cultivar (K 326 vs. K 346). Mechanical flower removal spreads *R. solanacearum* from infected plant tissue to healthy plants ($P < 0.001$) increasing the incidence and severity of disease. Host resistance (K346) did not reduce the spread of the disease through mechanical topping when compared to the susceptible control (K 326, $P = 0.05$).

The role of mechanical leaf harvesting on the spread of bacterial wilt was evaluated in randomized complete block factorial experiments. Main blocks were method of leaf removal (hand removal, simulated mechanical removal and simulated mechanical removal with slight injury to the stalk) and subplots were tobacco cultivar (K326 vs. K346). The bacterium was mechanically transmitted to healthy plants during hand and mechanical harvesting ($P < 0.001$). Transmission of the bacterium and infection of tobacco plants following leaf removal with *R. solanacearum*-contaminated hands or harvesting aids ranged from 47% to 83% of the planting (hand vs. mechanical harvesting, respectively). Infected plants remained symptomless for 3-6 weeks following infection and then wilted rapidly. Host resistance

(K346) did not reduce the spread of the disease through stalk injury (leaf removal) when compared to a susceptible control (K 326, $P = 0.05$). The presence of *R. solanacearum* was confirmed with a tetrazolium based selective medium, FAME analysis, and a tomato bioassay.

Introduction

Bacterial wilt is a destructive disease of flue-cured tobacco (*Nicotiana tabacum* L.) in the southeastern USA. During 1998, this disease accounted for over $39,260,000 in direct losses to North and South Carolina farmers (1,8). These losses do not take into account altered farming practices such as abandoned fields, losses due to gathering of unripe tobacco, lower yielding resistant varieties and the cost of extensive soil fumigation to aid in bacterial wilt suppression.

Bacterial wilt on tobacco traditionally has been a problem in the northern piedmont counties of North Carolina and has been limited to one or two counties of South Carolina; however every year tobacco in several fields in other counties are diagnosed with bacterial wilt. Although growers have adopted best management practices for disease control, disease losses within the Carolinas remain high (1,8). Newer varieties, such as K 149 and Ox 207, have improved bacterial wilt resistance but have failed to reduce disease losses (1,3). The rapid spread of bacterial wilt within South Carolina suggests that the organism is being spread in a more rapid and efficient manner than would be expected solely by the movement of soil on equipment.

Hollow stalk on tobacco is a disease caused by *Erwinia carotovora* subsp. *carotovora* (Jones) Bergey *et al.* where soft rot occurs on pith tissue exposed during hand flower removal (topping) (7). We have isolated *R. solanacearum*, the causal organism of bacterial wilt of tobacco, from many mechanically topped tobacco plants with hollow stalk-like symptoms. This suggests *R. solanacearum* may be spread during flower removal and may produce symptoms similar to hollow stalk. This investigation was undertaken to assess the level of bacterial wilt losses as influenced by consolidation of tobacco allotments, the role of mechanization in topping, and harvesting on the spread and severity of bacterial wilt.

Materials and Methods

DISEASE AND PRODUCTION SURVEYS

Losses reported in flue-cured tobacco caused by *R. solanacearum* were estimated based on the county agent's assessment of acreage affected within the county and average losses occurring among these problem sites based on a method previously described (2). Estimates of disease losses were made in 1981, and comparisons were based on losses occurring in that year. Disease loss was calculated with the following formula:

$$\text{Loss estimates} = [(n/\Sigma)(AXLY)/Ya + (n/\Sigma)(AXLY)] Z$$

where n, number of counties surveyed; A, acreage of tobacco within a county; X, percentage of tobacco acreage affected; L, average loss in an infested field; Y, statewide average yield per acre; Ya, actual reported yield within the state; and Z, state average price per pound. Yearly crop statistics were obtained from the South Carolina Agricultural Statistics (USDA NASS) and the Tobacco Situation Outlook (USDA ERS).

MECHANICAL TRANSMISSION IN FLOWER AND LEAF REMOVAL

Wilt induction by inoculation during flower removal. The test site was located at the Pee Dee Research and Education Center, Florence, South Carolina, on a Norfolk sandy loam (75% sand, 17% silt, 8% clay, 0.8% organic matter, pH 5.8) site. The field was fallow the year preceding the trial in 1996. Multipurpose soil fumigant 1,3-Dichloropropene (78%) + chloropicrin (17%), [98 liters/Ha (11.7 ml/m)] was applied with a positive pressure electric pump system and injected 15 cm deep with a single chisel placed in the center of a 60-cm-wide bed. Bedding disks were used to seal the chisel opening and form a 36-cm-high bed with fumigant placed 40 cm from the top of the bed. Plots consisted of a single row of plants, 12.2 m long, bordered by untreated rows with a 1.2-m row spacing. All treatments were replicated four times and arranged in a randomized complete block design. The tobacco cv. K 326 was grown using standard agronomic practices (3) and received irrigation as needed.

Bacterial cells from 48-hr old nutrient agar plates were suspended in sterile water (5 x 10^7 CFU/ml) and used as inoculum. Treatments included: bacteria atomized onto a steel cutter blade immediately prior to severing each tobacco flower, bacteria atomized onto a steel cutter blade prior to topping a plot row (20 plants), bacteria atomized on to the cut tobacco stalk immediately following mechanical topping, steel cutters disinfected with

70% ethanol and flowers removed, and a non-topped control row. Plants were assessed for disease symptoms 21-28 days following treatment.

Wilt resistance in tobacco cultivars inoculated during flower removal. The test site was located at the Pee Dee Research and Education Center, Florence, South Carolina, on Norfolk sandy loam soils (composition as above; pH 5.9-6.1). The field was planted in cotton the year preceding the trial (1997) and had no history of bacterial wilt. Multipurpose soil fumigants were applied as previously described. Tobacco cultivars K 326, and K 346 were transplanted in the test plots in mid-April 1998 and 1999. Plots were arranged in a randomized complete block 2x2 factorial design where main plots were topping method (hand vs. machine) and subplots were tobacco cultivar. The tobacco cultivars were selected based on their level of resistance to bacterial wilt and were classified as susceptible (K 326) or resistant (K 346) (3). Treatments were replicated four times and the test was repeated the next year. Each subplot consisted of a single row 1.2 m wide and 12.2 m long. A 1.4 m border separated each main block. Plants were assessed for disease symptoms 28 days following treatment.

Mechanical transmission during flower removal in large on-farm trials. Test sites were located in Horry County, near Bayboro, South Carolina, on Norfolk sandy loam soils (composition as above; pH 5.9-6.1). The fields were planted in corn the year preceding the trials in 1997 and 1998 and had a history of bacterial wilt. Tobacco cultivars K 326 and K 346 were selected based on their level of resistance as previously described. Multi-purpose soil fumigants were applied as previously described. Tobacco seedlings were transplanted in test plots in mid-April 1998 and 1999. Plots were arranged in a randomized complete block 2x2 factorial design and were replicated three times. Main blocks were topping method (machine vs. hand) and subplots were tobacco cultivar. Each subplot consisted of two rows 1.2 m wide and 104 m long. A 1.4 m border separated each main block. No *R. solanacearum* inoculum was applied to the machine topper prior to topping the field plots. Weed and insect control was maintained by standard agronomic practices and no supplemental irrigation was applied (3).

Mechanical transmission during leaf removal. The test site was located at the Pee Dee Research and Education Center, Florence, South Carolina, on a Norfolk sandy loam soil (composition as above; pH 5.9). The field was fallow the year preceding the trial in 1999 and had no history of bacterial wilt. Multipurpose soil fumigant was applied as previously described. Seedlings of tobacco cultivars K326 and K346 were trans-planted in test plots on 15 April 2000. Plots were arranged in a randomized complete block 3x2 factorial design where main blocks were leaf removal method and subplots were tobacco varieties. The tobacco cultivars were selected based on their level of resistance to bacterial wilt. Treatments were rep-

Table 1. Mechanical transmission of *Ralstonia solanacearum* on steel cutter blades during flower removal.

Flower removal	*R. solanacearum*	Inoculation Method	Percent Disease 21 days[a]	28 days
Uninoculated, uncut control (UTC)			0	2
Steel cutter		Uninoculated control	3	12
Steel cutter	+	Atomized on cut stem tissue after flower removal (Cs)	28	93
Steel cutter	+	Atomized on steel blade prior to cutting each stalk (Es)	57	100
Steel cutter	+	Atomized on steel blade prior to topping each plot (Ept)	55	100
Contrasts ($P \leq$ F)				
Cs vs Es 0.05			0.05	0.05
UTC vs Ept			0.001	0.001

[a] Interval following flower removal and inoculation.

licated four times. Each subplot consisted of a single row 1.2 m wide and 6.1 m long. A 1.4 m border separated each main block.

Data were analyzed using analysis of variance and factorial techniques (12). All calculations were performed with JMP Analysis System (SAS Institute, Cary, NC).

Results

DISEASE AND PRODUCTION SURVEYS

Bacterial wilt losses in South Carolina, expressed as the percentage of total crop production have increased from 0.2% in 1981 to 7.2% in 1998. Consolidation of tobacco allotments from 24,000 in 1981 to < 5000 in 1998 has resulted in larger farming units, and increased mechanization in topping and mechanical leaf removal. Disease losses have increased with bacterial wilt observed in fields with no previous history of this disease.

Wilt induction by inoculation during flower removal. R. solanacearum was atomized onto uninfected tobacco plants immediately following flower removal (topping). Within 28 days after inoculation, 93% of the tobacco plants showed typical bacterial wilt symptoms. Atomizing bacteria onto a steel cutter (topping blade) prior to topping was more effective in spreading the disease than atomizing the bacteria onto freshly cut tobacco stalks ($P <$ 0.05, Table 1). Atomizing the bacteria onto a tobacco topper (steel cutter blades) prior to topping a 20-plant plot resulted in 100% infection of the tobacco plants within 28 days following treatment (Table 1).

Wilt resistance in tobacco cultivars inoculated during flower removal. Contamination of steel cutter blades with a suspension of *R. solanacearum* (5×10^7 CFU/ml) resulted in 70-88% infection of tobacco plants following mechanical topping. Mechanical topping of healthy tobacco plants immediately following topping of bacterial wilt infected plants resulted in similar levels of disease (82-86%) following a 4-week incubation period (Table 2). No difference was observed between resistant and susceptible tobacco cultivars following mechanical transmission of the bacteria using bacterial suspensions or naturally occurring infected plant material (1998 and 1999). Some disease was observed in untreated plots in 1999 and a varietal effect was observed in non-inoculated plots (Table 2). Inoculation of the steel cutter blade with *R. solanacearum* immediately prior to topping caused soft rot like symptoms in tobacco similar to those caused by *E. carotovora.*

Mechanical transmission during leaf removal. R. solanacearum was transmitted from workers' hands or leaf removal aids (simulated mechanical harvester) to healthy tobacco during leaf removal when workers' hands or harvesting aids were contaminated with *R. solanacearum* (Table 4). Plants were symptomless for 3-4 weeks after which bacterial wilt developed

Table 2. Percent of tobacco plants infected with *ralstonia solanacearum* following mechanical flower removal with contaminated cutter blades.

		Percent diseased plants/20-plant plot			
		1998		1999	
Flower removal	Inoculation method[a]	K 326	K 346	K 326	K 346
---	None	1	1	25	19
Hand	None	2	0	10	8
Steel cutter	None	0	0	13	4
Steel cutter	Bacteria (B)	82	70	88	84
Steel cutter	Plant material (Pm)	85	86	82	85
$(P \leq F)$					
Treatments (trt)			0.001		0.001
Cultivar (Cv)			ns		0.01
Trt x Cv			ns		ns (0.12)

[a] B = Bacteria (5×10^7 CFU/ml) atomized onto steel cutter blade immediately preceding flower removal. Pm = mechanical topper driven through bacterial wilt diseased tobacco plants immediately prior to mechanically topping healthy tobacco plants.

Table 3. Effect of mechanical flower removal on the transmission of bacterial wilt in large-scale on-farm trials.

Flower removal[a]	Variety	R. solanacearum resistance	Percent disease 1998	Percent disease 1999
Hand	K 326	-	41	54
Mechanical	K 326	-	48	83
Hand	K 346	+	25	24
Mechanical	K 346	+	36	67
Contrasts				
	K 326 vs. K 346		0.02	0.09
	Hand vs. mechanical		0.08	0.01

[a] Fields were naturally infested with *R. solanacearum*. Each plot contained 350 plants and was replicated three times.

rapidly with typical bacterial wilt symptoms. Leaf removal with hands contaminated with *R. solanacearum* resulted in 47% of the planting showing symptoms of bacterial wilt. The percent disease increased with mild and severe stem abrasion (65% and 83% infection, respectively) during leaf removal. When averaged across treatments, the susceptible cultivar K 326 did not differ in percent disease from the resistant cultivar K 346 ($P = 0.05$, Table 4). The presence of *R. solanacearum* in plants showing signs of bacterial wilt was confirmed with a tetrazolium based selective medium, FAME analysis, and a tomato bioassay.

Discussion

The major components in a disease management program for endemic soilborne diseases such as bacterial wilt are crop rotation, host plant resistance, and soil fumigation with multipurpose fumigants containing chloropicrin. Normally, infection of tobacco in the field occurs through the root system. However, *R. solanacearum* can be transmitted from diseased to healthy Perilla (*Perilla crispa* Tanaka) plants during harvesting where leaves are removed with a mechanical steel cutter (4). Likewise, tomato can be inoculated with *R. solanacearum* during sucker removal and mechanical clipping (9,10). In banana, *R. solanacearum* infects roots slowly through root wounds, however, disease increases rapidly when bacteria are mechanically transmitted from diseased plants to healthy banana plants by pruning tools. Early reports on tobacco suggests that *R.*

Table 4. Effect of leaf removal with and without stalk injury on the mechanical transmission of bacterial wilt in field plants, 2000.

Leaf removal	R. solanacearum[a]	Percent disease[b]		Vascular necrosis	
		K 326	K 346	K 326	K 346
Hand	-	0	0	0	0
Hand	+	42	52	4.3	5.0
Blunt removal	-	0	0	0	0
Blunt removal	+	80	50	8.6	7.0
Scored stem	-	0	0	0	0
Scored	+	80	85	6.5	7.6
$(P \leq F)$					
Treatments (trt)		0.001		0.001	
Varieties (var)		ns		ns	
Trt x Var		ns		ns	

[a] Inoculum was prepared by placing 2-cm long R. solanacearum infected tobacco stalk sections into distilled water for 5 minutes. The solution was strained through cheesecloth and used as inoculum.

[b] K 326 = bacterial wilt susceptible cultivar, K 346 = bacterial wilt resistant cultivar.

R. solanacearum was confirmed in test plots by isolation on tetrazolium-based media, tomato bioassay and FAME analysis.

solanacearum can be spread during hand topping (11,13). Presumably the bacteria would be on workers' hands.

These studies show that R. solanacearum can be spread rapidly from a small number of infected plants to large areas of the field rendering standard disease management practices less effective. In order to obtain sufficient tobacco acreage, farmers frequently rent tobacco allotments across several farms. Farm machinery is then transported from farm to farm, potentially moving the organism to previously uncontaminated fields. The steady increase of bacterial wilt in South Carolina during the time of the increased role of mechanization suggests R. solanacearum is being transmitted on contaminated equipment, resulting in increased losses to bacterial wilt. Sterilization of contaminated tools or cutters is difficult and would pose a serious challenge to producers. Although the movement of contaminated machinery will be difficult to control, implementation of sound disease management strategies including equipment sanitation will minimize the impact of cross-contamination of fields with R. solanacearum. Disease management strategies need to be modified to account for the rapid spread of R. solanacearum on farm machinery.

Literature Cited

1. Fortnum, B.A. 2000. Disease management. Pages 38-59 in: South Carolina tobacco growers guide 2001. D.T. Gooden, ed. Clemson, SC Cooperative Extension Service, Clemson University.
2. Fortnum, B.A., Krausz, J.P., and Conrad, N. 1984. Increasing incidence of *Meloidogyne arenaria* on flue-cured tobacco in South Carolina. Plant Dis. 68:244-245.
3. Gooden, D.T., Christenbury, G.D., Fortnum, B.A., Manley, D.G., Rideout, J.W., and Sutton, R.W. 1996. South Carolina tobacco growers guide - 1997. Circular 569, Clemson University Cooperative Extension Service, Clemson.
4. Hsu, S.-T., W.-F., Tzeng, K.-C., and Chen, C.-C. 1993. Bacterial wilt of Perilla caused by *Pseudomonas solanacearum* and its transmission. Plant Dis. 77:674-677.
5. Kelman, A. 1953. The bacterial wilt caused by *Pseudomonas solanacearum*. N.C. Agric. Exp. Stn. Tech.Bull. 99.
6. Lucas, G.B. 1975. Diseases of Tobacco, 3rd ed. Biological Consulting Association, Raleigh, North Carolina. North Carolina Cooperative Extension Service., 1996. Flue-cured tobacco Information 1997. Bull. AG-187.
7. Lucas, G.B., and Shew, H.D. 1991. Hollow stalk, black leg, and barn rot. Pages 32-33 in: Compendium of Tobacco Diseases. H.D. Shew and G.B. Lucas, eds. American Phytopathological Society, St. Paul, MN.
8. Melton, T., Porter, D., and Broadwell A. 1999. Disease management. Pages 119-137 in: Flue-cured Tobacco Information, North Carolina Cooperative Extension Service Bull. AG-187. 165 p.
9. McCarter, S.M., and Jaworski, C.A. 1968. Greenhouse studies on the spread of *Pseudomonas solancearum* in tomato plants by clipping. Plant Dis. Rep. 52:330-334.
10. McCarter, S.M., and Jaworski, C.A. 1969. Field studies on spread of *Pseudomonas solanacearum* and tobacco mosaic virus in tomato plants by clipping. Plant Dis. Rep. 53:942-946.
11. Nakata, K., and Koba, S. 1936. On the relation between both bacterial wilt and hollow stalk and the topping operation. Phytopath. Soc. Japan Ann. 6:86-87.
12. Steel, R.G.D., and Torrie, J.H. 1960. Principles and procedures of statistics. McGraw-Hill, New York.
13. Thompson, A. 1934. Diseases of tobacco in Malaya. Malayan Agr. Jour. 22:263-269.

Processes in the Development of a Biocontrol Agent Against Bacterial Wilt

J.J. Smith[1], Z.K. Murimi[2], L.C. Offord[1], S. Clayton[1], N. Mienie[3], R. Gouws[3], S. Priou[4], M. Olanya[5], S. Simons[6], and G.S. Saddler[1]

[1] CABI Bioscience, UK Centre, TW20 9TY, UK; [2] Kenya Agricultural Research Institute, PO Box 14733, Kenya; [3] Potatoes South Africa, Potato Laboratory Services, Lynn East, Pretoria 0039, Republic of South Africa; [4] International Potato Centre, Apartado 1558, Peru; [5] International Potato Centre, P.O. Box 25171, Nairobi, Kenya; [6] CAB International Africa Regional Centre, PO. Box 633, Kenya

Potato is a critical component of farming systems in many developing countries. In Kenya potato cultivation is estimated at approximately 90,000 Ha, with neighboring Uganda cultivating approximately 60,000 Ha. The product of these cultivations is often critical to the food security and livelihood of small holder families, and it is therefore worrisome that these farms generally do not achieve the yields known to be possible under the prevailing climatic conditions (16). A primary reason for this discrepancy is poor seed management and farming practices, and a concomitant build-up of seed-borne disease and pest constraints, most notably bacterial wilt. Losses to bacterial wilt are frequently between 5-30 % (2,4) and in extreme cases may account for total crop failure (14).

In Kenya there is no extensive formal potato seed production system, and limited land is available for rotation (3). These factors compound, with farmers obliged to retain their own seed over many seasons and to cultivate land that has not been rested from potato. In addition, market pressure on ware biases seed selection towards the unmarketable fraction of the harvest, notably towards damaged tubers and tubers considered undersized for optimal on-farm ware seed (<25mm in diameter); these are more likely to be latently infected (24). This scenario is typical of many developing countries cultivating potato and requires a novel approach to break the bacterial wilt disease cycle.

Biological control of bacterial wilt by non-pathogenic mutants of the wild-type (WT) organism was reported at the 2nd IBWS in Guadeloupe as a promising control method in Kenya (22). These preliminary data were substantiated under contained-use conditions in the UK and Republic of

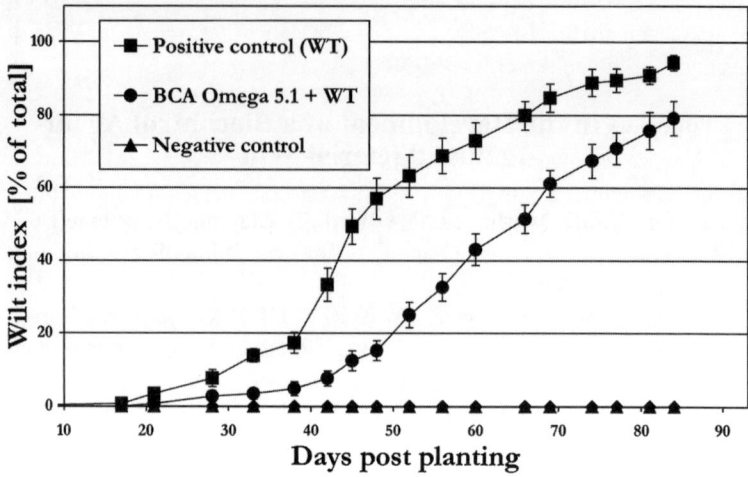

Fig. 1. BCA efficacy assessment against bacterial wilt.

South Africa (Fig. 1). This paper reports on studies of environmental impact of the biocontrol agent (BCA) and the identification of a niche within farmers' systems for its application. These studies have paved the way for the in-country testing for the BCA in Kenya, for which conditional approval has been obtained.

Addressing Environmental Impact

To address potential environmental impact of the BCA, we needed to develop methods for quantitative monitoring of the BCA population in other soil microbial communities in the soil (non-sterile environment). Key questions include the BCA's persistence in soils, interactions with crops and weeds commonly associating with potato and the stability of the BCA. In this paper we present some of the pilot data on BCA and WT *R. solanacearum* populations over time and in association with host and rotation crops. Ultimately, we expect these methods will be employed in the full risk assessment of the BCA in Kenya.

Monitoring BCA and WT R. solanacearum populations in soils. The BCA carries a kanamycin-resistance (kan) marker (10) and spontaneous rifampicin (rif) resistant mutants of WT *R. solanacearum* were isolated from rif-containing media (10ug ml^{-1}). Accordingly, SMSA^{kan}, and SMSA^{rif} media were used to monitor the BCA and WT populations, respectively, from a soil environment. The selectivity of this marker-based system was verified by taking a random sample of 50 isolates arising on

SMSA^{kan} and SMSA^{rif} plates inoculated with a soil sample that had previously been artificially inoculated. The bacterial identification was performed by fatty acid methyl ester (FAME) analysis (Microbial Identification System Inc. Delaware, USA). The minimum levels of detection were 10^3 CFU/cm^3 of soil for BCA or WT.

Two assessments were performed under contained-use conditions to determine 1) the interaction of the BCA with potato and 2) the interaction of the BCA with other crops commonly in rotation with potato. A WT population was always present to act as a control and to indicate the nature of the interaction with the crop. We postulated that a non-pathogenic interaction would generate similar responses by BCA and WT populations, whereas a pathogenic interaction would give rise to a differential response, with increased WT populations. It appeared that the BCA reacted neutrally to the presence of potato, decreasing over time (Fig. 2), but mimicked the WT population with respect to the rotation crops (Fig. 3). No apparent pathogenic interaction was evident, but there were significant differences in the supporting capacity of the rotation crops: compared to the fallow treatment, maize and bean supported approximately 200-300% more *R. solanacearum* CFU/g^{-1} of soil, whereas carrot appeared to depress populations by approx. 50% (Fig. 3). This latter observation has potential implications as to what is an appropriate rotation crop; unfortunately, the crops most commonly rotated with potato, namely maize and beans (*Vicea faba*), supported the highest populations of *R. solanacearum*. Clearly, we can-

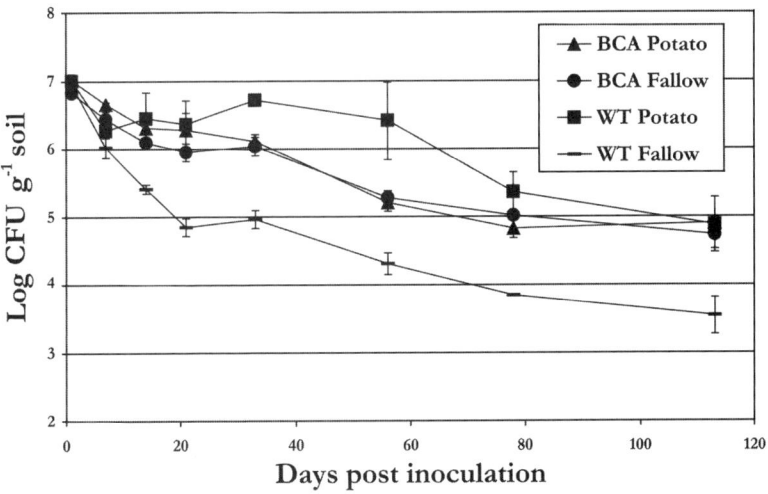

Fig. 2. BCA and WT survival with and without potato.

63

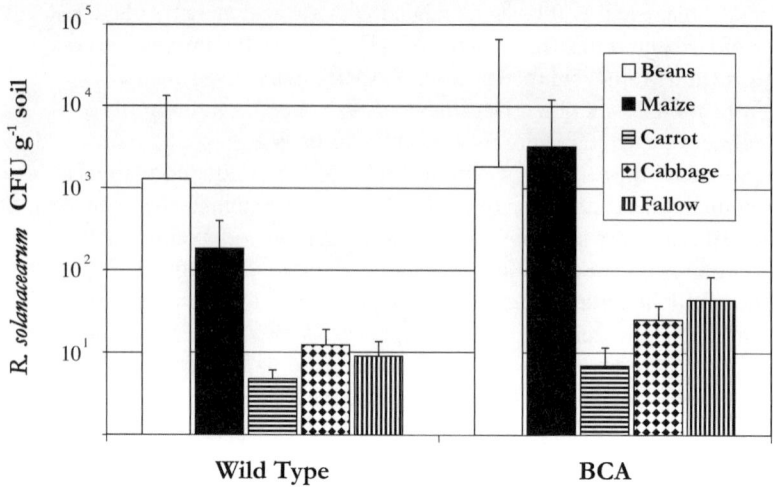

Fig. 3. Seasonal average pathogen populations for rotations on various crops.

not advise farmers not to plant maize or bean, but these crops should at least be avoided on land used for potato seed nursery.

Monitoring BCA stability in soil. The potential of the BCA to revert to the WT is of obvious concern. We speculated that such an event would occur at a very low frequency and would most probably be associated with the loss of the non-pathogenicity-inducing omega cassette and kanamycin resistance. Detecting a rare event that left no selectable marker would be virtually impossible. Therefore we used the potato plant itself to bait WT reversions, assuming that when the potato selects a WT strain from the soil, this will be visible as wilt disease. However, when soil inoculated with the BCA was repeatedly cultivated to potato under contained-use conditions, no WT reversion was observed.

Could the omega cassette transfer from the BCA to the WT population? BCA and rif-resistant WT populations were co-inoculated into soil then cultivated to potato. A transfer event would result in a rif/kan resistant mutant that could be selected for on SMSA$^{rif/kan}$ medium. To verify the parentage of any *R. solanacearum* rif/kan mutants that might arise, we used BCA and WT populations that had distinct DNA backgrounds (20). Based on the maximum population densities achieved in the soil, we estimated that each SMSA$^{rif/kan}$ plate tested 10^4 CFU BCA and WT. To date no rif/kan mutants have been isolated, however, this approach may not afford the sensitivity required to detect a rare transfer event.

Monitoring impact of the BCA on other microbial communities. This requires quantification of microbial species present and their abundance, and in an environment as complex as soil this is a very challenging task.

Media choices will bias those bacterial species recovered (1,8,13,17,23) and the work required in subsequent quantification and identification is substantial. Moreover, such an approach overlooks the majority of soil microbes, which are non-culturable. Rapidly improving DNA-based approaches present a real opportunity to study the microbial dynamics of complex environments (11,18,19,28). This is not to say that such methods are without bias (7,9,27), but they offer significant advantages in terms of practicality and are sensitive to non-culturables, including the recently proposed viable but non-culturable state of *R. solanacearum* (26).

At CABI we have started to develop one such DNA-based approach to address the impact of the BCA on the microbial community (19). We used GC-clamped universal 16S rRNA gene primers to amplify DNA fragments by PCR from all the microbial populations present in an environmental sample. The resulting single product (a species-composite of 16S rDNA fragments) is then analyzed by electrophoresis across a denaturation gradient that separates bands based on GC content rather than size (Density Gradient Gel Electrophoresis, DGGE). Under these conditions the respective 16S rDNA fragments of each of the bacterial species amplified are resolved according to small variations in their GC content. The identity of the bacterial species represented by a given DNA band can be ascertained by eluting and sequencing the band of interest. Lower order taxon-specific primers or primers to functional genes can be used for a more focused analysis of specific sub-populations (6,12).

We extracted total DNA from rhizosphere soils from crops inoculated with BCA and WT populations and performed 16S rDNA DGGE analyses. These profiles were reproducible between PCR runs and across replicate DNA extractions, with high microbial diversity associated with each of the crops and Rs-typical bands usually present in the rhizosphere soils. More significantly, rotation crops supported clearly different microbial populations. The complete results of these analyses may lead to a functional understanding of bacterial wilt suppressiveness, as apparently observed with carrot in these tests, as well as the biological impact of soil amendments (5,25,29).

A Niche within the Farming System to Apply the BCA

The primary constraints of seed and land and how these compound to exacerbate seed-borne tuber infection have been noted earlier (3). We proposed the idea of an on-farm nursery seed system in recognition of these limitations and to create a clear niche for application of the BCA. This system is described in detail by Kinyua *et al.* (this volume, 15), but briefly the Seed Plot Technique (SPT) is a small flat bed cultivation of potato planted at a high density that produces good quality seed for the subsequent ware season. The goal is to suppress large tubers by planting densely, thus maximizing tuber production of a size suitable for seed use.

Other attributes of the system were considered to be:

1. a small initial investment in seed by farmers, making more kinds of seed more affordable (linkage of formal and informal seed strengthened, and a flush-out mechanism for old seed);
2. a small amount for land required for crop rotation and other intensive disease and pest management practices, inclusive of the application of the BCA;
3. a clear differentiation in ware and seed management, resulting in improved seed health awareness.

In 1998 trials were set up to test these hypotheses. The comparison encompassed ware production from seed produced by the SPT and derived from Farmers' ware, with basic seed from Tigoni Potato Research Station acting as the ware control. The trial was conducted on-farm, comprising six farms (replicates), and proceeded for seven seasons (phases). Two varieties were evaluated: Tigoni and Roslin Tana. Land farmed with the SPT produced two to three times as much seed tuber as land under the Farmer's ware system (Fig. 4). We expected that differences in yield between the systems would become evident over cycles of multiplication due to declining seed health; however, the ware yields of the SPT and Farmers' derived seed remained similar to that of the control. Nevertheless, by ranking yields, SPT-derived seed performed better than Farmers' seed for both varieties in Phases 5, 6, 7, and 8 (Fig. 5) demonstrating SPT as an effective mechanism of managing on-farm seed. Further analyses revealed that the primary sources of variation were attributable to seasonal factors (rain) and farm fertility (Figs. 5 and 6), with disease pressure recorded as low. In one Tigoni farm, bacterial wilt was present within the seed plots and thus in the SPT-derived ware cultivations. From this farm extensive tuber sampling was conducted to monitor latent infection levels using the CIP NCM ELISA kit for bacterial wilt. We found a largely steady level of infection below the 3% level. The apparent effective management of bacterial wilt by the SPT system was encouraging, however, had bacterial wilt levels increased within the seed plots as visible by wilted plants then the harvest would have gone for consumption (not seed).

This visible seed health, which presents a buffer between the main ware cultivation and possible infection by latently infected tubers, is another positive attribute of the SPT system. The SPT has been seen as highly successful by the farmers and is now being promoted through donor

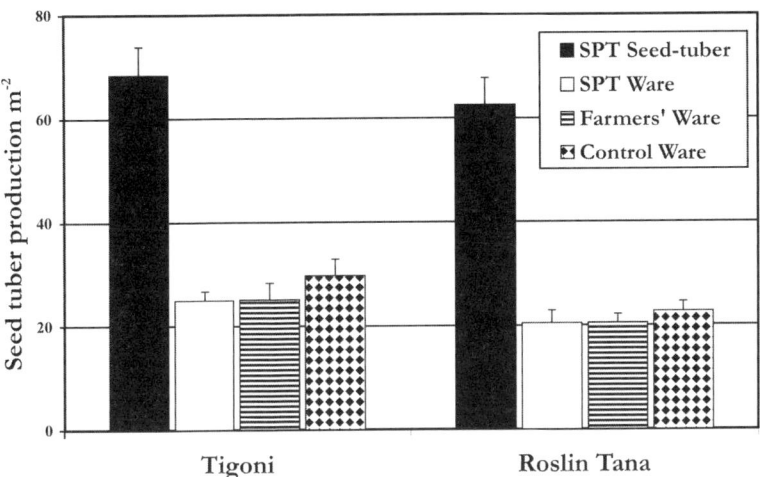

Fig. 4. Seed production per unit area of land between the nursery plot technique and various ware comparisons. (Average of six farms)

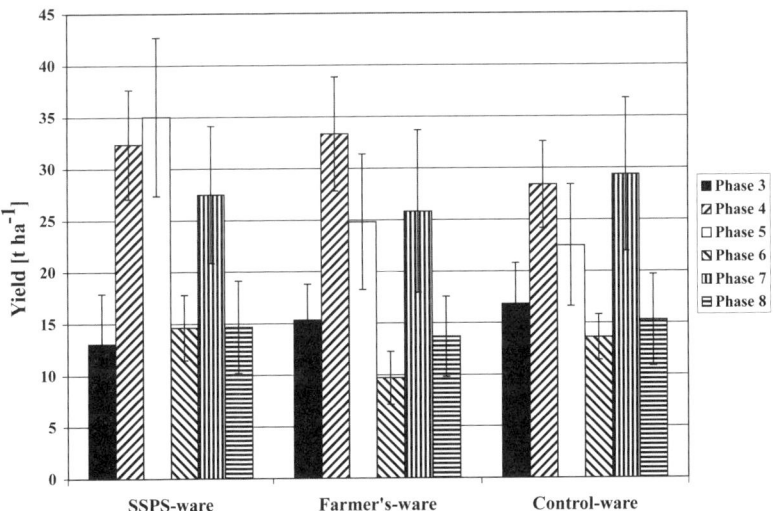

Fig. 5. Ware production over five seasons (phases). Seed derived from the SPT, Farmers' ware and Tigoni Potato Research Station (basic seed). (Average of six farms)

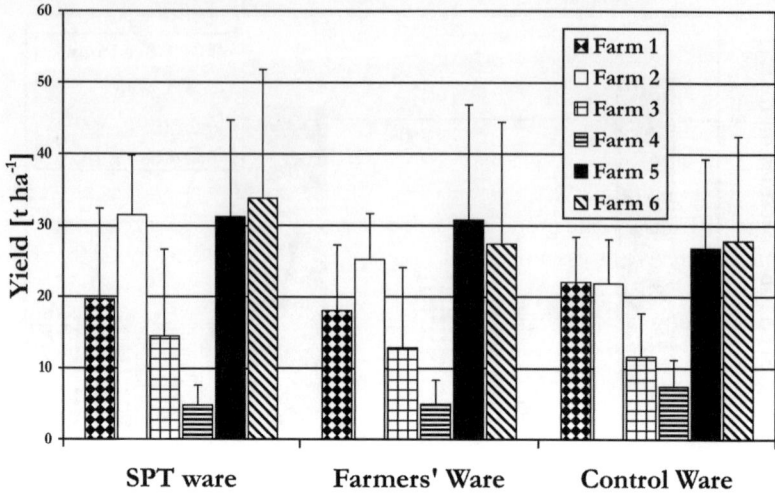

Fig. 6. Variation in ware production across six farms. Seed derived from the SPT, Farmers' ware and Tigoni Potato Research Station (basic seed). (Average of five seasons)

funding in Uganda, Bolivia and Peru. In Uganda in this growing season, some 75 SPT nurseries have been established by farmers, of which half have been undertaken wholly of the farmers' own motivation. Hence, the hypothesis can be accepted and improved farmer outreach for seed and a flush-out of old seed is being implemented.

Moreover, the SPT is evolving through farmer intervention; the width is narrowing from 2.0 to 1.6 m, soil hilling has been introduced with better results and mini-tubers are being used to plant the seed plots. Ultimately, though the seed produced by the formal sector must increase, with health-related quality guarantees in place.

Conclusions

Since the 2nd IBWS this project has developed a long way, not so much in the context of the BCA, although the data in support of its efficacy are now much more robust, but in the methods needed in the evaluation and adoption of the GM technology. It is of significance that these additional studies have had wider relevance than the BCA and are according benefit to farmers in the short-term today. I see this as a consequence of the high standards of research required when working with a GMO that has necessitated a meaningful exchange of ideas, research capacity and personnel between CABI and the national program staff in Kenya. The BCA is now critically positioned to go forward to a full evaluation in Kenya, however, donor funding is needed to see through this process.

The success of the SPT is particularly encouraging and has developed independently of the BCA with related activities underway in Uganda, Peru and Bolivia. However, whereas donors appear keen to fund this initiative, with its strong farmer visibility, it is unfortunate that the promotional phase of the SPT has to-date proceeded without strong backstopping research which I perceive as essential to its ultimate success. For example, the success of the SPT is dependent on accessing clean seed sources for farmers and providing farmers with proven recommendations on disease management. In the case of bacterial wilt neither of these requirements are in place, yet, as has been shown by aspects of the environmental impact assessment studies described here, such knowledge is achievable with today's improved research tools. It is a personal view, but the enthusiasm to work with farmers through farmers' field schools and the like is only as useful as the message you take and develop; if this message is not underpinned by sound scientific knowledge then these are just days spent hopefully in the sun.

Acknowledgements

This publication is the output of a research project funded by the United Kingdom Department for International Development (DFID) for the benefit of developing countries. The views expressed are not necessarily those of DFID.

Literature Cited

1. Aagot, N., Nybroe, O., Neilsen, P., and Johnsen, K. 2001. An altered *Pseudomonas* diversity is recovered from soil by using nutrient-poor *Pseudomonas*-selective soil extract media. Appl. Environ. Microbiol. 67: 5233-5239.
2. Ajanga, S. 1993. Status of bacterial wilt of potato in Kenya. Pages 338-340 in: Bacterial Wilt: Proceedings of an International Conference held in Kaohsiung, Taiwan, 28-30 October 1992 (ACIAR proceedings No. 45). G.L. Hartman and A.C. Hayward, eds. Australian Centre for International Agricultural Research, Canberra.
3. Barton, D., Smith, J.J., and Kinyua, Z.M. 1997. Socio-economic inputs to biological control of bacterial wilt disease of potato in Kenya. Pages

1-11 in: ODA RNRRS Crop Protection Project ZA0085. United Kingdom.

4. Berga, L., Kanzikwera, R., Kakuhenzire, R., Hakiza, J.J., and Manzi, G. 2001. The effects of crop rotation on bacterial wilt incidence and potato yield. African Crop Science Journal. 9: 267-278.

5. Berga, L., Sirri, D., and Ebanyat, P. 2001. Effect of soil amendments on bacterial wilt incidence and yield of potatoes in South Western Uganda. African Crop Science Journal. 9: 267-278.

6. De Oliveira, V.M., Coutinho, H.L.C., Sobral, B.M.S., Guimarães, J.D., Van Elsas, J.D., and Manfio, G.P. 1999. Discrimination of *Rhizobium tropici* and *R. leguminosarum* strains by PCR-specific amplification of 16S-23S rDNA spacer region fragments and denaturing gradient gel electrophoresis (DGGE). Lett. Appl. Microbiol. 28: 137-141.

7. Díez, B., Pedrós-Alió, C., Marsh, T., and Massana, R. 2001. Application of denaturing gradient gel electrophoresis (DGGE) to study the diversity of marine picoeukaryotic assemblages and comparison of DGGE with other molecular techniques. Appl. Environ. Microbiol. 67: 2942-2951.

8. Elliot, M.L., and Jardin, E.A.D. 1999. Comparison of media and diluents for enumeration of aerobic bacteria from Bermuda grass golf course putting greens. J. Microbial Meth. 34: 193-202.

9. Farrelly, V., Rainey, F.A., and Stackebrandt, E. 1995. Effects of genome size and rrn gene copy number on PCR amplification of 16S rRNA genes from a mixture of bacterialspecies. Appl. Environ. Microbiol. 61: 2798-2801.

10. Frey, P., Prior, P., Marie, C., Kotoujansky, A., Trigelet-Demery, D., and Trigalet, A. 1994. *Hrp* mutants of *Pseudomonas solanacearum* as potential biocontrol agents of tomato bacterial wilt. Appl. Environ. Microbiol. 60: 3175-3181.

11. Glandorf, D.C., Verheggen, P., Jansen, T., Jorritsma, J., Smit, E., Leeflang, P., Wernars, K., Thomashow, L. S., Laureijs, E., Thomas-Oates, J. E., Bakker, P.A.H.M., and van Loon, L.C. 2001. Effect of genetically modified *Pseudomonas putida* WCS358r on the fungal rhizosphere microflora of field-grown wheat. Appl. Environ. Microbiol. 67: 3371-3378.

12. Horz, H., Yimga, M.T., and Liesack, W. 2001. Detection of methanotroph diversity on roots of submerged rice plants by molecular retrieval of *pmoA*, *mmo*, *mxa*, and 16S rRNA and ribosomal DNA, including *pmoA*-based terminal restriction fragment length polymorphism profiling. Appl. Environ. Microbiol. 67: 4177-4185.

13. Johnson, K., and Nielson, P. 1999. Diversity of *Pseudomonas* strains isolated with King's B and Gould's S1 agar determined by repetitive extragenic palindromic-polymerase chain reaction, 16S rDNA,

sequencing and Fourier transformed spectroscopy characterisation. FEMS Microbial Lett. 173: 155-162.

14. Kakuhenzire, R., Alacho, F.O., Birikunzira, J., Turyamureeba, G., and Sikka, L. 1993. Progress in field evaluation for resistance to *Pseudomonas solanacearum* and cultural methods for control of bacterial wilt in Uganda. Pages 76-82 in: Proceedings of a workshop on bacterial wilt of potato caused by Pseudomonas solanacearum, Burundi, 22-26 February.

15. Kinyua, Z.M., Smith, J.J., Lung'aho, C., Olanya, M., and Priou, S. 2001. On-farm successes and challenges of producing bacterial wilt-free tubers in seed plots in Kenya. African Crop Science Journal. 9: 1-8.

16. Lung'aho, C., M'makwa, C., and Kidane-Mariam, H.M. 1997. Effect of source of mother plant, variety and growing conditions on the production of stem cuttings and subsequent yield of mini-tubers in the Kenyan potato programme. In *Proceedings of the Fourth Triennial Congress of the African Potato Association*, Pretoria, South Africa.

17. Martin, J.K. 1975. Comparison of agar media for counts of viable bacteria. Soil Biol. Biochem. 7: 401-402

18. Moënne-Loccoz, Y., Tichy, Hans-Volker., O'Donnell, A., Simon, R., and O'Gara, F. 2001. Impact of 2,4-diacretylphloroglucinol-producing biocontrol strain *Pseudomonas fluorescent* F113 on intraspecific diversity of resident culturable fluorescent Pseudomonads associated with the roots of field-grown sugar beet seedlings. Appl. Environ. Microbiol. 67: 3418-3425.

19. Muyzer, G., De Waal, E.C., and Uitterlinden, A.G. 1993. Profiling of complex microbial populations by denaturing gradient gel electrophoresis analysis of polymerase chain reaction-amplified genes coding for 16S rRNA. Appl. Environ. Microbiol. 59: 695-700.

20. Smith, J.J., Offord, L.C., Holderness, M., and Saddler, G.S. 1995. Pulsed-field gel electrophoresis analysis of *Pseudomonas solanacearum*. Bull. OEPP/EPPO Bull. 25: 163-167

21. Smith, J.J., Offord, L.C., Holderness, M., and Saddler, G.S. 1995. Genetic diversity of *Burkholderia solanacearum* (synonym *Pseudomonas solanacearum*) race 3 in Kenya. Appl. Environ. Microbiol. 61: 4263-4268.

22. Smith, J.J., Offord, L.C., Kibata, G.N., Murimi, Z. K., Trigalet, A., and Saddler, G.S. 1998. The development of a biological control against *Ralstonia solanacearum* race 3 in Kenya. Pages 337-342 in: Bacterial Wilt Disease: Molecular and Ecological Aspects. P. Prior, C. Allen, and J. Elphinstone, eds. Springer-Verlag, Berlin.

23. Sørheim, R., Torsvik, V.L., and Goksøyr, J. 1989. Phenotypical divergences between populations of soil bacteria isolated on different media. Microb. Ecol. 17: 181-192.
24. Steyn, M. 1997. The effect of seed size and population density on tuber distribution and yield. Pages 38-41 in: Potato production in South Africa with the emphasis on KwaZulu-Natal, ARC-Roodeplaat, Private Bag X293. Pretoria, RSA.
25. Terblanche, J., and de Villiers, D.A. 1998. The suppression of *Ralstonia solanacearum* by marigolds. Pages 359-374 in: Bacterial Wilt Disease: Molecular and Ecological Aspects. P. Prior, C. Allen, and J. Elphinstone, eds. Springer-Verlag, Berlin.
26. Van Elsas, J.D., Kastelein, P., van Bekkum, P., van derWolf, J.M., de Vries, P., and van Overbeek, L.S. 2000. Survival of *Ralstonia solanacearum* biovar 2, the causative agent of potato brown rot, in field and microcosm soils on temperate climates. Phytopathology 90: 1358-1366.
27. Von Wintzingerode, F., Goebel, U.B., and Stackebrandt, E. 1997. Determination of microbial diversity in environmental samples: pitfalls of PCR-based rRNA analysis. FEMS Microbiol. Rev. 21: 213-229.
28. Wieland, G., Neumann, R., and Backhaus, H. 2001. Variation of microbial communities in soil, rhizosphere and rhizoplane in response to crop species, soil type and crop development. Environ. Microbiol. 67: 5849-5854.
29. Yao, G., Zhang, F., and Li, Z. 1994. Control of bacterial wilt with soil amendment. Chin. J. Biol. Control 10: 106-109.

Colonization Capacity of *Ralstonia solanacearum* Tomato Strains Differing in Aggressiveness on Tomatoes and Weeds

J.-F. Wang and C.-H. Lin

Asian Vegetable Research and Development Center, 60 Yi Ming Liao, Shanhua, Tainan, Taiwan, R.O.C.

Ralstonia solanacearum is a complex species. Among the races of *R. solanacearum*, race 1 is the most diverse group (5), and large variation both in genotype and aggressiveness has been observed in several race 1 populations (7, 10). The location-specific nature of resistance in tomato to bacterial wilt (3) may be largely due to strain variation. A Taiwanese race 1 population isolated from tomatoes could be separated into six groups based on their interaction with tomato lines differing in bacterial wilt resistance (7). The most aggressive group overcame the resistance of Hawaii7996, a stable resistance source (13), while the least aggressive group caused low wilting incidence even on L390, a highly susceptible line. The ability to invade roots, colonize plants, and produce virulence factors is essential for *R. solanacearum* to cause disease in a susceptible host (13). To determine whether aggressiveness is related to the colonization capacity on host plants, we conducted a spatial and temporal monitoring of the internal bacterial density of *R. solanacearum* strains in resistant and susceptible tomato cultivars. Because association with weeds plays an important role in the survival and persistence of *R. solanacearum* (4), we also examined rhizosphere colonization of common tropical weed species by strains with different aggressiveness.

Materials and Methods

BACTERIAL STRAINS AND CULTURE CONDITIONS

R. solanacearum race 1 strains Pss190 (biovar 4), Pss186 (biovar 4), and Pss216 (biovar 3), were selected to represent high, moderate and low aggressiveness on tomato, respectively (7). Bacterial suspensions of $OD_{600} =$

0.3 (about 10^8 CFU/ml) were prepared as described (16) and diluted to desired density. A modified selective medium (SM-1) was used to enumerate *R. solanacearum* in soil and plant tissues (8).

PLANT MATERIALS, INOCULATION AND SAMPLING

Tomato cultivars used in this study were Hawaii7996 (H7996) and L390, bacterial wilt resistant and susceptible respectively (15). Soils infested with each strain to a density of 10^7 and 10^5 CFU per gram dry soil were prepared as described (7). Twenty-one-day-old seedlings were transplanted into ~300 ml plastic pots containing infested soils, arranged in a completely random design, and kept in growth chambers at 28°C/12h light. One experiment was sampled at 3 hours after inoculation (HAI) and at 1 day after inoculation (DAI), and a second duplicate experiment was sampled at 2, 4, and 7 DAI. Three common tropical weed species were used: nut sedge (*Cyperus rotundus*), Brazilian fireweed (*Erechtites valerianifolia*) and black nightshade (*Solanum nigrum*). Seeds or rhizomes (for nut sedge) were sown in Florabella peat moss, and six 1-month-old seedlings were transplanted into a plastic box (50cm L x 33cm W x 30cm H) containing 20 kg soil infested with individual bacterial strains at low (10^4 CFU per gram dry soil) density. A total of three boxes were prepared for each combination of weed species and strains and arranged in a CRD. Inoculated weeds were kept in a greenhouse at 28±2 C with natural light.

For tomato colonization experiments, a total of nine plants were randomly harvested from each treatment at each sampling time. Plants were uprooted, roots washed to remove soil, soaked in 70% alcohol for 3 to 5 min, rinsed in sterile water twice, and blotted dry on paper towels. Each plant was sectioned into root, a 2-cm collar section, mid-stem and top-stem. Each sample was weighed, macerated, and internal bacterial density was measured by direct plating. For the weed colonization experiment, three plants per weed species were randomly harvested from each treatment at 1, 3, and 5 weeks after inoculation (WAI). Plants were uprooted and shaken to remove most soil from the roots. Rhizosphere soil was collected from the root surface by shaking the plant roots in sterile water, and the bacterial population in the soil suspension was measured by direct plating on SM-1.

Results and Discussion

TOMATO COLONIZATION

Early infection of tomato by *R. solanacearum* involves root entry, mostly via lateral root emergence sites or wounds, and colonization of the intercellular spaces of the inner cortex and vascular parenchyma (14). At 3 HAI and 1 DAI at the 10^7 CFU/g soil inoculum, strains of different aggressiveness were detected at similar frequencies (>77%) and internal densities in roots and collars of resistant and susceptible tomato. The mean internal bacterial densities at 3 HAI (Log CFU/g fresh tissue) (L390/ H7996) were 5.1/4.7 in root and 3.9/3.5 in collar, and increased to 6.5/6.1 in roots and 5.8/5.1 in collars by 1 DAI. At the lower inoculum density (10^5 CFU), the least aggressive strain Pss216 colonized the resistant cultivar less well than the other strains, and its invasion of H7996 was slightly suppressed and delayed (Table 1).

No strain was detected at mid-stems and top-stems under low inoculum condition at this early stage. Since the sensory network that activates production of virulence factors is cell-density dependent (13), it is possible that resistance mechanisms against root invasion were masked under high inoculum densities. The lower inoculum density is a more natural condition. Thus, resistance expressed in roots may contribute partly to the overall resistance in tomato to bacterial wilt.

Table 1. Internal bacterial densities of *R. solanacearum* strains in tomato roots and collars 3 HAI and 1 DAI with 10^5-CFU per gram dry soil inoculum

Cultivar	Strain	3 HAI		1 DAI	
		Root	Collar	Root	Collar
L390	PSS190	2.9 A[a] (7)[b]	0.7 A (2)	2.9 A (6)	0.4 A (1)
	PSS186	3.0 A (7)	1.4 A (4)	2.8 A (6)	1.4 A (4)
	PSS216	0.8 B (2)	0.7 A (2)	2.5 A (6)	0.8 A (2)
H7996	PSS190	0.8 A (2)	0.0 A (0)	2.9 A (7)	1.5 A (4)
	PSS186	1.7 A (4)	0.7 A (3)	2.6 A (6)	2.8 A (6)
	PSS216	0.0 A (0)	0.0 A (0)	0.9 A (2)	0.0 A (0)

[a] Mean internal bacterial density presented as log (CFU/g fresh tissue) over nine plants. Mean comparisons were performed over strains by sampling time and plant sections, and means followed by the same letter were not significantly different according to DMRT ($P = 0.05$).

[b] Values in parentheses are the number of plants with positive pathogen detection.

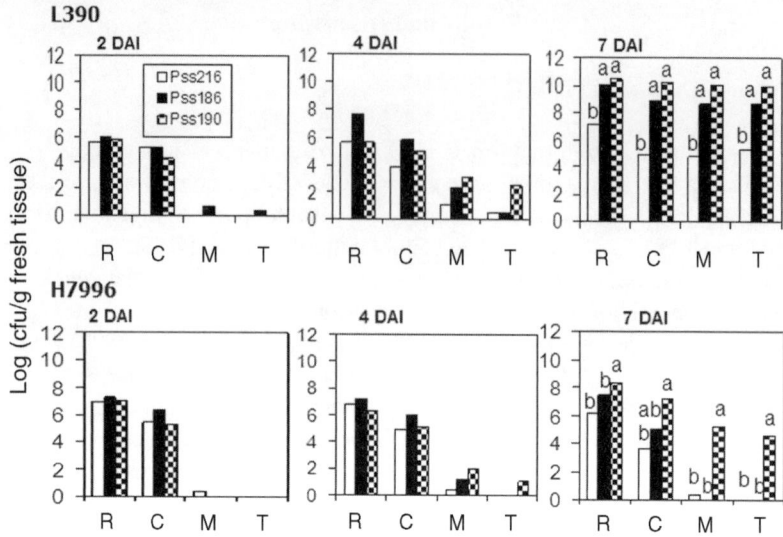

Fig. 1. Multiplication and spread of *R. solanacearum* strains in susceptible (L390) and resistant (H7996) tomato cultivars. The Y-axis indicates the mean internal bacterial density at root (R), collar (C), mid-stem (M), and top-stem (T) section over nine plants collected at 2, 4, and 7 DAI. Results of mean comparisons over strains by sampling time and plant section are indicated on top of columns when significant differences were observed.

In a compatible reaction, *R. solanacearum* invades and fills the xylem vessels, and travels rapidly to upper plant parts by 4 to 5 DAI (2,14). We observed differences among strains in tomato colonization by 4 DAI and these became significant by 7 DAI at the 10^7 CFU/g inoculum level (Figure 1). The aggressiveness expressed by the three strains in this study was similar to that observed previously (7). Mean percent wilting at 9 DAI on H7996 was 52.8, 0.0 and 0.0%, while that on L390 was 83.4, 69.4, and 11.1% % caused by Pss190, Pss186, and Pss216, respectively.

The internal bacterial density at 7 DAI was correlated well with the degree of disease severity. Although Pss216 had the lowest density in all plant parts, it was detected with similar frequencies (89 to 100%) as the other strains in all plant parts of L390. This indicates that the low aggressiveness of Pss216 was not due to the retarded upward movement, but more to its slower multiplication inside tomato tissues. Pss216 was detected in 11% of H7996 samples, compared to 0% for Pss186 and 67% for Pss190. The high bacterial density of Pss190 could result in greater expression of virulence factors, such as the high molecular mass acidic extracellular polysaccharide (EPS I) (12) and polygalacturonases (6), and thus the strain may be more efficient in horizontal movement by breaking and blocking vessels.

Using similar methods, the group of Prior found a direct relationship between levels of tomato resistance and the degree to which *R. solanacearum* colonized host stems (1,11).

Several mechanisms have been associated with bacterial wilt resistance in tomato, including formation of tyloses (1) and thickening of vessel pit membrane (9). Further molecular and histological studies are needed to understand the resistance-breaking process caused by Pss190 in H7996.

WEED COLONIZATION

Colonization capacity of *R. solanacearum* strains was examined on the rhizosphere of three weed species under low inoculum densities (10^4 CFU), individually. Pss216 was significantly poorer at colonizing black nightshade over the testing period (Table 2); however, the three strains had similarly poor colonization capacity on the other two weed species. This finding suggests that low aggressiveness of *R. solanacearum* strains on tomato was not related to their capacity for root invasion and upward movement, but more to internal multiplication and possibly horizontal movement among xylem vessels following inoculation at the 10^7 CFU level. The least aggressive strain Pss216 colonized tomato and black nightshade less well than the more aggressive strains under 10^4 to 10^5-CFU inoculum level.

Table 2. Bacterial density of *R. solanacearum* in rhizosphere soil of weeds at 1, 3, and 5 WAI at 10^4-CFU/g dry soil inoculum

Weed	Strain	1 WAI	3 WAI	5 WAI
Black nightshade	Pss190	5.2 A [a]	1.9 A	2.5 AB
	Pss186	6.2 A	1.6 A	3.8 A
	Pss216	1.2 B	0.0 A	0.0 B
	Pss186	2.5 A	0.0	0.0
Brazilian fireweed	Pss190	1.5 A	0.0	0.0
	Pss216	1.2 A	0.0	0.0
Nut sedge	Pss190	1.0	1.0	0.0
	Pss186	0.0	0.0	0.0
	Pss216	0.0	0.0	0.0

[a] Data were means of three plants as log (CFU/g dry soil). Mean comparisons were performed over strains by sampling time and weed species, and means followed by the same letter were not significantly different based on DMRT ($P = 0.05$).

This may explain why this type of strain accounts for a small proportion of the population in tomato production fields (7). On the other hand, it is puzzling that Pss190, being a good colonizer, was not a major part of the population. It is important to note that unlike the other strains, Pss190 was isolated from a highland location, where rotation with rice was not practiced as in the lowland tomato production area. The question of whether such an agro-ecosystem can support the persistence of strains like Pss190 remains for further investigations.

Acknowledgments

The authors would like to thank Ms. Chiou-fen Hsu for her technical assistance. This work was supported by the National Science Council, R.O.C. (NSC-2313-B-125-001).

Literature Cited

1. Grimault, V., Anais, G., and Prior, P. 1994. Distribution of *Pseudomonas solanacearum* in the stem tissues of tomato plants with different levels of resistance to bacterial wilt. Plant Pathol. 43:663-668.
2. Grimault, V., Gelie, B., Lemattre, M., Prior, P., and Schmit, J. 1994. Comparative histology of resistant and susceptible tomato cultivars infected by *Pseudomonas solanacearum*. Physiol. Mol. Plant Pathol. 44:105-123.
3. Hanson, P.M., Wang, J.-F., Licardo, O., Hanudin, Mah, S., Hartman, G.L., Lin, Y.C., and Chen, J.-T. 1996. Variable reaction of tomato lines to bacterial wilt evaluated at several locations in Southeast Asia. Hortscience 31:143-146.
4. Hayward, A.C. 1994. The hosts of *Pseudomonas solanacearum*. Pages 9-24 in: Bacterial Wilt: the Disease and its Causative Agent *Pseudomonas solanacearum*. A.C. Hayward and G.L. Hartman eds. Oxford, UK: CAB Int.
5. Hayward, A.C. 2000. *Ralstonia solanacearum*. Encycl. Microbiol. 4:32-42.
6. Huang, Q., and Allen, C. 2000. Polygalacturonases are required for rapid colonization and full virulence of *Ralstonia solanacearum* on tomato plants. Physiol. Mol. Plant Pathol. 57:77-83.
7. Jaunet, T.X., and Wang, J.-F. 1999. Variation in genotype and aggressiveness of *Ralstonia solanacearum* race 1 isolated from tomato in Taiwan. Phytopathology 89:320-327.

8. Michel, V.V., Hartman, G.L., and Midmore, D.J. 1996. Effect of previous crop on soil population of *Burkhoderia solanacearum*, bacterial wilt, and yield of tomatoes in Taiwan. Plant Dis. 80:1367-1372.

9. Nakaho, K., Hibino, H., and Miyagawa, H. 2000. Possible mechanisms limiting movement of *Ralstonia solanacearum* in resistant tomato tissues. J. Phytopathol. 148:181-190.

10. Prior, P., Steva, H., and Cadet, P. 1990. Aggressiveness of strains of *Pseudomonas solanacearum* from the French West Indies (Martinique and Guadeloupe) on tomato. Plant Dis. 74:962-965.

11. Prior, P., Bart, S., Leclercq, S., Darasse, A., and Anais, G. 1996. Resistance to bacterial wilt in tomato as discerned by spread of *Pseudomonas (Burkholderia) solanacearum* in stem tissues. Plant Pathol. 45:720-726.

12. Saile, E., McGarvey, J.A., Schell, M.A., and Denny, T.P. 1997. Role of extracellular polysaccharide and endoglucanase in root invasion and colonization of tomato plants by *Ralstonia solanacearum*. Phytopathology 87:1264-1271.

13. Schell, M.A. 2000. Control of virulence and pathogenicity genes of *Ralstonia solanacearum* by an elaborate sensory network. Annu. Rev. Phytopathol. 38:263-292.

14. Vasse, J., Frey, P., and Trigalet, A. 1995. Microscopic studies of intercellular infection and protoxylem invasion of tomato roots by *Pseudomonas solanacearum*. Mol. Plant-Microbe Interact. 8:241-251.

15. Wang, J.-F., Hanson, P., and Barnes, J. A. 1998. Worldwide evaluation of an international set of resistance sources to bacterial wilt in tomato. Pages 269-275 in: Bacterial Wilt Disease: Molecular and Ecological Aspects. P. Prior, C. Allen, and J. Elphinstone, eds. Springer-Verlag, Berlin, Germany.

16. Wang, J.-F., Oliver, J., Thoquet, P., Mangin, B., Sauviac, L., and Grimsley, N. H. 2000. Resistance of tomato line Hawaii7996 to *Ralstonia solanacearum* Pss4 in Taiwan is controlled mainly by a major strain-specific locus. Mol. Plant-Microbe Interact. 13:6-13.

Introduction to Europe of *Ralstonia solanacearum* Biovar 2, Race 3 in *Pelargonium zonale* Cuttings from Kenya

Jaap D. Janse[1], H.E. van den Beld[1], John Elphinstone[2], Sean Simpkins[2], Leon N.A. Tjou-Tam-Sin,[1] and Johan van Vaerenbergh[3]

[1] Department of Bacteriology, Plant Protection Service, Wageningen, The Netherlands; [2] Plant Health Group, Central Science Laboratory, York, UK; [3] Department of Crop Protection, Agriculture Research Center, Merelbeke, Belgium

Infections of *Ralstonia solanacearum* biovar 2, race 3 have recently been found on potato and tomato in several countries of the European Union. These findings have resulted in a control directive that is implemented in the European Union (2,7,22). Biovar 2, race 3 is usually restricted to the above-mentioned cultivated Solanaceae species, and has been reported occasionally on *Solanum melongena*, *Capsicum annuum* (24,4) and some solanaceous weeds. A number of additional symptomless weed hosts have been reported which may enable biovar 2, race 3 to survive in a latent form or in their rhizosphere, or which acted as hosts after artificial inoculation (Table 1).

Race 1 strains (biovars 1 and 3) have been found to occur on greenhouse ornamentals in the northern hemisphere. In a finding in 1979 of a strain of *R. solanacearum* from *Pelargonium x hortorum* (*P. zonale* hybrids or geranium) in the USA, race and biovar identification was unclear but pathogenicity tests showed that the isolates from *Pelargonium* failed to cause disease on tobacco, a trait of race 3 (39). More recently biovar 2, race 3 was diagnosed from *Pelargonium zonale* in Wisconsin (18,19,44). There are also some doubtful reports of findings of *R. solanacearum* in *Pelargonium* spp. from W. Australia (31) and Tanganika (45). The bacterium was also reported in *P. zonale* from Ohio (28) and Pennsylvania (2) in the USA. In these publications the race or biovar was not identified or reported, but there are indications that biovar 1, race 1 was involved (Hayward, pers. comm.). One case of infected *P. capitatum* from Reunion Is. Biovar 1, race 1 was noted (15). *R. solanacearum* was detected for the first time in December 1999 in the UK on imported *P. zonale* cuttings produced in Kenya for the European market. The following year symptoms of bacterial wilt were observed in several *Pelargonium* nurseries in Belgium and Germany. *R. solanacearum* biovar 2/race 3 was consistently isolated and identified. Surveys in Belgium, Germany and the Netherlands (where only latent infections were found) showed that the origin of the infection was cuttings produced in Kenya by several nurseries for export to associated companies in Belgium, Germany, the Netherlands and the UK for further propagation. We will present the results of surveys to trace the origin of infection and the control measures imposed to prevent spread and persistence of the organism in both Europe and Kenya. *R. solanacearum* isolates from *Pelargonium* were characterized on the basis of morphology, serology, PCR, RFLP, and fatty acid patterns. Symptoms in *Pelargonium*, results of isolate characterization and a proposed testing method for latent infections are also presented.

Material and Methods

BACTERIAL STRAINS

Reference strains. Strains PD (Culture Collection Plant Protection Service, Wageningen, NL) 4027 and 4052 isolated from *Pelargonium zonale* in the Netherlands, and strains PD 4116-4118 and 4124 isolated from *P. zonale* in Belgium were used in all identification and diagnostic tests mentioned below, except AFLP. Strain PD 2762 (biovar 2/race 3) from potato served as a positive control strain. Strain PD 4027 was used in all host studies performed by the PPS, Wageningen, NL. For fatty acid analysis and BOX PCR, we included a larger number of biovar 2/race 3 strains isolated from potato, tomato, water, *Solanum dulcamara* and surface water as well as some biovar 3/race 1 and biovar 1/race 2 strains present in the PD collection for comparison. For AFLP, we included similar control strains as well as strains NCPPB (National Collection of Plant Pathogenic Bacteria, CSL, York, UK) 4211 and 4212 isolated from *P. zonale* in Kenya and NCPPB 4213 and 4215 isolated from surface water in Kenya.

Isolation and identification. Methods, including pathogenicity tests, were those described by Wenneker *et al.* (47), using antiserum 2679/BE 21129 (Loewe Biochimika, Sauerlach, Germany) for indirect immuno-fluorescence test (IF). Fatty Acid Analysis (FAA) made use of the race-specific library developed at the PPS, Wageningen, NL (21). For routine PCR the primers of Seal *et al.* (35) were used. For biovar-specific PCR the primer pair and method of Fegan *et al.* (10) was used. BOX-PCR was performed according to Rademaker & De Bruijn (34). Quantitative PCR was also

Table 1. Hosts of *Ralstonia solanacearum* biovar 2, race 3 reported in literature

Natural host	Family	Occurrence	References and Remarks
Solanaceous crops			
Capsicum annuum	Solanaceae	rare, S. America	24
Lycopersicon esculentu	Solanaceae	widespread	many references
Solanum tuberosum	Solanaceae	widespread	many references
Solanum melongena (eggplant)	Solanaceae	rare, S. America, France	24
Solanum phureja	Solanaceae	rare, Colombia	5
Solanaceous weeds			
Cyphomandra betaceae	Solanaceae	2T? rare, Colombia	25
Datura stramonium*	Solanaceae	rare, Georgia, USA	6
Physalis sp*	Solanaceae	rare, Georgia, USA	6
Physalis angulatu	Solanaceae	rare, S. Africa	40
S. carolinens	Solanaceae	rare, Georgia, USA	6
S. cinereum	Solanaceae	Australia only	13
S. dulcamara (bittersweet)	Solanaceae	NW Europe	8, 9,22, 23, 29
S. nigrum (black nightshade)	Solanaceae	widespread, not common	17, 41
Non-solanaceous natural host plants			
Bidens pinnata*	Compositae	rare, Georgia, USA	6
Brassica rapa	Cruciferae	India	36
Chenopodium spp.	Chenopodiaceae	Nepal	33
Melampodium perfoliatum		Costa Rica	20
Momordica charantia (bitter gourd)	Cucurbitaceae	Philippines	42
Pelargonium zonale (= *P. x hortorum*)	Geraniaceae	USA	18, 19
Phaseolus vulgaris (string bean)	Leguminosae	Philippines	42
Portulaca oleracea	Portulacaceae	Kenya, Egypt Nepal	12; Janse, pers. comm, 33
Salvia reflex	Labiatae	Australia	16, under high inoculum
Natural latent hosts			
Cleome monophylla	Capparadidaceae	Kenya	14

Table 1 (continued). Hosts of *Ralstonia solanacearum* biovar 2, race 3 reported in literature

Natural Host	Family	Occurrence	References and Remarks
Natural latent hosts (continued)			
Galinsoga ciliata	Compositae	Nepal	33
Nicotiana glutinosa	Solanaceae		24, 27, symptoms with high inoculum in soil
Nicotiana rustica	Solanaceae		24, as for *N. glutinosa*
Polygonum capitata	Polygonaceae	Nepal	33
S. sisymbriifolium	Solanaceae	Brazil	12, host for biovar 2T
Urtica dioica	Urticaceae	Netherlands	47, rare, when roots exposed to high inoculation pressure from surface water, wilting under high temperature conditions in greenhouse
Root colonization or host with or without symptoms			
after artificial inoculation only			
Beta vulgaris	Chenopodiaceae	I	30
Brassica juncea, B. napus	Cruciferae	Nepal I, A, Sweden, S	30, 33
B. rapa	Cruciferae	I	3
Browallia specios	Solanaceae	I	30
Cerastium glomeratum	Caryophyllaceae	Nepal, S, A	33
Chenopodium abrosioides, C. amaranticolor, C. paniculatum	Chenopodiaceae	I	3
Cucurbita pepo	Cucurbitaceae	Japan	36
Drymaria cordata	Caryophyllaceae	Nepal, S	33
Erodium moschatum	Geraniaceae	I	3
Eupatorium cannabinum	Compositae	S	30
Galinsoga parviflora	Compositae	Nepal, N, A	33
Glycine max	Leguminosae	I	30

Table 1 (continued). Hosts of *Ralstonia solanacearum* biovar 2, race 3 reported in literature

Natural Host	Family	Occurrence	References and Remarks
Gnaphalium elegans	Compositae	I	3
Helianthus annuus	Compositae		27 showing stunting when grown in infested soil
Hordeum vulgare	Graminae	A	33
Hyoscyamus niger	Solanaceae	I	30
Ipomea sp.			48
Lycopersicon chilense	Solanaceae	I	30
Nicandra physaloides	Solanaceae	A, I	30, 33
Nicotiana alata	Solanaceae	I	30
Phaseolus vulgaris	Leguminosae	S, I	27, 30, stunting when planted in infected soils
P. multiflorus	Leguminosae		27, as for *P. vulgaris*
Physalis floridana	Solanaceae	Chile	11
Pisum sativum	Leguminosae	I	30
Rumex spp.	Polygonaceae	I	3, 48
Salpiglossis sinuata	Scrophulariaceae	S	29
Spergula arvensis	Caryophyllacae	I	3
Solanum capsisastrum	Solanaceae	Chile, S	11, 30
Solanun caripense	Solanaceae	Colombia, I	3
S. luteum	Solanaceae	S	29
S. sarrachoides	Solanaceae	Chile	11
S. xanthophyllum	Solanaceae	Nepal, I, A	33
Soliva anthemidifolia	Compositae	I	3
Tagetes sp.	Asteraceae		48
Tropaeolum majus	Tropaeolaceae	S	29
Verbena brasiliensis	Verbenaceae	I	3
Vicia faba	Leguminosae	I	30
Vigna sinensis	Leguminosae		26

* = On basis of data presented in publication doubtful if biovar 2, race 3 was involved.

N = natural, A = after artificial inoculation, S = through inoculum present in soil, I = stem inoculation.

performed on isolates obtained in the UK and Kenya using the Taqman assay of Weller *et al.* (46) with *R. solanacearum*-specific and biovar 2-specific probes. AFLP (43) was carried out using the primer combination *Eco*RI+C/*Mse*I+0 with analysis by the UPGMA method with Bionumerics software (Applied Maths, Belgium).

Host range tests. Young plants raised from cuttings of selected host plant species mentioned in Table 2 were grown at 75% RH, 25-23°C day/night air temperature during a 14 h photoperiod in a quarantine greenhouse. Inoculation was carried out by 1) micro-injection of 10 μl into the lower stem or 2) pouring 35 ml of bacterial suspension (10^7 CFU/ml^{-1}) of a 48h NA culture per plant (n=6) in soil around uninjured plants, according to the methods used by Wenneker *et al.* (47) for stinging nettle. Negative control plants were inoculated or drenched with sterile 0.01M PB only.

Surveys and method for detection of latent infections. Surveys were performed by sampling 200 stem parts (1cm in length) aseptically removed from the lower part of the stem or petiole of the lowest leaf per lot of *Pelargonium* cuttings. The samples were analyzed the same day in the laboratory. Stem parts were crushed in plastic bags (if necessary following a pre-wash and short disinfection in 70% alcohol and blotted dry). Thereafter 50 ml 0.05 M phosphate buffer (PB) was added and the homogenate incubated for 30 min at 100 rpm in a shaker at RT. The extract was then centrifuged for 15 min at 7000 g for subsequent testing (1,47).

Results

SYMPTOMS ON PELARGONIUM, ISOLATION AND IDENTIFICATION

Early symptoms were wilting of the lower leaves with rolling of the leaf margins (Color Plate 1). Subsequently leaves showed sectorial chlorosis and eventually papery, brown necrosis. Some stems showed brown to black discoloration, especially externally at the root-collar and when cut, showed brown watery discoloration of the vascular tissues. Sometimes only one part of the stem showed wilting symptoms.

All isolates formed *R. solanacearum*-typical pearly white, flat, irregular and fluidal colonies on YPGA and milky-white, flat, irregular and fluidal colonies with red coloured whorls in the centre on SMSA. All isolates from *Pelargonium* proved to be *R. solanacearum* in biochemical tests, PCR with all specific primer sets used, IF with specific sera, HR-reaction in tobacco and pathogenicity tests on tomato. All isolates from *Pelargonium* proved to be consistently biovar 2 by FAA, biovar 2-specific PCR and biochemical tests. Strains PD 4116-4118, 4124 and NCPPB 4211, 4212, 4213 and 4215 were also pathogenic to eggplant (*S. melongena* 'Black Beauty'), *S. nigrum*

Table 2. Results of host range pathogenicity tests by drenching (D) soil (35 ml) and stem inoculation (SI) with 10^7 CFU/ml of strain PD 4027 from *Pelargonium* and PD 2762 from potato

Host	D	SI
Pelargonium zonale	+	+
Tomato 'Moneymaker'	+	+
Portulaca oleracea	+	+
Petunia hybrid	latent	latent
Calibrachoa 'Million Bells'	latent	latent
Begonia sp.	-	-
Impatiens sp.	-	-*
Pointsettia sp.	-	-*
Saintpaulia sp.	-	-*

* Very low residual populations detected at site of inoculation after 28 days.

and potato. These strains were not pathogenic to tobacco after stem inoculation. Control strains of biovars 3 and 4 (race 1) and biovar 1 (race 2) always tested as expected. In BOX-PCR, biovar 2 strains from *Pelargonium* clustered with those isolated from other sources (Fig. 1). Only one strain showed a strong extra band, the significance of which was not apparent. In AFLP analysis, Kenyan strains from *Pelargonium* and surface water clustered with other reference strains belonging to biovar 2/race 3. Some other surface water strains clustered with biovar 3 strains and not with strains belonging to other biovar/race combinations. Amplified fragment length polymorphism (AFLP) analysis of *R. solanacearum* strains of different biovar/ race and origin revealed that Pelargonium strains and most irrigation water (Kenya) strains clustered together with known biovar 2, race 3 strains. Some water (Kenya) strains clustered with biovar 3 strains and one irrigation water (Kenya) strain was isolated.

HOST RANGE TESTS

Results of host tests are presented in Table 2. After challenge by stem inoculation or soil drenching (without wounding plants), *Pelargonium*, tomato and *Portulaca oleracea* showed typical wilting symptoms. *Petunia* and *Calibrachoa* showed latent populations of 10^5 CFU/ml^{-1} of tissue extract 28 days after stem inoculation and 10^3 CFU/ml^{-1} of root extracts 28 days after soil drenching.

Immediately after the finding in December 2000 of *R. solanacearum* biovar 2 in two nurseries in Belgium that received cuttings from a nursery in the Netherlands, which in turn had received its cuttings from a daughter nursery in Kenya, more than one hundred samples of 200 stem or petiole pieces were tested for latent infections. In one case the bacterium was found. Early in 2001, other Belgian and Dutch nurseries receiving cuttings from the Dutch nursery were checked for visual symptoms and latent infection. No further infections were found in Belgium, whereas one latently infected plant was found in one nursery in the Netherlands. In all other Dutch nurseries importing cuttings directly from Kenya no (latent) infections were found. In Kenya early in 2001, all mother material and cuttings from infected nurseries were checked and any infections found were destroyed. Usually infected plants in the nurseries involved showed symptoms and the number of latently infected plants was low.

A survey in the surroundings of one Kenyan nursery led to the detection of *R. solanacearum* biovars 2 and 3 in river water used for irrigation of *Pelargonium*. No infected weed hosts were found among several potential host species present. In the course of 2001 and 2002, following control measures mentioned below, no further infections were found upon visual inspections and testing for latency, in Europe or Kenya. The following control measures were imposed in Europe:

- Destruction of all plants of infected cultivars by burning or deep burial
- Disinfection of contaminated greenhouse (compartments), machines, tools and improved hygienic protocols
- Officially controlled delivery of all potentially infected lots, after testing, to local market only
- Tracing of all nurseries receiving material from Kenya
- Sampling and testing of all *Pelargonium* plants on contaminated nurseries and nurseries receiving propagating material from Kenya
- Prohibition of surface water for irrigation not only for potato and tomato, but also for *Pelargonium*, *Portulaca*, eggplant and *S. sisymbriifolium* in known contaminated surface water areas

In Kenya, plants of infected cultivars were destroyed by burning or controlled dedicated waste disposal areas. Contaminated greenhouses, machines and tools were disinfected and hygienic protocols were strengthened. Nurseries changed to the use of borehole water or disinfected surface water for irrigation (using combinations of filtration, UV irradiation, chlorine dioxide and/or hydrogen peroxide with peracetic acid). Furthermore, all production stock was discarded and the mother stock was tested (monitored) by IF or ELISA. Drainage systems were improved and discussions

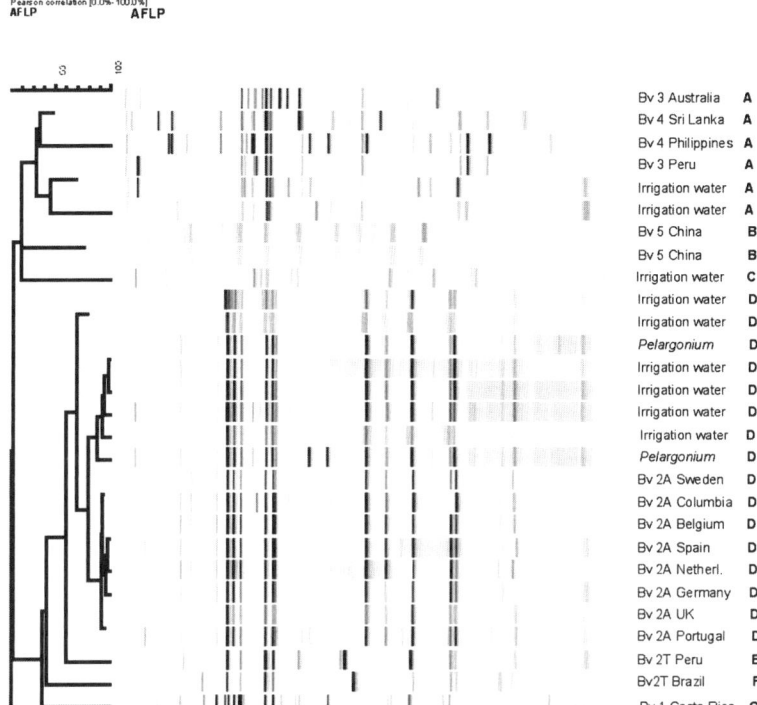

Pearson correlation [0.0%- 100.0%]
AFLP

Bv 3 Australia	A
Bv 4 Sri Lanka	A
Bv 4 Philippines	A
Bv 3 Peru	A
Irrigation water	A
Irrigation water	A
Bv 5 China	B
Bv 5 China	B
Irrigation water	C
Irrigation water	D
Irrigation water	D
Pelargonium	D
Irrigation water	D
Irrigation water	D
Irrigation water	D
Irrigation water	D
Pelargonium	D
Bv 2A Sweden	D
Bv 2A Columbia	D
Bv 2A Belgium	D
Bv 2A Spain	D
Bv 2A Netherl.	D
Bv 2A Germany	D
Bv 2A UK	D
Bv 2A Portugal	D
Bv 2T Peru	E
Bv2T Brazil	F
Bv 1 Costa Rica	G
Bv 1	H

Fig. 1. Dendrogram based on single linkage (Piersson correlation) of BOX-PCR patterns of *Ralstonia solanacearum* of different biotype/race and origin. *Pelargonium* strains group with known biovar 2, race 3 strains of different hosts and origin in one tight cluster.

were held with the Plant Protection Service in Kenya with a view to official monitoring of the control measures.

Discussion

Results of this study clearly show that *P. zonale* is a host for *R. solanacearum* biovar 2/race 3. Strains from *Pelargonium* matched perfectly with other strains of biovar 2/race 3 isolated from different hosts and habitats. In an early study on isolates from *Pelargonium* in the USA, race and biovar identification was unfortunately unclear but pathogenicity tests showed that the isolates from *Pelargonium* failed to cause disease on tobacco (39). The bacterium was also reported in *P. zonale* from Ohio (28) and Pennsylvania (2) in the USA. In all these cases the race or biovar was not identified, but there are indications that biovar 1/race 1 was involved (Hayward, pers. comm.). A more detailed report is from Hudelson (18), Hudelson *et al.* (19), and Williamson *et al.* (44) from Wisconsin USA, where introduction of *R. solanacearum* biovar 2/race 3 apparently took place through import of *Pelargonium* cuttings from Guatemala. The situation in Wisconsin is thus comparable to that in Europe (see below). In our study, strains from potato were pathogenic to *Pelargonium* and vice versa. *Pelargonium* appears not to be a very susceptible host. On contaminated nurseries in Kenya, spread from plant to plant only occurred in badly drained greenhouse compartments and most infected plants showed symptoms. Only very few plants were found to be latently infected. It was again demonstrated that *P. oleracea* is a host of *R. solanacearum* biovar 2/race 3, showing symptoms (for other reports see Table 1). *Petunia* and *Calibrachoa* were also found to act as latent hosts for this bacterium. *Calibrachoa* has never been reported before as a latent carrier of *R. solanacearum*. For *Petunia* hybrids there is only one report from the USA for race 3 (38).

Results also showed that the origin of the infection was contaminated surface water used for irrigation in *Pelargonium* nurseries producing cuttings in Kenya for the European market. The water may have become contaminated from infected potato crops known to be situated upstream. *R. solanacearum*, both race 1 and race 3, are widespread in Kenya (37). Unrooted cuttings from Kenya then contaminated a few nurseries in Europe. The following measures have been implemented at the Kenyan nurseries: 1) discontinued use of contaminated surface water for irrigation; 2) the destruction of infected production stocks, and 3) improved hygienic protocols. After taking these measures, no further infections have been found in propagation material.

Acknowledgements

The skillful technical assistance of P.P.M.A. Smits, M.S.W. Verdel and J.H.J. Derks, is greatly acknowledged; the authors also thank Dr. Chris Hayward, University of Queensland, Australia for carefully reading the manuscript and offering helpful suggestions.

Literature Cited

1. Anonymous, 1998. Interim testing scheme for the diagnosis, detection and identification of *Ralstonia solanacearum* (Smith) Yabuuchi *et al.*

in potatoes. Annex II to the Council Directive 98/57/EC of 20 July 1998 on the control of *Ralstonia solanacearum* (Smith) Yabuuchi *et al.* Publication 97/647/EC, Official Journal European Communities No. L 235: 8-39.

2. Anonymous, 1999. Southern bacterial wilt on geraniums. Pennsylvania Plant Pest Rep. 16(4).

3. Belalcazar, S., Uribe, G., and Thurston H.D. 1968. [Reconocimiento de hospedantes a *Pseudomonas solanacearum* (E.F. Sm.) en Colombia.] Revista ICA 3:37-46.

4. Caffier, D., and Herve, A. 1996. La pourriture brune de la pomme de terre, un nouveau risqué bacterien en Europe. La Pomme de Terre Française 492:20-23.

5. Ciampi, L., and Sequeira L. 1980. Influence of temperature on virulence of race 3 strains of *Pseudomonas solanacearum*. Am. Potato J. 57: 309-317.

6. Dukes, P.D., Morton, D.J., and Jenkins, S.F. 1965. Infection of indigenous hosts by *Pseudomonas solanacearum* in South Georgia. Phytopathology 55:1055.

7. Elphinstone, J.G. 1996. Survival and possibilities for extinction of *Pseudomonas solanacearum* (Smith) Smith in cool climates. Potato Res. 39:403-410.

8. Elphinstone, J.G., Hennessey, J.K., Wilson, J.K., and Stead, D.E. 1996. Sensitivity of different methods for the detection of *Ralstonia solanacearum* (Smith) Smith in cool climates. Bull. OEPP/EPPO Bull. 26:663-678.

9. Elphinstone, J.G., Stanford, H.M., and Stead, D.E. 1998. Detection of *Ralstonia solanacearum* in potato tubers, *Solanum dulcamara*, and associated irrigation water. Pages 133-139 in: Bacterial Wilt Disease: Molecular and Ecological Aspects. P. Prior, C. Allen, and J. Elphinstone, eds. Springer-Verlag, Heidelberg, Germany.

10. Fegan, M., Holoway, G., Hayward, A.C., and Timmis, J. 1998. Development of a diagnostic test based on the polymerase chain reaction (PCR) to identify strains of *R. solanacearum* exhibiting the biovar 2 genotype. Pages 34-43 in: Bacterial Wilt Disease: Molecular and Ecological Aspects. P. Prior, C. Allen, and J. Elphinstone, eds. Springer-Verlag, Heidelberg, Germany.

11. Fernandez, M.C. 1986. Some hosts of *Pseudomonas solanacearum* in Chile. Agric. Technica 46: 101-105.

12. Gillings, M., and Fahy, P. 1993. Genetic diversity of *Pseudomonas solanacearum* biovars 2 and N2 assessed using restriction endonuclease analysis of total genomic DNA. Plant Pathol. 42: 744-753.

13. Graham, J., and Lloyd, A.B. 1978. *Solanum cinereum*, a wild host of *Pseudomonas solanacearum* biotype II. J. Austr. Inst. Agric. Sci. 44: 124-126.

14. Harris, D.C. 1976. Bacterial wilt in Kenya with particular reference to potatoes. Pages 84-88 in: Proceedings of the First International Planning Conference and Workshop on the Ecology and Control of Bacterial Wilt Caused by *Pseudomonas solanacearum*. Raleigh, North Carolina, July 18-24. L. Sequeira and A. Kelman, eds.

15. Hayward, A.C. 1964. Characteristics of *Pseudomonas solanacearum*. J. Appl. Bacteriol. 2: 265-277.

16. Hayward, A.C. 1975. Biotypes of *Pseudomonas solanacearum* in Australia. Australian Plant Path. Soc. Newsletter 2: 9-11.

17. Hayward, A.C., and Fegan, M. 2001. Epidemiology detection and control of brown rot of potato in temperate regions. Pages 171-173 In: Proc. 2nd Australasian Soilborne Diseases Symp., Lorne, Victoria, Australia, 5-8 March, 2001. I.J. Porter *et al.,* eds.

18. Hudelson, B.D. 1999. Southern wilt. Univ. Wisconsin Garden Facts, May 11, 1999.

19. Hudelson, B.D., Williamson, L., Nakaho, K., and Allen, C. 2002. *R. solanacearum* race 3, biovar 2 strains isolated from geranium are pathogenic on potato. Page 14 in: Book of Abstracts, 3rd Int. Symp. Bacterial Wilt. Nelspruit, S.A., 4-8 February 2002.

20. Jackson, M.T., Gonzalez, L.C., and Aguilar, J.A. 1979. [Advances in controlling bacterial rot of potato in Costa Rica.] Fitopatologia 14: 48-53 (in Spanish).

21. Janse, J.D. 1991. Infra- and intraspecific classification of *Pseudomonas solanacearum* strains, using whole cell fatty analysis. Syst. Appl. Microbiol. 14: 335-345.

22. Janse, J.D. 1996. Potato brown rot in Western Europe – history, present occurrence and some remarks on possible origin, epidemiology and control strategies. Bull. OEPP/EPPO Bull. 26:679-695.

23. Janse, J.D., Arulappan, F.A.X., Schans, J., Wenneker, M., and Westerhuis, W. 1998. Experiences with bacterial brown rot *Ralstonia solanacearum* biovar 2, race 3 in The Netherlands. Pages 146-152 in: Bacterial Wilt Disease: Molecular and Ecological Aspects. P. Prior, C. Allen, and J. Elphinstone, eds. Springer-Verlag, Heidelberg, Germany.

24. Martin, C., and French, E.R. 1995. Covered-field host range test for *Pseudomonas solanacearum* race 3/biovar 2. ACIAR Bacterial Wilt Newsletter 12:9.

25. Martin, C., and Nydegger, U. 1982. Susceptibility of *Cyphomandra betaceae* to *Pseudomonas solanacearum*. Plant Dis. 66: 1025-1027.

26. Melo, M.S., Takatsu, A. 1998. Root colonization of non-susceptible hosts by *Ralstonia solanacearum*. In: Book of abstracts. 2nd Intern.

Bacterial Wilt Symposium, 22-27 June 1997, Guadeloupe, France. France: INRA.

27. Moraes, A. de M. 1947. [A bacterial wilt of potato due to *Bacterium solanacearum*.] Agron. Lusetania 9:277-328.

28. Nameth, S. 1999. Bacterial disease alert in geraniums. FlowerTECH 2(4):65-67.

29. Olsson, K. 1976a. Experience of brown rot caused by *Pseudomonas solanacearum* (Smith) Smith in Sweden. Bull. OEPP/EPPO Bull. 6: 199-207.

30. Olsson, K. 1976b. Overwintering of *Pseudomonas solanacearum* in Sweden. Pages 105-109 in: Int. Planning Conference and Workshop on the ecology and control of bacterial wilt caused by *Pseudomonas solanacearum*. L. Sequeira and A. Kelman, eds. North Carolina State University, Raleigh, USA.

31. Pittman, H.A. 1933. Bacterial wilt of tomatoes and other Solanaceous crops. West. Austral. Dept. Agr. J. (II)10: 373-374.

32. Pradhanang, P.M., Elphinstone, J.G., 1996. Identification of weed and crop hosts of *Pseudomonas solanacearum* race 3 in the hills of Nepal. Pages 39-49 in: Integrated management of bacterial wilt of potato: Lessons from the hills of Nepal. Proc. of a national workshop held at Lumle Agric. Res. Centre, Pokhara, Nepal, 4-5 November 1996. P.M. Pradhanang and J.G. Elphinstone, eds.

33. Pradhanang, P.M., Elphinstone, J.G., and Fox, R.T.V. 2000. Identification ofcrop and weed hosts of *Ralstonia solanacearum* biovar 2 in the hills of Nepal. Plant Pathol. 49: 403-413

34. Rademaker, J.L.W, and De Bruijn, F.J. 1997. Characterization and classification of microbes by rep-PCR genomic fingerprinting and computer assisted pattern analysis. Pages 151-171 in: DNA markers: Protocols, Applications and Overviews. Chapter 10. G. Caetano-Anollés and P.M. Gresshoff, eds. J. Wiley & Sons, New York (USA).

35. Seal, S.E., Jackson, L.A., Young, J.P.W., and Daniels, M.J. 1993. Detection of *Pseudomonas solanacearum*, *Pseudomonas syzygii*,, *Pseudomonas pickettii*, and Blood Disease Bacterium by partial 16S rRNA sequencing: construction of oligonucleotide primers for sensitive detection by polymerase chain reaction. J. Gen. Microbiol. 139: 1587-1594.

36. Singh, B. 1992. Rapeseed, mustard and cabbage new hosts for *Pseudomonas solanacearum*. Indian Phytopath. 45: 277.

37. Smith, J.J., Offord, L.C., Kibata, G.N., Murimi, Z.K., Trigalet, A., and Saddler, G.S. 1998. The development of a biological control agent against *Ralstonia solanacearum* race 3 in Kenya. Pages 337-342 in: Bacterial Wilt Disease: Molecular and Ecological Aspects. P. Prior, C. Allen, and J. Elphinstone, eds. Springer-Verlag, Heidelberg, Germany.

38. Smith, T.E. 1939. Host range studies with *Bacterium solanacearum*. J. Agric. Res. 6:429-440.
39. Strider, D.L., Jones, R.K., and Haygood, R.A. 1981. Southern bacterial wilt of geranium caused by *Pseudomonas solanacearum*. Plant Dis. 65: 52-53.
40. Swanepoel, A.E. 1992. Survival of South African strains of biovar 2 and biovar 3 of *Pseudomonas solanacearum* in the roots and stems of weeds. Potato Res. 35: 329-332.
41. Tomlinson, D.L., and Gunther, M.T., 1986. Bacterial wilt in Papua New Guinea. Pages 35-39 in: Bacterial wilt disease in Asia and the South Pacific. Proceedings of an International Workshop held at PCARRD, Los Baños, Philippines, 8-10 October 1985. G.J. Persley, ed. Canberra, ACIAR Proceedings 13.
42. Valdez, R.B. 1986. Bacterial wilt in the Philippines. Pages 49-56 in: Bacterial wilt disease in Asia and the South Pacific. Proceedings of an International Workshop held at PCARRD, Los Baños, Philippines, 8-10 October 1985. G.J. Persley, ed. Canberra, ACIAR Proceedings 13.
43. Vos, P., Hogers, R., Bleeker, M., Reijans, M., van de Lee, T., Hornes, M., Frijters, A., Pot, J., Peleman, J., Kuiper, M., and Zabeau, M. 1995. AFLP: a new technique for DNA fingerprinting. Nucleic Acids Res. 23: 4407-4414.
44. Williamson, L., Hudelson, B., Nakaho, K., and Allen, C. 2002. *Ralstonia solanacearum* race 3, biovar 2 strains isolated from geranium are pathogenic on Potato. Plant Dis. 86: 987-991
45. Wallace, G.B. 1934. Report of the mycologist for 1934. Tanganyika Dept. Agr. Ann. Rpt. For 1934: 90-93.
46. Weller, S.A., Elphinstone, J.G., Smith, N., Stead, D.E., and Boonham, N. 1999. Detection of *Ralstonia solanacearum* strains using an automated and quantitative fluorogenic 5' nuclease TaqMan assay. Appl. Environ. Microbiol. 66; 2853-2858.
47. Wenneker, M., Verdel, M.S.W., Groeneveld, R.M.W., Kempenaar, C., van Beuningen, A.R., and Janse, J.D. *Ralstonia (Pseudomonas) solanacearum* race 3 (biovar 2) in surface water and natural weed hosts: First report on stinging nettle (*Urtica dioica*). Eur. J. Plant Pathol. 105: 307-315.
48. Zambrano, B.Y.P. 1990. [Identification de hospedantes natives e introducidos de Pseudomonas solanacearum E.F. Smith en el Peru]. MSc thesis, Peru: Universidad Nacional Agraria La Molina.

Seeds from Infected Tomato Plants Appear to be Free from Contamination by *Ralstonia solanacearum* When Tested by PCR or Microbiological Assays

O.M. Martins, F. Nabizadeh-Ardekani, and K. Rudolph

Institute of Plant Pathology and Plant Protection, Georg-August University, Grisebachstrasse 6, 37077 Göttingen, Germany.
Current address of first author: EMBRAPA Clima Temperado, Cx. Postal 403, 96001-970 Pelotas, RS, Brazil.

Throughout the tropics and subtropics, tomatoes (*Lycopersicon esculentum* Mill.) are an important cultivated species in the field or under plastic. Both crop systems are subject to bacterial wilt caused by *Ralstonia solanacearum*, which constitutes a major limitation of production. For many phytobacterial pathogens, contaminated seed is a source of primary inoculum and pathogen dissemination. Although it is not considered a major route of transmission, there have been occasional reports of bacterial wilt transmission by seeds, through both natural contamination (groundnut) (7,8) and artificial contamination (capsicum, tomato) (14,19).

Seed assays for bacterial contamination involve soaking seeds in liquid for varying times and plating dilutions of liquid samples onto semi-selective agar media (15). With the advent of molecular biology, a new approach for diagnosis of bacterial diseases became feasible. Because *R. solanacearum* also causes serious losses in potato production worldwide, several sensitive detection methods have been developed (2,4,5,11). The polymerase chain reaction (PCR) has enabled the development of highly sensitive and accurate methods for detection of seedborne bacteria (13) and offers a powerful molecular technique for the selective amplification of *R. solanacearum* 16S rRNA sequences (2,11,17). For instance, a sensitive method known as Bio-PCR combines semi-selective media with serological tests, and also with PCR (2,5,6,9,11,12, 16,18). However, it has rarely been applied to detect *R. solanacearum* in tomato plants or seeds. Therefore, we evaluated a laboratory method for sensitive and reliable detection of *R. solanacearum* in plastic and field-grown tomatoes.

Material and Methods

Microbiological assays. Tomato plants 'Ontario 7710' were grown in the greenhouse (11-37°C) and inoculated at the size of four expanded true leaves. *R. solanacearum* biovars 1 and 3 were stem inoculated using an entomological needle inserted diagonally at the axil of the first true leaf, and depositing 10 µl of bacterial suspension (10^8 CFU/ml) with a pipette tip. Mature tomato plants were inoculated before and after flowering, and during fruit ripening with an inoculum concentration reduced to 10^6 CFU/ml to slow symptom development. Inoculum was deposited at the wounded axil of four different true leaves in the upper portion of the plants. Seed homogenates were prepared by soaking overnight in 0.01% Tween 20 (16). Aliquots (100 µl) were plated on the modified semi-selective SMSA medium (2,3) to check for the presence of viable cells. Additional aliquots were kept at $-20°$C and further tested by direct PCR. A bacterial suspension (10^8 CFU/ml) was added to seeds extracted from healthy control plants, and macerated. Homogenates were diluted 10-fold. Leaves, roots, stems, sepals, petals and fruits were weighed and homogenized by grinding in a mortar with the addition of TE buffer, pH 7.6, 1:4 (w/v). Bacterial populations were then enumerated after 48 h growth at $28°$C.

PCR amplification. The following PCR protocol was adapted from Nabizadech-Ardekani (10): 50-µl reaction mixture containing 0.2 mM of each dNTP, 1% (v/v) BSA (20 mg/ml), 0.01 mM 2-mercaptoethanol, 0.7 mM DMSO, 1% (v/v) Tween 20, 0.9 mM magnesium choride, 10% (v/v) 10 x PCR buffer (100 mM Tris-HCl pH 8.8 at $25°$C, 500 mM KCl, 0.8% Nonidet P40), 23.2 µl of bacterial suspension of each serial dilution as template DNA and 1 µM of each primer. Primers OLI 1 and Y2 (17) for amplification of the 16S rRNA region were synthesized by NAPS, Göttingen, Germany. The enzyme (4 U/µl) was diluted 1:10.5 (v/v) in 1 x PCR buffer separately from the master mix. The contents of each PCR tube were overlaid with 50 µl of sterile mineral oil. Negative as well as positive controls were designed to check the reaction. Amplifications were performed in a thermal cycler (Hybaid-OmniGene, Heidelberg, Germany) by programming a two step PCR made of a hot start PCR procedure followed by PCR cycling. At the first cycle template DNA were submitted to a 94°C-denaturing for 2 min followed by $85°$C for 8 min, in which 0.7 U *Taq* DNA polymerase was added to each reaction, with subsequent annealing at $59°$C for 2 min and extension at $72°$C for 30 s. The second stage was 36 cycles of denaturing at $94°$C for 1 min, and annealing and extension as described for the first stage. PCR products were resolved in 1.8% NEEO Ultra-Quality agarose gel in 0.5X TBE buffer.

Table 1. Concentration of *Ralstonia solanacearum* (CFU/ml) in different dilutions from tomato plant homogenates determined on the semi-selective SMSA medium

Samples	Undil	10^{-1}	10^{-2}	10^{-3}	10^{-4}	10^{-5}	10^{-6}	10^{-7}
Leaves	a	a	a	a	a	1.9×10^3	2.2×10^2	-
Roots	a	a	a	a	a	a	1.3×10^3	1.2×10^2
Sepals	a	a	a	a	a	5.8×10^2	1.1×10^2	-
Stems	a	a	a	a	a	a	2.4×10^3	1.6×10^2
Fruits	-	-	-	-	-	-	-	-
Petals	-	-	-	-	-	-	-	-
Seeds	-	-	-	-	-	-	-	-

[a] Uncountable colonies; - No bands were generated.

Results

PCR with primers OLI1 and Y2 yielded a single DNA fragment of approximately 288 bp (Figs. 1 and 2). These primers amplified products directly from plant homogenates in TE buffer. The sensitivity of the PCR technique was determined by assaying 10-fold dilution series of tomato tissue homogenates (Table 1). Detection limits for infected tomato tissue homogenates by the PCR assays were 2.2×10^2 /leaves, 1.2×10^2 /roots, 1.6×10^2 /stems and 1.1×10^2 CFU/ml /sepals (Fig. 2). No PCR product was generated from seeds, fruits or petals sampled from infected tomato plants. Microbiological assays revealed that these plant organs contained no detectable bacteria (Table 1). There were strong PCR inhibitors in raw homogenates as well as in the first dilution (1:10), so that no bands were visualized (Fig. 2, lanes 3 and 4). This effect was present in homogenates of tomato leaves, roots, sepals and stems, and also from spiked seeds (Fig. 1, lane 8).

Discussion

PCR assays have been used successfully to detect *R. solanacearum* in several instances (Poussier, this volume, 11) allowing detection of as few as 10^2 CFU/ml from homogenized tomato leaves, roots, stems and sepals. These results are far from those reported previously (17). Using the same primer pair, Seal *et al.* (17) could detect 1-10 cells after 50 cycles of amplification. Using the same primers, the standard PCR method lacked sensitivity for detecting *R. solanacearum* in potato tubers (2). Sensitivity increased 10-fold when Elphinstone *et al.* (2) used an enrichment procedure in SMSA broth medium and by boiling the tuber homogenates with 0.05 M NaOH prior to PCR. There were no inhibitory compounds in a 1:10 dilution of

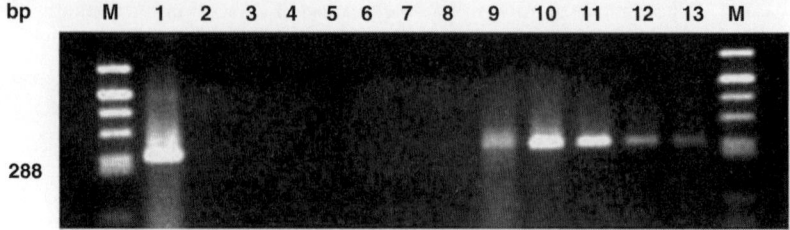

Fig. 1. Detection of *Ralstonia solanacearum* in tomato seeds by the PCR technique. M, shows the size of *Alu*I-digested pBR322 DNA marker in bp; lane 1, DNA control; lane 2, negative control; lanes 3 to 7, no DNA amplifications for seed samples from severely wilted tomato plants; lane 8, no DNA amplification for aliquot of undiluted bacterial suspension + healthy tomato seeds; lanes 9 to 13, positive signals for 10-fold serial dilutions (10^{-1} to 10^{-5}) from healthy seeds + bacterial suspension.

healthy tomato seeds macerated together with a bacterial suspension. However, inhibitory substances occurred in undiluted and 1:10 diluted homogenates of tomato plant tissues inoculated artificially. This inhibiting effect could be the result of phenolic compounds, possibly induced by anti-microbial defenses (1). Our results suggest that using spiked samples in PCR assays should be considered with caution, because the potentially in-hibitory compounds may not be expressed in the absence of the pathogen. In other words, the sensitivity of the PCR assay in spiked plant homogen-ates may be better than in infected tissues.

In our experimental conditions the absence of *R. solanacearum* in tomato fruits, petals and seeds from infected tomato plants was confirmed by both plating and PCR assays. Some reports have suggested that the bac-terium may survive and disseminate in tomato seeds (8). Earlier conflicting reports on the occurrence of seed transmission may have resulted from low numbers of bacteria on the seed surface and consequent difficulty in their detection by conventional methods (14). This may also explain the report from Vaughan (19) that apparently healthy tomato seedlings taken from infected seedbeds were responsible for dispersal of this bacterium when planted miles away. Some early evidence indicated that true seed could serve as a means of dispersal of the pathogen in the case of groundnut (*Arachis hypogaea* L.), but there are contradictory reports from Indonesia and the People's Republic of China regarding the occurrence of seed transmission for *R. solanacearum* (7,8).

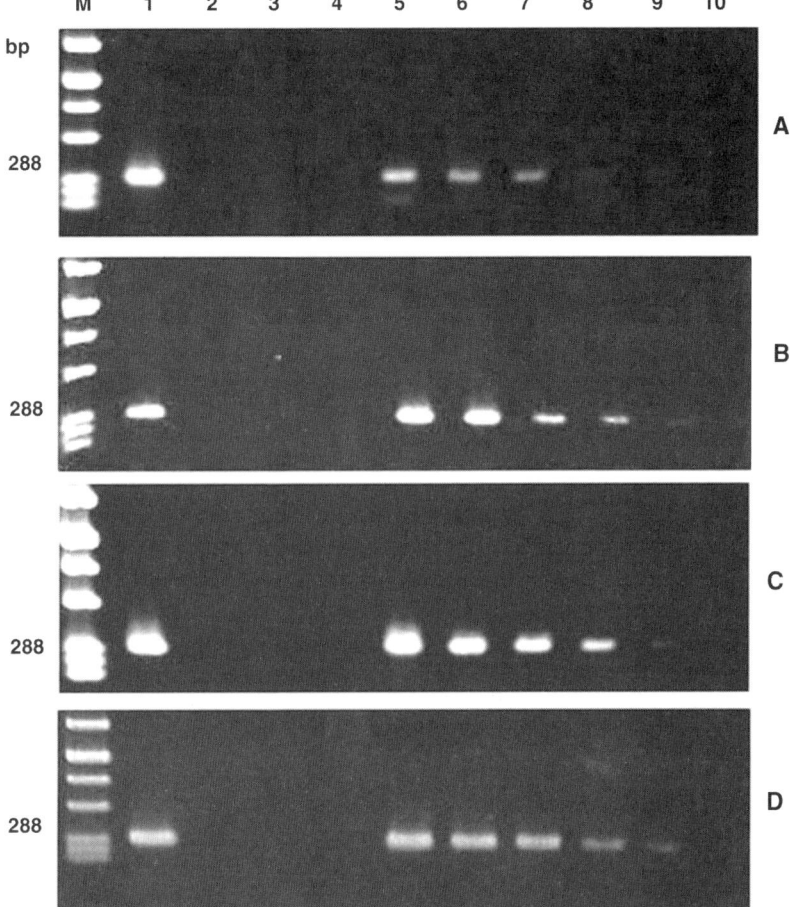

Fig. 2. Detection of *Ralstonia solanacearum* by standard PCR in homogenates from infected tomato plants. The marker (M) shows the size of *Alu*I-digested pBR322 DNA in bp; (1) DNA control; (2) negative control; (3) undiluted homogenate; (4 to 10) serial dilutions. Faint bands were visible for (**A**-9) 2.2 x 10^2 CFU/ml for leaves, (**B**-10) 1.2 x 10^2 CFU/ml for roots, (**C**-10) 1.6 x 10^2 CFU/ml for stems, (**D**-9) 1.1 x 10^2 CFU/ml for sepals. Bacterial concentrations were determined by using the modified semi-selective SMSA medium.

Acknowledgments

Scholarship from EMBRAPA, Brazil, to the first author is gratefully acknowledged. This paper is a portion of the first author's Ph.D. thesis, submitted to the Georg-August University, Göttingen.

Literature Cited

1. Barz, W. 1997. Phytoalexins. Pages 183-201 in: Resistance of Crop Plants against Fungi. H. Hartleb, R. Heitefuss, and H.-H. Hoppe, eds. Gustav Fisher Verlag.
2. Elphinstone, J.G., Hennessy, J., Wilson, J.K., and Stead, D.E. 1996. Sensitivity of different methods for the detection of *Ralstonia solanacearum* in potato tuber extracts. Bull. OEPP/EPPO Bull. 26:663-678.
3. Engelbrecht, M.C. 1994. Modification of a semi-selective medium for the isolation and quantification of *Pseudomonas solanacearum*. Bact. Wilt Newsl.10: 3-5.
4. Griep, R.A., van Twisk, C., van Beckhoven, J.R.C.M., van der Wolf, J.M., and Schots, A. 1998. Development of specific recombinant monoclonal antibodies against the lipopolysaccharide of *Ralstonia solanacearum* race 3. Phytopathology 88: 795-803.
5. International Potato Center (CIP). 1998. CIP NCM-ELISA kit for the detection of *Ralstonia solanacearum* in latently infected potato tubers - user manual. 21 pp.
6. Ito, S., Ushijima, Y., Fujii, T., Tanaka, S., Kameya-Iwaki, M., Yoshiwara, S., and Kishi, F. 1998. Detection of viable cells of *Ralstonia solanacearum* in soil using a semiselective medium and a PCR technique. J. Phytopathol. 146:379-384.
7. Kelman, A. 1953. The bacterial wilt caused by *Pseudomonas solanacearum*. N. C. Agric. Exp. St. Tec. Bull. 99.
8. Kelman, A., Hartman, G.L., and Hayward, A.C. 1994. Introduction. Pages 1-7 in: Bacterial Wilt: The Disease and its Causative Agent, *Pseudomonas solanacearum*. A.C. Hayward and G.L. Hartman, eds. CAB International.
9. Martins, O. M. 2000. Polymerase chain reaction in the diagnosis of bacterial wilt, caused by *Ralstonia solanacearum* (Smith) Yabuuchi *et al.*, Ph. D. Thesis, Georg-August University, Göttingen, Germany, 127 pp.
10. Nabizadeh-Ardekani, F. 1999. Nachweis bakterieller Krankheiten der Tomate durch die Polymerase-Kettenreaktion oder serologische Methoden und Bestimmung des Rassenspektrums von *Pseudomonas*

syringae pv. *tomato* in der Türkei. Ph. D. Thesis, Georg-August University, Göttingen, Germany, 118 pp.

11. Pradhanang, P.M., Elphinstone, J.G., and Fox, T.V. 2000. Sensitive detection of *Ralstonia solanacearum* in soil: a comparison of different detection techniques. Plant Pathol. 49:414-422.

12. Priou, S., Gutarra, L., Fernandez, H., and Aley, P. 1999. Sensitive detection of *Ralstonia solanacearum* (race 3) in soil by post-enrichment DAS-ELISA. Bact. Wilt Newsl. 16: 10-13.

13. Prosen, D., Hatziloukas, E., Schaad, N.W., and Panopoulos, N.J. 1993. Specific detection of *Pseudomonas syringae* pv. *phaseolicola* DNA in bean seed by polymerase chain reaction-based amplification of a phaseolotoxin gene region. Phytopathology 83:965-970.

14. Santos, M.S. 1997. The recurrence of *Burkholderia solanacearum* in Southern European countries. Pages 27-34 in: Seed Healthy Testing-Progress Towards the 21st Century. J.D. Hutchins and J.C. Reeves, eds. CAB International.

15. Schaad, N.W. 1982. Detection of seedborne bacterial plant pathogens. Plant Dis. 66:885-890.

16. Schaad, N.W., Cheong, S.S., Tamaki, S., Hatziloukas, E., and Panopoulos, N.J. 1995. A combined biological and enzymatic amplification (BIO-PCR) technique to detect *Pseudomonas syringae* pv. *phaseolicola* in bean seed extracts. Phytopathology 85:243-248.

17. Seal, S.E., Jackson. L.A., Young, J.P.W., and Daniels, M.J. 1993. Differentiation of *Pseudomonas solanacearum, Pseudomonas syzygii, Pseudomonas pickettii* and the blood disease bacterium by partial 16S rRNA sequencing: construction of oligonucleoide primers for sensitive detection by polymerase chain reaction. J. Gen. Microbiol. 139:1587-1594.

18. Van der Wolf, J.M., Van Bekkum, P.J., Van Elsas, J.D., Nijhuis, E.H., Vriend, S.G.C., and Ruissen, M.A. 1998. Immunofluorescence colony staining and selective enrichment in liquid medium for studying the population dynamics of *Ralstonia solanacearum* (race 3) in soil. Bull. OEPP/EPPO Bull. 28:71-79.

19. Vaughan, E.K. 1944. Bacterial wilt of tomato caused by *Phytomonas solanacearum*. Phytopathology 3:443-458.

The Viable but Non-culturable State in *Ralstonia solanacearum*: Is There a Realistic Threat to Our Strategic Concepts?

J.D. Van Elsas[1], L.S. Van Overbeek[1], and A. Trigalet[2]

[1] Plant Research International, Wageningen, The Netherlands;
[2] INRA/CNRS, Toulouse, France

About 20 years ago, Colwell and co-workers (8) postulated from their work with Gram-negative pathogens like *Escherichia coli* and *Vibrio cholerae* that these organisms might convert into cellular forms that were not (easily) culturable on plates, yet fully viable by a range of other metabolic criteria (32,47). They called this form the viable but non-culturable (VBNC) form. Moreover, in later work they indicated that a cellular population in the VBNC form is able to revert to fully culturable and aggressive forms after passage through the intestinal tract of susceptible host organisms (8, 32). Cells not able to grow directly on plates had, in fact, already been found long before in *E. coli* cultures, but their potential to be revived remained unexplored (14). The VBNC state was also found to occur in a wide range of other Gram-negative bacteria of hygienic importance: *Shigella dysenteriae* (13), *Salmonella typhimurium* (38), *S. enteritidis* (31), *Campylobacter jejuni* (15,29,30) and *Vibrio vulnificus* (45). The VBNC state has also been described in saprophytic, plant pathogenic and symbiotic bacteria, namely *Pseudomonas fluorescens* (5,22), *Agrobacterium tumefaciens* and *Rhizobium meliloti* (21), *R. leguminosarum* (1), *Xanthomonas campestris* pv *campestris* (10), and *Ralstonia solanacearum* (11,39,40). These observations indicate the wide distribution of the VBNC phenomenon among the Gram-negative bacteria. In fact, the VBNC form has been considered to represent some type of resting (spore or cyst-like) survival form that occurs in the non-differentiating bacteria (17,32), including Gram-negatives.

There has been fierce debate in the literature about the significance of VBNC forms and, in particular, the potential of such cells to revert to fully culturable forms (6,9,26,27). On the one hand, Bogosian et al (6) provided evidence that several strains of enteric bacteria including *E. coli*, in fact, merely entered a "pseudo"-VBNC state, defined as dead cells possessing residual enzymatic activity. This inference was made on the basis of the observation that resuscitation of VBNC cells could never have been shown, but that, instead, re-growth of a few culturable cells was involved in the putative resuscitation process. On the other hand, Oliver and co-workers (28), using extensive experimentation based on dilution series, showed that *V. vulnificus* VBNC cells were indeed able to revert to fully culturable organisms (27,28).

In order to meaningfully address the culturability versus viability issue, it is necessary to establish working definitions of the terms that are in place to describe the different physiological states of cells. We propose the use of definitions as in Table 1. Barer and Harwood (2) recently reviewed the viability versus culturability conundrum and suggested a number of plausible hypotheses to explain the VBNC status and the experimental findings with respect to resuscitation. First, they suggested that the VBNC form represented cells injured by stress, in particular as a result of the accumulation of reactive oxygen species, leading to damage to essential components of the cell. Second, cells might have lost their ability to grow or form colonies on

Table 1. Definition of terms according to Barer and Harwood (2)

Term	Definition
Culturable cell	Cell fully capable of growing (forming colonies on plates or dividing in liquid media) on selective or nonselective growth media
Viable cell	Cell able to maintain an energized membrane, to metabolize and to show the ability to respond to substrates; in principle viable cells maintain the capacity to divide
Dormant cell	Cell with drastically lowered metabolic activity; a physiological state which is reversible
Resting cell	Cell in non-growth (growth-arrested) stage
Dead cell	Cell with a non-energized membrane
Ghost cell	Cell with undetectable, or highly condensed, genome
Resuscitation	Transition from a state of non-culturability to one of culturability
Re-growth	Growth of a very small subpopulation of cells in a grossly VBNC population which leads to a larger population of fully culturable cells
Cryptic growth	Growth of a subpopulation of culturable cells in a population which cannot be measured by the techniques applied.

plates as a result of the lack of an essential factor which normally occurs when cells grow together (quorum-sensing-like). Third, there might be involvement of chromosomal suicide (*hok/sok* like) systems, and the lack of growth on plates might be linked to a imbalance in the levels of these toxins and antitoxins

Barer and Harwood (2), to avoid possible confusion between the terms culturable and viable, also proposed to rename the VBNC state to NIC, which stands for "not immediately culturable". For the purpose of this discussion, and in conformity with most of the literature, we prefer to stick to the use of the acronym VBNC.

In this chapter, we will discuss the current understanding of the VBNC status of *R. solanacearum,* with an emphasis on the experimental findings, the implications for practice and the potential strategies needed to further our understanding of this phenomenon.

Factors Inducing the VBNC Form in Bacteria

A range of factors that affect cellular growth, such as carbon starvation or limitation, extreme temperature, low water activity, oxygen depletion and the presence of noxious compounds, have been reported to trigger the VBNC state in Gram-negative bacterial cells (2,27). These conditions are common in most natural habitats like soil, water and at the surface of plants. It is, therefore, not surprising that most cells of non-differentiating bacterial species will rapidly become non-culturable when entering such environments. For instance, high levels of unculturable *P. fluorescens* cells were observed when exponentially-growing cells were introduced into two different soils (42). Although soil type affected the appearance of such cells, the adaptation to soil conditions was similar in both soils, as shown by exposure of cells to different stressors following their extraction from soil (41). Different conditions in the soil might have been responsible for the conversion of cells to unculturable forms. Mascher et al (22) later found, from *in vitro* experiments, that factors such as low redox potential, oxygen limitation and high NaCl levels could trigger the conversion of *P. fluorescens* cells to VBNC forms. In the following, we will briefly discuss the single factors that most likely induce the VBNC status in bacteria.

CARBON STARVATION

Induction of a carbon-limitation-responsive reporter gene in *P. fluorescens* R2f in soil indicated that carbon limitation was indeed a factor that affected the adaptation of this strain to soil conditions (42). A theoretical framework was postulated, in which the introduced *P. fluorescens* strain adapts, in different phases, to the conditions present in soil. During this process, cells would become progressively more resistant to different stressors and cellular morphology changes from the rod shape to small circular forms. Moreover, cells become less responsive to favorable circumstances like an adequate supply of nutrients and can thus turn into the VBNC state. However, it is doubtful that carbon limitation alone can trigger the conversion of *P. fluorescens* cells to VBNC forms, as the organism can survive long periods of time in, for instance, sterile carbon-deprived water. Hence, it is likely that the trigger lies in the combination of carbon starvation with some as-yet-undefined soil factor, which could well be osmotic or oxygen stress (22). Carbon starvation can also trigger the VBNC response in other organisms. For instance, *Listeria monocytogenes* VBNC cells were obtained by exposure to carbon deprivation, and then recovered from nonculturability in a DNA gyrase independent fashion (3).

COPPER

A key condition leading to VBNC cells in different bacterial species is enhanced copper ($CuSO_4$) concentration. *A. tumefaciens*, *R. leguminosarum* and *X. campestris* cells converted to the VBNC form at copper concentrations between 0.005 and 0.05 mM (1,10) and *E. coli* from 6 mM up (11). Although the VBNC status was, thus, triggered in taxonomically different groups of bacteria, the conditions for reaching this status differed by species or strain. The differences in copper concentrations needed may have been affected by the medium in which the cells were suspended. Moreover, not all bacterial species respond similarly to copper, which may be due to different intracellular mechanisms for coping with copper stress. This factor may be significant for *R. solanacearum,* as copper compounds are sometimes used to control bacterial plant diseases.

LOW TEMPERATURE

Low temperature, which is highly relevant under natural circumstances in many ecosystems, can stimulate bacterial cells to become VBNC (26,27). *V. vulnificus* cells were shown to become unculturable during incubation at temperatures below 15°C (27,28). Recovery from the VBNC status was observed after a temperature upshift (28,46). Moreover, *Aeromonas hydrophilia* cells reached the unculturable stage after exposure to 4°C, but colonies were again recoverable by plating onto media containing catalase or pyruvate. The data suggested that relief from oxidative stress was a prerequisite for the recovery of cells from the VBNC form. Most importantly, the finding that VBNC cells, e.g., of *V. vulnificus,* could thus be resuscitated by simple temperature increases has great impact on considerations of the potential risks to health posed by the aquatic systems in which these bacteria dwell.

HIGH OSMOLARITY OR LOW WATER ACTIVITY

Low water activity can be brought about by high solute concentrations or desiccation at surfaces, which are key processes in soil, at plant surfaces, but also in water systems. Bacterial cells exposed to low water activity will suffer from water deprivation which can result in a state of nonculturability (27). Different, successive, stages in cell physiology were observed in *S. typhimurium* cells following starvation in artificial seawater. Culturability, substrate responsiveness, respiratory activity, cytoplasmic permeability and cellular DNA content were measured (16). In total, six successive physiological states were defined, as follows: (i) culturable cells, (ii) unculturable cells with respiration activity, (iii) cells with respiratory activity, (iv) cells without respiration but possessing intact membranes, (v) cells that had lost membrane integrity, but with intact genomes, and (vi) cells which had partly or completely lost their genomes ("non-nucleoid" or "ghost" cells). Cells which lost their cytoplasmic membrane or genome integrity were considered to be non-recoverable from these stages and, thus, dying or dead. The different physiological states identified in the *S. typhimurium* cells covered the whole spectrum, from dividing and VNBC cells to dead cells. *E. coli* cells in the VBNC state resulting from exposure to saline, were retrieved from nonculturablity when the stress was relieved (25). Recovery from nonculturability was independent from DNA gyrase activity, indicating that these cells had truly been resuscitated and had not been recovered as a result of the outgrowth of a small subpopulation of culturable cells.

Moreover, *S. typhimurium* cells exposed to desiccation on solid surfaces lost both their culturability and their virulence (20). Genomic integrity was lost in some of the stressed cells, as determined by DAPI staining. This, in fact, indicated that this subpopulation represented ghost cells. The appearance of such ghosts may be a common phenomenon in prokaryotes, as these forms were also observed in marine bacterial populations (48), in *E. coli* introduced into river water (23) and in *V. vulnificus* upon starvation (44). *P. fluorescens* cells introduced into the rhizosphere of wheat presumably also turned largely into ghost forms, as evidenced by the absence of a PCR signal with targets from an abundant population of immunofluorescence-detectable cells (42). The terms ghost (or non- nucleoid) cells for cells devoid of any detectable DNA may be confusing, as it has never been confirmed whether these cells really lost their DNA or preserved it in a highly condensed form inaccessible to stains or replicating enzymes (2,44; see Table 1). Even though cell death may be inferred from the apparent absence of intact genomes in ghost cells, statements about the absence of revival and pathogenicity should be made with extreme care.

LOW OXYGEN TENSION

Low oxygen tension is a common condition in water and soil habitats. Reduced oxygen combined with low redox potential has been reported to induce VBNC forms in *Pseudomonas fluorescens* cells (22). The authors suggested that this combination of factors explained abundant *P. fluorescens* VBNC cells in waterlogged soil layers. Toffanin *et al.* (37) also showed that cells of other soil bacteria, *Sinorhizobium meliloti* and *Rhizobium "hedysari"*, converted into VBNC forms following exposure to low oxygen conditions coupled to low energy conditions. The presence of nitrogen oxides played a role in this conversion for the latter strain. The unifying concept in these findings is that in the absence of oxygen, cellular energy reserves were depleted, resulting in an enhanced conversion of cells to the VBNC state.

ROLE OF CYTOKINES

A possible role for small secreted molecules in controlling the cellular state and growth response of bacterial populations should also be considered (2). Circumstantial evidence suggests dependence of bacterial cells on specific compounds for the onset of growth, since a 17-kD protein in *Micrococcus luteus* was needed to induce *M. luteus* VBNC cells to growth (24). A cytokine-like factor has also been isolated and characterized from *Mycobacterium tuberculosis* and other high-G+C% Gram-positive bacteria (4). This compound, called the "resuscitation-promoting factor" (Rpf) controls the transition from unculturable to culturable forms of *M. tuberculosis*. This phenomenon is crucial and has large implications for the pathogenicity of this species after colonization of animal and human tissue (4). Although a proteinaceous factor like Rpf has not been found in Gram-negatives so far, similar or other factors, like those interfering with bacterial quorum sensing mechanisms, may play a role in the conversion of VBNC cells to culturability.

Factors Influencing the VBNC Form in *R. solanacearum*

Grey and Steck (11) recently indicated that large parts of a *R. solanacearum* cell population convert to VBNC forms after only 3 days in a sterilized soil system. They compared direct microscopic cell counts with counts obtained by plating (19) as well as the Live/Dead stain (Molecular

Probes, Oregon, USA). No clear explanation was given for the factors in soil that triggered this response, but any of the conditions known to influence the survival of bacteria, such as carbon availability, soil moisture, soil temperature, soil pH, and oxygen availability might have been involved. Toxic compounds released by soil autoclaving may have been involved. In addition to the conversion to the VBNC form in soil, the authors also provided evidence that *R. solanacearum* progressively turns VBNC *in planta*, concurrent with plant infestation. After 60 days, up to 99% of detectable cells were in the VBNC state (11). Unfortunately, no information on the plant factors that induce the conversion to VBNC forms was provided. In the following, we briefly discuss what is known about the single factors that trigger the conversion of *R. solanacearum* cells to VBNC forms.

CARBON STARVATION

Carbon starvation by itself is not likely to induce the VBNC status in *R. solanacearum*, as this organism is an excellent scavenger of scarce nutrients (40,43). When low numbers of *R. solanacearum* race 3 biovar 2 cells were introduced into water without added nutrients, growth ensued. This growth response could be repeated upon serial transfers to new lots of pure water, indicating the avidity of the organism to growth under conditions of extremely low nutrient (carbon/energy) supply. Bacterial survival in the pure water was also very good and cells remained mostly virulent. It is common practice in most laboratories to keep stocks of *R. solanacearum* in pure water. Moreover, upon long-term storage of *R. solanacearum* biovar 2 cells in pure water at room temperature, we have never observed the appearance of substantial numbers of VBNC cells (Van Elsas, unpublished). Thus, carbon limitation alone does not seem to be sufficient to trigger the conversion of *R. solanacearum* cells to VBNC forms.

COPPER

R. solanacearum strain AW1 showed an enhanced prevalence of VBNC cells in saline upon treatment with 0.005 mM and higher levels of $CuSO_4$ (11). At 0.05 mM, no CFU were recovered after 18 days of incubation. Also, the conversion of *R. solanacearum* cells to VBNC forms seemed to be accelerated in sterile soil (11). However, the conditions needed for reaching this state may differ by strain. For instance, *R. solanacearum* biovar 2 strain 1609 resisted copper concentrations of up to 25 mM for over 3 weeks (Van Overbeek, unpublished). Thus, exposure of *R. solanacearum* cells to a chemical trigger like copper can result in their conversion to

VBNC cells, but the level of the compound at which this conversion takes place and its progression, is probably strain-dependent.

LOW TEMPERATURE

Low temperature is an important factor that triggers the conversion of *R.. solanacearum* cells to the VBNC form. Recently, *R. solanacearum* biovar 2 was experimentally shown to become unculturable in two different soils during incubation at 4°C (39). Later, this observation was extended to water systems (40). As a criterion to define VBNC cells, we used: those cells unable to form colonies on commonly used agar plates, but still able to respond to the substrate - yeast extract – used in the DVC method (19) as well as maintain an energized membrane, as demonstrated by their ability to reduce the redox indicator 5-cyano-2,3-ditolyl tetrazolium chloride (CTC) (12). By these criteria, a high percentage of the unculturable cells induced by low temperature were, indeed, found to be in the VBNC form.

Although the conversion of *R. solanacearum* biovar 2 cells to VBNC forms at 4°C has, thus, been firmly established, we do not yet have data that fully explain the significance of this phenomenon. For instance, with the exception of the induction of *aphC*, we do not understand the molecular or physiological mechanisms that underpin the conversion. We speculate that due to some kind of interference with normal cellular metabolism, cells become progressively injured, leading to an impediment of their growth on common culture media.

LOW WATER ACTIVITY

R. solanacearum biovar 2 strain 1609 was affected in its survival upon incubation in water containing 100 mM NaCl, 10 mM CaCl$_2$ and 3.3 mM MgSO$_4$ (40). The concentrations of these salts were representative for sea-water and indicated that *R. solanacearum* cells are stressed by exposure to low water activity. However, in this study, we did not rigorously demonstrate the occurrence of VBNC forms. Van der Wolf (unpublished) showed the presence on metal surfaces of unculturable cells of *R. solanacearum* biovar 2 which were still stainable with SYTO9, the fluorescent compound of the Live/Dead stain used to discriminate viable cells. Desiccation on surfaces, thus, induces the VBNC state in *R. solanacearum* biovar 2. The presence of *R. solanacearum* VBNC cells in sterilized soil discussed in the foregoing (11) may also have been related to low water activity, which may have occurred locally in the soil used.

We have not been able to convert low-temperature-induced VBNC cells back to the fully culturable state simply by raising the temperature back to the original one - 20°C - (van Overbeek, unpublished), and this information is at present puzzling. In addition, addition of pyruvate or catalase to the growth medium did not facilitate this reversion. Since *R. solanacearum* VBNC cells may need specific plant-released compounds for their conversion, we also tested the effects of young tomato plants. Low-temperature-induced *R. solanacearum* biovar 2 strain 1609 VBNC cells could, indeed, infect tomato plants, although this did not lead to clear wilting (van Overbeek, unpublished). About 1% of the *R. solanacearum* cells extracted from infected plants could, again, form colonies on plates. However, none of the colonies tested so far was able to wilt susceptible tomato plants. This observation contrasts with Steck and Grey's finding that soil-induced VBNC cells of *R. solanacearum* were able to infect and wilt tomato plants (11). Research is in progress in our laboratory to further establish the virulence level of the colonies, as well as the factors that potentially triggered the resuscitation in the phytosphere (rhizosphere and/or vascular tissue) of the host plants.

Concept of Adaptation to Stress – Mild Stress Versus Severe Stress

It is plausible that bacteria in natural settings respond differentially to various different types of stress. Barer and Harwood (2) conceptualized the idea of different stressors leading to different outcomes into two broad categories, i.e. effects of mild stress versus those of severe stress. Figure 1 gives a visualization of this simple yet very useful concept. The conjecture here is that under conditions of mild stress, bacteria mount an adaptive response which enables them to trigger their cellular self-defense systems leading to cellular differentiation and adaptation to the stress. In contrast, under conditions of severe stress, the cellular response mechanisms may not be (fully) operational, the result being that cells are injured and turn non-culturable. Potentially, such cells maintain viability in the sense of recoverability and as defined by the working definition above. Cells in this state might be either on their way to cellular death (defined by the loss of membrane, or genomic, integrity, or both) or might be recoverable. The latter category of cells would be defined as "true" VBNC cells.

We propose that this simple concept is used as a working hypothesis to explain the VBNC conversion phenomena seen in *R. solanacearum*. An additional complication in this organism is its sophisticated yet genetically unstable machinery involved in plant pathogenesis. There has been long-standing speculation (see below) that survival forms of *R. solanacearum*, of any kind, may have developed compromised pathogenicity determinants, the nature of which is poorly understood. It is certainly a challenge for future research to attempt to link the mild/severe stress hypothesis to that of the injured pathogenicity traits.

Potential Strategies Needed to Further our Understanding of the VBNC Phenomenon in *R. solanacearum*

To unequivocally demonstrate the reversion from the VBNC status in *R. solanacearum*, a clear-cut distinction between re-growth and resuscitation needs to be made (Table 1). Both phenomena can convert a population of VBNC cells into a fully-grown population consisting largely of culturable cells, yet the two are fundamentally different. Three different approaches can discriminate re-growth from resuscitation: (1) Outdilution of culturable cells within populations that consist mainly of VBNC cells, (2) administration of DNA gyrase inhibitors and (3) separation of cells stained with SYTO9/Propidium Iodide-stained (of the Live/Dead staining kit) by flow cytometry. Rigorous exclusion of the possibility of re-growth is a critical part of sound evidence for reversion.

We further need to increase our knowledge about the gene(s) and subsequent molecular mechanism(s) involved in the entry into the VBNC state, and those potentially involved in resuscitation. As both the open natural environment (soil and water habitats) and the host plant apparently can play important roles, the focus should be on both types of systems. In the open habitats, low temperature may represent a more severe stress factor than the presence of e.g. copper, and we will need to focus on the similarities and differences between the cellular events induced by both types of stressors. In addition, another focus should be on plant-associated factors. Compounds either present in root exudates or within plants may mediate both conversion to, and reversion from, the VBNC state.

The extent to which loss of culturability takes place may relate to the severity (intensity and exposure time; Fig.1) of the stress to which the cells were exposed. Dissecting the molecular mechanisms that are responsible for stress responses is another challenge.

Is There a Link to Phenotypic Conversion?

Phenotypic conversion from the pathogenic, mucoid wild-type form to the non-pathogenic, rough phenotypically-converted (PC) form occurs spontaneously in unshaken liquid medium, suggesting that oxygen

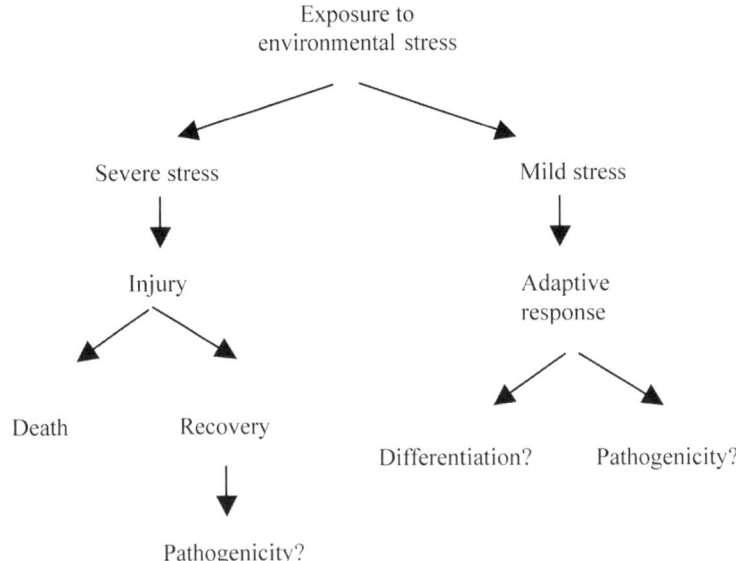

Fig. 1. Adaptation of *Ralstonia solanacearum* after exposure to environmental stress, after Barer and Harwood (2). Cells may differentiate and maintain virulence depending on the intensity of the stress. Interrogation marks indicate gaps in our knowledge.

limitation selects PC mutants due to their motility and positive aerotaxis (18). PC mutants appear spontaneously under prolonged culture on solid media, and can also be isolated from wilted plants or infested soils. This suggests that a variety of potential factors induce the shift (for instance, changes in temperature, pH, salinity, or starvation, UV radiation, plant molecules induced in the interaction with the bacterium, such as reactive oxygen species).

An as-yet unresolved question is whether different stresses, mild or severe, induce both the PC and VBNC forms, or specifically induce either one of these two forms. It is tempting to speculate that there is a link between the two forms, in particular in the light of the shared ecological triggers and (possible) ecological roles. Collaborative work between the authors is in progress to address this question.

Concluding Remarks

From all studies performed so far, *R. solanacearum* biovar 2 appears to be an organism with a remarkable genetic and physiological versatility. In addition to its sophisticated machinery involved in invasion of plant tissue (33,34), it possesses a surprising capacity to grow at very low substrate concentrations, as well as to convert to VBNC cells at low temperature. It is likely that these very divergent behavioral patterns evolved in the light of the multiphasic life strategy that the organism had to develop to successfully compete in its highly divergent habitats. We are looking forward to ecological studies with this organism to be performed with gene arrays exploiting the enormous information from the complete genomic sequence of strain GMI1000, which is now available (33).

However, because hardly anything is known about cellular mechanisms triggering cells to become unculturable (2), it is important to realize that different triggers may evoke different cellular responses that can finally lead to the same physiological condition, that is, the VBNC state. How cells are stressed or triggered may thus have consequences for resuscitation and/ or activation of virulence genes. Cells in natural environments will be provoked by different stress conditions. Therefore, it is expected that different mechanisms, in parallel, can contribute to nonculturability. The relevance of the unculturable or VBNC state for bacteria may be a philosophical question. Different functions have been proposed, ranging from degenerating (sublethally injured) cells (45) to specialized survival entities (27,44).

Is there a realistic challenge to our strategic concepts? Survival of *R. solanacearum* in natural settings has long been debated, and the most logical explanation for the long-term survival of *R. solanacearum* may be its association with plant roots (35). However, it should be stated that the pathogen is released into the environment from the wilted host-plant tissue in the pathogenic, mucoid form, then turned into the non-pathogenic, PC, form in soil or water systems *"where the bacteria survive as microcolonies with relatively low cell densities and slow rates of multiplication"*(7). Depending on whether different mild versus severe stress conditions are encountered in natural settings, the pathogen may turn into PC or VBNC forms, or even other adapted forms (Fig. 1).

Phase reversion from the non-pathogenic PC to the pathogenic wild-type form (Trigalet, this volume), as well as from the VBNC state to a pathogenic form (11) has been reported. The potential role of root exudates in survival of the pathogen may be more than just acting as food supply but could also be envisaged to trigger or to hinder the mechanism(s) by which the PC and/or VBNC forms revert to pathogenic forms. This speculation is worth addressing because the answer could suggest new approaches to control the disease by using simple agricultural practices to decrease the pathogenic form of the pathogen.

However, it is clear that we are only at the beginning of understanding the real ecological significance of the VBNC (as well as the PC) phenomenon in *R. solanacearum*. However, we foresee that, with the advent of bacterial genomics, and in particular the recent description of the full genome of *R. solanacearum* (33), this phenomenon will now be addressed at the very basic level of understanding, that is, at the level of cellular gene expression as a response to the triggers that are known to induce the conversions to VBNC/PC cells.

Acknowledgements

This work was supported by the EU FAIR Program (FATE project, contract no. 3832). We thank all participants to the Discussion session at the Nelspruit bacterial wilt meeting for their comments.

Literature Cited

1. Alexander, E., Pham, D., and Steck, T. 1999. The viable but nonculturable condition is induced by copper in *Agrobacterium tumefaciens* and *Rhizobium leguminosarum*. Appl. Environ. Microbiol. 65: 3754-3756.
2. Barer, M.R., and Harwood, C.R. 1999. Bacterial viability and culturability. Adv. Microb. Physiol. 41: 94-137.
3. Besnard, V., Federighi, M., and Cappelier, J.M. 2000. Development of a direct viable count procedure for the investigation of VBNC state in *Listeria monocytogenes*. Lett. Appl. Microbiol. 31: 77-81.
4. Biketov, S., Mukamolova, G.V., Potapov, V., Gilenkov, E., Vostroknutova, G., Kell, D.B., Young, M., and Kaprelyants, A.S. 2000. Culturability of *Mycobacterium tuberculosis* cells isolated from murine macrophages: a bacterial growth factor promotes recovery. FEMS Immunol. Med. Microbiol. 29: 233-240.
5. Binnerup, S., Jensen, D., Thordal-Christensen, H., and Sorensen, J. 1993. Detection of viable but non-culturable *Pseudomonas fluorescens* DF57 in soil using a microcolony epifluorescence technique. FEMS Microbiol. Ecol. 12: 97-105.
6. Bogosian, G., Morris, P.J.L., and O'Neill, J.P. 1998. A mixed culture recovery method indicates that enteric bacteria do not enter the viable-but-nonculturable state. Appl. Environ. Microbiol. 64: 1736-1742.

7. Denny, T., Brumbley, S., Carney, B., Clough, S., and Schell, M. 1994. Phenotype conversion of *Pseudomonas solanacearum*: its molecular basis and potential function. Pages 137-143 in: Bacterial Wilt: The Disease and its Causative Agent, *Pseudomonas solanacearum*. C. Hayward and G. Hartman, eds. CAB International.

8. Colwell, R.R., Brayton, P.R., Grimes, D.J., Roszak, D.B., Huq, S.A., and Palmer, L.M. 1985. Viable-but-nonculturable *Vibrio cholerae* and related pathogens in the environment: implications for release of genetically engineered microorganisms. BioTechnol. 3 : 817-820.

9. Dixon, B. 1998. Viable but nonculturable. ASM News 64: 372-373.

10. Ghezzi, J., and Steck, T. 1999. Induction of the viable but non-culturable condition in *Xanthomonas campestris* pv. *campestris* in liquid microcosms and sterile soils. FEMS Microbiol. Ecol. 30: 203-208.

11. Grey, B.E., and Steck, T.R. 2001. The viable but nonculturable state of *Ralstonia solanacearum* may be involved in long-term survival and plant infection. Appl. Environ. Microbiol. 67: 3866-3872.

12. Heijnen, C.E., Page, S., and Van Elsas, J.D. 1995. Metabolic activity of *Flavobacterium* strain P25 during starvation and after introduction into bulk soil and the rhizosphere of wheat. FEMS Microbiol. Ecol. 18: 129-138.

13. Islam, M.S., Hasan, M.K., Miah, M.A., Sur, G.C., Felsenstein, A., Venkatesan, M., Sack, R.B., and Albert, M.J. 1993. Use of the polymerase chain reaction and fluorescent anitbody methods for detecting viable but *nonculturable Shigella dysenteriae* type I in laboratory microcosms. Appl. Environ. Microbiol. 59: 536-540.

14. Jennison, M.W. 1937. Relations between plate counts and direct microscopic counts of *Escherichia coli* during logarithmic growth period. J. Bacteriol. 33: 461-469.

15. Jones, D.M., Sutcliffe, E.M., and Curry, A. 1991. Recovery of viable but non-culturable *Campylobacter jejuni*. J. Gen. Microbiol. 137: 2477-2482.

16. Joux, F., Lebaron, P., and Trousselier, M. 1997. Succession of cellular states in a *Salmonella typhimurium* population during starvation in artificial seawater microcosms. FEMS Microbiol. Ecol. 22: 65-76.

17. Kaprelyants, A.S., Gottschal, J.C., and Kell, D.B. 1993. Dormancy in non-sporulating bacteria. FEMS Microbiol. Rev. 104: 271-286.

18. Kelman, A., and Hruschka, J. 1973. The role of motility and aerotaxis in the selective increase of avirulent bacteria in still broth cultures of *Pseudomonas solanacearum*. J. Gen. Microbiol. 76: 177-188.

19. Kogure, K., Simidu, U., and Taga, N. 1979. A tentative direct microscopic method for counting living marine bacteria. Can. J. Microbiol. 25: 415-420.

20. Lesne, J., Berthet, S., Binard, S., Rouxel, A., and Humbert, F. 2000. Changes in culturability and virulence of *Salmonella typhimurium* during long-term starvation under desiccating conditions. Int. J. Food Microbiol. 60: 195-203.

21. Manahan, S., and Steck, T. 1997. The viable but nonculturable state in *Agrobacterium tumefaciens* and *Rhizobium meliloti*. FEMS Microbiol. Ecol. 22: 29-38.

22. Mascher, F., Hase, C., Moënne-Loccoz, Y., and Dëfago, G. 2000. The viable-but-nonculturable state induced by abiotic stress in the biocontrol agent *Pseudomonas fluorescens* CHA0 does not promote strain persistence in soil. Appl. Environ. Microbiol. 66: 1662-1667.

23. Muela, A., Arana, I., Justo, J.I., and Barcina, I. 1999. Changes in DNA content and cellular death during a starvation-survival process of *Escherichia coli* in river water. Microb. Ecol. 37: 62-69.

24. Mukamolova, G., Kaprelyants, A., Young, D.I., and Young, M. 1998. A bacterial cytokine. Proc. Natl. Acad. Sci. 95: 8916-8921.

25. Ohtomo, R., and Saito, M. 2001. Increase in the culturable cell number of *Escherichia coli* during recovery from saline stress: possible implication for resuscitation from the VBNC state. Microb. Ecol. 42: 208-214.

26. Oliver, J.D. 1993. Formation of viable but nonculturable cells. Pages 239-272 in: Starvation in Bacteria. S. Kjelleberg, ed. Plenum Press, New York.

27. Oliver, J.D. 2000. Problems in detecting dormant (VBNC) cells, and the role of DNA elements in this response. Pages 1-15 in: Tracking Genetically-Engineered Microorganisms. J.K. Jansson, J.D. van Elsas, and M.J. Bailey, eds. Landes Bioscience, Georgetown, TX, USA.

28. Oliver, J.D., Hite, F., McDougald, D., Andon, N.L., and Simpson, L.M. 1995. Entry into, and resuscitation from, the viable but nonculturable state by *Vibrio vulnificus* in an estuarine environment. Appl. Environ. Microbiol. 61: 2624-2630.

29. Oyofo, B.A., and Rollins, D.M. 1993. Efficacy of filter types for detection of *Campylobacter jejuni* and *Campylobacter coli* in environmental water samples by polymerase chain reaction. Appl. Environ. Microbiol. 59: 4090-4095.

30. Rollins, D.M., and Colwell, R.R. 1986. Viable but non-culturable stage of *Campylobacter jejuni* and its role in surival in the natural environment. Appl. Environ. Microbiol. 52: 531-538.

31. Roszak, D.B., Grimes, D.J., and Colwell, R.R. 1984. Viable but non-recoverable stage of *Salmonella enteritidis* in aquatic systems. Can J. Microbiol. 30: 334-338.

32. Roszak, D.B., and Colwell, R.R. 1987. Survival strategies of bacteria in the natural environment. Microbiol. Rev. 51: 365-379.

33. Salanoubat, M., Genin, S., Artiguenave, F., Gouzy, J., Mangenot, S., Arlat, M., Billault, A., Brottier, P., Camus, J.C., Cattolico, L., Chandler, M., Choisne, N., Claudel-Renard, C., Cunnac, S., Demange, N., Gaspin, C., Lavle, M., Moisan, A., Robert, C., Saurin, W., Schiex, T., Sguier, P., Thèbault, P., Whalen, M., Wincker, P., Levy, M., Weissenbach, J., and Boucher, C.A. 2002. Genome sequence of the plant pathogen *Ralstonia solanacearum*. Nature 415: 497-502.

34. Schell, M. 2000. Control of virulence and pathogenicity genes of *Ralstonia solanacearum* by an elaborate sensory network. Ann. Rev. Phytopathol. 38: 263-292.

35. Sequeira, L. 1993. Bacterial Wilt: Past, Present and Future. Pages 12-21 in: Bacterial Wilt. G.L. Hartmann and C.A. Hayward, eds. ACIAR Proceedings No 45.

36. Tholozan, J.L., Cappelier, J.M., Tissier, J.P., Delattre, G., and Federighi, M. 1999. Physiological characterization of viable-but-nonculturable *Campylobacter jejuni* cells. Appl. Environ. Microbiol. 65: 1110-1116.

37. Toffanin, A., Basaglia, M., Ciardi, C., Vian, P., Povolo, S., and Casella, S. 2000. Energy content decrease and viable-but-nonculturable status induced by oxygen limitation coupled to the presence of nitrogen oxides in *Rhizobium "hedysari"*. Biol. Fertil. Soils 31: 484-488.

38. Turpin, P.E., Maycroft, K.A., Rowlands, C.L., and Wellington, E.M.H. 1993. Viable but non-culturable salmonellas in soil. J. Appl. Bacteriol. 74: 421-427.

39. Van Elsas, J.D., Kastelein, P., Van Bekkum, P., Van der Wolf, J.M., de Vries, P.M., and Van Overbeek, L.S. 2000. Survival of *Ralstonia solanacearum* biovar 2, the causative agent of potato brown rot, in field and microcosm soils in temperate climates. Phytopathology 90: 1358-1366.

40. Van Elsas, J.D., Kastelein, P., de Vries, P.M., and Van Overbeek, L.S. 2001. Effects of ecological factors on the survival and physiology of *Ralstonia solanacearum* biovar 2 in agricultural drainage water. Can. J. Microbiol. 47: 842-854.

41. Van Overbeek, L.S., Eberl, L., Givskov, M., Molin, S., and Van Elsas, J.D. 1995. Survival of, and induced stress resistance in, carbon-starved *Pseudomonas fluorescens* residing in soil. Appl. Environ,. Microbiol. 61: 4202-4208.

42. Van Overbeek, L.S., Van Elsas, J.D., and Van Veen, J.A. 1997. Induced reporter gene activity, enhanced stress resistance, and competitive ability of a genetically modified *Pseudomonas fluorescens* strain released into a field plot planted with wheat. Appl. Environ. Microbiol. 63: 1965-1973.

43. Wakimoto, U. I., Matsuo, N., and Hayashi, I. 1982. Multiplication of *Pseudomonas solanacearum* in pure water. Ann. Rev. Phytopathol. Soc. Japan 48: 620-627.
44. Warner, J.M., and Oliver, J.D. 1998. Randomly amplified polymorphic DNA analysis of starved and viable but nonculturable *Vibrio vulnificus* cells. Appl. Environ. Microbiol. 64: 3025-3028.
45. Weichart, D., Oliver, J.D., and Kjelleberg, S. 1992. Low temperature induced nonculturability and killing of *Vibrio vulnificus*. FEMS Microbiol. Lett. 79: 205-210.
46. Whitesides, M.D., and Oliver, J.D. 1997. Resuscitation of *Vibrio vulnicus* from the viable but nonculturable state. Appl. Environ. Microbiol. 63: 1002-1005.
47. Xu, H.-S., Roberts, N., Singleton, F.L., Attwell, R.W., Grimes, D.J., and Colwell, R.R. 1982. Survival and viability of non-culturable *Escherichia coli* and *Vibrio cholerae* in the estuarine and marine environment. Microb. Ecol. 8: 313-323.
48. Zweifel, U.L., and Hagström, Å. 1995. Total counts of marine bacteria include a large fraction of non-nucleoid-containing bacteria (ghosts). Appl. Environ. Microbiol. 61: 2180-218.

Management of Bacterial Wilt Disease

G.S. Saddler

Scottish Agricultural Science Agency, East Craigs, Edinburgh, Scotland

Bacterial wilt, which is caused by *Ralstonia solanacearum*, remains one of the most intractable plant diseases known. An incomplete understanding of infraspecific diversity, coupled with gaps in knowledge on dissemination and infection has hampered the development of effective disease management strategies (38). Species ecology is highly diverse and as a consequence no universal control measures exist. As with other bacterial plant diseases, breeding for host resistance remains one of the most promising avenues for control (Liao, this volume). Resistance breeding has been effective with tobacco and groundnut, but success with solanaceous crops appears to be regional or linked to climatic conditions (13,17). Resistance, or more accurately tolerance as asymptomatic infections are commonplace with solanaceous hosts, can be neutralized by the actions of other pests, namely nematodes (54). Despite the less than universal success achieved breeding for disease resistance this avenue remains the most likely route for achieving long-term, disease control. However, effective and long-term control will only be achieved if the deployment of resistant/tolerant varieties takes place as part of an integrated pest management strategy. To date, a wide range of disease management and control methods have been studied. Many have been studied in isolation, however increasingly combinations are being applied and many of these are amenable for use in conjunction with resistant/tolerant varieties.

Plant Health and Quarantine Measures

The movement of infected, generally asymptomatic, planting material represents the most significant route by which the disease has spread on a global scale. The regulation and supervision of trade in commodities and seed delineates the frontline defense against the continued disease spread. To this end, quarantine regulations against the possible introduction of *R. solanacearum* are enforced in many regions of the world. Seed and plants for planting are generally the subject of rigorous inspection to ensure material is pathogen-free. Methods range from visual inspection of material, to sampling backed-up with laboratory diagnosis or the imposition of post-entry quarantine measures to ensure freedom from disease. International trade in seed potatoes is possibly the most heavily regulated in terms of attempting to control the further spread of bacterial wilt disease (López, this volume, 51). Within the European Union quarantine procedures are enforced and legislation provides for the establishment of a demarcated zone wherever the pathogen is located. The imposition of measures to prevent spread and eradicate the outbreak involve the enforcement of quarantine measures on infected fields and farms, crop rotation, control of weed hosts and volunteer plants, avoidance of surface water for irrigation, and education. Similar strategies have been adopted elsewhere to control the spread of disease, in particular with infected *Heliconia* plants in Cairns, Australia (18). Rapid quarantine action involved the destruction of imported plants, treatment of infested sites and restrictions on movement of plant material. This was followed up by extensive surveys at the site of importation over an extended period to ensure that the pathogen did not remerge.

Cultural Control

In regions where the disease is endemic cultural control methods have the potential to ameliorate its worst excesses. Frequently these methods require simple inputs, facilitating their uptake by resource-poor farmers. Crop rotation can be particularly effective especially when attempting to control pathogenic races that exhibit a narrow host range, namely race 3 on potato. In this regard, 3-year rotations with faba beans, garlic, maize, soya-bean or wheat were effective at reducing disease incidence (1). Rotation length varies, but short-term rotations involving one intermediary crop appear to be ineffective (7) and significant disease reduction can only be achieved using rotations of two (22) to five years (50). In the latter study a rotation involving potato-wheat-lupin-maize-potato was found to reduce disease incidence from more than 80% to less than 10%. Intercropping has also been shown to be effective for small farmers and cultivation of beans or maize can significantly reduce disease incidence (6). It should be stressed that as race 3 is not thought to persist in soil without an appropriate host for extended periods it is vital that rotation is applied only in conjunction with disease-free seed (Kinyua and coworkers, Mienie and Theron, this volume) and appropriate weed management strategies to ensure that the disease cycle is broken.

Controlling the actions of pathogenic races that exhibit a wider host range through crop rotation is more problematic. This is particularly true of tomato bacterial wilt, though there is some evidence that disease severity can be reduced by a rotation system using maize, okra and cowpea (3). Rice, but not eggplant, can also be effective at reducing wilt incidence (27). The pathogenic population was also found to decline somewhat after the soil was left fallow, indicating that a suitable host plant is required to maintain pathogen numbers. Monitoring the population of *R. solanacearum* in soil used for tomato cultivation would suggest that a rotation involving greater than two non-host crops is effective at reducing incidence (2). As with potato, intercropping tomato with Chinese chive (56) or cowpea (28) has been shown to significantly suppress bacterial wilt.

Rotation has also been used effectively with other wilt sensitive hosts. Rice, maize, wheat, sorghum and sugarcane have all proved effective at reducing disease incidence and severity in groundnut. In tobacco, disease incidence was reduced and the yield increased using a one-year rotation with maize, fescue (*Festuca* sp.) or soybeans (26). Similarly, French marigolds (*Tagetes patula*) may also serve as an appropriate rotation crop (46).

In conjunction with crop rotation, weed control can be effective at reducing disease incidence. In a comprehensive study of common weeds found in Taiwan, 12% of the weed species surveyed were found to harbour *R. solanacearum*. All were symptomless carriers that have the potential to serve as disease reservoirs (23). Similar results were found studying weeds commonly associated with rice grown in rotation with potato (32, 33).

Chemicals and Soil Treatments

In addition to cultural methods, chemicals and other forms of treatments, in particular treatment of soil infestations has been investigated as a means of controlling bacterial wilt disease. In general, chemical control is difficult to apply and some soil fumigants showed either slight or no effect. Application of stable bleaching powder gave disease suppression of 70-89% in greenhouse and field trials in Nepal (11). Similar results were obtained in an Indian study when applied in conjunction with deep ploughing (20). However, contrasting results would suggest that effects can be soil dependent and that soil disinfection is not universally applicable (29).

Studies on the mixed application of organic amendments and plant products with chemical fertilizers (NPK) clearly revealed that a combined application of compost and NPK was most effective in reducing the disease intensity on banana (36). It has also been suggested that control of bacterial wilt of tomato plants may be possible by supplying acidified nutrient solution (55). Soil amendments, similar to S-H mixture (containing, bagasse, rice husk powder, oyster shell powder, urea, etc.) have been used to reduce disease incidence by more than 60% in naturally infested fields of tobacco and tomato (53). It is interesting to note that control was reduced if the amendment mixture was heat treated prior to application, suggesting that control derived from an element that was biological in its origin.

Solarization has also been studied and some workers have noted a decline in the number of *R. solanacearum* cells in soil as a result (31). This method is frequently used with other control strategies such as; the application of soil warming in greenhouse soils (45), in combination with soil amendments such as bleaching powder, lime or mustard cake (10,39), with fumigants such as Dazomet (52) or with biological control agents (4). The application of such treatments however is clearly not universal; other studies have shown little effect on *R. solanacearum* numbers in soil when soil solarization and a variety of fumigants are applied (8).

Finally, there is a great deal of anecdotal evidence suggesting that certain soils are suppressive to bacterial wilt disease. As yet the nature of this suppression remains a matter for speculation. Shiomi *et al.* (40) investigated suppressive soils and identified a link between the diversity of the bacterial population and the degree of suppression. The results imply that it is difficult for the pathogen to dominate when a highly diverse rhizobacterial community is present. Attractive though this hypothesis undoubtedly is, other studies suggest that the presence of other bacteria has a limited affect on *R. solanacearum* numbers (47).

Biological Control

Biological control has been investigated extensively as a means of controlling bacterial wilt. In the vast majority of studies promising results generated under controlled conditions have failed to be replicated in the field. There is no single explanation as to why success has been so limited. However, whilst knowledge of the pathogen, its ability to colonize and induce disease and its soil/rhizosphere interactions remains so limited, effective deployment of a biological control agent is unlikely to be achieved in the near future. Not withstanding this lack of field success and the paucity of quality data on the disease, sufficient evidence does exist to indicate that control might yet be achieved if effective mechanisms of delivery, linked to good persistence of the control agent can be obtained. To date, a number of bacteria antagonistic towards *R. solanacearum* have been isolated from various sources and evaluated as control agents (Table 1). All of these studies have shown encouraging results in the greenhouse or in strictly controlled field tests. None have managed to progress beyond this evaluation phase. Largely as a consequence of the limited success achieved using saprophytic bacteria to control bacterial wilt a number of studies have focused on the use of antagonists that are closely related to or derived from the wild type pathogen itself. In general, this approach is based on the belief that these microorganisms are adapted to survive in the same plant microenvironment in which the pathogen operates. The use of such antagonists is thought to have several advantages, principally that the antagonist will be able to exploit conditions which favor the pathogen and, that once established, may be able to persist and thereby provide continuous protection. In essence, the ideal antagonist must be able to colonize and survive asymptomatically on the host under all the varying conditions in which the host is grown, without reducing yield.

Spontaneous avirulent mutants of *R. solanacearum*, deficient in exopolysaccharide (EPS) production that are able to colonize the host, albeit in a limited capacity, have been known for some time (21). Using avirulent *R. solanacearum* strains, some of which also produced bacteriocins, protection has been achieved with tobacco (9,44), tomato (24,35) and potato (25,34). In general, mutants that did not produce bacteriocins were only partially effective at halting the development of disease symptoms and protection was heavily dependent on environmental conditions, amongst other things

Table 1. Saprophytic bacteria that have been studied as biological control agents against bacterial wilt[a]

Bacteria	Host
Pseudomonas aeruginosa, P. fluorescens, Burkholderia glumae, Bacillus spp., *B. polymyxa, B. subtilis, Streptomyces mutabilis,* actinomycetes[1]	Tomato
P. fluorescens, Bacillus sp., *B. subtilis, B. cereus, Actinomycetes*	Potato
Corynebacterium sp.[†], *Bacillus* spp.[†], *Escherichia* sp.[†], *Serratia* sp.[†], *Pseudomonas* sp.[†],	Pepper
P. fluorescens, Bacillus spp.	Banana, Eggplant, Tomato
Bacillus spp.	Tobacco
Ectomycorrhizal fungi[#]	Eucalyptus

[a] Adapted from Smith and Saddler (43). Additional references: ([†], 16; [*], 41; [‡], 30; [#], 15).

ambient CO_2 levels (19). In general, systemic spread was restricted and numbers declined as host defense mechanisms took effect (37). Although promising under controlled conditions none of these attempts have proven universally effective in the natural environment. In most cases field experiments were too limited and protection was insufficient to warrant commercial development (5,44). Equally, in some cases protection failed because root colonization of the biocontrol agent was poor (9), or was highly dependent on environmental conditions (25).

A more recent, sophisticated and alternative approach has centered on the use of *hrp*O mutants of *R. solanacearum* generated by inserting a nontransposable omega interposon encoding for kanamycin resistance (14) into the wild-type pathogen's genome. Such strains possess the same level of ecological 'fitness' as the pathogen and, with the sole exception of the ability to cause disease, all other cellular functions are retained intact. Colonization and biological control assays have been conducted using *hrp*O⁻ on tomato (48,49) and potato (42,43) using challenge inoculation tests. In the former study, avirulent mutants were able to colonize taproot and collar tissues, but did not reach the fruits and fruit production was unaffected. In the latter study, mutants could only be detected in the root system and not the stem. In both cases, inoculation with avirulent mutants correlated with a significant reduction in the onset of disease and disease severity when plants were subsequently challenged with a pathogenic strain. In the tomato study the link between xylem colonization and the efficiency of control was highlighted (12). Virulent bacteria were still able to multiply in protected tissues, attaining population levels five to six orders of magnitude greater than those attained by the avirulent strain. These data indicate that protection was unlikely to have resulted from the general exclusion of the virulent strain. It seems likely that control is achieved through competition for space or nutrients, as no evidence of direct antagonism was found. Certainly, these data confirm that prior root inoculation with *hrp*O⁻ mutants limits disease development upon subsequent inoculation with virulent *R. solanacearum*, even under conditions most favorable for disease.

Taken together, it is clear that the use of *hrp*O⁻ mutants confers protection against bacterial wilt disease under greenhouse conditions. However, much work remains to be done as appropriate delivery mechanisms have yet to be developed, both agents have to be fully evaluated under true field conditions and the exact mechanism of control has yet to be elucidated.

Conclusions and Future Prospects

In the last twenty years numerous reports have described the development of control strategies against bacterial wilt disease and its causative organism *R. solanacearum*. Set against the background of our restricted knowledge of the pathogen it is perhaps unsurprising that few of these studies have generated control strategies that are 100% effective. Yet despite the lack of progress generating robust control methods, these studies have produced substantial quantities of information on the mechanism of host colonization and infection, disease development and spread, and highlighted links between symptom expression and environmental and nutritional conditions. This substantial body of work has also facilitated the growing sense that a more holistic approach is required if effective control of bacterial wilt is to be achieved in areas where the disease is endemic. In the immediate future, rather than absolute disease control, reducing the impact of the disease region by region is probably a more achievable and appropriate goal. In this regard, disease free planting material, when used with crop rotation and good field sanitation may keep the worst excesses of the disease at bay (Kinyua, this volume). Clearly in the longer term, benefits derived from genomic studies on both the pathogen and its hosts are likely to enable the production of more effective resistant varieties or more targeted and ecologically active biological agents. It will be at this point that the true benefits of the years of research into disease management will be realized, as it will form the foundations onto which an integrated management strategy for bacterial wilt disease can be constructed.

Literature Cited

1. Abd El-Ghafar, N.Y. 1998. Control of potato bacterial wilt using crop rotation. Ann. Agric. Sci. (Cairo) 43:575-587.
2. Abdullah, H., and Sijam, K. 1992. Effect of selected vegetable crops on bacterial wilt pathogen population and their use in crop rotation programmes for bacterial wilt disease control. Acta Hortic. 292:161-165.
3. Adhikari, T.B., and Basnyat, R.C. 1998. Effect of crop rotation and cultivar resistance on bacterial wilt of tomato in Nepal. Can. J. Plant Pathol. 20:283-287.
4. Anith, K.N., Manomohandas, T.P., Jayarajan, M., Vasanthakumar, K., and Aipe, K.C. 2000. Integration of soil solarization and biological control with a fluorescent *Pseudomonas* sp. for controlling bacterial wilt *Ralstonia solanacearum* (E.F. Smith) Yabuuchi *et al.* of ginger. J. Biol. Control 14:25-29.
5. Anuratha, C., and Gnanamanickam, S. 1990. Biological control of bacterial wilt caused by *Pseudomonas solanacearum* in India with antagonistic bacteria. Plant Soil 124:109-116.

6. Autrique, A., and Potts, M.J. 1987. The influence of mixed cropping on the control of potato bacterial wilt. Ann. Appl. Biol. 111:125-133.

7. Arthy, J., and Akiew, S. 1999. Effect of short term rotation on *Ralstonia solanacearum* populations in soil. ACIAR Bacterial Wilt Newsl. No.16:13-14.

8. Chellemi, D.O., Olson, S.M., Mitchell, D.J., Secker, I., and McSorley, R. 1997. Adaptation of soil solarization to the integrated management of soilborne pests of tomato under humid conditions. Phytopathology 87:250-258.

9. Chen, W., and Echandi, E. 1984. Effects of avirulent bacteriocin-producing strains of *Pseudomonas solanacearum* on the control of bacterial wilt of tobacco. Plant Pathol. 33:245-253.

10. Chowdhury, A.K., Mitra, P., Panja, B.N., Chakraborty, A., Roy, S., and Laha, S.K. 2000. Effects of soil amendments and chemicals on bacterial wilt of tomato caused by *Pseudomonas solanacearum*. Environ. Ecol. 18:476-478.

11. Dhital S.P., Thaveechai N., Kositratana W., Piluek K., and Shrestha S.K. 1997. Effect of chemical and soil amendment for the control of bacterial wilt of potato in Nepal caused by *Ralstonia solanacearum*. Kasetsart J. (Natural Sci.) 31:497-509.

12. Etchebar, C, Trigalet-Demery, D., van Gijsegem, F., Vasse, J., and Trigalet, A. 1998. Xylem colonization by an *HrcV⁻* mutant of *Ralstonia solanacearum* is a key factor for the efficient biological control of tomato bacterial wilt. Mol. Plant-Microbe Interact. 11:869-877.

13. French, E.R. 1994. Strategies for integrated control of bacterial wilt of potatoes. Pages 199-207 in: Bacterial Wilt: The Disease and its Causative Agent, *Pseudomonas solanacearum*. A.C. Hayward and G.L. Hartman, eds. CAB International, Wallingford, Oxon, UK.

14. Frey, P., Prior, P., Marie, C., Kotoujansky, A., Trigelet-Demery, D., and Trigalet, A. 1994. *Hrp* mutants of *Pseudomonas solanacearum* as potential biocontrol agents of tomato bacterial wilt. Appl. Environ. Microbiol. 60:3175–3181.

15. Gong, M.Q., Chen Y., Wang F.Z., and Chen Y.L. Inhibitory effect of ectomycorrhizal fungi on bacterial wilt of Eucalyptus. 1999. For. Res. (Beijing) 12:339-345.

16. Guo, J.H., Guo, Y.H., Zhang, L.X., Qi, H.Y., and Fang Z.D. 2001. Screening for biocontrol agents against *Ralstonia solanacearum*. Chin. J. Biol. Control 17:101-106.

17. Hayward, A.C. 1991. Biology and epidemiology of bacterial wilt caused by *Pseudomonas solanacearum*. Annu. Rev. Phytopathol. 29:65-87.

18. Hyde, K.D., McCulloch, B., Akiew, E., Peterson, R.A., and Diatloff, A. 1992. Strategies used to eradicate bacterial wilt of *Heliconia* (race 2) in

Cairns, Australia, following introduction of the disease from Hawaii. Australas. Plant Pathol. 21:29-31.

19. Kim, D.H. and Misaghi, I.J. 1996. Biocontrol performance of two isolates of *Pseudomonas fluorescens* in modified soil atmospheres. Phytopathology 86:1238-1241.

20. Kishore, V., Shekhawat, G.S., and Sunaina, V. 1996. Cultural practices to reduce *Pseudomonas solanacearum* in the infested soil. J. Indian Potato Assoc. 23:130-133.

21. Kelman, A. 1954. The relationship of pathogenicity in *Pseudomonas solanacearum* to colony appearance on a tetrazolium medium. Phytopathology 44:693-695.

22. Lemaga, B., Kanzikwera, R., Kakuhenzire, R., Hakiza, J.J., and Manzi, G. 2001. The effect of crop rotation on bacterial wilt incidence and potato tuber yield. Afr. Crop Sci. J. 9:257-266.

23. Lin, J.C., Hsu, S.T., and Tzeng, K.C. 1999. Weed hosts of *Ralstonia solanacearum* in Taiwan. Plant Prot.Bull. (Taichung) 41:277-292.

24. Luo, K., and Wang, Z. 1983. Study of bacterial wilt (*Pseudomonas solanacearum*) controlled by antagonistic and avirulent *P. solanacearum*. Acta Phytopathol. Sin. 13:51-56.

25. McLaughlin, R., and Sequeira, L. 1988. Evaluation of an avirulent strain of *Pseudomonas solanacearum* for biological control of bacterial wilt of potato. Am. Potato J. 65:255-268.

26. Melton, T.A., and Powell, N.T., 1991. Effects of two-year crop rotations and cultivar resistance on bacterial wilt in flue-cured tobacco. Plant Dis. 75:695-698.

27. Michel, V.V., Hartman, G.L., and Midmore, D.J. 1996. Effect of previous crop on soil populations of *Burkholderia solanacearum*, bacterial wilt, and yield of tomatoes in Taiwan. Plant Dis. 80:1367-1372.

28. Michel, V.V., Wang, J.F., Midmore, D.J., and Hartman, G.L. 1997. Effects of intercropping and soil amendment with urea and calcium oxide on the incidence of bacterial wilt of tomato and survival of soil-borne *Pseudomonas solanacearum* in Taiwan. Plant Pathol. 46:600-610.

29. Michel, V.V., and Mew, T.W. 1998. Effect of a soil amendment on the survival of *Ralstonia solanacearum* in different soils. Phytopathology 88:300-305.

30. Moura, A.B., and da Romeiro, R.S. 2000. Use of actinomycetes pre-selected for the control of *Ralstonia solanacearum* as tomato plant growth promoters. Rev. Ceres 47:613-626.

31. Pradeep K., and Sood, A.K. 2001. Integration of antagonistic rhizobacteria and soil solarization for the management of bacterial wilt

of tomato caused by *Ralstonia solanacearum*. Indian Phytopathol. 54:12-15.

32. Pradhanang, P.M., Elphinstone, J.G., and Fox, R.T.V. 2000. Identification of crop and weed hosts of *Ralstonia solanacearum* biovar 2 in the hills of Nepal. Plant Pathol. 49:403-413.

33. Pradhanang, P.M., and Momol, M.T. 2001. Survival of *Ralstonia solanacearum* in soil under irrigated rice culture and aquatic weeds. J. Phytopathol. 149:707-711.

34. Quezado-Soares, A.M., and Lopes, C.A. 1994. Lack of biological control of potato bacterial wilt by avirulent mutants of *Pseudomonas solanacearum* and by fluorescent pseudomonads. ACIAR Bacterial Wilt Newsl. No. 11:3-5.

35. Ren, X.Z., Shen, D.L., and Fang, Z.D. 1988. Preliminary studies on control of bacterial wilt of tomato (*Pseudomonas solanacearum*) by avirulent bacteriocin-producing strain MA-7. Chin. J. Biol. Control 4:62-64.

36. Roy, S., Ojha, P.K., Ojha, K.L., Upadhyay, J.P., and Jha, M.M. 1999. Effect of mixed application of fertilizers and organic amendments on the disease intensity of wilt complexes in banana (*Musa* sp.). J. Appl. Biol. 9:84-86.

37. Sequeira, L. 1982. Determinants of plant response to bacterial infection. Pages 85-102 in: Active Defense Mechanisms in Plants. R.K.S. Wood, ed. Plenum Press, New York, USA.

38. Sequeira, L. 1994. Epilogue: Life with a 'mutable and treacherous tribe'. Pages 235-247 in: Bacterial Wilt: The Disease and its Causative Agent, *Pseudomonas solanacearum*. A.C. Hayward and G.L. Hartman, eds. CAB International, Wallingford, Oxon, UK.

39. Sharma, J.P., and Kumar, S. 2000. Management of *Ralstonia* wilt through soil disinfectant, mulch, lime and cakes in tomato (*Lycopersicon esculentum*). Indian J. Agric. Sci. 70: 17-19.

40. Shiomi, Y., Nishiyama, M., Onizuka, T., and Marumoto, T. 1999. Comparison of bacterial community structures in the rhizoplane of tomato plants grown in soils suppressive and conducive towards bacterial wilt. Appl. Environ. Microbiol. 65: 3996-4001.

41. Singh, D., and Rana, S.K. 2000. Biocontrol of bacterial wilt/brown rot (*Ralstonia solanacearum*) of potato. J. Mycol. Plant Pathol. 30:420-421.

42. Smith, J.J., Offord, L.C., Kibata, G.N., Murimi, Z.K., Trigalet, A., and Saddler, G.S. 1998. The development of a biological control against *Ralstonia solanacearum* race 3 in Kenya. Pages 337-342 in: Bacterial Wilt Disease: Molecular and Ecological Aspects. P. Prior, C. Allen and J. Elphinstone, eds. Springer-Verlag, Berlin, Germany.

43. Smith, J.J., and Saddler, G.S. 2001. The use of avirulent mutants of *Ralstonia solanacearum* to control bacterial wilt disease. Pages 159-176 in: Biotic interactions in plant-pathogen associations. M.J. Jeger and N.J. Spence, eds. CABI Publishing, Wallingford, UK

44. Tanaka, H., Negishi, H., and Maeda, H. 1990. Control of tobacco bacterial wilt by an avirulent strain of *Pseudomonas solanacearum* M4S and its bacteriophage. Ann. Phytopathol. Soc. Jpn 56:243-246.

45. Tanaka, T., Chikawa, K., Matsusaki, M., and Sakai, K. 2000. Effect of soil disinfection using solar heating with soil warming system to *Meloidgyne* sp. and *Ralstonia solanacearum*. Res. Bull. Aichi-ken Agric. Res. Cen. No.32:105-110.

46. Terblanche, J., and de Villiers, D.A. (1998). The suppression of *Ralstonia solanacearum* by marigolds. Pages 325-331 in: Bacterial Wilt Disease: Molecular and Ecological Aspects. P. Prior, C. Allen and J. Elphinstone, eds. Springer-Verlag, Berlin, Germany.

47. Toyota, K., and Kimura, M. 2000. Suppression of *Ralstonia solanacearum* in soil following colonization by other strains of *R. solanacearum*. Soil Sci. Plant Nutr. 46:449-459.

48. Trigalet, A., Frey, P., and Trigalet-Demery, D. 1994. Biological control of bacterial wilt caused by *Pseudomonas solanacearum*: State of the art and understanding. Pages 225-233 in: Bacterial Wilt: The Disease and its causative agent, *Pseudomonas solanacearum*. A.C. Hayward and G.L. Hartman, eds. CAB International, Wallingford, Oxon, UK.

49. Trigalet, A., Trigalet-Demery, D., and Prior, P. 1998. Elements of biocontrol of tomato bacterial wilt. Pages 332-336 in: Bacterial Wilt Disease: Molecular and Ecological Aspects. P. Prior, C. Allen, and J. Elphinstone, eds. Springer-Verlag, Berlin, Germany.

50. Verma, R.K., and Shekhawat, G.S. 1991. Effect of crop rotation and chemical soil treatment on bacterial wilt of potato. Indian Phytopathol. 44:5-8.

51. Wright, A.J. 1998. Legislative measures to prevent the introduction and spread of *Ralstonia solanacearum* in the European Union. EPPO Bull. 28:513-518.

52. Yamada, M., Nakazawa, Y., and Kitamura, T. 1997. Control of tomato bacterial wilt by dazomet combined with soil solarization. Proc. Kanto-Tosan Plant Prot. Soc. No.44:75-78.

53. Yao, G., Zhang, F., and Li, Z. 1994. Control of bacterial wilt with soil amendment. Chin. J. Biol. Control 10:106-109.

54. Yen, J.H., Chen, D.Y., Hseu, S.H., Lin, C.Y., and Tsay T.T. 1997. The effect of plant parasitic nematodes on severity of bacterial wilt in solanaceous plants. Plant Pathol. Bull. (Taichung) 6:141-153.

55. Yi Y.K., and Sul K.C. 1998. Control strategy of acidified nutrient solution on bacterial wilt of tomato plants. Korean J. Plant Pathol. 14:744-746.

56. Yu J.Q. 1999. Allelopathic suppression of *Pseudomonas solanacearum* infection of tomato (*Lycopersicon esculentum*) in a tomato-Chinese chive (*Allium tuberosum*) intercropping system. J. Chem. Ecol. 25:2409-2417.

Management of Bacterial Wilt in Tomato with Essential Oils and Systemic Acquired Resistance Inducers

P.M. Pradhanang[1], M.T. Momol[1], S.M. Olson[1], and J.B.Jones[2]

[1]North Florida Research and Education Center (NFREC), University of Florida, Quincy, FL 32351; [2]Plant Pathology Department, University of Florida, Gainesville, FL 32611

Due to the limited efficacy of the current integrated management strategies, bacterial wilt caused by *Ralstonia solanacearum* continues to be economically important for field-grown, fresh-market tomato production in the southeastern United States and many subtropical and tropical areas of the world.

Essential oils and extracts, usually from medicinal plants, have been recognized as having good fungicidal effects (10), but their efficacy as biofumigants on *R. solanacearum* had not been studied prior 1999. Preliminary *in vitro* and greenhouse experiments conducted with several plant essential oils showed that some essential oils have significant efficacy against *R. solanacearum* (5) and against several soilborne fungi of tomato (6). Recently, several formulated botanical extracts including essential oils were shown to effectively reduce soil populations of *Fusarium oxysporum* and reduce wilt incidence on muskmelon (1).

The natural protection of plants against pathogens when expressed systemically in tissues remote from the initial treatment is termed systemic acquired resistance (SAR) (9). Recently, products called "plant activators" that induce SAR in plants were identified. One such compound, acibenzolar-S-methyl (Actigard 50 WG, Bion 50 WG, Syngenta, Basel, Switzerland), showed activity against bacterial spot of tomato (4). Similarly the harpin protein isolated from *Erwinia amylovora* (Messenger, Eden Bioscience, WA, USA), the elicitor of hypersensitive responses in a non-host, has been shown to induce host resistance in tomato to bacterial wilt in a preliminary study (7).

The objectives of this study were to further evaluate the effects of plant essential oils on population density of *R. solanacearum* in soil and on incidence of bacterial wilt, and to investigate effect of SAR inducers against bacterial wilt on susceptible and moderately resistant tomato cultivars in the greenhouse.

Materials and Methods

BACTERIAL STRAIN AND INOCULUM

R. solanacearum (biovar 1, race 1), tomato strain Rs5 isolated in Quincy, Florida was used in these studies. The bacterium was grown overnight (18 h) in casamino acid peptone glucose (CPG) broth on a shaker (200 RPM) at 28°C. The concentration of the inoculum was estimated by absorbance at 590 nm.

ESSENTIAL OILS

R. solanacearum suspensions were incorporated into soil (potting mixture) at an inoculum density of 6.5×10^7 CFU/cm^3 of soil. After thoroughly mixing in closed polyethylene bags and incubation for 1 h, soil was treated by incorporating 0.7 g or 0.4 g thymol (2-Isopropyl-5-methylphenol, Sigma, St. Louis, MO, USA) (aqueous emulsion of thymol prepared in 6.3 ml of 70% ethanol) into 1 L of soil. Soil kept in closed bags was mixed thoroughly daily to allow fumigation in the dark at room temperature for 3 days, followed by aeration for 4 days to remove excess essential oils. An untreated water control consisted of the same amount of ethanol as above. Palmarosa (*Cymbopogon martini*), tea tree (*Melaleuca alternifolia*), and lemongrass (*Cymbopogon flexuosus*) oils (Prima Fleur, CA, USA) (0.7 ml or 0.4 ml) were mixed with one liter soil and incubated as described above.

Seven days after essential oil treatments, *R. solanacearum* population density was determined from each replicated bag separately by culturing 1:9 serial dilutions on modified SMSA agar (2,3). Subsequently, 10-cm pots were filled with treated soil and a tomato seedling cv. Equinox (5-6 leaf stage) transplanted into each pot. Bacterial wilt incidence was recorded until four weeks after transplanting. Plants that did not develop wilt symptoms were tested for latent infection by macerating 1 cm section of the basal stem in one ml sterile deionized water and streaking a loopful on SMSA agar.

INDUCED RESISTANCE

Acibenzolar-S-methyl (Actigard 50WG) was used as a soil drench and foliar spray, whereas harpin protein (Messenger) was applied as seed treatment, soil drench, and foliar spray. Actigard was applied at 6 µg /ml before

134

transplanting and increased to 60 μg/ml after transplanting, whereas Messenger was applied at 600 μg/ml concentration. Seeds were soaked in a messenger suspension and sown in a soil-less medium in trays made of expanded polystyrene beads. The initial foliar application was applied 14 days after seed germination. For soil drenching, 5 ml of Actigard and Messenger were poured into each cell five days prior to inoculation. Plants were also sprayed until run off with both products on the day of soil drenching. Seedlings were inoculated by drenching soil with *R. solanacearum* at 5 ml per cell (8). Inoculum concentration was 1.2×10^7 CFU/ml.

Seedlings were transplanted into 10-cm pots filled with soil-less medium 3 days after inoculation. All experiments were randomized complete blocks with five replications and four plants per replication. Observations for wilt incidence and latent infection were conducted as described above.

Results

ESSENTIAL OILS

Seven days after essential oil application (high concentration), the bacterium was not detected in thymol, palmarosa, or lemongrass oil-treated soil, whereas a high *R. solanacearum* population was recovered from tea tree oil-treated and untreated control soils. Plants grown potting soil amended with the high concentration of thymol, palmarosa, and lemon grass oil were free from wilt, and only 10% of the plants in palmarosa and lemongrass oil- treated soil produced latent infections. Disease incidence was highest (75%) in tea tree oil-treated soil. Although the pathogen was not detected in the potting mixture treated with a low concentration of thymol, 10% of the tomatoes planted in the soil wilted. Significantly more wilt occurred in tomato plants grown in soil treated with low concentration of palmarosa and lemongrass oils than the higher concentrations (Table 1).

INDUCED RESISTANCE

None of the Actigard-treated, bacterial wilt-resistant tomato (cv. Neptune) plants were wilted, whereas 20% of the non-treated Neptune plants developed wilt symptoms (Table 2). The trend of wilt suppression was similar on BHN 466 and between Actigard treated and non-treated plants. Bacterial wilt-susceptible cv. Equinox rapidly developed wilt symptoms in 95% of the plants irrespective of Actigard application. Latent infection detection was determined one month after inoculation. All apparently healthy plants (all cultivars) were systemically infected by *R. solanacearum*.

Table 1. Effect of essential oils on bacterial wilt incidence

| | Concentration of essential oil | | | |
| | High[a] | | Low[b] | |
Treatment	% Bacterial wilt	% Latent infection	% Bacterial wilt	% Latent infection
Thymol	0	0	10	0
Palmarosa oil	0	10	40	10
Tea tree oil	75	10	100	0
Lemongrass oil	0	10	65	0
Untreated control[c]	100	0	100	0
LSD (0.05)			30.63	

[a] 0.7 g Thymol or 0.7 ml of plant oils / 6.3 ml of 70 % ethanol/L of soil.
[b] 0.4 g Thymol or 0.4 ml of plant oils / 3.6 ml of 70 % ethanol/L of soil.
[c] 6.3 or 3.6 ml of 70 % Ethanol/L of soil.

Discussion

The results presented above show that thymol, palmarosa and lemon grass oils effectively reduced bacterial wilt incidence and *R. solanacearum* populations in soil. However, their effectiveness was reduced when application rates were lowered. Lack of effectiveness of tea tree oil shows that all essential oils are not bactericidal to *R. solanacearum*.

SAR inducers did not induce resistance against bacterial wilt in a susceptible tomato cultivar. Actigard effectively reduced bacterial wilt incidence but only on moderately resistant cultivars (Table 2). Actigard reduced bacterial wilt by 20% and 25% in Neptune and BHN 466, respectively. Actigard elevated the level of resistance in Neptune and BHN 466 from moderate resistance to a high level of resistance. Messenger was not effective at the concentration used in these experiments or against the *R. solanacearum* strain (Rs5) used in this study.

In warm sub-tropical and tropical parts of the world it is not economical to grow tomatoes in *R. solanacearum*-infested soils unless plants are resistant to bacterial wilt. However, bacterial wilt resistant cultivars were not accepted by the commercial tomato industry in the southeastern U.S. due to several factors. It can be beneficial if the effect of Actigard shown in this study can be used to enhance the level of resistance in moderately resistant or highly resistant cultivars. Therefore, those cultivars may gain market acceptance by increasing the level of resistance.

Table 2. Bacterial wilt incidence as affected by Actigard

Treatment	Bacterial wilt incidence (%)		
	BHN 466[a]	Neptune[a]	Equinox[a]
Actigard	5	0	95
No Actigard	30	20	95
Chi-square(X^2)	6.03[b]	8.16[b]	

[a] Cultivars BHN 466 and Neptune are moderately resistant. Equinox is susceptible to bacterial wilt.
[b] X^2 value, significant at 0.05.

Acknowledgements

This research was sponsored in part by the SR-IPM and T-STAR programs of USDA. We thank J.J. Marois for statistical advice.

Literature Cited

1. Bowers, J.H., and Locke, J.C. 2000. Effects of botanical extracts on the population density of *Fusarium oxysporum* in soil and control of Fusarium wilt in the greenhouse. Plant Dis. 84: 300-305.
2. Engelbrecht, M.C. 1994. Modification of a semi-selective medium for the isolation and quantification of *Pseudomonas solanacearum*. ACIAR Bacterial Wilt Newsl. 10: 3-5.
3. Elphinstone, J.G., Hennessy, J., Wilson, J.K., and Stead, D.E. 1996. Sensitivity of detection of *Ralstonia solanacearum* in potato tuber extracts. EPPO Bull. 26: 663-678.
4. Louws, F.J., Wilson, M., Campbell, H.L., Cuppels, D.A., Jones, J.B., Sahin, F., and Miller, S.A. 2001. Field control of bacterial spot and bacterial speck of tomato using a plant activator. Plant Dis. 85:481-488.
5. Momol, M.T., Momol, E.A., Dankers, W.A., Olson, S.M., Simmons, J.A., and Rich, J.R. 1999. Evaluation of selected plant essential oils for suppression of *Ralstonia solanacearum* and *Meloidogyne arenaria* on tomato. Phytopathology 89: S54.
6. Momol, M.T., Mitchell, D.J., Rayside P.A., Olson S.M., and Momol, E.A. 2000. Plant essential oils as potential biofumigants for the management of soilborne pathogens of tomato. Phytopathology 90: S127.

7. Qui, D., Wei, Z.-M., Bauer D.W., and Beer, S.V. 1997. Treatment of tomato seed with harpin enhances germination and growth and induces resistance to *Ralstonia solanacearum*. Phytopathology 87: S80.
8. Somodi, G.C., Jones, J.B., and Scott, J.W. 1992. Comparison of inoculation techniques for screening tomato genotypes for bacterial wilt resistance. Pages 120-123 in: Bacterial Wilt: Proceedings of an International Conference held at Kaohsiung, Taiwan, 28-31 October 1992. G.L. Hartman and A.C. Hayward, eds. ACIAR Proc. No.45, 381p.
9. Sticher, L., Mauchmani, B., and Metraux, J.P. 1997. Systemic acquired resistance. Annu. Rev. Phytopathol. 35:235-270.
10. Wilson, C.L., Solar, J.M., El Ghaouth, A., and Wisniewsky, M.E. 1997. Rapid evaluation of plant extracts and essential oils for antifungal activity against *Botrytis cinerea*. Plant Dis. 81:204-210.

Monitoring of Bacterial Wilt in Potato Propagation Material: A Success Story

N.J.J. Mienie and D.J. Theron

Potatoes South Africa, Potato Laboratory Services, Lynn East, Pretoria 0039, Republic of South Africa

Bacterial wilt, caused by *R. solanacearum* (Smith) Yabuuchi *et al.* on potatoes, was first reported during 1914 in South Africa (4). In South Africa, *R. solanacearum* biovar 2, race 3 is mainly associated with bacterial wilt of potatoes, however, biovar 3, race 1 was also isolated from wilted potato plants (9). After serious outbreaks of bacterial wilt in some of the important seed production areas during the 1980's, the importance of infected propagation material as the primary source of the disease was realized. Consequently an ELISA test for the detection of *R. solanacearum* was developed by the University of Stellenbosch (1), which enabled the screening of large amounts of seed tuber samples in commercial laboratories. Testing of seed tubers of generations G1 to G4 was implemented in 1991. Generations G5 to G8 were not subjected to testing, except when bacterial wilt infection was suspected. Reliance on visual inspections was found to be unreliable due to latent infections and in 1995 compulsory testing of all registered seed tuber plantings (G1 to G8) was implemented. Additional control measures were also implemented in cases of confirmed infection. Since 1996, compulsory testing of mini tubers (G0) was implemented and the following year all *in vitro* plantlets were also subjected to testing. In South Africa, *R. solanacearum* is considered a prohibited organism according to the Agricultural Pest Act, 1983 (Act 36 of 1983) and a zero tolerance for bacterial wilt in potato propagation material is applied.

Control Measures Implemented

All *in vitro* plantlets are subjected to extensive screening for *R. solanacearum*, *Erwinia* spp. and internal contamination. Mini tubers (G0) produced from *in vitro* plants are screened for *R. solanacearum* and *Erwinia* spp. Tubers (G1 to G8) are screened for *R. solanacearum* only.

FIELD INSPECTIONS

All fields registered for seed tuber production are plotted with a GPS. Relevant information on origin and pedigree of the seed tubers planted is kept in a database. This enables Certification Services to record all confirmed infections and facilitates the tracing of the origin and possible dissemination of infected tubers. The registration of fields, or fields planted with seed that seems risky, can be withheld. All registered seed tuber plantings (G0 to G8) are subjected to two visual inspections, the first 30 days after emergence, and the second during the full-flowering stage. All plants showing wilt symptoms during these inspections are sampled and tested for bacterial wilt.

LABORATORY TESTING

Sampling method. In vitro plants are sampled prior to planting in the green houses. Tuber samples (one tuber per plant) are taken at random after natural senescence or artificial killing of the foliage prior to harvesting. Sample size (Table 1) was based on the statistical model of Clayton and Slack (2) with a 99% probability of detection if 0.1% disease incidence should occur and the planting is 10 Haand is cultivated as a unit.

In vitro plantlets. These plantlets are aseptically removed from the containers in which they have been cultivated and batched into sub-samples of 50 plantlets each. Sub-samples are placed separately in a sterile plastic bag (BIOREBA) and homogenized with a BIOREBA hand held homogeniser. Sterile distilled water (10 ml) is added to the contents of the bag (10^{-1} dilution), diluted to 10^{-4}, and an aliquot of 0.2 ml is plated on tetrazolium chloride (TZC) and crystal violet pectate (CVP) media (3) and incubated at 30°C for 48 h (5,7). TZC plates are visually evaluated for typical *R. solanacearum* colonies. If *R. solanacearum* is suspected, it was further identified by means of a series of biochemical and physiological tests (6)

Table 1. Samples for bacterial wilt testing

Generation	Number of plants or tubers
In vitro plants	1 plant / container / clone
G0	4 tubers / 100 plants / cultivar
G1	1 tuber / 10 m plant row / cultivar
G2-G8	4605* tubers / unit

* Based on the statistical model of Clayton and Slack (2).

and pathogenicity was tested on tomato seedlings (Koch's postulates). CVP plates are inspected for deep pits due to the presence of pectolytic *Erwinia* spp. Pure cultures are identified by means of a series of biochemical tests for the presence of *E. c.* subsp. *carotovora*, *E. c.* subsp. *atroseptica* and *E. chrysanthemi* (8).

Internal contamination. This is tested by adding 0.2 ml of the 10^{-2} dilution into nutrient broth and incubating at 30°C for 48 h. Development of turbidity in the medium indicates internal contamination.

Mini tubers. Sub-samples of 50 tubers are batched. A 15 mm slice from the stolon and apical end of the tuber are sliced and batched together. The slices are washed three times with sterile tap water after which 100 ml of sterile distilled water is added and the contents homogenized in a commercial Waring blender. The pulp is left for three minutes for diffusion of any bacteria and thereafter drained through a sieve (1 mm). Of the filtrate, 1 ml is used in a dilution series up to the 10^{-5} dilution. Of the 10^{-5}, 10^{-4}, 10^{-3} and 10^{-2} dilutions, 0.2 ml is spread on selective media for *R. solanacearum* and *Erwinia* spp. and treated as described above.

Tuber samples. Tubers (4,605) are washed and sub-sampled as 100 tuber lots. Lots are placed in plastic crates to dry. Tubers were peeled at the stolon-end side and a piece (0.5 mm^3) of the vascular tissue was removed from each tuber. Pieces from each sub-sample are homogenized in a commercial Waring blender and left for 3 min to allow diffusion of bacteria from the tissue and then drained through a sieve (1 mm). Filtrates of the 46 sub-samples are routinely tested for *R. solanacearum* cells by using ELISA (1). All filtrates are maintained at 4°C until completion of the ELISA test. Sub-samples giving positive ELISA readings (absorbancy value ≥ 0.15 at $OD_{405\,nm}$), are further evaluated to confirm identity as previously mentioned and tested for pathogenicity on tomato.

Additional Control Measures

Identification of *R. solanacearum* in a registered seed tuber planting results in immediate withdrawal of registration, and cultivation of seed tubers in that specific location is not allowed for a ten year period when contaminated with biovar 2 race 3, or indefinitely in the case of biovar 3 race 1. A special bacterial wilt investigation committee has been established, made up of experts on the disease and representatives from Certification Services and the Department of Agriculture, which investigates each contamination case. When necessary, this committee may decide to visit the farm in question to familiarise themselves with the situation. They will then also advise the producer on crop rotation, quarantine and sanitation practices and determine the probability of infection of adjacent fields and how to prevent it. They will also determine the distance surrounding the infection site, where cultivation of potatoes will be prohibited.

Results and Conclusions

From 1997, when the compulsory testing of *in vitro* plantlets was introduced, until 2001, only one sample of the 1235 samples tested has tested positive for *Erwinia* sp. None of these samples tested positive for *R. solanacearum* (Table 2). This is a clear indication that, at present, the nuclear stock material of the potato industry is disease-free.

No *R. solanacearum* has been detected in the G0 material since 1996, when compulsory testing was introduced. However, of the 2737 samples tested, *Erwinia* spp. were detected in 97 of these samples (Table 3). Since the introduction of compulsory testing of all registered seed tuber plantings

Table 2. *In vitro* plantlet samples tested for *R. solanacearum* and *Erwinia* spp.

Year	Samples Tested	*R. solanacearum* positive	*R. solanacearum* positive (%)	*Erwinia* positive	*Erwinia* positive (%)
1997	455	0	0	1	0.22
1998	141	0	0	0	0
1999	220	0	0	0	0
2000	199	0	0	0	0
2001	220	0	0	0	0
Total	1,235	0	0	1	0.08

Table 3. Mini tuber samples tested for *R. solanacearum* and *Erwinia* spp.

Year	Samples Tested	*R. solanacearum* positive	*R. solanacearum* positive (%)	*Erwinia* positive	*Erwinia* positive (%)
1996	364	0	0	0	0
1997	185	0	0	0	0
1998	776	0	0	29	3.7
1999	265	0	0	16	6.0
2000	664	0	0	28	4.2
2001	483	0	0	24	4.9
Total	2,737	0	0	97	3.5

Table 4. Seed tuber samples (4605 tubers per sample) tested for *R.. solanacearum*

Year	Samples tested	*R. solanacearum* positive	*R. solanacearum* positive (%)
1995	464	20	4.3
1996	690	24	3.5
1997	728	6	0.8
1998	786	4	0.5
1999	715	10	1.4
2000	328	1	0.3
2001	557	0	0.0
Total	4,268	65	1.52

(G1 - G8) in 1995, 65 of the 4268 statistically-based tuber samples tested positive for *R. solanacearum*. No visible bacterial wilt symptoms were detected during field inspections in these cases. These results indicate that if these plantings had not been tested, 1.52% of the seed tubers offered for certification over the past seven years, would have been infected and there-fore would not only have seriously hampered yield and quality but also would have spread the disease to previously uninfected locations (Table 4).

There has been a definite downward trend in the number of bacterial wilt cases since the introduction of compulsory testing, and it is believed that the control measures implemented by the South African Potato Certification Schemes are not only beneficial in the control of the disease, but essential for the survival of the potato industry in South Africa.

Literature Cited

1. Bellstedt, D.U., and Van der Merwe, K.J. 1989.The development of ELISA kits for detection of *Pseudomonas solanacearum* bacterial wilt in potatoes. First International Research Symposium. S. Afr. J. Sci. 85: 672-676.
2. Clayton, M.K., and Slack, S.A. 1988. Sample size determination in zero tolerance circumstances and the implications of stepwise sampling: Bacterial ring rot as a special case. Am. Potato J. 165: 711-723.
3. Cuppels, D., and Kelman, A. 1974. Evaluation of selective media for the isolation of soft-rot bacteria from soil and plant tissue. Phytopathology 64: 468-475.

4. Doidge, E.M. 1914. Some diseases of the potato. Union S. Afr. Agric. J. 7: 698-703.
5. Elphinstone, J.G., Hennessy, J., Wilson, J.K., and Stead, D.E. 1996. Sensitivity of different methods for the detection of *Ralstonia solanacearum* in potato tuber extracts. EPPO Bull. 26: 663-678.
6. Hayward, A.C.1976. Some techniques of importance in the identification of *Pseudomonas solanacearum*. Pages 137-142 in: Proceedings of the International Planning Conference and Workshop on Ecology and Control of Bacterial Wilt Caused by *Pseudomonas solanacearum*. Raleigh, North Carolina 18-24 July. L. Sequeira and A. Kelman, eds.
7. Kelman, A. 1954. The relationship of pathogenicity in *Pseudomonas solanacearum* to colony appearance on a tetrazolium medium. Phytopathology 44: 693-695.
8. Serfontein, S., Logan, C., Swanepoel, A.E., Boelema, B.H., and Theron, D.J. 1991. A potato wilt disease in South Africa caused by *Erwinia carotovora* subspecies *carotovora* and *E. chrysanthemi*. Plant Pathol. 40: 382-386.
9. Swanepoel, A.E., and Young, B.W. 1988. Characteristics of South African strains of *Pseudomonas solanacearum*. Plant Dis. 72:403-404.

Integrated Control of Potato Bacterial Wilt in Eastern Africa: The Experience of African Highlands Initiative

Berga Lemaga[1], R. Kakuhenzire[2], Bekele Kassa[3],
P.T. Ewell[4], and S. Priou[5]

[1]PRAPACE, Kampala, Uganda; [2]National Agricultural Research Organization, Uganda; [3]Ethiopian Agricultural Research Organization, Addis Ababa, Ethiopia; [4]CIP, Nairobi, Kenya; [5]CIP, Lima, Peru

Introduction

The potato (*Solanum tuberosum L*) is an important food security and cash crop in the highlands of eastern and central Africa, and it is expanding to the lowlands. However, the national yields average less than 7 t/Ha, which are very low compared with the world average of 16.3 t/Ha and the Africa average of 11.5 t/Ha (6). Factors such as diseases, insects, weather, declining soil fertility and inadequate farmer knowledge and practice contribute to the low yields.

Bacterial wilt of potato caused by *Ralstonia solanacearum* is, after late blight, the most important biotic constraint to potato production in eastern Africa. Yield losses due to bacterial wilt are estimated as high as 50% in ware and 75% in seed potatoes in Kenya (1) and over 30% in Uganda (2) with occasional losses of 100% (9,17). In Ethiopia, the disease has been observed at altitudes higher than 3,000 meters. Race 3 is the major cause of bacterial wilt in the region, although race 1 is also present in the lowlands of Kenya and Uganda and biovar 2-T has been reported in Kenya (17,21). Past experience has shown that *R. solanacearum* race 3 can be successfully controlled by integrated disease management (IDM) practices. The most important components of IDM include bacterial wilt-free seed (4), crop rotation (8,15), use of less susceptible varieties (22), and pathogen-free soil. The successful control of bacterial wilt by small-holder farmers in the region is a challenge because of small and fragmented landholdings that limit crop rotation, intensively cultivated landscapes with declining soil fertility, presence of a variety of weed hosts and different *R. solanacearum* biovars.

145

Research to control bacterial wilt in the region was undertaken between 1995 and 1999 by the African Highlands Initiative, an Eco-regional program of the CGIAR affiliated with the Association of Strengthening Agricultural Research in East and Central Africa (ASARECA) and the Global Mountain Program, in collaboration with the Uganda National Agricultural Research Organization (NARO). The research focused on testing various sets of IDM options and identification of IDM components, some of which are reported here. The objectives of the research presented in this paper were to (a) identify biovars of *R. solanacearum* in Uganda, (b) provide potato producers with pragmatic and economically viable IDM options for the control of bacterial wilt and (c) determine the effects of various control components on bacterial wilt incidence and tuber yields.

Materials and Methods

BIOVAR IDENTIFICATION

A total of 106 samples of infected tubers were collected from plants exhibiting bacterial wilt symptoms at altitudes ranging from 1200 m to 2500 m in Uganda. Bacterial exudates were removed from the tubers and suspended in sterilized distilled water in Uganda and biovar identification was done at the International Potato Center (CIP), Lima. Isolations for the determination of *R. solanacearum* were made on Kelman's TZC medium (10) directly from tuber oozing extracts or after enrichment in M-SMSA (5). The determination of biovars of *R. solanacearum* was based on the utilization of two disaccharides: lactose and maltose, and the oxidation of two hexose alcohols: mannitol and sorbitol (7) [Editor's note: according to the original publication of Hayward, biovar classification should also include cellobiose and dulcitol]. The differentiation of biovar 2 phenotypes 2-A and 2-T [Editor's note; biovar 2-T also named biovar N2 in the literature] was based on the utilization of D (-) ribose, D (+) trehalose, L (-) tryptophan and L (+) tartrate (7).

OPTIONS FOR INTEGRATED CONTROL OF BACTERIAL WILT

Research on the integrated control of potato bacterial wilt was conducted in Uganda and Ethiopia using a farmer participatory approach. This paper will focus on results from Uganda, where research was conducted in Kabale, a major potato-growing district in the southwest, for five seasons between 1995 and 1997, while in Ethiopia it was done in 1997 in the surroundings of the Plant Protection Research Center. The selection of participating farmers and communities was based on the presence of bacterial wilt in the field plots to be used and farmers' willingness to provide land for the experiment, perform recommended cultural practices for IDM, and harvest the crop at maturity.

The management options assessed were (a) improved package consisting of a less susceptible variety, Victoria (CIP-381381.20), bacterial wilt-free seed, planting in rows at a spacing of 75 x 30 cm; hilling at planting; roguing of volunteer potatoes; sanitation; and minimum post-emergence cultivation, (b) the farmer package consisting of farmers' variety, farmers' seed and farmers' cultural practices, (c) bacterial wilt-free seed of var. Victoria planted under farmers' cultural practices and (d) farmers' variety and seed planted under improved cultural practices. Within a season, each farmer's field (farm) was considered as a replication; the number of farmers per season averaged 14. For each plot, the soil type and history of crop rotation were recorded. Plots were assessed at weekly intervals to determine days to onset of first wilt symptoms. Subsequent counts of wilted plants were made at two-week intervals. At each assessment, all plants that showed either complete or partial wilting were considered wilted and staked. The counts of wilted plants were expressed as a percent of the total number of plants that emerged. Late blight was controlled with three to four sprays of Dithane M45, starting from the first visible symptoms. Farmers participated in collecting disease data, harvesting and in discussions to evaluate the options. Data on bacterial wilt incidence were subjected to square root transformation before analysis using Genstat 4.23. This paper presents the results of IDM experiments in Uganda; these were fairly similar to the results obtained in Ethiopia.

ECONOMIC ANALYSIS

Analyses of partial budget and marginal rates of return were done in Uganda for each of the IDM options to select those that are economically beneficial. Twenty-two farmers who participated in on-farm integrated bacterial wilt control experiments in 1997 were also involved in this study. The costs of different inputs and cultural practices that varied for each option were obtained from the farmers and from the National Potato Program. The income generated from each option varied according to the proportions of produce sold as seed or as ware and also the location of sale (market or farm gate), all of which were taken into consideration. Net benefits were calculated by subtracting total costs from gross income. The exchange rate in 1997, US$1= UgSh 1050, was used. Marginal rates of return were analyzed to determine the benefits farmers gained in return to their investment by changing from their traditional practice to each of the management options.

SOIL AMENDMENTS

This study was conducted in the 1998A, 1998B, and 1999A seasons at Kachwekano Agricultural Research and Development Center (KARDC) in southwest Uganda. The soils at Kachwekano are generally deficient in nitrogen and are acidic. The experiment was laid out in a randomized complete block design with three replications. Disease-free Victoria potato seed pieces were planted in plots amended with either organic materials from *Sesbania sesban* (Sesbania) or *Leucaena diversifolia* (leucaena), inorganic fertilizers nitrogen (N), phosphorus (P), potassium (K), or with different combinations of these organic and inorganic fertilizers. Fresh sesbania and leucaena leaves and twigs were incorporated into soil a week before planting in amounts required to supply 100 kg N/Ha. Inorganic fertilizers N, P, and K were side-dressed at rates of 100 kg/Ha each as urea, triple super phosphate (TSP), and murate of potash (KCl), respectively. Full doses of TSP and KCl were applied at planting, while urea was split-applied in equal halves at planting and one month after planting. The control of late blight and methods used to assess and collect data on bacterial wilt incidence, yields, and statistical analyses were similar to those used in the IDM experiment.

CROP ROTATION

Rotation experiments were conducted between the 1995B and 1999A seasons at KARDC, Uganda. Fields that showed uniform bacterial wilt incidence before the experiment were used to conduct one- and two-season rotation trials. The one-season rotation trial was conducted in a field that exhibited an initial bacterial wilt incidence of 15–20% (mildly infested), while the two-season trial was conducted in a field that exhibited an initial bacterial wilt incidence of over 90% (heavily infested). Crops that are commonly grown in the area were included in the rotation treatments. Plots were laid out in a randomized complete block design with three replications for the one-season experiment and four replications for the two-season experiment. In the two-season experiment, either two different rotational crops or the same crop were grown in two consecutive seasons. bacterial wilt-free seed of the potato variety Victoria was used for both trials, and local varieties were used for the rotation crops. All the crops were planted at their recommended spacing. Control of late blight, data collection and analysis were similar to the other two experiments.

Results and Discussion

BIOVAR IDENTIFICATION

Of the 106 samples sent to Lima, *R. solanacearum* could be isolated by direct plating on Kelman's medium from only 21 samples because of delays in transport and custom clearance in Lima, where the tests were conducted. However, the post enrichment procedure increased the number of isolations to 68 samples from which 66, all collected from the highlands of southwest Uganda, belonged to biovar 2. Two isolates obtained at an altitude of 1224 m in central Uganda, near Kampala, belonged to biovar 3. This is in agreement with the findings of Opio (17) who reported the presence of race 1 biovar3 strains in the same location. The phenotypic differentiation of biovar 2 isolates revealed that they all belonged to 2-A indicating the absence of 2-T in the sampled areas. Smith *et al.* (21), however, reported the presence of 2-T in western Kenya so it may be important to include areas bordering Kenya before it is concluded that biovar 2-T is absent in Uganda.

OPTIONS FOR INTEGRATED CONTROL OF BACTERIAL WILT RACE 3

The incidence of bacterial wilt varied with the seasons (Table 1) due to variations in weather conditions, particularly rainfall and soil populations of *R. solanacearum*. Wilt incidence was higher during the seasons that had more rainfall. Regardless of seasons, the lowest wilt incidence was recorded under improved package and the highest under farmer package with differences being significant most of the time. Tuber yields were significantly higher with improved package than with farmer package, and yields of the other two options were intermediate.

The results of this study suggest that bacterial wilt-free seed is an important component of IDM of bacterial wilt substantiating those of Berrios and Rubirigi (4) in Burundi. In the region, shortage of bacterial wilt-free seed is the leading constraint to potato production, and farmers usually buy seed of unknown origin. This increases the chances of bacterial wilt dissemination through latently infected tubers (23). CABI Bioscience, CIP, and their national partners in Kenya have developed a technology to produce bacterial wilt-free seed at higher densities in small nursery beds that are bacterial wilt-free (11). This technology is being promoted by NARO, the NGO Africare, CIP and PRAPACE using the farmer field schools (FFS) approach funded by IFAD. This together with the informal farmer-based bacterial wilt-free seed production initiated by CIP will help partially solve the seed problem. In this experiment, since bacterial wilt-free seed of a less susceptible variety Victoria was used, we anticipate that host

Table 1. Effects of bacterial wilt management options on wilt incidence, total and marketable yields during seasons 1996A, 1996B, and 1997A, Kabale, Uganda

Options	Wilt incidence[a] (%)	Total yield (t/Ha)	Marketable yield (t/Ha)
1996A			
Improved package	5.3	17.1	16.5
Farmer package	13.4	12.1	12.3
Improved variety and bacterial wilt-free seed under farmer cultural practices	9.7	14.6	14.1
Farmer variety and seed under improved cultural practices	11.0	10.1	10.4
$LSD_{0.05}$	NS	3.2	4.1
1996B			
Improved package	15.8b	15.8	14.8
Farmer package	27.8a	10.8	9.9
Improved variety and bacterial wilt-free seed under farmer cultural practices	20.7b	11.7	10.8
Farmer variety and seed under improved cultural practices	24.1b	13.5	12.1
$LSD_{0.05}$		2.3	2.3
1997A			
Improved package	6.1b	10.4	10.1
Farmer package	20.7a	7.6	7.3
Improved variety and bacterial wilt-free seed under farmer cultural practices	9.9b	7.9	7.7
Farmer variety and seed under improved cultural practices	17.1a	9.7	9.3
$LSD_{0.05}$		1.9	2.0

[a] NS = not significant. Means followed by the same letter in columns are not significantly different at $P < 0.05$ by Duncan's Multiple Range test. Extracted from Lemaga (13).

resistance might have contributed to reducing wilt, as reported by Tusiime *et al.* (22). Although improved cultural practices did not significantly reduce wilt in this experiment, they contributed to the overall good performance of improved package. Indeed best results were obtained when a less susceptible variety, bacterial wilt-free seed and improved cultural practices were combined in an IDM option.

The improved package resulted in the highest net benefit of US$3347/Ha followed by the package consisting of a less susceptible variety and bacterial wilt-free seed planted under farmer cultural practices and farmer variety and seed planted under improved cultural practices, whose net benefits were $2547 and $1889, respectively.

ECONOMIC ANALYSIS

All the three options resulted in higher economic benefits than the farmer package despite the lowest variable cost of the latter (Table 2).

The difference in benefits between the last two options was not due to differences in yields, but in amounts sold as seed and ware with the seed fetching more money. Results of marginal rates of return (MRR) showed that the benefits of changing from farmer package to the improved package, less susceptible variety and bacterial wilt-free seed planted under farmer cultural practices and to farmer variety and seed-planted under improved cultural practices were 1034%, 805% and 634%, respectively.

All these values are much higher than the 100% MRR usually accepted to be high enough to recommend a given technology for adoption. Thus, all

Table 2. Analysis of partial budget and marginal rates of return for farmer and improved management options

| Components | Bacterial wilt management options | | | |
	Improved package	Farmer package	Less susceptible cv. and bacterial wilt-free seed in farmers' cultural practices	Farmer cv. and seed in improved cultural practices
Yield (t/Ha)	13.9	9.4	11.3	11.7
Income from seed*	3,386	1,206	2,621	1,286
Income from ware*	848	981	782	1,371
Gross income*	4,233	2,187	3,382	2,657
Costs that vary*	884	69	836	768
Net benefit*	3,347	1,483	2,547	1,889
Marginal rates of return (%)	1,034	-	806	634

* Values in US$/Ha.

Extracted from Lemaga (13).

the options can be recommended, with the improved package being the best.

SOIL AMENDMENTS

Soil amendments significantly affected mean bacterial wilt incidence and both total and marketable tuber yields (Table 3). Wilt incidence was lowest with the treatment *Sesbania* + phosphorus + potassium, which differed significantly from all other treatments except for the treatment NP. Well-nourished plants can better withstand disease organisms than poorly nourished ones (16) probably because of absorption of adequate nutrients through a well-established root system. Earlier studies indicated a negative relationship between the population of *R. solanacearum* race 3 and soil nitrogen content (19). In the current study, however, adding the green manures alone did not necessarily reduce wilt incidence, but when they were added together with inorganic fertilizers, they became useful. The discrepancy can partly be explained by differences in supressiveness, moisture and NPK contents of the different soils used.

Table 3. Effect of soil amendments on mean bacterial wilt incidence, potato yields over three seasons (1998A, 1998B and 1999A), Kabale

Treatments[a]	Bacterial wilt incidence (%)	Total yield (t Ha^{-1})	Marketable yield (t Ha^{-1})	Relative increase in marketable yield (%)
Sesbania (S)	27.8ab	18.1b	16.6b	71.6
Leucaena (L)	30.3ab	16.8bc	14.9bc	54.1
S+PK	19.1c	22.4a	20.8a	114.6
L+PK	26.2ab	18.8b	16.4b	69.7
SP	26.0a	17.1bc	15.2bc	56.9
LP	27.1ab	15.4c	13.3c	37.4
NPK	22.8ab	18.8b	16.9b	74.6
NP	16.2bc	16.6bc	15.2bc	56.9
Control	32.2a	11.2d	9.7d	-
%CV	22.3	14.0	16.7	

[a] N = nitrogen, P = Phosphorus, K = Potassium. Means followed by same letters in columns are not statistically different at $P < 0.05$. Most data adopted from Lemaga *et al.* (14).

152

Soil amendments significantly increased both total and marketable tuber yields when compared with the control (Table 3). Adding sesbania alone was as effective as application of NPK or application of leucaena + phosphorus + potassium. The highest total and marketable yields of 22.4 t/Ha and 20.8 t/Ha, respectively were obtained from a combined application of sesbania and PK and both yields differed significantly from all other treatments. This could be attributed to a better nutrient balance achieved when both organic and inorganic sources are used, as organic residues improve nutrient availability and nutrient use efficiency (18).

While adding phosphorus did not increase yield, potassium was found to be useful for both reducing bacterial wilt incidence and increasing tuber yields, which is contrary to the general belief that east African soils are rich in potassium. The results of this experiment suggest that the use of both organic and inorganic soil amendments is a better option than using either of them. In this study, sesbania performed better than leucaena perhaps because of its lower polyphenol content.

CROP ROTATION

A one-season rotation with cereals, pulses, vegetables and root crops in a mildly infested field (15-20% infestation) significantly decreased bacterial wilt incidence ($P < 0.05$) and significantly increased tuber yields ($P < 0.01$) when compared with the control (Table 4A). The various rotation treatments, however, did not differ form each other. This substantiates the findings of Kloos et al. (12), who reported significant wilt reductions after a one-season rotation. The table also shows that although rotations with millet and sweet potatoes resulted in the lowest wilt incidences, the corresponding tuber yields were lower than those obtained after rotations with onions and carrots that had relatively high wilt incidences. This may be attributed to the higher nutrient removal from the soil by sweet potatoes and millets as compared to shallow-rooted carrots and onions. It is thus important to also consider the soil fertility aspect when crops are selected for rotation with potatoes. Gunadi et al. (8) also obtained high tuber yields in a rotation following carrots. Sweet potato, which is an important food crop in the region, can be a good rotation crop for potatoes in areas prone to bacterial wilt. This is in agreement with the findings of Kloos et al. (12), Bang and Wiles (3) and Priou (pers. comm.).

A two-season rotation with cereals and beans in a heavily infested (>90% incidence) field reduced wilt incidence to less than 50%, which was significant compared to a wilt incidence of over 80% recorded under the control monocrop (Table 4B). Wilt reductions were greatest where two different crops were planted in succession rather than the same crop in two

Table 4. Effect of one-season (A) and two-season (B) crop rotation on wilt incidence and tubers yields, Kabale, Uganda[a]

Treatment	Bacterial wilt incidence (%)	Total yield (t Ha⁻¹)	Marketable yield (t Ha⁻¹)
A. One-season			
Potato (Pot)-onions-pot	12.4b	20.4a	20.0a
Pot-peas-pot	5.0b	18.6a	18.5a
Pot-cabbage-pot	6.9b	17.7a	17.6a
Pot-sweet potato-pot	3.8b	16.4ab	16.4a
Pot-millet-pot	3.2b	16.7ab	16.7a
Pot-carrots-pot	11.0b	20.4a	20.4a
Pot-beans-pot	7.4b	18.1a	18.1a
Pot-pot-pot	62.2a	12.4b	11.1b
B. Two-season			
Pot-beans-wheat-pot	36.4bcd	9.27a	7.40a
Pot-beans-maize-pot	21.9d	10.37a	9.00a
Pot-wheat-maize-pot	25.2cd	10.7a	8.90a
Pot-beans-beans-pot	40.3bc	8.92a	6.68a
Pot-maize-maize-pot	49.4b	10.15a	8.40a
Pot-wheat-wheat-pot	40.0bc	10.73a	9.23a
Pot-pot-pot-pot	81.1a	3.20b	1.85b
LSD $_{(0.05)}$		2.72	2.41

[a] Means followed by the same letters in columns are not significantly different at 5% probability level. Extracted from Lemaga *et al.* (15).

consecutive seasons. This result supports the findings of Bang and Wiles (4), who reported that in a two-season rotation, a higher reduction in wilt was obtained with the treatment maize-sweetpotato than with sweetpotato-sweetpotato. Interestingly, bean, which is a symptomless carrier of *R. solanacearum*, can be a good rotation crop if it is followed or preceded by a cereal in a potato rotation sequence. This is important because beans are a cheap source of protein for the poor in the region.

Conclusion

Research reported here suggests that *R. solanacearum* biovar 2-A can be satisfactorily controlled in Sub-Saharan Africa by the combined use of bacterial wilt-free seed of a less susceptible variety and improved cultural practices. The use of bacterial wilt-free seed of a less susceptible variety under the farmer cultural practices or the use of improved cultural practices with the existing farmer varieties has the potential to significantly reduce wilt and increase yield. All three options are easy to adopt and utilize and are economically beneficial based on partial budget analysis. Bacterial wilt-free seed proved to be a very important component of IDM and its production on small plots using the FFS approach needs to be enhanced. Moreover, the seed health status in relation to latent infections should be monitored with CIP serological kits (19).

Crop rotation, another important component of IDM, significantly reduced wilt and increased yield even under serious bacterial wilt infestations. Generally, cereals proved to be better than pulses as rotation crops for potatoes in bacterial wilt infested soils. An important crop in the region, sweet potato, also proved to be a good rotation crop. In a two-season rotation, planting two different crops in succession is better than planting the same crop in two consecutive seasons. Control measures become more effective under good soil management, preferably fertilized with a combination of organic and inorganic sources. However, more work needs to be done in the validation of these options in soils infested with other biovars of *R. solanacearum*, production of bacterial wilt-free seed and application of good quarantine measures both within and between countries. A community-based approach that intensively involves women farmers can bring about a successful control of bacterial wilt using the IDM components mentioned above.

Literature Cited

1. Ajanga, S. 1993. Status of bacterial wilt of potato in Kenya. Pages 338-340 in: Bacterial Wilt. ACIAR Proc. No. 45, G.L. Hartman and A.C. Hayward, eds. Canberra, Australia.
2. Alacho, F.O., and Akimanzi, D.R.. 1993. Progress achievements and constraints on bacterial wilt control in Uganda. Pages 32-41 in: Workshop on Bacterial Wilt of Potato Caused by *Pseudomonas solanacearum*, Bujumbura, Burundi, Feb. 22-26, 1993.
3. Bang, S.K., and Wiles, G.C. 1996. Control of bacterial wilt (*Pseudomonas solanacearum*) in potato by crop rotation, Final Report. Pages 79-86 in: SAPPRAD on the fourth year of phase III. Selected research papers. Vol. 1: Potato. E.T. Rasco, Jr. and F.B Aromin, eds. South Asian Program for Potato Research and Development, Manila, Philippines.
4. Berrios, D.E., and Rubirigi, A. 1993. Integrated control of bacterial wilt in seed production by the Burundi national Potato Program. Pages

284-288 in: Bacterial Wilt. ACIAR Proc. No. 45. G.L. Hartman and A.C. Hayward, eds. Canberra, Australia.

5. Elphinstone, J.G., Hennessy, J., Wilson, J.K., and Stead., D.E. 1996. Sensitivity of different methods for the detection of *Pseudomonas solanacearum* (Smith) in potato tuber extracts. EPPO Bull. 26: 663-678.

6. FAO. 2001. Production yearbook. Food and Agricultural Organization of the United Nations, Rome, Italy.

7. French, E.R., Gutarra, L., Aley, P., and Elphinstone, J. 1995. Culture media for *Pesudomonas solanacearum*: isolation, identification and maintenance. Fitopatologia. 30: 126-130.

8. Gunadi, N., Chujoy, E., Kusmana, M., Surviani, I., Gunawan, O.S., and Sinung-Basuki, R. 1998. Pages 58-61 in: Effect of crop rotation patterns on *Ralstonia solanacearum* population in the soil. Potato research in Indonesia. CIP Working Paper Series. CIP/RIV.

9. Kakuhenzire, R., Alacho, F., Birikunzira, J., Turyamureeba, G., and Sikka, L. 1993. Progress in field evaluation for resistance to *Pseudomonas solanacearum* and cultural methods for control of bacterial wilt in Uganda. Pages 76-82 in: Workshop on Bacterial Wilt of Potato Caused by *Pseudomonas solanacearum*, Bujumbura, Burundi, Feb. 22-26, 1993.

10. Kelman, A. 1954. The relationship of pathogenicity in *Pseudomonas solanacearum* to colony appearance on tetrazolium medium. Phytopathology. 44: 693-695.

11. Kinyua, Z.M., Smith, J.J., Lung'aho, C., Olanya, M., and Priou., S. 2001. On-farm success and challenges of producing bacterial wilt-free tubers in seed plots in Kenya. Afr. Crop Sci. J. 9: 279-285.

12. Kloos, J.P., Fernandez, B.B., Tumapon, A.S., and Villanueva, L. 1991. Effects of crop rotation on incidence of potato bacterial wilt caused by *Pseudomonas solanacearum* E.F. Smith. Asian Potato J. 2: 1-3.

13. Lemaga , B. 2001. Integrated control of potato bacterial wilt in Kabale district, southwestern Uganda. Pages 129-141 in: Scientist and Farmer: Partners in research for the 21st Century. CIP Program Report 1999-2000.

14. Lemaga, B., Siriri, D., and Ebanyat, P. 2001a. Effect of soil amendments on bacterial wilt incidence and yield of potatoes in southwestern Uganda. Afr. Crop Sci. J. 9: 267–278.

15. Lemaga, B., Kanzikwera, R., Kakuhenzire, R., Hakiza, J.J., and Manzi, G. 2001b. The effect of crop rotation on bacterial wilt incidence and potato tuber yield. Afr. Crop Sci. J. 9: 257–266.

16. Muchovej, V.V., Muchovej, R.C.M., Dingra, O.D., and Majia, L.A. 1980. Suppression of anthracnose of soybeans by calcium. Plant Dis. 64: 1088–1089.

17. Opio, A.F. 1988. Host range and biotypes of *Pseudomonas solanacearum* E.F. Smith in Uganda: A preliminary study. Paper

presented at the 15th Int. Congr. Plant Pathol., Kyoto, Japan, 20-27 August 1988.

18. Palm, C.A., and Rowland, A.P. 1997. Chemical characterisation of plant quality for decomposition. Pages 379-392 in: Driven by Nature: Plant Litter Quality and Decomposition. G. Cadish and K.E. Giller, eds. CAB International, Wallingford, UK.

19. Prior, P., Beramis, M., Clairon, M., Quiquampoix, H., Robert, M., and Schmit, J. 1993. Contribution to integrated control against bacterial wilt in different pedoclimatic situations: Guadeloupe Experience. Pages 294-304 in: G.L. Hartman and A.C. Hayward , eds. Bacterial wilt. ACIAR Proc. No. 45, Canberra, Australia.

20. Priou, S., Gutarra, L., and Aley, P. 1999. Highly sensitive detection of *Ralstonia solanacearum* in latently infected potato tubers by post-enrichment ELISA on nitrocellulose membrane. EPPO Bull. 29: 117-125.

21. Smith, J.J., Saddler, G.S., Holderness, M., and Offord, L.C. 1996. Biological control of *Pseudomonas solanacearum*: Causative organism of bacterial wilt disease. International Mycological Institute. ODA RNRRS Contract R5310 (NRI: EMC X0194), Report for the period 1 February- 31 March 1996.

22. Tusiime, G., Adipala, E., Opio, F., and Bhagsari, A.S. 1996a. Screening *solanum* potato genotypes for resistance to *Pseudomonas solanacearum* in Uganda. Afr. J. Plant Prot. 6: 96-107.

23. Tusiime, G., Adipala, E., Opio, F., and Bhagsari, A.S. 1996b. Occurrence of *Pseudomonas solanacearum* latent infection in potato tubers and weeds in highland Uganda. Afr. J. Plant Prot. 6: 108-118.

Using *Brassica* spp. as Biofumigants to Reduce the Population of *Ralstonia solanacearum*

J.R. Arthy[1], E.B. Akiew[1], J.A. Kirkegaard[2], and P.R. Trevorrow[1]

[1]Queensland Department of Primary Industries, Mareeba, Queensland, Australia, 4880; [2]Commonwealth Scientific and Industrial Research Organisation, Acton, Canberra, Australia, 2601

Bacterial wilt caused by *Ralstonia solanacearum* (biovar 3) is a major disease affecting vegetable production in central and north Queensland. Biovar 2 has only been recorded on potatoes grown in the Atherton Tablelands region of north Queensland and is less economically important than biovar 3. Bacterial wilt (biovar 3) causes significant losses in the tomato, capsicum, chili, eggplant, potato, and tobacco industries of the region. Unfortunately the options for control are very limited and the most common recommendations to growers are to use a two- to three-year rotation or grow a non-host crop. These options are not possible in some cropping systems due to resource and financial constraints and therefore management of this disease requires further investigation.

In 1995, biocidal compounds released from decomposing *Brassica* plant tissue were found to reduce the population of *R. solanacearum* in inoculated soil *in vitro*. These preliminary findings formed the basis for the concept of using biofumigation to control bacterial wilt in the field. Biofumigation in this instance describes the process of using *Brassica* green manure crops to control soil-borne diseases of other crops. In the field a 77% reduction in bacterial wilt infection in tobacco was achieved by using a commercially available Indian mustard variety *(Brassica juncea)* (2). Based on encouraging preliminary results, small laboratory trials were established to test the effects of 45 different *Brassica* varieties on the population of a rifampicin-resistant strain of *R. solanacearum*. The results of these trials indicated that *Brassica* spp. differ in their ability to reduce the population of the bacterium.

The culmination of over three years of research into the use of *Brassica* plants as biofumigation crops has resulted in a project titled 'Evaluating biofumigation for soil-borne disease management in tropical vegetable production' funded by the Australian Centre for International Agricultural

Research (ACIAR). Until recently all experiments involving biofumigation and the monitoring of *R. solanacearum* populations have been carried out in the laboratory. This paper describes an experiment designed to test the effectiveness of the *Brassica* plants in reducing the population of *R. solanacearum* under field conditions.

Biofumigation Using *Brassicas*

GLUCOSINOLATES AND ISOTHIOCYANATES

Cruciferous plants, which include crops such as canola, fodder rape, radish and mustard synthesize amino acid-derived compounds called glucosinolates (10). Brassica and radish plants contain significant quantities of glucosinolates in all parts of the plant, however the type and concentration of these compounds varies between species and varieties (7). When the myrinase enzyme hydrolyses glucosinolates during cell rupture or decomposition, isothiocyanates, nitriles or thiocyanates are formed (7). The volatile isothiocyanates (ITCs) are responsible for the strong flavour of mustards and radishes and have also been shown to have anti-microbial activity. The effects of green manure *Brassica* plants on other plant pathogens has been reported by Mojtahedi *et al.* (6) and Chan *et al.* (4). Chan *et al.* reported an average 41% reduction in the disease severity index of *Aphanomyces* root rot of peas. Mojtahedi *et al.* studied the effects of decomposing *Brassica* tissue on nematode population density and found a significant reduction using rapeseed as a green manure. Akiew *et al.* (2) found that Indian mustard and black mustard were more effective than other brassicas in reducing the population of *R. solanacearum* in the field.

Isothiocyanates are also the active ingredients of commercially available soil fumigants such as Basamid and Metham sodium, however in these products the concentration of ITC is much higher than is present in *Brassica* leaf tissue. For example, the concentration of methyl isothiocyanate in Basamid is 1500 nmoles/g and, depending on the method of incorporation, the release from incorporating *Brassica* leaf could range from 50-1000 nmoles/g of tissue (3).

BIOFUMIGATION IN THE FIELD

In the field situation, the concept of biofumigation can be tailored to suit the crop being grown. The use of biofumigation to control *R. solanacearum* in north Queensland, Australia can be applied to many different cropping systems, however the concept is generally the same for all crops. The biofumigant crop is grown up until early flowering stage at 8-10 weeks and it is at this time that the concentration of glucosinolates is at its highest (8). Once the crop has reached early flowering, a rotary hoe is used to incorporate the crop to a depth of approximately 15 cm. To increase the degree of tissue maceration, two or more passes of the rotary hoe are recommended. The field/seed bed is watered to provide a seal and left undisturbed for a period of 4 weeks to allow for complete breakdown of the plant material. After this withholding period, the land is prepared and the commercial crop is sown. Recent experiments by the CSIRO team have demonstrated that much higher release of ITCs can be achieved using mulching prior to incorporation and/or irrigation following incorporation.

Combined Laboratory and Field Experiment

MATERIALS AND METHODS

The nine *Brassica* varieties representing five *Brassica* spp. (*B. napus, B. carinata, B. juncea, B. nigra,* and *B. oleraceae*) and one radish variety (*Raphanus sativus*) used in the experiment were grown under shade cloth until the plants reached early flowering. At this time, the leaves and shoots were harvested, chopped finely and incorporated at a rate of 5% fresh weight (FW) into 500g of field soil previously inoculated with a rifampicin resistant strain of *R. solanacearum* (biovar 3) to a level of 7.5×10^7 colony forming units (CFU)/g soil. The control treatments included were tobacco (host crop), forage sorghum (non-host crop) at 5% FW and soil with no amendments.

The inoculated soil and plant material were mixed thoroughly and placed onto two layers of cheesecloth material; the bundles were then tied and buried at a trial site to a depth of 20cm. There were 13 treatments altogether with three replicates of each treatment arranged in blocks. The soil was sampled at three different times: 10, 20 and 30 days after burial. The bacteria were recovered on casamino acid glucose peptone agar (bactopeptone 10g/L, caseinamino hydrolysate 1g/L, bacto-agar 15g/L and glucose 5g/L) (5) containing tetrazolium chloride (5ml of a 1% solution per L), cycloheximide (100mg/L) and rifampicin(100mg/L).

At each sample time 10g of soil were removed from the overall sample and diluted in 90ml of sterile water. The samples were re-buried after each sub sample. The serial dilution plating method was used to determine bacterial populations with $100\mu L$ of each dilution plated and plates were incubated at 30°C for 48 h. A log(x+1) transformation was applied to the data and ANOVA was used to analyse the data for each sample time. Frozen samples of the plant tissue used in this experiment were analysed for glucosinolate concentration.

The population counts for Days 10 and 30 are presented in this paper; Day 20 population counts do not reveal any trends or differences not explained by Day 10 and 30 counts.

RESULTS

At each sample time significant differences were found between treatments (Tables 1 and 2). On Day 10 (Table 1), the only treatment with a significantly lower bacterial population than the unamended soil control was variety number 29. All other treatments with the exception of tobacco could not be separated statistically from the unamended soil only control. The varieties with the highest glucosinolate concentration (29, 23, 38, 24, and 90) all recorded lower population counts than the unamended soil control; however, these were not significant in most cases. Variety number 60 has a very low glucosinolate concentration (0.6 μmoles/g tissue) when compared with the other varieties listed in the top half of the table.

Table 1. Effect of soil amendment with *Brassica, Raphanus,* and other plant species on *R. solanacearum* population 10 days after amendment

Variety No/ Species	Mean CFU[1]/g soil (back transformed)	LSD group (5%)	Glucosinolate Concentration (μmoles/g tissue)
29/*Brassica nigra*	1371	a	42.4
23/*B.carinata*	1394	ab	25.5
38/*B.juncea*	2427	abc	13.6
24/*B.carinata*	2880	abc	29.0
60/*B.napus*	3662	abcd	0.4
90/*Raphanus sativus*	4225	abcde	16.2
Soil (Control)	10403	bcdef	0.0
Broccoli/*B.oleraceae*	13426	cdefg	2.4
Forage sorghum	15183	cdefg	0.0
Cabbage/*B.oleraceae*	23812	defg	3.7
58/*B.napus*	30363	efg	3.0
57/*B.napus*	38753	fg	6.4
Tobacco	82124	g	0.0

[1] Colony forming units.

On Day 30 (Table 2), a similar trend exists within the data (as seen on Day 10) however there are some marked differences. At this sample time, variety number 29 and the tobacco control had significantly less population levels than all other treatments. All varieties with the exception of cabbage reduced the population significantly when compared with the unamended soil control and the forage sorghum control. Once again, the varieties with the highest glucosinolate concentration fall in the top half of the table; however, this trend is not as clear as at Day 10 and the appearance of tobacco at the top of the table requires some explanation.

A difference in the speed with which the leaf material of the different varieties decomposes was also observed for the first time. At 10 days after burial there was little or no evidence of the leaf material incorporated in the following treatments 29, 23, 24, and 38. In all other treatments with the exception of the unamended soil control, the leaf material remained intact with little or no degradation apparent, and was yellow in color. It can be speculated that those treatments, in which the leaf material decomposed very rapidly, would have completed their biofumigation activity by Day 10.

Table 2. Effect of soil amendment with *Brassica, Raphanus,* and other plant species on *R. solanacearum* population 30 days after amendment

Variety Number/ Species	Mean CFU[1]/g soil (back transformed)	LSD group (5%)	Glucosinolate Concentration (μmoles/g tissue)
Tobacco	2.36	a	0.0
29/*B.nigra*	3.88	a	42.4
Broccoli	4.42	ab	2.4
38/*B.juncea*	12.4	abc	13.6
23/*B.carinata*	13.2	abc	25.5
24/*B.carinata*	15.3	abc	29.0
60/*B.napus*	21.1	abc	0.4
57/*B.napus*	40.1	bcd	6.4
90/*R.sativus*	43.7	cd	16.2
58/*B.napus*	47.3	cd	3.0
Cabbage	292	de	3.7
Soil (Control)	562	e	0.0
Forage sorghum	836	e	0.0

[1] Colony forming units.

Discussion

The results of this experiment have further confirmed the relationship between isothiocyanates released from *Brassica* plant tissue and a reduction in *R. solanacearum* populations. On both Day 10 and 30, variety number 29 (*B. nigra*) performed significantly better than the forage sorghum and unamended soil controls. This variety also has the highest glucosinolate concentration (42.4 µmoles/g) in the leaf tissue. This is 32% more than the next highest concentration of 29 µmoles/g recorded for variety number 24.

It appears that the results at Day 10 more strongly relate to the glucosinolate concentration than the results at day 30. This can be expected considering that other work has shown that 80-90% of ITCs are released within two to three days (Dr John Kirkegaard, personal communication). The mode of action of ITCs in relation to the bacterial cell is not known; however, other work has suggested that certain types of isothiocyanates and possibly other breakdown products of cruciferous plants interfere with bio-chemical reactions causing a decline in cell metabolism or death. (2) The reduction in *R. solanacearum* population after Day 10 is likely to be due to a combination of factors rather than just ITCs. This is evident in the tobac-co result at Day 30, and it is probable that other non-volatile toxic compounds or anti-microbial proteins (1,9) found in the tobacco *(Nicotiana tabacum)* leaf are responsible for this result. In hindsight using tobacco leaves was probably not the best option for a host control treatment. In future experiments tobacco roots will be used considering this is the preferred location for *R. solanacearum* in the tobacco plant. It is also probable that in the presence of decaying plant material the population of saprophytic microorganisms increases dramatically providing competition for the bacterial cells.

Based on the findings of this experiment it would be highly informative to monitor the population of *R. solanacearum* intensively over the first ten days of the experiment to further prove or disprove the relationship between ITCs and a reduction in population. This is of increased importance following the discovery that the majority of ITCs are released from *Brassica* tissue in the first two to three days after incorporation. Biofumigation research would also benefit from research into the mode of action of ITCs against the bacterial cell.

Acknowledgements

The continuing support of Dr Tony Fischer (ACIAR) and the financial support of the Australian Centre for International Agricultural Research is gratefully acknowledged.

Literature Cited

1. Abad, L.R., D'Urzo, M.P., Liu, D., Narasimhan, M.L., Reuveni, M., Kang Zhu, J., Niu, X., Singh, N.K., Hasegawa, P.M., and Bressan, R.A. 1996. Antifungal activity of tobacco osmotin has specificity and involves plasma membrane permeabilization. Plant Science 118:11-23.
2. Akiew, S., Trevorrow, P.R., and Kirkegaard, J. 1996. Mustard as green manure reduces bacterial wilt. ACIAR Bacterial Wilt Newsletter 13:5-6.
3. Brown, P.D., and Morra, M.J. 1997. Control of soil-borne plant pests using glucosinolate-containing plants. Advances in Agronomy 61:167-231.
4. Chan , M.K.Y., and Close, R.C. 1987. *Aphanomyces* root rot of peas 3. Control by the use of cruciferous amendments. N.Z. J. Agric. Res. 30:225-233.
5. De Boer, S.H., and Kelman, A. 2001. II. Gram-negative bacteria B-2 *Erwinia* soft rot group. Pages 56-72 in: Laboratory Guide for Identification of Plant Pathogenic Bacteria. N.W. Schaad, J.B. Jones, and W. Chun, eds. The American Phytopathological Society, St. Paul, Minnesota.
6. Mojtahedi, H., Santo, G.S., Hang, A.N., and Wilson, J.H. 1991. Suppression of root-knot nematode populations with selected rapeseed cultivars as green manure. Journal of Nematology 23:170-174.
7. Sang, J. P., Minchinton, I. R., Johnstone, P. K., and Truscott, R. J. W. 1984. Glucosinolate profiles in the seed, root and leaf tissue of cabbage, mustard, rapeseed, radish and swede. Canadian Journal of Plant Science 64:77-93.
8. Sarwar, M., and Kirkegaard, J.A. 1998. Biofumigation potential of brassicas. II. Effect of environment and ontogeny on glucosinolate production and implications for screening. Plant and Soil 201:91-101.
9. Sela-Buurlage, M.B., Ponstein, A.S., Bres-Vloemans, S.A., Melchers, L.S., van den Elzen, P.J.M., and Cornelissen, B.J.C. 1993. Only specific tobacco *(Nicotiana tabacum)* chitinases and β-1,3-glucanases exhibit antifungal activity. Plant Physiology 101:857-863.
10. Vierheilig, H., Bennett, R., Kiddle, G., Kaldorf, M., and Ludwig-Muller, J. 2000. Differences in glucosinolate patterns and arbuscular mycorrhizal status of glucosinolate-containing plant species. New Phytologist 146: 343-352.

Seed-Plot Technique: Empowerment of Farmers in Production of Bacterial Wilt-Free Seed Potato in Kenya and Uganda

Z.M. Kinyua[1], M. Olanya[2], J.J. Smith[3], R. El-Bedewy[2], S.N. Kihara[1], R.K. Kakuhenzire[4], C. Crissman[2], and B. Lemaga[5]

[1]Kenya Agricultural Research Institute, Nairobi, Kenya; [2]International Potato Center, Sub-Saharan Africa Region, Nairobi, Kenya; [3]CABI-Bioscience, U.K. Centre (Egham), United Kingdom; [4]National Agricultural Research Organization, Uganda; [5]PRAPACE Network, Kampala, Uganda

Introduction

Bacterial wilt (caused by *Ralstonia solanacearum)* is a major constraint to potato production in Kenya, Uganda and other Sub-Saharan African countries, especially in small-holdings that are intensively cultivated (3,7,10). Yield losses attributable to the disease in Kenya are estimated at 50%, occasionally reaching about 75% (1) while over 30% yield loss, with an extreme of 100%, has been recorded in Uganda (2,6,10). Such losses are of great economic importance to countries like Kenya and Uganda, where the total land area under potato cultivation every year is estimated to be at least 96,000 and 60,000 Ha, respectively (3,10). The losses result from inadequate disease control occasioned by insufficient land for rotation and unavailability of certified potato seed tubers (3,7,14). Farmers commonly overcome the shortage or unavailability of healthy potato seed by planting tubers retained from their own previous crop harvests or purchased from 'neighbors' or markets (3). Such tubers may often be infected by *R. solanacearum*, and might play a major role in the spread of the pathogen (9), thus contributing significantly to this vicious disease. Planting bacterial wilt-free seed has been reported to be a key component of bacterial wilt management, with significant increases in potato yields in many instances (4,5,6,16,17). However, the availability of good quality seed potato is far below on-farm seed requirements in Kenya and Uganda (3,10).

Therefore, there is a clear demand for technologies to increase the availability of "high-health" seed potato and to enhance adoption of integrated bacterial wilt management strategies among farmers. One such technology is a seed plot technique, which focuses on maximizing tuber production per unit area of limited, disease-free land through high-density planting (8). Opportunities offered by the seed plot technique (9) have been utilized and attempts made to overcome on-farm seed-health challenges through farmer groups in Kenya and Uganda.

Principles of the Seed-plot Technique

The seed-plot technique separates seed production from ware production and maintains a good health status of seed tubers through intensive control of pests and diseases. Bacterial wilt-free tubers should be obtained from a reliable source, preferably a seed production center or a recognized potato seed dealer. To reduce risks of bacterial wilt infection, the system requires that tuber multiplication plots be established on land with no history of potato production or other solanaceous crops and exempt from inflow of runoff water.

The soil is loosened sufficiently to a satisfactory depth before applying diammonium phosphate (DAP) fertilizer (N:P:K = 18:46:0) at the rate of about $60g/m^2$ by broadcasting on a fine-tilth flat bed, followed by raking to mix with the soil. Planting holes are then made at a spacing of 20cm by 20cm on the flat bed by pushing a dibber (spade handle without a blade or a similar tool) through the soil to a depth of about 15cm; the holes are easily made if the soil is moist. Well-sprouted tubers are planted in each hole. Hand weeding is recommended and ordinary soil hilling is not necessary provided an appropriate planting depth is adopted. Foliar pesticides should be applied at regular intervals to control fungal diseases and arthropod pests.

On-Farm Trials

Individual-farm trials were initiated in Nyandarua and Meru regions of Kenya, which had been surveyed earlier and known to have bacterial wilt-infested farms, in order to compare tuber yields and bacterial wilt control potential at seed-plot (20cm x 20cm spacing) and ware-plot (75cm x 30cm spacing) densities. Certified seed tubers of varieties 'Tigoni' and 'Roslin Tana' were used in Nyandarua and varieties 'Asante' and 'Kerr's Pink' were used in Meru. Preference for potato skin color was the key selection criterion in the two regions. Six farm sites were established in each region and management of the plots was the responsibility of the respective farm owners.

Subsequent trials were carried out through farmer groups in order to disseminate the technology more widely. Three farmer groups were formed at Marimba, Katheri and Kaugu in Meru district, Kenya and two existing farmer groups at Nyabyumba and Rosanghati in Kabale district, Uganda were introduced to the seed-plot technique. The groups utilized land belonging to public institutions such as schools or plots made available by some group members. The groups were first trained/refreshed on the mechanisms of bacterial wilt spread and persistence and disease management options in a simple language that they could understand. The farmers were then asked to identify land that they considered to be free from *R. solanacearum* infestation on the basis of the land's cropping history and location relative to agents of pathogen spread such as surface runoff and kitchen waste. Certified or 'high-health' seed tubers of variety 'Asante' (Kenya) / 'Victoria' (Uganda) [CIP 381381.20] were planted in flat-bed plots (seed plots) at a close spacing of 20cm by 20cm in comparison to the wide spacing of 75cm by 30cm (Kenya) or 70cm by 30cm (Uganda) for ware potato production. Technical assistance and seed tubers were provided by researchers while the farmer groups contributed land, labor and other plot management logistics.

Data taken included bacterial wilt incidence and tuber yields in the experimental plots; the surrounding farmer-planted ware fields were also observed for disease incidence. Harvested tubers were analyzed for latent infection by enzyme-linked immunosorbent assay on nitrocellulose membranes, NCM-ELISA (15). Data from planting to harvesting were analyzed by farmers, extension agents and researchers to reach a common understanding.

The Seed-Plot Technique Experience

TUBER MULTIPLICATION AND LAND PRODUCTIVITY

Land productivity for total and seed-size tubers was significantly higher under seed-plot (close spacing) than under ware-plot (wide spacing) density for all the tested varieties across all the sites. The ratios of seed tuber yield at seed density to the yield at ware density ranged from 1.87 (variety 'Victoria' at Rosaghati) to 3.55 for variety 'Tigoni' in Nyandarua (Table 1). Consequently, the proportion of land under potato cultivation required for seed production was significantly reduced by planting at seed density, the land requirement being 4.18-9.43% in comparison to 11.71-19.02% needed under ware density planting. Hence, the seed-plot system can utilize less than 50% of the land committed to seed production under the ware production system to meet on-farm seed tuber requirements. It is recommended

Table 1. Tuber multiplication, land requirements and bacterial wilt incidence in seed and ware potato production plots* in Kenya and Uganda

Variety – Site	Planting density	Land productivity (tubers/m²)		Percentage seed-size tubers	Land productivity ratio (seed:ware)		% Potato land for seed production[a]	Bacterial wilt incidence (%)	
		Seed-size	Total		Seed-size	Total		Field incidence	Latent infection
Tigoni–Nyandarua[b]	Seed	95.6	115.4	82.8	3.55		4.65	1.8	2.9
	Ware	26.9	43.2	62.3		2.67	16.54	0.9	5.7
R. Tana–Nyandarua[b]	Seed	73.5	96.6	76.1	2.83		6.05	0.0	0.0
	Ware	26.0	31.7	82.0		3.05	17.12	0.0	0.0
[c]Asante –Meru	Seed	62.0	77.2	80.3	2.09		7.18	1.1	2.1
	Ware	29.6	37.7	78.5		2.05	15.03	1.4	3.7
K. Pink-Meru	Seed	106.5	125.0	85.2	2.80		4.18	1.2	4.1
	Ware	38.0	46.6	81.5		2.68	11.71	9.1	29.6
[c]Victoria-Nyabyumba	Seed	69.7	96.0	72.6	2.98		6.38	0.0	-[d]
	Ware	23.4	45.4	51.5		2.11	19.02	0.0	-[d]
[c]Victoria-Rosanghati	Seed	47.2	90.2	52.3	1.87		9.43	0.0	-[d]
	Ware	25.2	36.9	68.3		2.44	17.66	0.0	-[d]
LSD[0.05]		27.9	32.2	11.2			5.34		

*All values are means of six replicates (farms) except for Nyabyumba and Rosanghati, which had one farm site each; [a]Figures were calculated on the basis of a ware plant population of 44,500 plants/Ha at a spacing of 75cm by 30cm; [b]Pooled means for 5 consecutive seasons. [c]Varieties 'Asante' and 'Victoria' are the same genotype (CIP 381381.20); [d]NCM-ELISA was not done but a few tubers had bacterial wilt symptoms despite the absence of field symptoms.

that the 'freed' land be managed as next season's seed plot by leaving it fallow or planting a short season non-solanaceous crop. This practice would encourage a crop rotation program to prevent the build-up of pests and diseases, some of which contribute to poor seed tuber quality.

On the basis of group-managed plots, high tuber yields were realized from both Kenyan and Ugandan seed plots; the yields ranged from 42.5 (Rosaghati, Uganda) to 119.4 t/Ha at Kaugu, Kenya (Fig. 1) and averaged about 74 t/Ha. This wide range in yield might be attributed to soil and other environmental differences, in part, but a major contribution could have been differences in seed-plot management among the farmer groups; Ugandan farmers were introduced to the seed-plot technique for the first time during these trials. These factors had been recognized elsewhere (9), and appear to be inevitable during the early stages of introduction of the technique to farmers. Given that the proportion of seed-size tubers was above 50% at all the sites, the mean yield for seed potato would translate to above 37 t/Ha, which is substantially higher than the Kenyan national average yield of below 10t/Ha at ware planting density (12). This indicates high land productivity potential for seed tubers, which can benefit farmers with small pieces of land. Promotion of the seed-plot technique would, therefore, alleviate the persistent problem of seed tuber unavailability among farmers in intensively cultivated potato regions. The high land productivity also increases the feasibility of rotation of seed production plots because smaller portions of land, which are easier to get, would be needed to satisfy on-farm demand for disease-free tubers than if seed production was carried out at ware plant spacing.

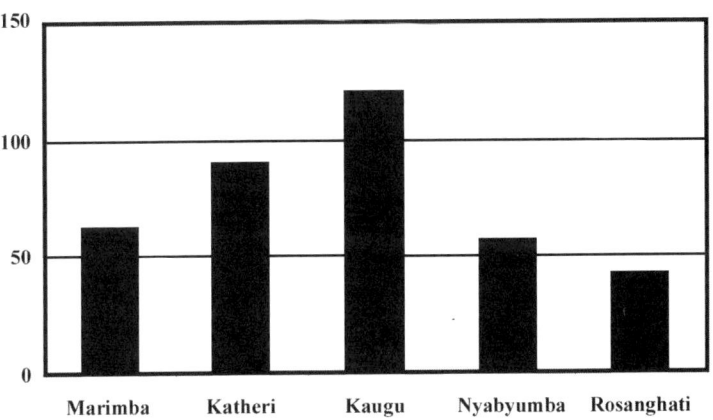

Fig. 1. Tuber yields for variety 'Asante'/'Victoria' at five sites in Kenya and Uganda (March-July 2001 season).

Initial trials in Kenya. Bacterial wilt was experienced in only one among the six experimental sites in Nyandarua during five consecutive seasons; the other sites remained free from the disease despite its existence in the farmer-planted ware fields. However, field disease incidence at the said farm was substantially reduced, averaging below 2%, and latent infection levels hardly reached 6% (Table 1). Infection of plants could have resulted from previously infested soils (no soil inoculum test was done) or introduction through farm implements. The farmer was encouraged to observe good field sanitation and to rogue and destroy diseased plants as soon as they were noticed to prevent increases in disease levels over the seasons. This also helped to prevent the disease spread to other plots, given that only one variety ('Tigoni') was affected (Table 1). The ability to maintain disease-free potato plots on a bacterial wilt-infested farm marked a key achievement of the seed-plot technique.

In Meru, bacterial wilt was observed in both seed and ware plots, the latter exhibiting a higher disease incidence especially with variety 'Kerr's Pink' (Table 1). Tubers from such plots should not be used as seed in order to prevent new land infestations and potential disease 'explosion'. Instead, farmers should start afresh with disease-free tubers on bacterial wilt-free land. In some instances, the disease was observed at the periphery or from only one side of the plots, indicating inoculum introduction through infested feet/shoes and farm implements or contaminated runoff water. Therefore training of farmers on field sanitation/hygiene is an important requirement for success of the seed-plot technique.

Group seed-plot trials. Bacterial wilt was not noticed in experimental plots at Marimba, Kaugu, Nyabyumba and Rosanghati. However, a cumulative field disease incidence of 5.1% was recorded at Katheri and latent infection analysis of harvested tubers revealed that 35% of the sampled tubers harbored *R. solanacearum*. These results were consistent with the initial trials observation that bacterial wilt can occur and render the seed-plot technique ineffective if care is not taken in site selection and in preventing inoculum introduction.

Tubers sampled from the symptomless plots at Nyabyumba and Rosanghati had obvious bacterial wilt symptoms such as oozing from tuber 'eyes' and vascular browning. This points to the need for keen observation on seed plots in order to avoid possible spread of the pathogen through tubers from such multiplication plots. Visual inspection also needs to be supplemented with laboratory analyses such as NCM-ELISA. However, this demands the goodwill of farmers, agricultural extension agents and facilitating institutions such as seed quality inspection and research organizations.

Conclusions and Recommendations

The seed-plot technique can help in satisfying on-farm seed potato requirements through its potential of high tuber output per unit area. It also acts as a window for the promotion and application of intensive bacterial wilt management strategies such as bacterial wilt-free field selection, sanitation, seed selection and rotation of seed production plots. Therefore, the technique needs to be promoted among farmers for wide-scale adoption, making the necessary adjustments to suit various local environments.

Acknowledgements

The authors acknowledge the facilitation of research activities by the Kenya Agricultural Research Institute (KARI), International Potato Center (CIP), CAB International, National Agricultural Research Organization (NARO) and Africare–Uganda. Financial support from the Department for International Development (DFID) of the United Kingdom, CIP, Africare and others is highly appreciated.

Literature Cited

1. Ajanga, S. 1993. Status of bacterial wilt of potato in Kenya. Pages 28-31 in: Bacterial Wilt. Proceedings of an international conference held at Kaohsiung, Taiwan, 28-31 October, 1992. ACIAR Proc. No. 45. G.L. Hartman and A.C. Hayward, eds. Canberra, Australia.
2. Alacho, F.O., and Akimanzi, D.R. 1993. Progress, achievements and constraints on bacterial wilt control in Uganda. Pages 32-41 in: Proceedings of a Workshop on Bacterial Wilt of Potatoes Caused by *Pseudomonas solanacearum*. 22-26 February 1993. Bunjumbura, Burundi.
3. Barton, D., Smith, J.J., and Kinyua, Z.M. 1997. Socio-economic inputs to Biological Control of Bacterial Wilt Disease of Potato in Kenya. ODA RNRRS Crop Protection Project R6629. NR International, United Kingdom.
4. Berrios, D.E., and Rubirigi, A. 1993. Integrated control of bacterial wilt in seed production by the Burundi National Potato Program. Pages 284-288 in: Bacterial Wilt. Proceedings of an international conference held at Kaohsiung, Taiwan, 28-31 October, 1992. ACIAR Proc. No. 45. G.L. Hartman and A.C. Hayward, eds. Canberra, Australia.
5. French, E.R. 1994. Strategies for integrated control of bacterial wilt of potatoes. Pages 199-204 in: Bacterial wilt: the disease and its causative

agent, *Pseudomonas solanacearum*. A.C. Hayward and G.L. Hartman, eds. CAB International, UK.

6. Kakuhenzire, R., Alacho, F., Birikunzira, J., Turyamureeba, G., and Sikka, L. 1993. Progress in field evaluation for resistance to *Pseudomonas solanacearum* and cultural methods for control of bacterial wilt in Uganda. Pages 76-82 in: Proceedings of a Workshop on Bacterial Wilt of Potatoes Caused by *Pseudomonas solanacearum*. 22-26 February 1993. Bunjumbura, Burundi.

7. Kinyae, P.M., Lung'aho, C., Kanguha, E., and Njenga, D.N. 1994. The status of seed potato in Meru, Nyambene, Nyandarua and Laikipia Districts. Second KARI/CIP Technical Workshop on collaborative research, Nairobi. January 1994.

8. Kinyua, Z.M., Smith, J.J., Oduor, G.I., and Wachira, J.N. 2001. Increasing the availability of disease-free potato seed tubers to small-hold farmers in Kenya. Pages 494-499 in: Proc. Seventh Symposium Int. Soc. for Tropical Root Crops - Africa Branch; 12-16 October, 1998. Cotonou, Benin.

9. Kinyua Z.M., Smith, J.J., Lung'aho, C., Olanya, M., and Priou, S. 2001. On-farm successes and challenges of producing bacterial wilt-free tubers in seed plots in Kenya. Afr. Crop Sci. J. 9: 279-285.

10. Lemaga, B., Hakiza, J.J., Alacho, F.O., and Kakuhenzire, R. 1997. Integrated control of potato bacterial wilt in Southwestern Uganda. Pages 188-195 in: Proc. Fourth Triennial Congr. Afr. Potato Assoc. Pretoria, South Africa.

11. Low, J.W. 1997. Potato in southwestern Uganda: Threats to sustainable production. Afr. Crop Sci. J. 5: 295-312.

12. Lung'aho, C., M'makwa, C., and Kidane-Mariam, H.M. 1997. Effect of source of mother plant, variety and growing conditions on the production of stem cuttings and subsequent yield of mini-tubers in the Kenyan potato programme. Pages 275-283 in: Proc. Fourth Triennial Congr. Afr. Potato Assoc. Pretoria, South Africa.

13. Nyangeri, J.B., Gathuru, E.M., and Mukunya, D.M. 1984. Effect of latent infection on the spread of bacterial wilt of potatoes in Kenya. Trop Pest Manag. 30: 163-165.

14. Opio, A.F. 1988. Host range and biotypes of *Pseudomonas solanacearum* E.F. Smith in Uganda: A preliminary study. Paper presented at the 15th Int. Congr. Plant Pathol.; 20-27 August 1988, Kyoto, Japan.

15. Priou, S., Gutarra, L., Fernandez, H., and Aley, P. 1999. Sensitive detection of *Ralstonia solanacearum* in latently infected potato tubers and soil by post-enrichment ELISA. Pages 111-121 in: CIP Program Report 1997-98. International Potato Center, Lima, Peru.

16. Saumtally, S., Autrey, L.J.C., Ferre, P., and Dookun, A. 1993. Disease management strategies for the control of bacterial wilt disease of potato in Mauritius. Pages 289-293 in: Bacterial Wilt.Proceedings of an international conference held at Kaohsiung, Taiwan, 28-31 October 1992, ACIAR Proc. No. 45. G.L. Hartman and A.C. Hayward, eds. Canberra, Australia.

17. Shekhawat, G.S. 1995. Effect of changes in seed sources on potato bacterial wilt. Pages 79-86 in: Integrated Management of Bacterial Wilt. Proceedings of an international workshop, New Delhi, India, 11-16 Oct. 1993. B. Hardy and E.R. French, eds. CIP.

18. Tusiime, G., Adipala, E. Opio, F., and Bhagsari, A.S. 1996. Occurrence of *Pseudomonas solanacearum* latent infection in tubers and weeds in highland Uganda. Afr. J. Plant Prot. 6: 108-118.

Primary Bacterial Wilt Study on Tomato in Vegetable Areas of Ho Chi Minh City, Vietnam

M.T. Vinh[1], T.T. Tung[2], and H.X. Quang[1]

[1]Institute of Agricultural Sciences of South Vietnam (IAS), HCMC;
[2]Pesticide Center, Plant Protection Department, HCMC, Vietnam

Abstract

Bacterial wilt of tomato (*Lycopersicum esculentum* L.) is one of the most noticeable diseases in vegetable-production areas of Ho Chi Minh City, Vietnam. Among eight isolates of *Ralstonia solanacearum*, six were identified as biovar 3 and two as biovar 5. The disease was more severe in Cu Chi, an area of intensive vegetable production, than in Hoc Mon, which has an annual rotation with rice (disease incidences were 100% and 3.6%, respectively). Among nine tomato hybrid varieties, only Red Crown 25 was relatively tolerant to bacterial wilt. Soil amended with 300 kg N and 1500 kg CaO could partly control the disease. Soil solarization using transparent plastic mulches for 60 days prior to planting of tomato reduced bacterial wilt incidence. Integrated disease management resulted in lower disease incidence (from 43 to 63.3 %) and grower profits were higher (from 5.2 to 14 millions Vietnam dong per hectare, equivalent to 369 to 998 US$).

Introduction

Ho Chi Minh City (HCMC), Vietnam, covers an area of 2,095 km^2. Vegetables are grown in the outskirts of the city in a harvested area of 12,000 Ha annually which meets about 40-50% of the public demand. Bacterial wilt caused by *Ralstonia solanacearum* on solanaceous crops (8) is the most important constraint, which reduces tomato yield about 35 to 100 %, in the HCMC vegetable area. Chemical control is not effective. Farmers are not familiar with the use of resistant tomato cultivars. Alternative strategies such as grafting of commercially valuable tomatoes on resistant rootstocks are only just beginning to be developed. In such an unfavourable agronomic situation, cultural practices are essential compo-

177

nents of integrated bacterial wilt management (IBWM). No study on this aspect has been carried out in the vegetable area of HCMC, Vietnam in recent years. The objectives of our study were to investigate the severity of bacterial wilt, the resistance of some popular tomato varieties and to develop IBWM based on cultural practices to support farmers in reducing yield loss.

Materials and Methods

During 1997 and 1999, an investigation of bacterial wilt severity was carried out in Binh Chanh and Hoc Mon Districts, where tomato crops are rotated with rice annually and in Cu Chi District which is an area of intensive vegetable production. Five fields (1,000 m^2) were selected at each District. *R. solanacearum* was isolated from the bacterial exudate flowing from a segment of the lower-stem of a wilted plant in sterile distilled water. Extracts were plated on tetrazolium agar (TTC). These TTC agar plates were incubated at 28-30°C for two-three days before single fluidal, virulent, colonies were further purified. Isolates were identified based on cultural, morphological and biochemical characteristics, and the biovar was determined (5,12).

Nine tomato hybrid varieties (F$_1$) commonly used by farmers were tested for resistance to bacterial wilt, from June to September 1998 in Cu Chi. Red Crown 250, NS-Swaraksha, NG1, L 520, Venus, 2100 and TN 49 were F$_1$ hybrid varieties, KBT $_4$ (OP) was used as a local check and L 390 (OP) as susceptible check. The plant density was 20,000 plants per hectare; 25,000 kg of manure and 1,000 kg of coconut cake were amended to each one-hectare. The fertilizer formula was N:P:K = 115:105:150. The experiment was designed in RCBD with three replications. The percentages of wilted plants were recorded at one-week intervals.

The soil amendment experiment included in the main plot treatments 100 kg, 200 kg and 300 kg of nitrogen fertilizer per hectare and the subplot treatments were no CaO, 1000 kg CaO and 1500 kg CaO. Urea and dehydrated lime were applied to the soil two weeks before transplanting. A split-plot design was used with three replications in Cu Chi District, during July - December 1998. The percentage of surviving tomato plants was noted at seven-day intervals. Data were analysed using the MSTATC program.

Soil solarization consisted of three treatments: untreated control and covering the soil with transparent polyethylene mulch 30 and 60 days before transplanting tomato. Soil was thoroughly moistened by furrow irrigation before being covered. A large-plot design was used without

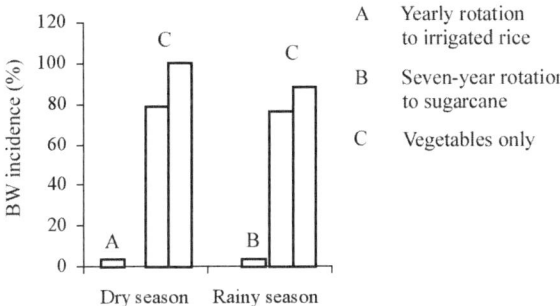

Fig. 1. Bacterial wilt incidence on tomato after different crop rotation.

replication from March to July 1999. Surviving plants were counted at seven-day intervals. Data were statistically analyzed by a T test.

Demonstration of IBWM was done during the rainy season from 1998-2001. Planting tomato with some degree of resistance to bacterial wilt was combined with cultural methods to reduce *R. solanacearum* in soil (4,6). Four fields were successively designed in Cu Chi District, HCMC. The experimental unit was 1000 m². Cultural practices of IPM fields were as follows: seed treatment with hot water at 50°C for 30 min; soil for seedlings taken from rice fields; tomato field rotated with rice annually; urea and dehydrated lime applied two weeks before transplanting; transparent polyethylene mulch for 30-60 days as soil solarization; burning diseased plants; black polyethylene mulch used as weed control; and treating soil with Vimoca (Nematicide). Bacterial wilt incidence, yield and economic efficiency were calculated and compared with farmers' fields. T test was used for statistical analysis.

Results and Discussion

Yearly rotation with rice in the rainy season or long-term rotation with another non-host plant (sugarcane) significantly decreased bacterial wilt severity compared to mono-cropping of vegetables (Fig. 1). This is consistent with reports that short-term rotations are insufficient to control *R. solanacearum* (1). Pradhanang (9) showed that soilborne infection was absent after a rotation period of 2.5 years. It has been reported that high temperature and rainfall promote bacterial wilt development. However, our results showed that tomato bacterial wilt was severe in both dry and rainy seasons in the vegetable area of HCMC.

The isolates were all gram-negative, non-fluorescent, short rods that reduced nitrate, failed to hydrolyze starch, and were catalase and oxidase

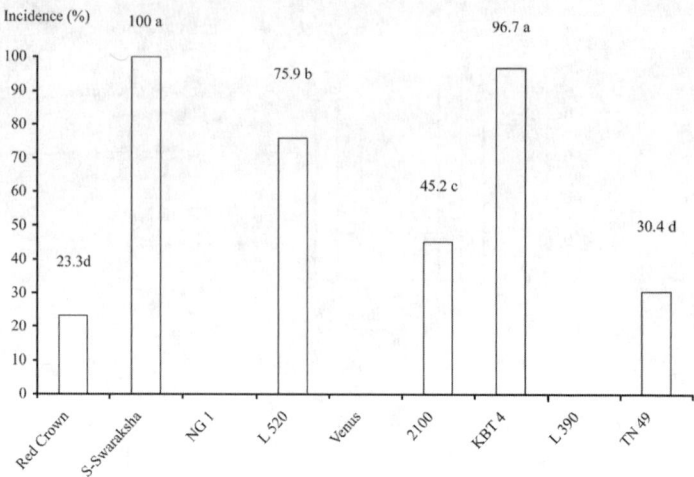

Fig. 2. Bacterial wilt incidence of tomato varieties in Cu Chi. Numbers followed by the same letters are not significantly different at P=0.05.

positive. There was growth at 37°C; no growth occurred in a 5 % sodium chloride medium. All of these properties are consistent with *R. solanacearum*. Of the eight isolates, six were typed as biovar 3 and two as biovar 5 (12).

Resistant varieties are the most efficient method for disease control. In the HCMC vegetable areas, F_1 commercial hybrids are most commonly grown as well as some local varieties. Among nine tested tomato varieties, only Red Crown had a significantly lower disease incidence at P=0.05 (Fig. 2), at 55 days after transplanting (DAT).

Soil amended with urea together with lime reduced the *R. solanacearum* populations in the soil and disease incidence in the field (3,4,8). The suppressive effects of the soil amendment on populations of *R. solanacearum* and disease incidence were probably due to the production of one or several toxic substances during the transformation of urea in the presence of CaO (7). Lime was also necessary to increase pH of the soil. Michel and Mew (7) showed that soil with low pH did not accumulate nitrite and the *R. solanacearum* population did not decline.

Soil amendment with 300 kg N and 1,500 kg of lime significantly reduced the percentage of bacterial wilt plants at 30 DAT (Fig. 3). Chellemi *et al.* (2) concluded that bacterial wilt incidence was not affected by soil treatments. Soil solarization for 8 and 10 weeks increased wilt incidence in comparison to non-solarization (11). The use of a clear plastic sheet to cover moist soil for six weeks gave some control (10). However, our results showed that the incidence of bacterial wilt on tomato decreased significant-ly after 60 days of solarization before transplanting in HCMC (Table 1).

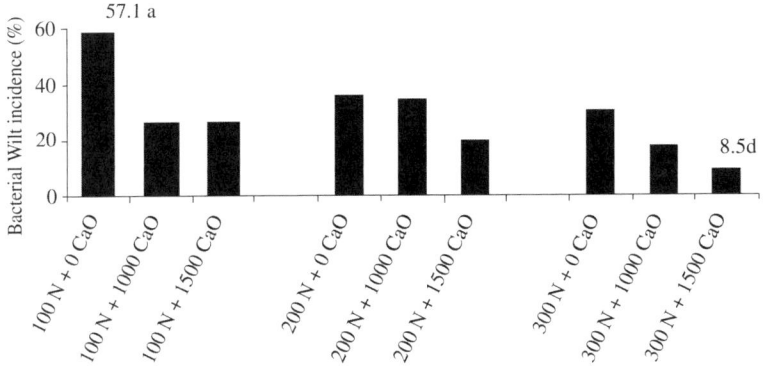

Fig. 3. Bacterial wilt incidence (%) of tomato with soil amendment of nitrogen and lime on 30 DAT. Numbers followed by the same letters are not significantly different at P=0.05.

Table 1. Effect of soil solarization on incidence of bacterial wilt in tomato (*R. solanacearum*) in Cu Chi, HCMC vegetable area.

Treatment	Bacterial wilt incidence (%)
No covering	65.8 [a]
Soil solarization 30 days	59.4
Prob (t)	0.18 ns
No covering	65.8
Soil solarization 60 days	59.4
Prob (t)	0.00*
Soil solarization 30 days	59.4
Soil solarization 60 days	59.4
Prob (t)	0.00*

[a] 60 days after transplanting

In demonstrating IBWM, cultural methods were the most important. Our results showed that bacterial wilt incidence in tested fields was significantly lower in comparison to farmers' fields. Disease management technologies helped increase the yield and the profit (Table 2). This is the first research on bacterial wilt on tomato in the vegetable areas of HCMC, Vietnam. Results showed that integrated disease management could reduce wilt

Table 2. Economic efficiency of IBWM on tomato in HCMC vegetable areas, in rainy seasons of 1999 and 2000.

Treatment	Yield (T/Ha)	Income (1,000d/Ha)	Outcome (1,000d/Ha)	Profit (1,000d/Ha)	Benefit index
1999					
Test field	22.6	72,448	25,200	47,248	1.87
Farmer field	16.5	52,800	19,560	33,240	1.69
2000					
Test field	17.9	23,300	14,000	9,300	0.66
Farmer field	11.6	15,100	11,000	4,100	0.37

$1US equivalent to 14,030 and 14,086 VN dong at harvesting time.

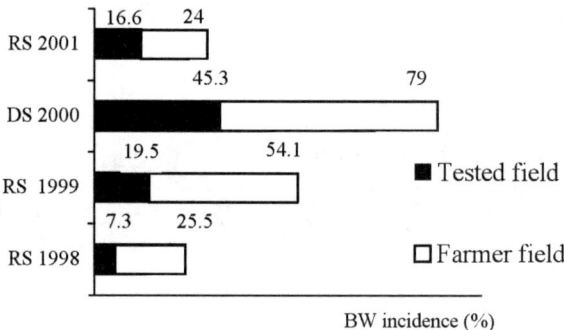

Fig. 4. Disease incidence (%) of tested fields and farmer fields from 1998-2001. DS dry season, RS rainy season.

incidence. However, further research is required on hosts, pathogen population, and environment of these vegetable areas.

Acknowledgements

Appreciation is expressed to Prof. Dr. P.V. Bien, IAS, Prof. Dr. W.H. Schnitzler, TUM, for their encouragement and support, and to Dr. J.F. Wang, AVRDC and CIRAD for help and provision of travel funds.

Literature Cited

1. Arthy, J., and Akiew, S. 1999. Effect of short-term rotation on *Ralstonia solanacearum* populations in soil. ACIAR Bacterial Wilt Newsl. 16: 13-14.

2. Chellemi, D.O., Olson, S.M., Michelle, D.J., Secker, L., and McSorley, R. 1997. Adaptation of soil solarization to the integrated management of soil borne pests of tomato under humid conditions. Phytopathology 97: 250-258.
3. Dhital, S.P., Thaveechai, N., Kositratana, W., Pluek, K., and Shrestha, S.K. 1997. Effect of chemical and soil amendment for the control of bacteria wilt of potato in Nepal caused by *Ralstonia solanacearum*. Kasetsart J.(Natural Sci.) 31: 497-509.
4. Elphinstone, J.G., and Aley, P. 1993. Integrated control of bacterial wilt of potato in the warm tropics of Peru. Pages 276-283 in: Bacterial Wilt. Proceedings of an International Conference held at Kaohsiung, Taiwan, 28-31 October 1992. ACIAR Proc. No. 45. G.L. Hartman and A.C. Hayward, eds.
5. Hayward, A.C. 1964. Characteristics of *Pseudomonas solanacearum*. J. Appl. Bacteriol. 27: 265-277.
6. Michel, V.V., Wang, J.F., Midmore, D.J., and Hartman, G.L. 1997. Effect of intercropping and soil amendment with urea and calcium oxide on the incidence of bacterial wilt of tomato and the survival of soil borne *Pseudomonas solanacearum* in Taiwan. Plant Pathol. 46: 600-610.
7. Michel, V.V., and Mew, T.W. 1998. Effect of a soil amendment on the survival of *Ralstonia solanacearum* in different soils. Phytopathology 88: 300-305.
8. Persley, G.J. 1986. Bacterial wilt disease in Asia and the South Pacific. Proceedings of an international workshop held at PCAARD, Los Banos, Philippines, 8-10 October 1985. ACIAR Proc. No. 13.
9. Pradhanang, P.M. 1998. Bacterial wilt of potato caused by *Ralstonia solanacearum* biovar 2A: a study of ecology and taxonomy of the pathogen in Nepal. PhD thesis, University of Reading, UK.
10. Saumtally, S., Autrey, L.J.C., Ferre, P., and Dookun, A. 1992. Disease management strategies for the control of bacterial wilt disease of potato in Mauritius. Pages 289-293 in: Bacterial Wilt. Proceedings of an International Conference held at at Kaohsiung, Taiwan, 28-31 October 1992. ACIAR Proc. No. 45. G.L. Hartman and A.C. Hayward, eds.
11. Sood, A.K., Kalha, C.S., and Parashar, A. 1998. Ecofriendly method for the management of bacterial wilt of tomato caused by *Ralstonia solanacearum*. ACIAR Bacterial Wilt Newsl. 15: 7.
12. Thaveechai, N. 1996. Laboratory course on bacterial wilt of tomato. Kasetsart University, Thailand.

Rhizome Solarization and Microwave Treatment: Ecofriendly Methods for Disinfecting Ginger Seed Rhizomes

A. Kumar, M. Anandaraj, and Y.R. Sarma

Indian Institute of Spices Research (ICAR), PB No. 1701,
Marikunnu PO, Calicut - 673 012, Kerala, India

Abstract

Bacterial wilt caused by *Ralstonia solanacearum* biovar 3 (Smith) Yabuuchi is one of the important rhizome borne diseases affecting ginger (*Zingiber officinale* Rosc) crop in the field. We explored the possibilities of using heat treatment through rhizome solarization and microwave exposure of rhizomes to contain the disease by reducing the primary source of inoculum. Initially, the thermal death point of the pathogen was identified as 47°C for 30 min of exposure in a water suspension and the optimum period of solarization and microwave treatment of ginger rhizomes was later standardized to attain the determined rhizome temperature without affecting germination, by duly exposing the rhizomes packed in sealed polythene bags. The rhizomes (250 g) reached a temperature of 50°C when solarized for 2 h (9:00 to 11:00 a.m.) without significant reduction in germination. When the rhizomes were exposed to microwaves for a period 30 s, rhizome temperature of 45°C was recorded. Since significant reduction in rhizome germination was observed beyond 50 s of exposure, the optimum microwave exposure was determined as 30 s. When artificially inoculated rhizomes were solarized for 2 or 4 h the developing ginger plants were free from bacterial wilt disease, indicating the effectiveness of rhizome solarization as a method of disinfecting seed rhizomes. When such rhizomes were tested for *R. solanacearum* using post enrichment NCM-ELISA, none of the treated rhizomes gave a positive reaction with antibodies specific for the pathogen, which indicates the effectiveness of solarization in inactivating seedborne infection. A trial conducted in farmers' fields showed that solarization of rhizomes for 2 h (9:00 to 11:00 a.m.) resulted in negligible disease incidence (< 1%) and another treatment with 2 h of solarization from 10 am-12 noon was completely free from disease after three months of planting as compared to unsolarized rhizomes where 33.6% of the emerged plants succumbed to bacterial wilt. In greenhouse trials using different microwave exposures ranging from 0-100 s, plants emerged from rhizomes that had been treated for 30 s were free from bacterial wilt infection. Rhizomes subjected to pulse microwaving involving 4-5 cycles of 10 s, at intervals of 5 s between cycles, also confirmed the effectiveness of microwave disinfection. However, these heat treatments recorded marginal reduction in germination. This incidentally is the first report of disinfection of ginger from bacterial wilt pathogen using solar energy or microwaves.

Introduction

Though first reported from Southern India in 1941 (12, 16) bacterial wilt of ginger has since been reported from many other ginger growing states such as Himachal Pradesh, West Bengal, Sikkim and all other north eastern states (13). The disease is widespread in other ginger growing countries such as China, Indonesia, Philippines and Hawaii (5). Under favorable conditions the crop loss is total. *R. solanacearum* is known to be transmitted through latently infected ginger seed rhizomes (7) as in potato tubers (14), as well as being soil borne. The latent infection of ginger by *R. solanacearum* has been reported and confirmed by indirect ELISA (15). The occurrence of bacterial wilt in ginger planted in virgin soils clearly points to the rhizome-borne nature of the bacterial pathogen. It has been suggested to produce and plant pathogen free seed rhizomes to ensure a healthy crop of ginger (8). Though seed monitoring techniques are available, applicability of these tests for large scale seed testing has practical limitations. Among the methods of rhizome disinfection through heat or antibiotics (4, 8), hot water treatment of ginger rhizomes is reported to inactivate the deep-seated *Ralstonia* in rhizomes (17) and also to eliminate root knot nematode infection (1). However, its practical applicability for large volumes of seed rhizomes severely limits its utility as a method for seed disinfection. Microwave ovens have been used as a research tool in several different investigations including pathogen disinfection in soil and true seed (2, 9). In the present work, we report, for the first time, cheap and very practical methods for disinfecting seed rhizomes from *R. solanacearum* by heat induction using two non conventional methods *viz.*, solar energy and microwaves.

Materials and Methods

Effect of heat or microwaves on survival and pathogenicity of R. solanacearum. Cells of *R. solanacearum* strain GRS Tms, biovar 3 were exposed to varying temperatures (40-55°C) for 30 to 60 min. or exposed to different durations of microwaving viz., 0-30 s with 5 s increment in a microwave oven (BPL; Model BMC-900T; 2450MHz; 36.8 L; 1350W) and plated for enumeration and calculation of per cent death. After heat or microwave treatment, about 100 µl of suspension was inoculated in ginger by stem inoculation method and plants were observed for wilt incidence.

Effects of solarization on heat build-up in seed rhizome and on physical status of seed rhizomes. Sprouted seed rhizomes (25-30 g each) packed in 250 g batches in transparent polypropylene bags (200 gauge) of size 30x20cm were sealed and exposed to sunlight from 9:00 a.m. to 5:00 p.m. during the first fortnight of May 2000. A thermometer was kept in one of the bags to record internal air temperature and the mercury end of another thermometer was inserted in the rhizome at a depth of 2 cm to record rhizome temperature. Rhizome and air temperatures were recorded at hourly intervals. In a parallel experiment, seed rhizomes contained in sealed polypropylene bag were exposed to sunlight for 2 days (16 h) from 9:00 a.m. on first day to 5:00 p.m. on next day and the rhizomes were examined for any damage on sprouts.

Effects of continuous microwaving on heat build up in rhizomes of ginger. Rhizome temperature upon microwave treatment was recorded after exposing the rhizomes (250 g) to microwaves for 0-100 s at increments of 10 s. Rhizome temperature upon microwaving was recorded immediately by inserting the mercury end of the thermometer into the rhizome.

EFFECT OF RHIZOME SOLARIZATION OR MICROWAVING ON GERMINATION, VIABILITY OF GINGER RHIZOMES AND BACTERIAL WILT INCIDENCE

Greenhouse trial. Rhizome sprouts inoculated with *R. solanacearum* were exposed to sunlight from 9:00 a.m. to 1:00 p.m. for two days. After every 2 h one of the bags was transferred to room temperature (28°C). In another experiment, ginger rhizomes (250 g) inoculated with *R. solanacearum* were exposed to microwaves for different durations 0-100 s at increments of 10 s. Another batch of ginger rhizomes was exposed to pulse microwaving for 10-50 s at increments of 10 s. After every 10 s, the exposure was interrupted for 10 s for 10, 2x10, 3x10, 4x10 and 5x10 s of microwaving. The treated rhizomes were planted in pots and observed for germination and bacterial wilt incidence.

Field evaluation of rhizome solarization for management of bacterial wilt of ginger. A field trial was conducted in farmers' fields in Kothamangalam, Eranakulam District of Kerala state for management of bacterial wilt by rhizome solarization. Fifty beds of 3x1 m size were prepared in a location with no history of bacterial wilt of ginger. Fifty kilograms of ginger seed rhizomes (*cv. Himachal*) (25 g each) were packed in 1 kg quantities in a polypropylene bag (200 gauge) of size 30x20 cm and solarized as described above. Rhizome and air temperatures were recorded every 30 min. The solarized rhizomes were planted at the rate of 40 pieces per bed and standard agronomic practices were followed. The data on germination were recorded after two months of planting and the disease incidence was recorded four months after planting.

Detection of R. solanacearum *in plants emerged from solarized rhizomes.* The non-symptomatic plants surviving after 60 days of planting were removed and the ginger rhizome extract was tested for presence of the bacterium using NCM-ELISA (10).

Results and Discussion

EFFECT OF HEAT ON SURVIVAL AND PATHOGENICITY OF *R. SOLANACEARUM*

The optimum temperature for growth of *R. solanacearum* is reported to be 28°C. At 37°C few strains grew and at 41°C only one strain exhibited slight growth (6). Reduction in survival of *R. solanacearum* was observed when the cells were exposed to higher temperatures. As the temperature increased, the survival of the bacteria decreased. When the bacterium was exposed for 30 min at 46°C, 98.0% cell death was recorded, whereas 100 percent death could be observed upon longer (60 min) exposure. Thus the thermal inactivation point of *R. solanacearum* was estimated to be 30 min at 47°C. It was further confirmed with microwaves: a temperature of 48°C was recorded after 15 s of exposure and complete death of bacterial cells occurred. Microwaves either directly or indirectly kill bacterial cells by heat induction. The effectiveness of microwaves for sterilization and disinfection has been well established by numerous recent studies (3,11). When the heat-exposed cells (40 and 45°C) were inoculated, the expression of the wilting symptom was delayed for 2 days compared to the check (30°C), where wilting was seen after 6 days. When exposure temperature was above 45°C, the pathogen could no longer cause a wilt, obviously due to complete death of all the cells at this temperature. Microwave or heat exposed bacterial cells could not induce wilt, which could be due to heat inactivation of virulent cells or could be attributed to direct killing of cells.

TEMPERATURE BUILDUP IN RHIZOME UPON SOLAR
OR MICROWAVE HEATING

Rhizome temperatures recorded after exposure to sunlight are shown in Fig. 1 and Fig. 2. Before exposure, the rhizome temperature was 30°C, reaching 53°C after 2 h of exposure. There was a drop in temperature after

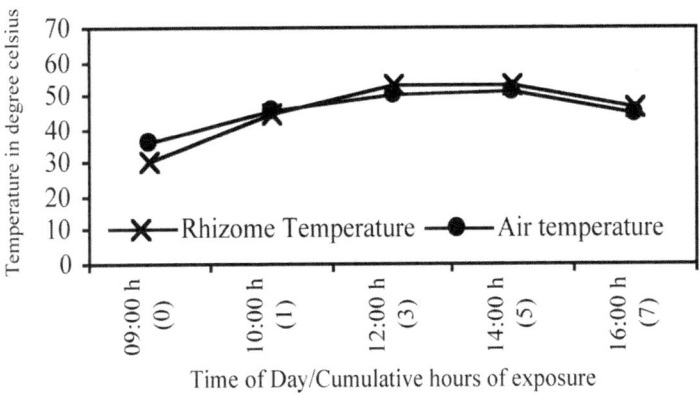

Fig. 1. Mean temperatures recorded in seed rhizome during solarization (May 21-28, 2000).

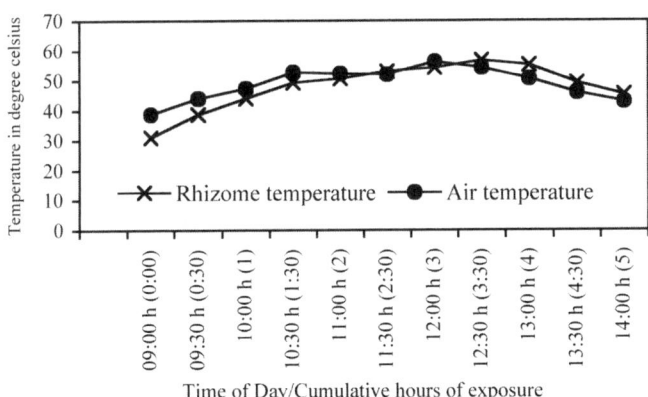

Fig. 2. Effect of rhizome solarization on heat build up in rhizome (Kothamanagalam on 24 April 2001).

1:30 p.m., largely because of pre-monsoon clouds, which clearly indicates the need for bright sunlight at least for two hours (Fig. 2). The buildup of heat in the rhizome could be due to the smaller seed pieces (25 g) used in the present study, which are widely used by the farmers in India. The relationship between rhizome size and heat build up has been reported (17).

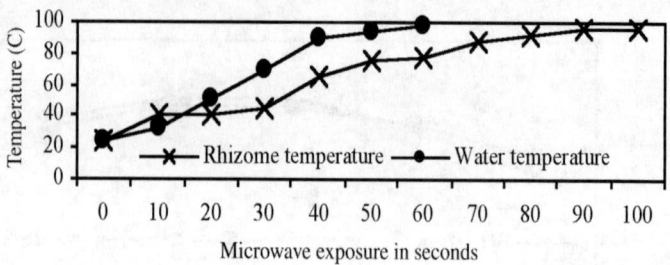

Fig. 3. Mean temperature recorded in bacterial suspension/seed rhizome after microwaving.

Based on the thermal inactivation temperature of *R. solanacearum,* the optimum duration for solarization was set at 2 h. Since it is known that the plant offers protection to the bacteria from external temperature and other environmental conditions, the prolonged exposure to sunlight was chosen. Relationship between microwave exposure and heat build up in rhizome is presented in Fig. 3. A temperature of 48°C was recorded in the bacterial suspension exposed for 15 s of microwaving. To achieve this temperature in rhizomes the duration of microwave exposure was determined to be 30 s.

EFFECT OF RHIZOME SOLARIZATION ON SEED VIABILITY

When the seed-rhizomes were exposed to solarization for 28 days (8 to 224 h of day light exposure), sprouts were burnt and rhizomes turned soft and rotten, which could be due to heat injury (above 50°C). This indicates that an extended period of rhizome solarization has detrimental effect on rhizomes and germination. Even after 8 h of solarization, sprouts were completely burnt and rhizomes were rotten following one week of storage.

Prolonged exposure to heat has been shown to be detrimental to germination of ginger (17). An exposure period of 2 to 4 h did not cause any abnormalities in sprouts and rhizomes, whereas after 6 h sprouts were completely burnt. Above 30 s of microwave exposure, the germination was significantly reduced, which could be due to heat injury to rhizomes at extended durations of exposure to microwaves. Temperatures of 59-95°C were recorded when the rhizomes were exposed to microwaves for a duration of 40-100 s (Table 1).

EVALUATION OF RHIZOME SOLARIZATION AND MICROWAVE TREATMENT FOR BACTERIAL WILT MANAGEMENT

Having generated the basic information on thermal inactivation point of *R. solanacearum* and chosen the '*modus operandi*' of raising the

Table 1. Effect of microwave on ginger germination and bacterial wilt incidence

Exposure (second)	°C	Sprouts	Height (cm)	Plant stand*	Wilt (%)*	Plant stand**	Wilt (%)**
UT	-	6.00^{ab}	11.5^{abcd}	8.0	0.0	10.0	0.0
0	26	5.7^{ab}	15.3^{abc}	8.3	8.3	7.0	26.7
10	40	3.0^{bcd}	17.7^{a}	5.3	0.0	5.0	0.0
20	40	4.3^{abc}	17.2^{ab}	7.3	0.0	8.7	0.0
30	45	6.3^{a}	9.1^{bcde}	6.3	0.0	7.3	0.0
40	59	2.3^{cd}	7.3^{cdef}	3.0	0.0	3.0	0.0
50	74	0.7^{d}	2.3^{ef}	0.7	0.0	1.0	0.0
60	75	0.0^{d}	0.0^{f}	0.0	0.0	0.0	0.0
70	88	1.0^{d}	6.5^{def}	1.0	0.0	1.0	0.0
80	89	0.0^{d}	0.0^{f}	0.0	0.0	0.0	0.0
90	96	0.0^{d}	0.0^{f}	0.0	0.0	0.0	0.0
100	95	0.0^{d}	0.0^{f}	0.0	0.0	0.0	0.0

* -45 Days after planting; **- 60 Days After Planting
UT- Untreated; Data with same letter designation are not significantly different
   (Duncan's Multiple Range Test at P=0.05%)

temperature of seed rhizomes by solar energy or microwaves, a series of experiments was conducted to test efficiency of methods for disinfecting seed rhizomes. In order to eliminate the deep-seated *R. solanacearum*, the sunlight/microwave exposure should be long enough to generate the lethal temperature inside the rhizomes. However, a longer exposure should not be injurious to seed pieces.

For total elimination of bacteria from seed pieces, a longer exposure to heat is needed because bacteria not only contaminate external tissue but are also located deep inside the rhizomes (17). Artificially infected rhizomes of ginger were solarized for a period of 2 and 4 h in day-light (8 h) and in another experiment the exposed rhizomes were once again solarized for the same duration next day to ensure complete inactivation of bacterial cells. A temperature of 55°C was achieved inside the rhizomes within 2 h of exposure from 9:00 a.m. to 11:00 a.m. on a bright sunny day. Two and 4 h of rhizome solarization did not significantly affect the germination of sprouts though there is a numerical inferiority in the 4 h solarized rhizomes. The data on plant stand also did not differ significantly. Wilt incidence was recorded after 45 days of planting and 35% of the plants emerged from unsolarized seed pieces expressed wilting symptoms after 60 days. Incidence was 75% on the 90th day and none of the plants survived after 100 days of planting (Table 2). When the surviving plants were tested for the presence of *R. solanacearum* using NCM-ELISA, none of the samples yielded a positive reaction, clearly indicating the effectiveness of rhizome solarization in eliminating the seed borne bacterium.

It is clear from the data presented in Table 1 that microwave treatment above 30 s of continuous exposure is detrimental to germination. The fact that none of the plants emerged from continuous microwave-exposed rhizomes expressed wilting indicated the effectiveness of the treatment in inactivating the bacterial cells in rhizomes. However, when pulse microwaving was used bacterial wilt could be observed even after 3 pulses of 10 s of exposure (42°C), revealing the difference between continuous and discontinuous microwaving in disinfecting the ginger rhizomes from bacterial wilt (Table 3). None of the plants that emerged from discontinuously microwaved rhizomes after 4 (45°C) or 5 (47°C) pulses of 10 s developed bacterial wilt.

EFFECT OF RHIZOME SOLARIZATION ON BACTERIAL WILT INCIDENCE IN FIELD

It is clear that rhizome solarization had direct effects on germination and disease incidence (Table 4). The germination of solarized rhizomes were 85.4% and 83.7%, whereas germination of the unsolarized rhizomes was 93%. However, the incidence of bacterial wilt was significantly reduced in solarized rhizomes. Bacterial wilt was observed in 33.8% of plants that emerged from unsolarized rhizomes, whereas wilt incidence was negligible

Table 2. Effect of rhizome solarization on germination and bacterial wilt incidence of ginger.

Treatment	Sprouts per pot	Plant height (cm)	Plant stand*	Wilt (%)*	Plant stand**	Wilt (%)**
No solarization	5.3^a	0.0^{ab}	5.0^c	35.3	1.1^d	75.5
2h from 9 a.m.	8.0^a	57.9^{ab}	12.3^{ab}	0.0	15.3^{abc}	0.0
4h from 9 a.m.	6.7^a	56.3^{ab}	10.3^{abc}	0.0	10.3^{abc}	0.0
2h from 9 a.m. during 2 days	6.3^a	61.7^a	10.7^{abc}	0.0	9.7^{bc}	0.0
4h from 9 a.m. during 2 days	7.3^a	53.3^b	13.3^{ab}	0.0	14.7^{abc}	0.0

Data with same letter designation are not different significantly according to Duncan's Multiple Range Test (P = 0.05); *60 Days After Planting; **90 Days After Planting in plants emerged from solarized rhizomes. This could be due to heat inactivation of bacterial cells upon solarization.

It is also interesting to note that wilt development was delayed for 30 days in solarized rhizomes, where 14 plants succumbed to the disease. This could be due to a low level of inoculum that escaped because of possible differences in the size of rhizomes used for planting. Alternately, it could be due to lateral spread of inoculum from untreated beds, which indicates the need for alternative strategies for checking the plant to plant spread of bacterial wilt in field. However, this aspect needs to be further investigated using NCM-ELISA or PCR with antibodies or primers specific for *R. solanacearum*. This work shows the effectiveness of rhizome solarization and rhizome microwaving for management of bacterial wilt of ginger.

Table 3. Effect of discontinuous microwaving on bacterial wilt of ginger

Microwave Treatment (10 s pulse)	Temperature (°C)	*Cumulative wilt incidence (%)
Unexposed	26	0.0
0	27	57.0
1	30	26.7
2	35	13.2
3	42	19.1
4	45	0.0
5	47	0.0

* Total numbers of plants wilted during 120 Days After Planting

Table 4. Effect of rhizome solarization on germination and bacterial wilt incidence of ginger in field

Rhizome solarization	Germination (%)	Days to express wilting symptom	*Wilt (%)
No solarization	93.0 (75.95)[a]	80	33.8 (32.1)[a]
2 h from 9-11am	85.4 (68.96)[b]	110	0.93 (6.1)[b]
2 h from 10-12 am	82.0 (67.08)[b]	–	0.0 (4.5)[b]

*-120 Days After Planting; Data with same letter designation are not different significantly according to Duncan's Multiple Range Test (P = 0.05); Figures in the parentheses are angular transformed values.

Acknowledgements

NCM-ELISA kit supplied by Dr. Sylvie Priou, Bacteriologist, CIP, Lima, Peru is gratefully acknowledged. We thank Prof. Chris Hayward for his critical comments and suggestions while preparing the manuscript.

Literature Cited

1. Colbran, R.C., and Davis, J.J. 1969. Studies on hot water treatment and soil fumigation for control of root knot of ginger. Qld J. Agric. Sci. 26: 439-445.
2. Ferris, R.S. 1984. Effect of microwave oven treatment on microorganisms in soil. Phytopathology 74: 121-126.
3. Goldblith, S.A., and Wang, D.I.C. 1967. Effect of microwaves on *Escherichia coli* and *Bacillus subtilis*. Appl. Microbiol. 15: 1371-1375.
4. Hartati, S.Y., and Supriadi. 1994. Systemic action of bactericide containing oxytetracycline and streptomycin sulphate in treated ginger rhizomes. J. Spices Med. Crops 3: 7-11.
5. Hayward, A.C., Moffett. M.L., and Pegg, K.G. 1967. Bacterial wilt of ginger in Queensland. Qld. J. Agric. Anim. Sci. 24:1-5.
6. He, L.Y., Sequeira, L., and Kelman, A. 1983. Characteristics of strains of *Pseudomonas solanacearum* from China. Plant Dis. 67: 1356-1361.
7. Indrasenan, G., Kumar, K.V., Mathew, J., and Mammen, M.K. 1982. Reaction of different types of ginger to bacterial wilt caused by *Pseudomonas solanacearum* (Smith) Smith. Agric. Res. J. Kerala 20:73-75.
8. Ishii, M., and Aragaki, M. 1963. Ginger wilt caused by *Pseudomonas solanacearum* E. F. Smith. Plant Dis. Rep. 47: 710-713.
9. Jolicoeur, G., Hackham, R and Tu, J.C. 1982. The selective inactivation of seed borne soybean mosaic virus by exposure to microwaves. J. Microw. Power 10:341-344.
10. Priou, S., Gutarra, L., and Aley, P. 1999. Highly sensitive detection of *Ralstonia solanacearum* in latently infected potato tubers by post-enrichment ELISA on nitrocellulose membrane. EPPO Bull. 29: 117-125.
11. Sanborn, M.R., Wan, S.K., and Bulard, R. 1982. Microwave sterilization of plastic tissue culture vessels for reuse. Appl. Environ. Microbiol. 44: 960-964.
12. Sarma, Y.R., Indrasenan, G., and Rohini Iyer, R. 1978. Bacterial wilt of ginger (*Zingiber officinale*). Indian Arecanut Spices Cocoa J. 2: 29-31.

13. Sharma, B.K., and Rana, K.S. 1999. Bacterial wilt: a threat to ginger cultivation in Himachal Pradesh. Plant Dis. Res. 14: 216-217.
14. Sunaina, V., Kishore, V., and Shekhawat, G.S. 1989. Latent survival of *Pseudomonas solanacearum* in potato tubers and weeds. J. Plant Dis. Prot. 96: 361-364.
15. Supriadi, Elphinstone, J.G., and Hartati, S.Y. 1995. Detection of latent infection of *Pseudomonas solanacearum* in ginger rhizomes and weeds by indirect ELISA. J. Spices Med. Crops 3: 5-10.
16. Thomas, K.M. 1941. Detailed Administration Report of the Government Mycologist for the year 1940-41. pp: 153-154.
17. Tsang, M.M.C., and Shintaku, M. 1998. Hot air treatment for control of bacterial wilt in ginger root. Appl. Eng. Agr. 14: 159-163.

Management of Bacterial Wilt of Potato Using One-Season Rotation Crops in Southwestern Uganda

M. Katafiire[1], E. Adipala[1], B. Lemaga[2], M. Olanya[3], R. El-Bedewy[3], and P. Ewell[3]

[1]Makerere University, P.O Box 7062, Kampala, Uganda.; [2]PRAPACE, P.O Box 22274, Kampala, Uganda; [3]International Potato Centre (CIP), P.O Box 25171, Nairobi, Kenya.

Bacterial wilt of potato, caused by *Ralstonia solanacearum,* is an important seed- and soil-borne disease in southwestern Uganda. In this region, potato is ranked as the number one cash crop and the fourth most important food crop. Adipala (1) and Berga *et al.* (5) reported that more than 70% of the potatoes grown in Uganda are produced in this area (2,4). The same authors also reported that the region where 70% of the farming community are subsistence growers, is characterized by a high population density, with severe land shortage and declining soil fertility (1,5), and that most of the households survive on less than one hectare while others depend on rented land for cultivation (1,6). Hence continuous cultivation of potato is common and results in increased incidence of various diseases, particularly bacterial wilt caused by *R. solanacearum* E. F. Smith (7,11). A number of authors including Berga *et al.* (5) reported that bacterial wilt accounts for about 30% potato yield loss in southwestern Uganda, (4,7,22). Tusiime *et al.* (24) reported that the use of resistant cultivars has not been consistently effective for the control of bacterial wilt due to the resistance of available cultivars breaking down quickly (11,23). A number of scientists have reported that chemical management is not practical due to the variable nature of the pathogen and its ability to survive for a long time in soil and the rhizosphere of non-host plants which would bring in cost implications (2,5,24). Moreover many herbaceous weeds are latently infected with the bacterium thus increasing its survival in the absence of potatoes (8,23). Several research scientists have recommended crop rotation as an effective method for reducing or even eradicating potato bacterial wilt due to rhizosphere suppression of *R. solanacearum* (5,7,8). Some non-host crops aggressively suppress *R. solanacearum* in the soil within a relatively short time (8,11,21). Berga *et al.* (5) and French (8) recommend crop rotation as a component of integrated disease management (IDM). Murithi (16) reported that crop rotation led to higher potato yields in the presence of bacteria wilt in Kenya. In Indonesia, rotation of potato with pulses, cereals and root crops for two seasons led to significant reduction of potato wilt and in-creased both total yield and the ratio of marketable tubers to total yield compared to the potato repeat (7,8). Therefore this study was set up to identify multipurpose rotation crop(s) that would in the subsequent season a) delay onset of wilt, b) reduce wilt incidence, c) reduce latent infections, d) reduce *R. solanacearum* populations in the soil and e) increase tuber size and yield.

Materials and Methods

Studies were conducted between 2000 and 2001, in Kachwekano Agricultural Research and Development Centre (01° 16'S, 29° 57'E) located at 2200 m elevation. The experiments were conducted for three consecutive seasons in bacterial wilt-infested plots. Plots measuring 6x4m with 1m alley between plots were laid out in a randomized complete block design with three replicates. The initial experiment was conducted during the first rains of 2000 (noted 2000A), the second experiment was during the second rains of 2000 (noted 2000B), and the third experiment was during the first rains of 2001. Prior to planting the experiment for the rains of 2000, experimental plots were planted with the highly susceptible tomato variety 'Money-maker' in an attempt to generate a uniform disease inocu-lum pressure. Plants that had not wilted by 28 days after planting (DAP) were artificially infected using a stem-puncture procedure with a pure cul-ture of *R. solanacearum*. That culture was obtained from bacterial ooze collected on infected tubers and cultured in the laboratory on the modified Kelman's medium.

During 2000A's rains, potato was grown in all plots to simulate the shortened rotation existing in the region and create uniform field conditions. In the second rains 2000B, experimental plots were planted to sorghum, wheat, maize, finger millet, sweet potato, carrots, beans, and potato – food crops that are commonly grown in the highlands of southwestern Uganda. In the first rain 2001 season potato was again grown in all the study plots to test the effect of the rotation crops on the subsequent potato crop.

During these three seasons, soil fertility of experimental plots was improved using urea, single super phosphate and muriate of potash ac-cording to Berga *et al.* (5). The most common pests and diseases (i.e. potato aphids and late blight) were controlled using Ambush CY and Ridomil MZ, 63.5 respectively. During seasons 2000A and 2001, plots were sprayed twice and during rains of 2000B plots were sprayed three times according to manufacturers' instructions. Data were collected as percentage of wilted plants on a weekly basis, starting from the onset of wilt symptoms. Plants were considered wilted when partially or completely diseased and were staked to avoid confusion in the subsequent recording and also to avoid missing data from the plants that died early in the season. Final wilt incidence for each treatment was calculated as percentage of total number of plants emerged.

Harvesting of tubers was done when about 75% of the plants reached senescence. Weights of ware tubers, seed size and bacterial wilt infected tubers were also recorded separately at harvest (5). Indicator plant/pathogenicity test was used to test R. solanacearum inoculum levels in the soil (23) before and after each season. Latently infected tubers were determined in sterile soil tests with incubation at high temperature for 6 weeks and detection of R. solanacearum using CIP's NCM-ELISA (18). Incubated tubers were observed for bacterial wilt ooze weekly during the first four weeks and daily during the last two weeks. Tubers used for the sterile soil tests were first stored until they sprouted before they were planted out in the sterile soil medium loaded in plastic trays of 30x60 cm. After emergence, plants were observed for wilt symptoms on a daily basis. In both latent infection tests, tubers that did not show disease symptoms were recorded separately from infected tubers and the latter were disposed of carefully. Latent infection in stems and root segments of rotation crops was determined using NCM-ELISA kit (18). Percentage values were log_{10} transformed before analysis of variance using Genstat 4.32 statistical package.

Results and Discussion

The plots that had been under sorghum, wheat, finger millet, and maize during 2000B had lower wilt incidences than those that had been under sweet potatoes, carrots, beans, and continuous potato. Continuous potato cropping had the highest wilt incidence (72%) at the end of the three seasons. Sorghum, wheat, maize, and finger millet had the lowest R. solanacearum inoculum level in the soil compared to other crops under evaluation during this study. Continuous potato cultivation increased potato tuber latent infection and lowered the shelf life (Table 1). Potatoes following sorghum, wheat, finger millet and maize had higher tuber weights and higher ratio of marketable tubers to total yield compared to the control plots (Table 2).

During the 2001 season, NCM-ELISA tests detected latent infections in potato tubers from plots that had been under beans, carrots, and sweet potato. The tubers from continuous potato cropping had clear bacterial ooze

Table 1. Effect of rotation crops grown during the second rains 2000 on the soil and tuber latent infections of potato crop during the first rains 2001

Plot rotation	Pathogenicity Test (12/00)	Wilt Onset (DAP[a])	Wilt (%)	Sterile soil test	Incubation test
Sweet potato/potato	8	28	26	74	60.2
Wheat/potato	17	42	6.0	55	33.9
Potato/potato	88	21(45[b])	72(20)	87(80)	70.1(100)
Maize/potato	10	35	8.0	57	40
Millet/potato	11	35	8.0	64	40.2
Carrots/potato	17	28	16	79	60.5
Sorghum/potato	7	45	4	68	30.8
Phaseolus beans/ potato	8	28	26	55	33.9
LSD$_{(0.5)}$	21.3	5.2	9.2	9.2	7.5
CV %	19.1	13.3	30.5	15.5	13.0

[a] Days after planting.
[b] Figures in brackets are data for second rainy season 2000.

symptoms, whereas the tubers from plots previously under cereals (sorghum, wheat, maize and finger millet) were tested negative. Incubation of potato tubers of the subsequent crop provided a higher estimate of *R. solanacearum* levels than sterile soil tests and NCM-ELISA, which could be attributed to the duration and the high temperature which offers a conducive environment for *R. solanacearum* to express itself.

Conclusions

The rotation crops sorghum, wheat, maize and finger millet were effective in delaying the onset of wilt, reducing wilt incidence, increasing tuber yields and improving potato tuber shelf-life. This study showed that growing any of the evaluated rotation crops was better than the continuous cropping of potato and the latter should therefore be avoided. Low wilt incidence in the field cannot be relied on as an indicator of low level of the bacterium in the soil as shown by the high percentage infection obtained from incubated and sterile soil samples. Although incubation takes longer, it is simple and practically feasible for farmers in Uganda.

Table 2. Effect of rotation crops grown during the second rains of 2000 on the yield of the potato crop during the first rains of 2001

Plot rotation	Yield (tons/Ha)			
	Ware	Seed tuber	Diseased tuber	Total tuber
Sweet potato/potato	5.6	4.6	2.6	12.8
Wheat/potato	9.5	4.5	0.6	14.5
Potato/potato	1.1(29.9[a])	1.0(1.7)	8.3(6.3)	10.5(37.9)
Maize/potato	8.6	3.8	0.1	13.1
Millet/potato	8.3	3.3	0.7	12.2
Carrots/potato	6.3	2.7	4.5	13.5
Sorghum/potato	9.4	2.3	0.5	12.6
Phaseolus beans/potato	2.5	2.8	6.4	11.8
$LSD_{(0.5)}$	1.4	1.2	0.2	1.5
CV %	16.1	28.7	22.6	15.7

[a] Figures in brackets are data for second rainy season 2000.

Literature Cited

1. Adipala E., 1999. Potato Production in Uganda. A survey perspective. Makerere University, Kampala.
2. Adipala, E., Namanda, S., Mukalazi, J., Abalo, G., Kimoone, G., and Hakiza, J.J., 2000. Understanding farmer's perception of potato production constraints and responses to yield decline in Uganda. Afr. Potato Assoc. Conf. Proc. 5: 429-438.
3. Berga Lemaga, Hakiza J.J., Alacho F.O.A., and Kakuhenzire R, 1997. Integrated control of potato bacterial wilt in south western Uganda. Pages 188-195 in: Proc. 4th Triennial Conf. Afr. Potato Assoc. Pretoria, South Africa, 23-28 February 1997.
4. Berga Lemaga, Hakiza J.J., Bariyanga J., and Ewell P.T., 1999. Potato production and importance of bacterial wilt in Kabale district – Uganda. A farm survey report. African Highlands Initiative/ International Potato Center.
5. Berga Lemaga, Kanzikwera, R., Hakiza, J.J., Kakuhenzire, R., and Manzi, G. 2001. The effect of crop rotation on bacterial wilt incidence and potato tuber yield. Afr. Crop Sci. J. 9: 257-266.
6. CIP/CIAT/IFPRI/IITA/IPGRI, 2000. Roots and Tubers in the Global Food System: A Vision Statement to the year 2020. Lima, Peru.

7. Devaux, A., Michelante, D., and Bicamumpaka, M. 1987. Combination of rotation and resistance to control bacterial wilt (*Pseudomonas solanacearum*) in Rwanda. Pages 100-1 in: European Assoc. Potato Res. Abstracts 10th Triennial Conf., Aolborg, Denmark.

8. French, E.R. 1994. Strategies for integrated control of bacterial wilt of potatoes. Pages 199-207 in: Bacterial Wilt: The Disease and its Causative Agent *Pseudomonas solanacearum*. A.C. Hayward and G.L. Hartman, eds. CAB International, Wallingford, UK.

9. Hakiza, J.J., Turyamureeba, G., Kakuhenzire, R.M., Odong, B., Mwanga, R.M., Kanzikwera, R., and Adipala, E. 2000. Potato and sweet potato improvement in Uganda: A historical perspective. Afr. Potato Assoc. Conf. Proc. 5:47-58.

10. Hayward, A.C. 1991. Biology and epidemiology of bacterial wilt caused by *Pseudomonas solanacearum*. Annu. Rev. Phytopathol. 29: 65-87.

11. Hayward, A.C. 1994. The hosts of *Pseudomonas solanacearum*. Pages 9-24 in: Bacterial Wilt: The Disease and its Causative Agent *Pseudomonas solanacearum*. A.C. Hayward and G.L. Hartman, eds.. CAB International, Wallingford, UK.

12. Hayward, A.C. 1986. Bacterial wilt caused by *Pseudomonas solanacearum* in Asia and Australia: An overview. Pages 15-24 in: Proceedings of an International Workshop on Bacterial Wilt Disease in Asia and the South Pacific. ACIAR Proc. No. 13. G.J. Persley, ed.

13. International Potato Center. 2000. Annual Report. (CIP) Lima, Peru.

14. Kakuhenzire, R., Hakiza, J.J., Berga Lemaga, Tusiime, G., and Alacho F., 2000. Past, present and future strategies for integrated management of potato bacterial wilt disease in Uganda. Afr. Potato Assoc. Conf. Proc. 5:353-360.

15. Low, J. W. 1997. Potato in southwestern Uganda: Threats to sustainable production. Afr. Crop. Sci. J. 5:22–28.

16. Muriithi, L.M.M. 2000. Farmer participation in management of potato bacterial wilt in central and eastern Kenya. Afr. Potato Assoc. Conf. Proc. 5: 361-368.

17. OEPP/EPPO 1996. Data sheets on Quarantine Pests: *Ralstonia solanacearum*. CABI and EPPO 90/399003.

18. Priou, S., and Gutarra, L. 1998. NCM-ELISA kit for the detection of *Ralstonia solanacerum* in latently infected potato tubers. International Potato Centre (CIP). Lima, Peru.

19. Ricaud, C. 1990. Seed potato for warm tropics: constraints and options. Pages 22-28 in: Production, Post-harvest Technology and Utilisation of Potato in the Warm Tropics. Proceedings of a workshop held in Reduit, Mauritius 23-27 July 1990.

20. Skoglund, L.G., Berrios, D.E., and Rubirigi, A. 1993. Study of latent infection of potato tubers by *Pseudomonas solanacearum* in Burundi. Pages 46-53 in: Proceedings of the workshop on bacterial wilt of potato caused by *Pseudomonas solanacearum*. Bujumbura, Burundi, February 22-26.

21. Terblanche, J., and De Villiers, D., 1999. Marigolds as biological control for bacterial wilt. Afr. Crop. Sci. Conf. Proc. 4: 523-525.

22. Tusiime, G., Adipala, E., Opio, F., and Bhagsari, A.S. 1996. Occurrence of *Pseudomonas solanacearum* latent infection in potato tubers and weeds in highland Uganda. Afr. J. Plant Prot. 6: 108-118.

23. Tusiime, G., Adipala, E., Opio, F., and Bhagsari, A.S., 1996. Screening solanum potato genotypes for resistance to *Pseudomonas solanacearum* in Uganda. Afr. J. Plant Prot. 6: 96-107.

24. Tusiime, G., and Adipala, E. 2000. Management of bacterial wilt of potato: approaches, limitations and the role of stakeholders. Afr. Potato Assoc. Conf. Proc. 5: 347-352.

25. Van Der Zaag, P. 1994. Seed potato production in Uganda: present status and future direction. Presented to International Potato Centre and National Agricultural Research Organisation. Pages 24-37. CIP, Lima, Peru.

26. Yabuuchi, E., Kosaka, Y., Oyaizu, H., Yano, I., Hotta, H., and Nishiuchi, Y. 1995. Transfer of two *Burkholderia* and an *Alcaligenes* species to *Ralstonia* gen. nov.: Proposal of *Ralstonia pickettii* (Ralston, Palleroni and Doudoroff 1973). and *Ralstonia eutropha* (Davis 1996) comb. nov. Microbiol. Immunol. 39:897-904.

Potato Bacterial Wilt Management: New Prospects for an Old Problem

María M. López and Elena G. Biosca
Instituto Valenciano de Investigaciones Agrarias, IVIA,
Apartado Oficial 46113, Moncada, Valencia, Spain

Potato Is One of the Favorite Hosts of *Ralstonia solanacearum*

Since 1896, when the bacterium was identified by E.F. Smith on potato for the first time, *R. solanacearum* has become a major threat to potato cultivation worldwide. Potato strains of *R. solanacearum* can belong to biovars 1, 2, 2T, 3 and 4, but at present only biovar 2 is adapted to cool temperate zones, while the other three biovars are found in subtropical or tropical areas [Editor's note: according to Fegan and Prior, this volume, biovar 2 are Phylotype II sequevars 1 and 2]. Numerous outbreaks due to biovar 2 strains have been reported in the last ten years in Europe, where it is considered a quarantine bacterium (2). The distribution of potato brown rot in Europe has been reported (6,15,31,69) and for an exhaustive review see Elphinstone (this volume). *R. solanacearum* may infect potato as a soil-borne, water-borne or tuber-borne organism (5,10,26,30). Volunteer plants or weeds are considered to be plant reservoirs for contamination when potato crops are planted in the same field in successive growing seasons. The bacterium may spread from these sources during cultivation and harvesting operations. Insect pests have been considered as a means of dissemination of the pathogen but this is not established and further research is required. Inoculum of *R. solanacearum* may also be disseminated by contaminated equipment.

In 1994, Sequeira (59) pointed out that "the ecology was the forgotten element in bacterial wilt research and that the dearth of information was related to the lack of adequate methodology". Eight years later, new techniques were developed (4,7,8,45,46,54,75,79) which improved our knowledge on survival of the pathogen (van Elsas *et al.* this volume, 15,16,17, 21,27,33,49,50,67,68,69,76), but there are still many unanswered questions remaining on the long-term survival of the bacterium and its reservoirs.

There is no universal control strategy for potato bacterial wilt. This could be explained by different soils and ecological conditions for potato cultivation, and the different nature and behavior of strains of *R. solanacearum* affecting this host. Recommended control was based on an integrated strategy consisting of cumulative effects of complementary measures as described by French (23): healthy seed planted in pathogen free soil, or in plots with agronomic practices to decrease populations of the pathogen. However, a century after the discovery of the bacterium it is still necessary to avoid planting of potato in heavily infested soils. In such situations the use of new cultivars with durable resistance is still a priority. Control of potato bacterial wilt is difficult and requires a multidisciplinary approach and efficient technology transfer to the growers. In this context, we present here some relevant data or relatively new factors that may help in controlling this devastating pathogen on potato. Also, comments and discussions from participants at the "Special session on brown rot of potato" organized during 3rd IBWS are reported. Because there is a chapter devoted to bacterial wilt management in this volume, only bacterial wilt of potato caused by *R. solanacearum* biovar 2 is covered.

How to Prevent Potato Bacterial Wilt

Preventive measures are essential to maintain countries, areas or plots free of bacterial wilt. Among them are the use of healthy seed, shown to be free of the pathogen in statistically controlled tests and produced in pathogen-free areas, combined with irrigation using water known to be free of *R. solanacearum*. Imported ware potatoes are a major potential means of introduction of *R. solanacearum* to new areas (31). For this reason the European Union (EU) member states conduct annual surveys of potato seed and surface water (2). In addition, ware potatoes imported from developing countries are tested for brown rot, when they come from areas where the disease has been reported.

CLEAN SOIL

It is well known that *R. solanacearum* is a soil-borne bacterium (5,30) that is endemic in most tropical lands (5). There may be prolonged survival of the bacterium in soils, water, and plant material. The bacterium can survive for many years in the soil when potatoes or other hosts are cultivated but survival has not always been fully evaluated after rotations or fallow periods, in naturally infested soils. The nutritionally most versatile biovar 3 strains are believed to have a greater capacity for survival in soil than biovar 2. However, this is not consistent with repeated outbreaks due to biovar 2 strains in some Asian and African countries (50). In Europe biovar 2 strains have been shown to survive for at least one year in soil in the Neth-

206

erlands (68). Soil temperature and moisture are key factors in survival (30,47). High soil temperatures (43°C for four days) decrease population of *R. solanacearum*. Long-term survival in deeper soil layers is probably a function of lower soil temperatures (30). Survival of this bacterium is greater in wet but well-drained soils than in soil after desiccation or flooding (5,30,47,64). Reports indicate population levels of 1 x 10^4 to 10^6 CFU/g of soil in the Netherlands (69) and in Nepal (50). An accelerated decline of the culturable form of the bacteria was detected at 4°C, a condition that induced the viable but nonculturable (VBNC) state (69). Some soils seem to be conducive to bacterial wilt and others suppressive (23,30). Nevertheless, systematic study of the biotic and abiotic factors responsible for suppressiveness is lacking.

Although the reversible phenotype conversion in *R. solanacearum* has only been observed when the bacterium is growing *in vitro*, it is possible that similar behavior may also occur in natural settings such as soil (11). A reduced production of extracellular proteins and exopolysaccharides should conserve energy and resources, thus enhancing survival. However the experiments supporting this hypothesis have not yet been performed. The numbers of culturable cells of *R. solanacearum* was much higher in the rhizosphere of potato plants than in the soil in naturally infested fields (Vicedo *et al.*, unpublished data); one possible explanation is that the bacterium is attracted by root exudates or other root components by chemotaxis.

Exact knowledge of the survival strategies and the life cycle of the bacterium in soil requires quantitative analysis with accurate detection techniques. Major difficulties in detection of the bacterium in soil are related to the heterogeneous nature of soil, the irregular distribution of the pathogen, the lack of efficient soil sampling procedures and the presence of inhibitors and competitors. The comparative evaluation of sensitivity and specificity of different techniques to detect *R. solanacearum* in soil, shows that dilution plating on a modified SMSA medium (19) is most sensitive, whereas tomato bioassay and ELISA were less efficient for low bacterial populations (51, López *et al.*, unpublished data). Immunofluorescence colony staining (69), enrichment-ELISA using specific monoclonal antibodies (8) and enrichment-PCR with specific primers (51) are also reliable techniques.

In spite of the high sensitivity of some methods, recovery of *R. solanacearum* from naturally infested soils is frequently negative, even in presence of symptomatic host plants (Vicedo *et al.*, unpublished data). This could be related to either the low numbers of pathogenic *Ralstonia*, its irregular distribution in the soil, the population of antagonists, the VBNC state of *R. solanacearum* cells, the extent of enrichment or presence of inhibitors of PCR, or a combination of all or several factors. It is more reliable to take representative soil samples, plant susceptible tomato seedlings (such as varieties Roma or Moneymaker) in them and inspect weekly for the development of wilt symptoms (López *et al.*, unpublished data). Negative results do not guarantee that the soil is free of *R. solanacearum* but are at least indicative of low populations of the pathogen. Bacteriophages able to lyse *R. solanacearum* have been found in soil without wilted plants (71), which may also be indicative of the presence of the bacterium in the soil. This could be another approach for the indirect detection of the pathogen in soil.

CLEAN SEED

To produce clean potato seed it is obvious that the mother tubers should be free of *R. solanacearum* and that they should be produced in a pathogen-free area or multiplied *in vitro* (Mienie, this volume, 77). In some areas it is difficult to ensure that such tubers can be produced because of insufficient land and frequent exchange of machinery, laborers etc, between infested and uninfested land. The pathogen can be present on the surface, lenticels and vascular tissue of latently infected potato tubers (10,30) but the possibility of spread on true seeds is unclear (30). Tolerant potato selections or susceptible cultivars grown under conditions unfavorable for disease expression can act as a vehicle of *R. solanacearum,* with the result that the disease is disseminated on latently infected but healthy-appearing planting material (30).

R. *solanacearum* is considered a quarantine pathogen in the EU and by the European and Mediterranean Plant Protection Organization (EPPO), which has necessitated specific legislation and protocols for detection in potato tubers and of measures to apply following a new outbreak (2,20). The aim is to detect and eradicate outbreaks surveyed in the different countries and to limit the spread of the bacterium through latently infected tubers. These measures enabled national surveillance of imported stocks and required surveys of home production, with inspection for symptoms and analysis for latent infections. Increased trade in seed potatoes throughout the EU, together with outbreaks found in many EU countries has increased the need for disease monitoring (2,7,77).

The official EU protocol for detection of latent infections requires the examination of at least 200 tubers per lot of potato of 25 metric tons or less (2). This allows the detection of at least one infected tuber with a 87% probability in a lot showing 1% infection rate. In other countries like South Africa, the sample size is 4605 tubers per registered planting unit, based on a statistical model for zero tolerance (Mienie, this volume). The sampling methodology plays a major role in the reliability of the final results, but this aspect has not been analysed in different practical situations. However the results of an SMT project funded by the EU (van Vaerenbergh and

Elphinstone, pers. comm.) support the proposed EU methodology. This project has set up several protocols for detection and identification of *R. solanacearum* in potato tubers (7,18,45,46,75) based on enrichment, the use of specific monoclonal antibodies and new PCR primers that provide better sensitivity and specificity than those previously available. Optimised protocols to detect the target in soil, water, sewage sludge, waste water, etc, have also been proposed and after consideration by the Standards Committee for Plant Health of the EU Commission could be implemented in place of existing legislation.

The application of the recommended EU measures (2) and the annual analysis of more than 60,000 potato lots since 1995 in the Netherlands has resulted in a reduction in the number of potato lots found positive, but not the eradication of the disease as a whole (34). Similar measures have been applied in recent years in Egypt with good results (J. Janse, pers. comm.). The declaration of pathogen-free areas is necessary in countries where the disease is not widespread but present in some zones. The free area can also be a whole country, even if some outbreaks were found, provided that eradication measures were taken.

Dissemination of *R. solanacearum* may be reduced by disease surveys; success depends on effective survey design, the use of the most appropriate methodology for analysis (8,16), the relationship between the number of people involved in the surveys, and the number of fields to visit and/or tons to analyse. In this context, potato growers should be well informed and trained for symptom detection and motivated to send the suspected samples to the laboratory. An important requirement for successful eradication is the need to compensate the growers when outbreaks of the disease are found. In addition, in countries like the Netherlands insurance against potato brown rot is more and more frequent because only insured growers are compensated if an outbreak of the bacterium is detected. According to EU legislation (2) when an infected lot is confirmed, infected material should be incinerated, buried deep in places without risk of dissemination, processed for industry under official control, or be used as animal feed after heat treatment.

The methods for producing seed potato free from *R. solanacearum* should be adapted to the particular situation of the potato farms in the different zones. The most convenient preventive measures, cultural practices and treatments should be explained to the farmers by using experimental plots and by training campaigns adapted to their education level and available resources (13). Simple methods such as the use of disease-free nurseries (Lemaga *et al.*, this volume), the seed-plot technique (Kinyua *et al.*, this volume) or more sophisticated technology like *in vitro* propagation (Mienie, this volume, 77) and analysis by sensitive and specific techniques (2,7,17, 18,45,46,53,58,75) have greatly improved the health status of the potato in some countries and have reduced the presence of *R. solanacearum* in the seed tubers.

CLEAN WATER

The role of water as a reservoir and vehicle of transmission of bacterial wilt was underestimated until potato irrigation became popular in Northern Europe in the 1990s. It is now accepted in most EU countries, that water-borne *R. solanacearum* biovar 2 was at the origin of most outbreaks, with involvement of the weed *Solanum dulcamara* as a reservoir of the pathogen, in Sweden (43), the United Kingdom, Belgium, The Netherlands, France (31) and Spain (44). Irrigation of potato fields was soon related to these outbreaks. Some European rivers or channels were shown to maintain live populations of *R. solanacearum* biovar 2 at certain locations. The available data suggest that the bacterium entered the river with rotten potatoes discarded by the growers, with sewage sludge and/or industrial or domestic residues from contaminated tubers imported from African or Asian countries and processed several years earlier. Thus potato process water and sewage effluents must be taken into account and analyzed (2,21, 31). In spite of its importance as an inoculum source (16,17,33) the fate of *R. solanacearum* biovar 2 in aquatic environments of temperate regions is still poorly understood (68). The concentration of *R. solanacearum* biovar 2 in different European water systems could be highly variable. The most intensive studies have been performed in the United Kingdom and The Netherlands where notably high populations (1×10^6 CFU/L) were detected during the summer (16,17,33). However, populations were very low in most of the water samples when the water temperature was below 15°C (4,33). As total bacterial populations in water are usually around 1×10^4 CFU/L (33), and taking into account the number of litres used for irrigation by spraying or flooding of crops, this represents a massive density of bacteria arriving to potato roots. Populations of *R. solanacearum* were higher in water surrounding latently infected *S. dulcamara* plants and its persistence is clearly enhanced by the presence of this semi-aquatic weed (16,17,33). Nevertheless, under natural conditions this weed usually shows no symptoms.

In other countries the relationship between *R. solanacearum* occurrence, *S. dulcamara* distribution and contaminated water has not been established. In Australia or Egypt (21), where *S. dulcamara* is not present, other weeds and other abiotic or biotic factors may be responsible for persistence of the pathogen in surface water. However, the warmer temperatures of the rivers in these areas may favor pathogen survival in the absence of alternative host plants and it may also persist in ditch sediments or biofilms that may protect bacteria from detrimental environmental conditions.

Early detection of *R. solanacearum* biovar 2 in surface irrigation water is essential to prevent introduction to new areas and irrigation water should be routinely analyzed every year, at least in summer months when water temperatures exceed 15°C. It is not known whether the bacterium can survive in the long-term in water by adopting a starvation-survival state, or if they lose culturability on artificial media (VBNC state) when exposed to low winter temperatures (4,33,68). These cells would escape current detection methods based on direct isolation on SMSA (19) or even by PCR (5, 45,46) when present at low density. The inability to grow VBNC cells on solid media mirrors the development of a form with altered nutritional or physicochemical requirements that might need special conditions for culture as suggested by Weichart *et al.* (72). In fact, VBNC cells respond to the addition of nutrients provided in liquid form, as in the Kogure method (39) currently used for direct viable counts, during a longer period than on solid standard media (4). Further, the most probable number (MPN) method is an alternative for quantifying viability via growth in liquid media (56) that can assist detection. We have devised an enrichment in modified Wilbrink broth (7) for 72h at 35°C and use of the MPN method, that can be combined with DASI-ELISA (Biosca *et al.*, this volume, 8) or PCR (4,45,46,58) to detect both starved and stressed cells in watercourses during winter. Lytic bacteriophages for *R. solanacearum* biovar 2 were easily isolated from river water. They could be used for indirect detection of the pathogen from water samples (Biosca *et al.*, unpublished data). These methodologies may help to improve our knowledge of the ecology and waterborne transmission of the pathogen and aid in development of new control strategies.

How to Control Potato Bacterial Wilt in Endemic Areas

Bacterial wilt may be endemic in some potato growing areas where *R. solanacearum* persists naturally in several environmental niches (soil, water, weeds, non-hosts) and/or may disseminate from these sites through contaminated plant materials.

CHEMICAL CONTROL

Commercial chemicals, including antibiotics, copper compounds, fungicides, soil fumigants and many other products, have been extensively evaluated in the past without gaining acceptance for eradication of *R. solanacearum* from soil, to prevent or to cure diseased potato (29). Furthermore, the use of chemicals like antibiotics to control plant pathogens has been seriously questioned because of development of resistant strains and bears a hazard to human health and the environment. Difficulties in control were related to survival of the bacterium in the deeper soil layers and its localization in the xylem vessels of plants. Nevertheless the fumigant chloropicrin was successfully used in the southern USA and Japan (23).

Bacterial wilt is more severe when the root-knot nematode (*Meloidogyne* spp.) occurs concomitantly (30,36,74). Disease incidence was reduced by widening the spacing between liquid fertilizer chisels to minimize root damage. Soil fumigation with 1,3-D or metam sodium, oxamyl or ethroprop reduces the incidence and severity of bacterial wilt (73). New products that show no effect *in vitro* but are known to stimulate host defenses have been registered in some countries against bacterial diseases. They are based on harpin (Actigard and Messenger) or benzothiodiazol (Bion). Pradhanang *et al.* (52) have shown that Actigard enhances resistance in naturally resistant tomato cultivars, but efficacy on potato was not tested.

CULTURAL PRACTICES

Changes in cultural practices for potato production may reduce severity of but not eradicate bacterial wilt. Effective cultural control practices must be adapted to each specific area; whether they reduce pathogen populations and/or symptom expression is unclear. In several areas in Colombia and Costa Rica the disease has disappeared for years without any scientific explanation, but this does not indicate that the bacterium has really declined to extinction. By contrast, in other areas bacterial wilt can increase exponentially when cultural practices are modified, for example by use of nitrogen fertilizers or cutting of mother tubers. In the production of ware potatoes, losses could be reduced by modifying planting date to seasons that are less conducive for symptom expression (30), but this does not reduce the incidence of latent infections. Soil treatments like $CaCO_3$, sea-shell grit (42% CaO) or urea have been used with variable effectiveness but they can affect the soil quality for potato cultivation (Siverio *et al.* unpublished data, 30). Traditional farmer's manure or compost may reduce bacterial wilt, but results are quite variable (van Elsas *et al.*, this volume; Hernández *et al.* unpublished data). Solarization assays have demonstrated some efficacy against soilborne *R. solanacearum* biovar 2, but not against other biovars (23). However, solarization alone was not sufficient for full control. Compost or biofumigant combined with solarization decreased pathogen population in soil (van Elsas *et al.*, this volume). However, the real impact of these measures on the potato crop has not been evaluated. Inundation was used in Thailand with apparently good results, probably due to the anaerobic conditions that affect survival of *R. solanacearum*.

Cropping systems. The effectiveness of short-term rotations (1-2 years) to control bacterial wilt was limited by survival of *R. solanacearum* in soil, even in the absence of susceptible hosts. Continuous cropping of a susceptible host leads to increased populations of the pathogen. The effectiveness of different crop rotations has been reported (Katafiire *et al.*, Lemaga *et al.*, this volume). One season rotations are insufficient to eradicate the pathogen, but partial control of bacterial wilt should be further evaluated. Cereals (12) and crops like onion, pea, cabbage, cowpea or bean generally provide acceptable control (1,23,30), alone or in different combinations. In some Asian countries rotation using rice has shown efficacy in decreasing inoculum (13). The variable results obtained using crops like maize or sweet potato may be a reflection of the differences in interactions between microbial communities in soil, populations of *R. solanacearum* and distinct soil microbiota. The ideal crop for rotation should be not only immune to *R. solanacearum* but also able to produce root exudates toxic for the bacterium. The role of crop residues has not been extensively studied (26) and should be evaluated.

Bare fallow. In the absence of an ideal, universal, non-host, candidate crop for rotations extended fallow periods have some advantages, especially in dry areas with irrigated fields. Populations of *R. solanacearum* may drop to undetectable levels after the dry season and longer periods (Vicedo *et al.*, unpublished data, 5,23,30,49,64). However the bacterium may also concentrate in hot spots for long-term survival under suitable conditions such as in the deep moist layer of the soil (30). The bacterium may also shift to a VBNC state but this has not yet been proven. Nevertheless it is clear that measures should be taken to eliminate volunteer potato plants that have been shown to act as an inoculum source. The EU legislation (2) includes three years without cultivation or cultivation of non-host crops (cereals) among the measures that must be taken in the EU countries in response to an outbreak of bacterial wilt. Wherever reduction of bacterial wilt incidence is a priority, technical people and farmers should realize that this is a difficult and long term task. When possible, economically unprofitable decisions but proven effective methods should be taken, such as bare fallow for 3-5 years in infested plots.

Weeds. The range and variety of weeds that are hosts of *R. solanacearum* have increased every year since the monograph of Smith in 1896 (62). However, their significance varies greatly in different areas and most are asymptomatic carriers. The role of the weed rhizosphere as a shelter for pathogenic cells has been demonstrated for several *Solanum* species such as *S. dulcamara*, *S. cinereum*, *S. nigrum*, *S. carolinense* and for many species of other genera (30). Recent findings confirm that members of different botanical families may host the pathogen. *R. solanacearum* was detected in naturally infected *Erechthites hieracifolia* (61) in Brasil and in *Urtica dioica* in the Netherlands (76). In Nepal the bacterium was isolated from *Galinsoga parvifolia*, *G. ciliata*, *Polygonum capitata*, *Oxalis* sp. and *Fagopyrum* sp. (49). In Cuba it was found on *Milleria quinqueflora* and

Parthenium hysterophorus (64) and in Uganda on *Amaranthus* sp., *Bidens pilosa, G. parvifolium, Oxalis latifoliae, Spergula arvensis, Rumex abyssinicum, Polygonum nepalense, Tagetes minuta, Stellaria sennii, Leucas martinicensis, Erigeron floribundus* and *Ageratum conyzoides* (67). These studies show that low numbers of *R. solanacearum* may be released from symptomless infected weeds, and such weed hosts should play a major role in survival of the pathogen in the absence of a susceptible host. *R. solanacearum* can infect a large number of weeds upon artificial inoculation; whether they act as hosts under natural conditions is unknown, but successful colonization of these species suggests this potential. *Bidens pilosa* (found as a host in Uganda), *Galinsoga parviflora, Brachiaria plantaginea* and *Digitaria horizontalis* (61) are some of the weed reservoirs recognized in the past ten years. Pradhanang and Elphinstone (49) reported successful root colonization of *S. xanthophyllum, Brassica juncea, Drymaria cordata, Cerastium glomeratum, Nicandra physaloides, Polygonum capitata* and *Portulaca oleracea*. Similar results were obtained with *Physalis philadelphica* (Palacio *et al.*, unpublished data). Consequently, herbicide treatment is recommended in eradication programs or in fields used for potato production.

Irrigation water. Long term survival of *R. solanacearum* in water makes necessary its disinfection in dry areas where irrigation of potato is required. Although there are few reports comparing the efficacy of different treatments, water disinfection by ozonization for 60 min has been reported to reduce the numbers of bacterial cells (80). The efficacy of chlorine, hydrogen peroxide and, more recently, calcium hypochlorite (35) has also been assessed. The newly developed compounds percarbonic acid (Clarmarin) and peracetic acid (Degaclean) (42) combined with a catalase inhibitor have shown efficacy in eradicating *R. solanacearum* biovar 2 from sewage water containing solid and potato debris; they are environmentally acceptable and easily degraded, but need to be tested under field conditions. Nevertheless, true eradication of the pathogen from waterways in many areas can only be achieved by elimination of *S. dulcamara*. Glyphosate treatments at the beginning and the end of a warm period gave a significant reduction of pathogen population in Scottish waterways (78), but there have been environmental problems in other areas. In other countries mechanical removal of this weed has been effective as a key measure in bacterial wilt eradication (48).

BIOLOGICALLY BASED METHODS

Chemical treatments are potentially harmful to the environment and their efficacy for control of bacterial wilt is low. This led to development of alternative control strategies acceptable to the environment as well as for human nutrition. Biocontrol agents tested so far like Hrp⁻ mutants of *R. solanacearum,* and *Pseudomonas fluorescens, P. glumae, Burkholderia cepacia, Bacillus* sp. and *Erwinia* sp. were not highly effective when tested under natural conditions. This may be due to poor competitive ability with the indigenous rhizosphere microbiota and poor edaphic adaptation (24).

Recent studies have shown the potential value of some promising antagonists for controlling bacterial wilt (Smalla *et al.*, unpublished data, 70) but they have not been tested on potato. Further, Sunaina *et al.* (65) have reported control of bacterial wilt in naturally infested soils in India by applying *Bacillus subtilis* strain B5 to potato tubers before planting. The potential of avirulent Hrp⁻ mutants of *R. solanacearum* biovar 2 against potato wilt was first reported by Smith *et al.* (63) and Kinyua *et al.* (38); a consistent 30% reduction in disease incidence was obtained. However, field experiments in different naturally infested soils still have to be done and biocontrol mechanisms investigated. Short and long term environmental impact should be further considered.

Previous studies have demonstrated inhibition of *R. solanacearum* by extracts of *Casuarina* sp. (28), the major antibacterial component being a flavonoid. The resistance of many plant species against a wide range of pathogens was related to the production of such compounds, with beneficial effects on human health. Thus, future research could explore the role of flavonoids in potato plant resistance. Other plant-derived extracts and essential oils, that may inhibit the chemotactic response of the pathogen to the host, have been shown to reduce populations of *R. solanacearum* in soil (3,52).

Biological control of *R. solanacearum* biovar 2 in water has not been reported, but biological control of *S. dulcamara* using Biochon has been tested (37). Early studies have shown that phages can be useful for control of plant diseases (66) and lytic phages could provide a natural, nontoxic, feasible approach to biological control.

HOST RESISTANCE AND INTEGRATED CONTROL

The most effective control strategy for *R. solanacearum* remains the use of cultivars showing durable resistance combined with agronomic traits acceptable to the market. Nevertheless, there is a risk in using varieties of low susceptibility or tolerance because they can shelter virulent bacteria without showing disease symptoms (53). The high genetic variability of strains within the *R. solanacearum* species complex poses major problems in obtaining such cultivars resistant to bacterial wilt. This may explain the failure to obtain universally resistant potato material. Most of the cultivars obtained have shown unstable resistance (29). Selection of cultivars with durable resistance across all agro-ecological zones is difficult (41).

Combining resistance to bacterial wilt and root-knot nematode is an interesting approach for some zones and new technologies are now available such as somatic hybridization of transgenic cultivars (22,40). Transgenic potato plants showing bactericidal activity due to T4 lysozyme have been obtained (14). The effects of T4 lysozyme produced and released by transgenic plants on bacterial rhizosphere communities were reported to be negligible relative to natural factors (32), but more research is needed. In the context of an EU project, selected T4 lysozyme, cecropin and/or attacin-containing transgenic potato plants (Sessitsch, pers.comm.), as well as novel *hrp* mutants are under investigation, for their impact on the indigenous soil microbiota and their efficacy for control of bacterial wilt of potato in EU countries (van Elsas *et al.*, unpublished data).

Effective control of bacterial wilt requires an integrated management program. High-quality pathogen-free potato seed with an acceptable level of resistance, combined with multiyear rotational cropping schemes, should be effective in limiting pathogen populations. Fumigants and chemical treatments are still used in some situations, but increasing public concern may limit their use in the future, and biocontrol agents might be the alternative. Cultural practices are an important component; planting and harvest dates may be timed to minimize losses, and management of irrigation and soil fertility also will be important. Vine removal or burning may be appropriate to minimize incorporation of inoculum, although this is likely to be limited by legal and practical considerations. Integrated control needs to be adapted to the cultural practices prevalent in each zone with particular attention to the endemic strains of *R. solanacearum*; whether biovar 2 of restricted host range or isolates with wider host range and higher optimum temperature (23,55). In Brazil, Mauritius or Nepal different integrated approaches are recommended (13,60).

Knowledge of the Enemy

Effective control of a "mutable and treacherous tribe" as defined by Sequeira (59) requires imaginative and creative research. Certain aspects of biology and behavior of the pathogen are still not understood, including: survival in water and soil, mechanism of latency, adaptation to new hosts and genetic determinants of host specificity, inoculum sources and dissemination pathways. Rapid sensitive and specific methods for detection of *R. solanacearum* were developed recently and should be used to process large numbers of samples not only from tubers or plants, but from complex environments like soil, water or sewage sludge. It is likely that DNA microarray technology combined with recent advances in the knowledge of the genome of *R. solanacearum* strain GMI 1000 (57), and improved under-

216

standing of pathogenicity mechanisms (25) may help to reveal the hidden life of the bacterium and provide a basis for pathologists and breeders to develop new strategies for control of bacterial wilt. Additional research needs to investigate ways of improving plant resistance of the economically important cultivars, without environmental risk.

Improved cultural practices, including crop rotation, are probably essential for sustainable potato bacterial wilt management programs in many countries. New strategies including biological control and acquired systemic resistance with chemicals may be combined. We need to increase our knowledge of the role of natural or genetically modified enemies of *R. solanacearum* and the mechanisms they use against this bacterium including risk assessment. However given the diversity of bacterial wilt problems on potato worldwide, integrated management programs should be tailored specifically to each growing region.

Acknowledgments

We would like to thank B. Vicedo, L. Gallo, F. Siverio, A. Hernández, B. A. Espino, J.L. Palomo, and P.G. Benavides for providing data about *R. solanacearum* survival and control experiments. We are also grateful to the coordinators and partners of the SMT, FAIR and QLK3 projects for unpublished data. Our work on *R. solanacearum* detection and ecology was financed by EU-SMT program (CT 97-2179), EU-FAIR program (PL 97-3632) and EU-QLK3 program (CT 00-01598)

Literature Cited

1. Akiew, E., and Trevorrow, P.R. 1994. Management of bacterial wilt of tobacco. Pages 179-198 in: Bacterial Wilt: The Disease and its Causative Agent, *Pseudomonas solanacearum*. CAB International, Wallingford, UK. A.C. Hayward and G.L. Hartman, eds.
2. Anonymous. 1998. Council Directive 98/57/EC of 20 July 1998 on the control of *Ralstonia solanacearum* (Smith) Yabuuchi *et al.* Off. J. Eur. Comm. L235, 1-39.
3. Arthy, J.R., Akiew, E.B., and Kirkegaard, J.A. 2002. Using *Brassica* spp. as biofumigants to reduce the population of *Ralstonia solanacearum*. Abstracts of the 3rd IBWS, South Africa.
4. Boudazin, G., Le Roux, A.C., Josi, K., Labarre , P., and Jouan, B. 1999. Design of division specific primers of *Ralstonia solanacearum* and application to the identification of European isolates. Eur. J. Plant. Pathol. 105: 373-380.

5. Buddenhagen, I., and Kelman, A. 1964. Biological and physiological aspects of bacterial wilt caused by *Pseudomonas solanacearum*. Annu. Rev. Phytopathol. 2: 203-230.

6. CABI/EPPO. 1998. *Ralstonia solanacearum* race 1 and race 3. Pages 274-276 in: Distribution maps of quarantine pest for Europe. CABI Publishing, CAB International, Wallingford, UK.

7. Caruso, P., Gorris, M.T., Cambra, M., Palomo, J.L., Collar, J., Carbonell, E., and López, M.M. 2002. Enrichment DAS-ELISA for sensitive detection of *Ralstonia solanacearum* in asymptomatic potato tubers using a specific monoclonal antibody. Appl. Environ. Microbiol. 68: 3634-3638.

8. Caruso, P., Gorris, M.T., Vicedo, B., Ferre, A., Lastra, B., Cambra, M., and López, M.M. 2000. Pages 87-89 in: Sensitive and specific detection of *Ralstonia solanacearum* by enrichment-ELISA in plant material and environmental samples. Proc. 5th Congr. Eur. Foundn Plant Pathol.

9. Caruso, P., Llop, P., Palomo, J.L., García, P., Morente, C., and López, M.M. 1998. Evaluation of methods for detection of potato seed contamination by *Ralstonia solanacearum*. Pages 128-132 in: Bacterial Wilt Disease. Molecular and Ecological Aspects. P. Prior, C. Allen, and J.G. Elphinstone, eds. Springer Verlag, Berlin.

10. Ciampi, L., and Sequeira, L. 1980. Multiplication of *Pseudomonas solanacearum* in resistant potato plants and the establishment of latent infections. Am. Potato J. 57: 319-329.

11. Denny, T.P., Brumbley, S.M., Carney, B.F., Clough, S.J., and Schell, M.A. 1994. Phenotype conversion of *Pseudomonas solanacearum*: its molecular basis and potential function. Pages 137-144 in: Bacterial Wilt: The disease and its causative agent, *Pseudomonas solanacearum*. A.C. Hayward and G.L. Hartman, eds. CAB International, Wallingford, U.K.

12. Devaux, A., Michelante, D., and Bicamumpaka, M. 1987. Combination of rotation and resistance to control bacterial wilt (*Pseudomonas solanacearum*) in Rwanda. Pages 100-101 in: Eur. Assoc. Potato Res. Abstract 10th Triennial Conference, Aalborg, Denmark.

13. Dhital, B.K., Ghimire, S.R., and Pradhanang, P.M. 1996. Sustainable production of *Pseudomonas solanacearum* free seed potatoes to manage bacterial wilt of potato. Lessons from the hills of Nepal. Proc. Natl. Workshop Lumle Agric. Res. Cent., Nepal.

14. Düring, J., 1996. Genetic engineering for resistance to bacteria in transgenic plants by introduction of foreign genes. Mol. Breed. 2: 297-305.

15. Elphinstone, J.G. 1996. Survival and possibilities for extinction of *Pseudomonas solanacearum* (Smith) Smith in cool climates. Potato Res. 39: 403-410.

16. Elphinstone, J.G., Standford, H., and Stead, D.E. 1998a. Detection of *Ralstonia solanacearum* in potato tubers, *Solanum dulcamara* and associated irrigation water. Pages 133-139 in: Bacterial Wilt Disease: Molecular and Ecological Aspects. P. Prior, C. Allen, and J.G. Elphinstone, eds. Springer-Verlag, Berlin.

17. Elphinstone, J.G., Standford, H., and Stead, D.E. 1998b. Survival and transmission of *Ralstonia solanacearum* in aquatic plants of *Solanum dulcamara* and associated surface water in England. EPPO Bull. 28: 93-94.

18. Elphinstone, J.G., Stead, D.E., Caffier, D., Janse, J.D., López, M.M., Mazzucchi, U., Müller, P., Persson, P., Rauscher, E., Schiessendoppler, E., Sousa Santos, M., Stefani, E., and van Vaerenbergh, J. 2000. Standarization of methods for detection of *Ralstonia solanacearum* in potato. EPPO Bull. 30: 391-395.

19. Englebrecht, M.C. 1994. Modification of a semi-selective medium for the isolation and quantification of *Pseudomonas solanacearum*. ACIAR Bacterial Wilt Newsl. 10: 3-5.

20. EPPO. 1990. Quarantine procedures no. 26. *Pseudomonas solanacearum*. EPPO Bull. 20: 255-262.

21. Farag, N., Stead, D.E., and Janse, J.D. 1999. *Ralstonia (Pseudomonas) solanacearum* race 3 biovar 2 detected in surface (irrigation) water in Egypt. J. Phytopathol. 147: 485-487.

22. Fock, I., Purwito, A., Luisetti, J., Souvannavong, V., Vedel, F., Servaes, A., Ambroise, A., Kodja, H., Ducreux, G., Sihachakr, D., and Collonnier, C. 2000. Resistance to bacterial wilt in somatic hybrids between *Solanum tuberosum* and *S. phureja*. Plant Sci. 160: 165-176.

23. French, E.R. 1994. Strategies for integrated control of bacterial wilt of potato. Pages 199-207 in: Bacterial wilt: the disease and its causative agent, *Pseudomonas solanacearum*. CAB International, Wallingford, U.K. pp. 199-207.

24. Frey, P., Marie, C., Kotoujansky, A., Trigalet-Demery, D., and Trigalet, A. 1994. Hrp⁻ mutants of *Pseudomonas solanacearum* as potential biocontrol agents of tomato bacterial wilt. Appl. Environ. Microbiol. 60: 3175-3181.

25. Genin, S., and Boucher, C. 2002. *Ralstonia solanacearum:* secrets of a major pathogen unveiled by analysis of its genome. Mol. Plant Pathol. 3:111-118.

26. Graham, J., Jones, D.A., and Lloyd, A.B. 1979. Survival of *Pseudomonas solanacearum* race 3 in plant debris and in latently infected potato tubers. Phytopathology 69: 1100-1103.

27. Grey, B.E., and Steck, T.R. 2001. The viable but nonculturable state of *Ralstonia solanacearum* may be involved in long-term survival and plant infection. Appl. Environ. Microbiol. 67: 3866-3872.

28. Guo, Q., and Liang, Z.C. 1985. Inhibition of bacterial growth by extracts from beef wood tissues and its relation to bacterial wilt resistance. J.South Chin. Agric. Univ. 6: 49-57.

29. Hartman, G.L., and Elphinstone, J.G. 1994. Advances in the control of *Pseudomonas solanacearum* race 1 in major food crops. Pages 157-178 in: Bacterial wilt: the disease and its causative agent, *Pseudomonas solanacearum*. A.C. Hayward and G.L. Hartman, eds. CAB International, Wallingford, U.K.

30. Hayward, A.C. 1991. Biology and epidemiology of bacterial wilt caused by *Pseudomonas solanacearum*. Annu. Rev. Phytopathol. 29: 65-87.

31. Hayward, A.C., Elphinstone, J.G., Caffier, D., Janse, J., Stefani, E., French, E.R., and Wright, A.J. 1998. Round table on bacterial wilt (brown rot) of potato. Pages 420-430 in: Bacterial wilt disease. Molecular and Ecological Aspects. P. Prior, C. Allen, and J.G. Elphinstone, eds. Springer-Verlag, Berlin. pp. 420-430.

32. Heuer, H., Kroppenstedt, R.M., Lottmann, J., Berg, G., and Smalla, K. 2002. Effects of T4 lysozyme release from transgenic potato roots on bacterial rhizosphere communities are negligible relative to natural factors. Appl. Environ. Microbiol. 68: 1325-1335.

33. Janse, J.D., Araluppan, F.A.X., Schans, J., Wenneker, M., and Westerhuis, W. 1998. Experiences with bacterial brown rot *Ralstonia solanacearum* biovar 2, race 3 in The Netherlands. Pages 146-152 in: Bacterial wilt disease. Molecular and Ecological Aspects. P. Prior, C. Allen, and J.G. Elphinstone, eds. Springer-Verlag, Berlin. pp.146-152.

34. Janse, J.D., and Schans, J. 1998. Experiences with the diagnosis and epidemiology of bacterial brown rot (*Ralstonia solanacearum)* in The Netherlands. EPPO Bull. 28: 65-67.

35. Kelaniyangoda, D.B. 2002. Bacterial wilt (*Ralstonia solanacearum* E.F. Smith) management in potato rooted stem cuttings in the net-house. Abstracts of the 3rd IBWS, South Africa.

36. Kelman, A. 1953. The bacterial wilt caused by *Pseudomonas solanacearum*. N.C. Agric. Exp. Stn. Tech. Bull. 99.

37. Kempenaar, C., Groeneveld, R.M.W., Scheepens, P.C., Zwerdee, W., van der Lotz, L.A.P., and van der Zwerde, W. 1997. Ecology and biological control of bittersweet (*Solanum dulcamara*). Rep. Res. Inst. Agrobiol. Soil Fert. 86: 1-23.

38. Kinyua, Z.M., Offord, L.C., Mienie, N., Gouws, R., Priou, S. Olanyo, M., Simons, S., Saddler, G.S., and Smith, J.J. 2002. Fate of a non-

pathogenic mutant of *R. solanacearum* in soil: risk assessment of a putative biocontrol agent. Abstracts of the 3rd IBWS, South Africa.

39. Kogure, K., Simidu, U., and Taga, N. 1979. A tentative direct microscopic method for counting living marine bacteria. Can. J. Microbiol. 25: 415-420.

40. Laferriere, L., Helgeson, J.P., and Allen, C. 1999. Fertile *Solanum tuberosum* X *S. commersonii* somatic hybrids as sources of resistance to bacterial wilt caused by *Ralstonia solanacearum*. Theor. Appl. Genet. 98:1272-1278.

41. Mendoza, H.A. 1994. Development of potatoes with multiple resistance to biotic and abiotic stresses: the International Potato Center approach. Pages 627-642 in: Advances in Potato Pest Biology and Management. G.W. Zehnder, M.L. Powelson, and R. Jansson, eds. APS Press, St Paul, MN.

42. Niepold, F. 1999. Efficiency surveys of the peracids Degaclean and Clarmarin in combination wilth the catalase inhibitor KH10 from the Degussa company for eradicating the two quarantine bacteria *Clavibacter michiganensis* subsp. *sepedonicus* and *Ralstonia solanacearum* in an aqueous suspension and in the sewage water of the starch industry. J. Phytopathol. 147: 625-634.

43. Olsson, K. 1976. Experience of brown rot caused by *Pseudomonas solanacearum* in Sweden. EPPO Bull. 6:199-207.

44. Palomo, J.L., Caruso, P., Gorris, M.T., López, M.M., and Garcia-Benavides, P. 2000. Comparación de métodos de detección de *Ralstonia solanacearum* en aguas superficiales. Page 120 in: X Congreso de la Sociedad Española de Fitopatología. Valencia.

45. Pastrik, K.H., Elphinstone, J.G., and Pukall, R. 2002. Sequence analysis and detection of *Ralstonia solanacearum* by multiplex PCR amplification of 16S-23S ribosomal intergenic spacer region with internal positive control. Eur. J. Plant Pathol. 108: 831-842.

46. Pastrik, K.H., and Maiss, E. 2000. Detection of *Ralstonia solanacearum* in potato tubers by polymerase chain reaction. J. Phytopathol. 148: 619-626.

47. Pereira, L.V., and Normando, M.C.S. 1993. Sobrevivência de *Pseudomonas solanacerum* raça 2 em solos de terra-firme do Estado do Amazonas. Fitopatol. Bras. 18:137-142.

48. Persson, P. 1998. Successful eradication of *Ralstonia solanacearum* from Sweden. EPPO Bull. 28: 113-119.

49. Pradhanang, P.M., and Elphinstone, J.G. 1996. Identification of weed and crop hosts of *Pseudomonas solanacearum* race 3 in the hills of Nepal. Pages 39-49 in: Integrated management of bacterial wilt of potato. Lessons from the hills of Nepal. Proc. Natl Workshop, Lumle Agric. Res. Cent. Nepal.

50. Pradhanang, P.M., Elphinstone, J.G., and Fox, R.T.V. 1998. Relative importance of latent tuber infection and soil infestation by *Ralstonia solanacearum* on the incidence of bacterial wilt of potato. Pages 403-409 in: Bacterial wilt disease. Molecular and Ecological Aspects. P.Prior, C.Allen, and J.G.Elphinstone, eds. Springer-Verlag, Berlin.

51. Pradhanang, P.M., Elphinstone, J.G., and Fox, R.T.V. 2000. Sensitive detection of *Ralstonia solanacearum* in soil: comparison of different detection techniques. Plant Pathol. 49: 414-422.

52. Pradhanang, P.M., Momol, M.T., Olson, S.M., and Jones, J.B. 2002. Management of bacterial wilt in tomato with essential oils and systemic acquired resistance inducers. Abstracts of the 3rd IBWS, South Africa.

53. Priou, S., Gutarra, L., and Aley, P. 1999. Highly sensitive detection of *Ralstonia solanacearum* in latently infected potato tubers by post-enrichment enzyme-linked immunosorbent assay on nitrocellulose membrane. EPPO Bull. 29:117-125.

54. Robinson-Smith, A., Jones, P., Elphinstone, J.G., and Forde, S.M.D. 1995. Production of antibodies to *Pseudomonas solanacearum*, the causative agent of bacterial wilt. Food Agric. Immunol. 7: 67-79.

55. Rueda, J.L. 1990. Seed potato improvement under bacterial wilt (*Pseudomonas solanacearum* E.F. Smith) pressure: an integrated approach. Ph. D. Thesis, University of Reading, U.K.

56. Russek, E., and Colwell, R.R. 1979. Computation of Most Probable Numbers. Appl. Environ. Microbiol. 45: 1646-1650.

57. Salanoubat, M., Genin, S., Artiguenave, F., Gouzy, J., Mangenot, S., Arlat, M., Billault, A., Brottier, P., Camus, J.C., Cattolico, L., Chandler, M., Choisne, N., Claudel-Renard, C., Cunnac, S., Demange, N., Gaspin, C., Lavle, M., Moisan, A., Robert, C., Saurin, W., Schiex, T., Sguier, P., Thëbault, P., Whalen, M., Wincker, P., Levy, M., Weissenbach, J., and Boucher, C.A. 2002. Genome sequence of the plant pathogen *Ralstonia solanacearum*. Nature 415: 497-502.

58. Seal, S.E., Jackson, L.A., Young, J.P.W., and Daniels, M.J. 1993. Detection of *Pseudomonas solanacearum*, *Pseudomonas syzygii*, *Pseudomonas pickettii* and Blood Disease Bacterium by partial 16S rRNA sequencing: construction of oligonucleotide primers for sensitive detection by polymerase chain reaction. J. Gen. Microbiol. 139: 1587-1594.

59. Sequeira, L. 1994. Epilogue: life with a "mutable and treacherous tribe" Pages 235-247 in: Bacterial wilt: the disease and its causative agent, *Pseudomonas solanacearum*. A.C. Hayward and G.L. Hartman, eds. CAB International, Wallingford, U.K.

60. Shrestha, S.K. 1996. Bacterial wilt of potato in Nepal: spread, losses and magnitude of disease. Pages 11-18 in: Integrated management of bacterial wilt of potato: Lessons from the hills of Nepal. Proc. Natl.

Workshop. P.M. Pradhanang and J.G. Elphinstone, eds. Lumle Agric. Res. Cent., Nepal.

61. Silveira, N.S.S., Michereff, S.J., and Mariano, R.L.R. 1996. *Pseudomonas solanacearum* no Brasil. Summa Phytopathol. 22: 97-111.

62. Smith, E.F. 1896. A bacterial disease of the tomato, eggplant and Irish potato. U.S.D.A. Bull. No 12. 1-28. Div. Veg. Phys. and Pathol. Govt Printing Office, Washington, DC.

63. Smith, J.J., Offord, L.C., Kibata, G.N., Murimi, Z.K., Trigalet, A., and Saddler, G.S. 1998. The development of a biological control agent against *Ralstonia solanacearum* race 3 in Kenya. Pages 337-342 in: Bacterial wilt disease. Molecular and Ecological Aspects. P. Prior, C. Allen, and J.G. Elphinstone, eds. Springer-Verlag, Berlin.

64. Stefanova, M. 1998. Current situation of bacterial wilt (*Ralstonia solanacearum* Smith) in Cuba. Pages 364-368 in: Bacterial wilt disease. Molecular and Ecological Aspects. P. Prior, C. Allen, and J.G. Elphinstone, eds. Springer-Verlag, Berlin.

65. Sunaina, V., Kishore, V., and Shekhawat, G.S. 2002. Evaluation of *Bacillus subtilis* B5 for biological control of bacterial wilt of potato. Abstracts of the 3rd IBWS, South Africa.

66. Tanaka, H., Negishi, H., and Maeda, H. 1990. Control of tobacco bacterial wilt by an avirulent strain of *Pseudomonas solanacearum* M4S and its bacteriophage. Ann. Phytopathol. Soc. Jpn. 56: 243-246.

67. Tusiime, G., Adipala, E., Opio, F., and Bhagsari, A.S. 1998. Weeds as latent hosts of *Ralstonia solanacearum* in highland Uganda: implications to development of an integrated control package for bacterial wilt. Pages 413-419 in: Bacterial wilt disease. Molecular and Ecological Aspects. P. Prior, C. Allen, and J.G. Elphinstone, eds. Springer-Verlag, Berlin.

68. van Elsas, J.D., Kastelein, P., de Vries, P.M., and van Overbeck, L.S. 2001. Effects of ecological factors on the survival and physiology of *Ralstonia solanacearum* bv. 2 in agricultural drainage water. Can. J. Microbiol. 47: 842-854.

69. van Elsas, J.D., Kastelein, P., van Bekkum, P., van der Wolf, J.M., de Vries, P.M., and van Overbeek, L.S. 2000. Survival of *Ralstonia solanacearum* biovar 2, the causative agent of potato brown rot, in field and microcosm soils in temperate climates. Phytopathology 90: 1358-1366.

70. van Overbeek, L.S., Cassidy, M., Kozdroj, J., Trevors. J.T., and van Elsas, J.D. 2001. A polyphasic approach for studying the interaction between *Ralstonia solanacearum* and potential control agents in the tomato rhizosphere. J. Microbiol. Methods 48: 69-86.

71. Wall, G.C., and Sanchez, J.L. 1993. A biocontrol agent for *Pseudomonas solanacearum*. Pages 320-321 in: Bacterial wilt. Proceedings of an international conference held at Kaohsiung, Taiwan, 28-31 October 1992. G.L. Hartman and A.C. Hayward, eds. ACIAR Proc. No. 45, Canberra.

72. Weichart, D., Oliver, J.D., and Kjelleberg, S. 1992. Low temperature induced non-culturability and killing of *Vibrio vulnificus*. FEMS Microbiol. Lett. 100: 205-210.

73. Weingartner, D.P., and McSorley, R. 1994. Management of nematodes and soil borne pathogens in subtropical potato production. Pages 202-213 in: G.W. Zehnder, M.L. Powelson, R.K. Jansson, and K.V. Raman (eds). Advances in Potato Pest Biology and Management. APS Press, St. Paul, MN, USA.

74. Weingartner, D.P. and Shumaker, J.R. 1990. Effects of soil fumigants and aldicarb on bacterial wilt and root-knot nematodes in potato. J. Nematol. (Suppl.) 22: 681-688.

75. Weller, S.A., Elphinstone, J.G., Smith, N., and Stead, D.E. 2000. Detection of *Ralstonia solanacearum* from potato tissue by post enrichment TaqManPCR. EPPO Bull. 30: 381-384.

76. Wenneker, M., Verdel, M.S.W., Groeneveld, R.M.W., Kempenaar, C., van Beuningen, A.R., and Janse, J.D. 1999. *Ralstonia* (*Pseudomonas solanacearum*) race 3 (biovar 2) in surface water and natural weed hosts; first report on stinging nettle (*Urtica dioica*). Eur. J. Plant. Pathol. 105: 307-315.

77. Wood, J.R., and Breckenridge, K. 1998. Maintaining Scottish seed potato production free from *Ralstonia solanacearum*. Pages 410-412 in: Bacterial wilt disease. Molecular and Ecological Aspects. P. Prior, C. Allen, and J.G. Elphinstone, eds. Springer-Verlag, Berlin.

78. Wood, J.R., Breckenridge, K., and Chard, J.M. 2002. Eradicating *Ralstonia solanacearum* from Scottish rivers. Abstracts of the 3rd IBWS, South Africa.

79. Wullings, B.A., van Beuningen, A.R., Janse, J.D., and Akkermans A.D.L. 1998. Detection of *Ralstonia solanacearum*, which causes brown rot of potato, by fluorescent in situ hybridization with 23S rRNA-targeted probes. Appl. Environ. Microbiol. 64: 4546-4554.

80. Yamamoto, H., Terada, T., Naganawa, T., and Tatsuyama, K. 1990. Disinfectious effect of ozonation on water infested with several root-infecting pathogens. Ann. Phytopathol. Soc. Jpn 56: 250-251.

A Broad Review and Perspective on Breeding for Resistance to Bacterial Wilt

Liao Boshou

Oil Crops Research Institute, Chinese Academy of Agricultural Sciences, Wuhan, Hubei, 430062, China

Introduction

It is universally recognized that the most effective and practical way to control bacterial wilt caused by *Ralstonia solanacearum* in various crops of economic importance is to plant cultivars with suitable resistance. As a result, genetic enhancement for host plant resistance has been one of the most important research activities for scientists fighting this disease. Variation in reaction to bacterial wilt among host plant genotypes was observed soon after the disease was reported in 1896. For example, resistant peanut or groundnut (*Arachis hypogaea* L) materials were known by 1910 even though the disease had been reported in peanut only in 1905 (29, 32). Thus, bacterial wilt-resistant varieties have been in use for disease control for over 90 years. Worldwide, breeding for resistance to bacterial wilt has been concentrated on crops of wide economic importance such as tomato (*Lycopersicum esculentum* L.), potato (*Solanum tuberosum* L.), tobacco (*Nicotiana tabacum* L.), eggplant (*Solanum melongena* L.), peppers (*Capsicum* spp.) and peanut. As with many other plant diseases, breeding for resistance to bacterial wilt has usually been influenced by factors like availability of resistance sources and their diversity, genetic linkage between resistance and other agronomic traits, differentiation and variability in pathogenic strains, the mechanism of plant-pathogen interactions, and breeding or selection methodology. In several crops, generating effective resistance has proven to be difficult while in certain crops the development of useful resistant cultivars has been quite successful. This chapter attempts to give an overall review of the recent status and perspectives on crop genetic enhancement for resistance to bacterial wilt worldwide.

Genetic Resources and Breeding Progress Towards Resistant Cultivars

Because genetic resources containing resistance to *R. solanacearum* are the basis of resistance breeding, extensive efforts have been made in many countries and international organizations to screen such resources for bacterial wilt resistance in crops of economic importance. Resistance to *R. solanacearum* in most host plant species has been defined and evaluated as high survival percentage under infection pressures. Naturally-infested fields or nurseries with high and uniform infection pressure are generally necessary for large-scale germplasm evaluation and breeding selection. In most host crops, reliable techniques for screening for resistance by artificial inoculation, mostly in the seedling stage, have also been established and extensively applied. In this way, sources of resistance have been identified in many crops and their wild relatives. Systematic evaluation of crop germplasm for bacterial wilt resistance has been conducted by the International Potato Center (CIP) for potato, Asian Vegetable Research and Development Center (AVRDC) in Taiwan for solanaceous vegetables, Oil Crops Research Institute (OCRI) of the Chinese Academy of Agricultural Sciences (CAAS) in China for peanut, and numerous national programs for these crops.

The first successful attempt to breed or select for resistance to *R. solanacearum* was conducted in peanut in the 1910s in Indonesia (32). Breeding for resistance to bacterial wilt has been conducted for many years in important crops such as tomato, potato, eggplant, tobacco, pepper and peanut (15). In most cases, conventional sexual hybridization approaches have been employed in breeding to create wilt-resistant and agronomically acceptable cultivars of various crops.

Eggplant

Resistance sources in eggplant were first reported from Puerto Rico (33). Extensive screening has been conducted in India in recent decades. Several eggplant (brinjal) varieties including Surya, Swetha, Haritha and Neelima were identified as resistant to bacterial wilt in south India. Chaudhary (2000) reported that eggplant genotypes including Arka Kesav, Arks Neelkanth, Arka Nidhi and SM 6-6 with good agronomic traits were resistant to bacterial wilt in India. Ten brinjal genotypes resistant to bacterial wilt were evaluated for three years in infested fields. Cultivars Surya, Swetha and SM 141 showed low wilt incidences (9.9%, 7.3% and 11.2%, respectively); Surya and Swetha have been recommended for large-scale cultivation in India (4).

At AVRDC, sources of resistance in eggplant are available and are being tested in multilocation trials to judge the stability of resistance before they are recommended for use in breeding programs. A total of 344 accessions were screened, mainly from Indonesia, Malaysia, Thailand, and India. After confirmation, 17 accessions with different fruit types showing consistent resistance were selected (44). Resistance to *R. solanacearum* in eggplant is thought to actually be tolerance, since the bacteria colonize the plants without causing noticable wilting. This phenomenon of latent infection has been observed in other hosts, such as potato, tomato, pepper and peanut. As an aside, breeders should be aware that such resistant hosts may suffer significant yield losses to bacterial wilt even though they show no symptoms (12, 26,34).

In eggplant, several wild species were identified as highly resistant or even immune to some strains (2), and resistant progenies from interspecific hybrids were obtained (3). Somatic hybrids between *S. melongena* and two groups of *S. aethiopicum* were also produced by electrofusion of mesophyll protoplasts, producing plants with vigorous and intermediate morphological traits. Encouragingly, all somatic hybrids tested were as tolerant to a race 1, biovar 3 strain of *R. solanacearum* as the wild species (5).

Peanut

Worldwide, over 170 genotypes comprising considerable genetic diversity in the cultivated peanut and its related wild species have been identified as resistant to bacterial wilt. As early as the 1920s, Schwarz 21 was the first peanut genotype identified with a high level of resistance to *R. solanacearum*. During the past three decades, germplasm evaluation for bacterial wilt resistance in peanut has been conducted extensively in China. Resistant genotypes have been identified in all the four botanical types of *A. hypogaea* (Virginia, Spanish, Valencia, and Chinese dragon). In China, Xiekangqing and Taishan Sanlirou have been the two resistant genotypes most extensively and successfully used in breeding programs (Liao et al, this volume). Recently, considerable progress has also been made in evaluating peanut germplasm for resistance in Vietnam. Three elite germplasm lines, including Gie Nho Quan, have been identified (17).

It is interesting to note that many Chinese dragon-type peanuts collected from south China, where bacterial wilt has long been prevalent, have been identified as highly resistant; however, no Chinese dragon-type landrace collected from north China has good bacterial wilt resistance, indicating that the resistance might have evolved in response to natural selection pressure (8). Bacterial wilt resistance in peanut has been more stable than resistance in other agronomically important hosts of *R.solanacearum*. For example, the resistant genotype Schwarz 21, developed 80 years ago, is still resistant across different regions. In the cultivated peanut, the resistance is controlled by a few major genes (24). Recent evidence of bacterial wilt resistance transfer from diploid wild species into the tetrapliod cultivated peanut without any obvious undesirable genetic linkage verified that resistance to bacterial wilt in some wild species might be controlled by major genes (25).

During the past ten years, seven new peanut cultivars with high levels of bacterial wilt resistance and improved agronomic traits have been developed and released to production in China. These have been extensively applied in production. In peanut, only a few lines have been used successfully as resistance donors in breeding programs even though many resistant landraces have been identified. In Indonesia, only Schwarz 21 and its derivatives have been used as resistant parents. In China, most bacterial wilt - resistant peanut cultivars were developed by using Xiekangqing and Taishan Sanlirou belonging to the subspecies *fastigiata*, even though many other resistant lines of subspecies *hypogaea* have been unsuccessfully used in breeding programs. Due to undesirable genetic linkages, the agronomic traits derived from the subspecies *hypogaea* did not perform well in central and southern China where bacterial wilt is generally serious, even though the bacterial wilt resistance in the progenies was often high. Thus, there is an undesirably narrow genetic background among the available bacterial wilt-resistant peanut cultivars. Further broadening the genetic base for resistance and adaptation to the environments in diseased areas should be a priority.

Pepper

Resistance sources in peppers have been reported in several countries and in different types of pepper (14,31,44). In Brazil and Taiwan, the *Capsicum* breeding line MC-4 was found to be very resistant to various isolates of biovars 1 and 3, and is being recommended for breeding programs in Brazil (C. Lopes, personal communication). In Japan, India and Taiwan, other sources of resistance have been identified in sweet peppers. Highly resistant accessions have been found in sweet pepper and some commercial F_1 cultivars. A resistant variety, Mie-Midori and its derived progenies have been used extensively in the breeding of Japanese green pepper cultivars. *Capsicum* germplasm resources originally from Asian countries like Japan and China were found to be moderately or highly resistant to bacterial wilt, while those from American or European countries were more susceptible (37). At AVRDC, screening mostly hot pepper germplasm has resulted in identification of some quite resistant lines (44).

Potato

Bacterial wilt in potato is caused by both race 1 and race 3 of *R. solanacearum* (15). Resistance to race 1, race 3, and to both has been identified or improved even though the genetic background of bacterial wilt resistance in *S. tuberosum* had been thought to be narrow. Desirable resistance has been identified from several related species of potato including *S. chacoense, S. microdontum, S. phureja, S. sparsipilum,* and *S. stenotomum.* Among these, high level resistance in *S. phureja* to different strains of *R. solanacearum* identified in late 1960s was thought to be a milestone for bacterial wilt resistance enhancement in potato (39).

However, the performance of bacterial wilt resistance in potato seems relatively unstable across locations. Several controlled-environment studies have shown that high temperature was the most important factor causing the breakdown of resistance in potato (10). In addition, resistance was better expressed at high light intensities at 24°C and 28°C, while decreased light intensity and photoperiod reduced resistance in some lines (39).

Breeding for resistance to bacterial wilt in potato is generally assessed as moderately successful. Some researchers have observed differences in potato wilt caused by race 1 and race 3. In addition, researchers from several countries have noted differing behavior of resistance to *R. solanacearum* in the same potato lines under different environmental conditions (15). The relatively narrow host range and genetic diversity of race 3 *R. solanacearum* strains should make it an easier resistance breeding target than race 1, where bacterial wilt resistance must be combined with heat adaptation in potatoes for the lowland humid tropics (11).

A number of potato varieties with resistance to bacterial wilt have been developed using resistant accessions of *S. phureja* originating in Colombia (11,28,38,39,42). Achat is a popular German cultivar grown in Brazil with desirable resistance to bacterial wilt. However, its acceptance has considerably dropped in the last few years due to its poor cooking qualities. With the objective of developing a bacterial wilt -resistant cultivar to replace Achat, genotype selection for bacterial wilt resistance began in 1987 through a cooperative project with the International Potato Center (CIP), and several new potato clones with high level resistance to bacterial wilt have been developed. Among them, MB-03 showed resistance to both races 1 and 3 (Priou *et al.*, this volume. Because latently-infected seed potatoes are a common source of inoculum, resistance to latent infection by *R. solanacearum* has been recommended as an important new criterion for potato breeders (Priou *et al.*, this volume). A recent pre-breeding program at CIP has been initiated to evaluate wild species of potatoes for resistance to bacterial wilt, giving emphasis to resistance to latent infection in stems and tubers using CIP's detection tools (Priou et al, 1997). This novel screening procedure and the fact that the germplasm accessions tested are new specimens never before screened for bacterial wilt resistance should lead to promising identification of higher levels of resistance (Priou, personal communication).

Extensive efforts have been made to transfer bacterial wilt resistance from various wild potato relatives. Disappointingly, hybrids of potato with resistant genotypes of *S. chacoense*, *S. sparsipillum* and *S. multidissectum* showed wild traits and usually moderate resistance. Fock et al (9, and Fock et al, this volume) reported that somatic hybrids of *S. phureja* and *S. stenotomum* with cultivated potato resulted in lines with enhanced resistance to race 1 of *R. solanacearum*. Similar race 3-resistant lines were reported using *S. tuberosum* x *S.commersonii* somatic hybrids, which retained their resistance even at high temperatures (23). Limited efforts were also made to select bacterial wilt resistance from somatic variation *in vitro* for potato (21).

Tobacco

In tobacco, the line T.I.448A, originating from Colombia, was an important genotype with bacterial wilt resistance, and many resistant cultivars, including NC95, Coker 347, and Speight G-140, were developed from it (1). In recent years, very limited work has been done for tobacco in screening for resistance to bacterial wilt. It was reported that improved bacterial wilt resistance was selected from somaclonal variants of tobacco (6). Recently, three tobacco lines, namely G3, Fandi and G6, were identified as resistant to three strains of *R. solanacearum* in Fujian Province of China (Xu et al, personal communication).

Breeding efforts are underway to improve resistance to bacterial wilt in flue-cured and Burley cultivars by enhancing levels of resistance, identifying useful sources of resistance, improving selection efficiency, and improving yield and quality characteristics of highly resistant lines. Developed via pedigree selection in a single cross between Coker 319 and K399, Oxford 207 is a flue-cured tobacco cultivar released in 1997 with high resistance to the major soilborne diseases (*R. solanacearum*, *Phytophthora nicotianae*, *Meloidogyne incognita* and *Fusarium oxysporum*) combined with good yield and quality characteristics (40).

Tomato

Tomato has attracted extensive research efforts with respect to germplasm identification, breeding, and molecular markers for resistance to bacterial wilt (12,13,14,42). Hawaii 7996 has been reported as highly resistant to bacterial wilt, and its resistance appears most durable among tomato varieties (42). Many resistant tomato germplasm accessions are available for breeding programs in several countries. In general, AVRDC has taken a leading role in evaluating tomato germplasm for bacterial wilt resistance. Most AVRDC advanced breeding lines carry a good level of resistance, and these sources of resistance are available and utilized in breeding programs. Desirable resistant germplasm accessions, including some improved varieties, have been identified in India, Indonesia, the Philippines, Thailand and USA.

As with potato, resistance to bacterial wilt in tomato has occasionally proved unstable. In order to test the stability of available resistance sources across varying conditions and regions, AVRDC organized a coherent international evaluation in 11 infested fields in 10 countries of a set of 35 resistant tomato lines and accessions collected from various breeding programs worldwide. Among the entries tested, Hawaii 7996 appeared to be the most stable resistant line with the highest survival (96.9%) over all locations (45). Other resistant lines with relatively better stability included BF-Okitsu 101, Hawaii 7997, Hawaii 7998, CRA 66, Tml 114-48-5-N-spreading, Tml 46-N-12-N-early N.T., R-3034-3-10-N-UG, and F7-80-465-10-pink (45). The stability of a resistance source and its derived breeding lines could be similar or different depending on the genetic basis of resistance and the genetic background into which it was transferred.

Breeding in tomato has been focused on development of varieties that combine bacterial wilt resistance with heat tolerance and desirable agronomic features. In the Philippines, tomato lines TML 114 and TML 216 have been developed with resistance to three biovars of *R. solanacearum* and they were also heat-tolerant (Deanon *et al.*, this volume). Research efforts have been made in developing a bacterial wilt -resistant tomato with quality suitable for processing in India (Gopalakrishnan *et al.*, this volume). In Brazil, some tomato progenies obtained from crossing IPA-5 (susceptible) and CL5915-93 (resistant) were evaluated for resistance to bacterial wilt (Lopes et al, this volume).

Mandal (1999) reported somaclonal variations induced from several tomato varieties. Somaclones were screened for bacterial wilt resistance in disease nurseries. Marked variation in resistance was noted in comparison to the parental populations, and a few useful lines with bacterial wilt resistance were selected (30).

Several researchers have reported molecular markers of bacterial wilt resistance in tomato (7, 41,46). Quantitative trait loci (QTL) related to bacterial wilt resistance have been identified on chromosomes 6,7 and 10 in a cross between L285 (resistant) and a susceptible genotype (7). In another study using Hawaii 7996, Wang *et al.* (2000) found a major QTL on chromosome 12, which seems to be specific to the Taiwanese strain used (46). Balatero *et al.* (this volume) continued to work on F6 recombinant inbred lines of the same population. Based on single marker analysis on 80 markers, they identified at least seven AFLP and one resistance gene analog (RGA) markers clustered in at least two genomic regions putatively associated with resistance to *R. solanacearum*. The identification of these PCR-based DNA markers could facilitate marker-assisted breeding and selection for bacterial wilt resistance in tomato (Balatero et al, this volume).

Other Crops

Several resistant clones of cassava (*Manihot* spp.) were identified in Indonesia, but the expression of the resistance varied across locations (29). In a study conducted in India, a cultivated sesame (*Sesamum indicum* L.) variety Pb Til No. 1 showed lowest wilt incidence (15.1%) among the genotypes tested. Research has been done to identify resistance in banana, ginger, eucalyptus, and other plant species with limited progress.

Genetic Transformation for Improved Wilt Resistance

The Biotechnology Research Center of the Chinese Academy of Agricultural Sciences (CAAS) has introduced a synthetic gene for an anti-bacterial peptide into a major potato cultivar extensively planted in China and obtained transgenic potato lines with improved resistance to several diseases, including bacterial wilt (19,20). These anti-bacterial peptide genes have been supplied to several research institutes for bacterial wilt resistance improvement in potato, peanut, and tomato and resistance to other diseases including Chinese cabbage soft rot. Peptides isolated from *Hylophora cecropia* and *Antheraea pernyi* can inhibit growth of bacteria, including *R. solanacearum,* by digesting the cell wall. Resistance to bacterial wilt was enhanced by expression of a cecropin lytic peptide in transgenic tobacco (18). At the Guangdong Acdademy of Agricultural Sciences, China, isolated genes for cecropin B and cecropin D have been successfully transferred into pepper through Agro-infection of pepper cotyledons *in vitro*. Encouragingly, improved resistance to bacterial wilt has been identified among the regenerated plantlets. However in general, creation of transgenic plants to improve resistance to bacterial wilt is not yet well advanced, possibly because of political opposition to GMOs in the developed world. It is to be hoped that there will be more research effort in this area in the near future.

Constraints Facing Resistance Breeders

The progress of plant breeding for resistance to bacterial wilt varies enormously among different crops. These uneven achievements may reflect variations in breeding efforts and their success. However, in some important crops, such as banana, the slow progress towards development of resistant cultivars is due to lack of stable breeding programs rather than the practical difficulties of the breeding. Of course, the most important problem that the breeders face is the lack of desirable resistant germplasm sources for several important host crops. In solanaceous crops, some useful resistance has been found, but not enough. The widely used criterion for resistance scoring is survival ratio under infection pressures, but unfortunately this means that in most cases latent infection/colonization of the bacteria in plants cannot be taken into account in resistance evaluation. Plant genotypes with high survival percentage may in fact merely be disease-tolerant if their latent infection level is high. Reaction to latent infection is genotype-dependent, but variation of latent infection reaction has not been carefully evaluated in most crops. This is important because latent infection of supposedly resistant genotypes can lead to hidden yield losses, as well as the undesirable increase of population levels and spread of inoculum. Resistance to bacterial wilt in crops such as tomato and potato has been found to be unstable, probably because of complex interactions between *R. solanacearum*, host genotypes, and the environment. As understanding of the pathogen-plant interaction is still limited, approaches for improving resistance stability are not yet available. One approach that may help breeders achieve more stable bacterial wilt resistance is the use of a "cocktail" of diverse *R. solanacearum* strains during resistance screening, since some data suggest that the high diversity of pathogen strains may explain the variability of resistance in different locations. Finally, to some extent, resistance to bacterial wilt in many crops is negatively correlated with yield and quality. Thus, released resistant cultivars may be poor in other agronomic traits and are not widely accepted by farmers or consumers.

Perspectives

More research efforts are needed to screen additional desirable germplasm lines for resistance to bacterial wilt in various crops. Even though the extent of genetic diversity of resistance to bacterial wilt in different crops may vary, it is likely that more resistant materials could be found if local landraces or germplasm materials were extensively and systematically evaluated, especially in areas where the cultivated crops originated. Special emphasis should be given to the wild relative species of the important crops.

Reaction to latent infection should be intensively evaluated in several crops in which germplasm with resistance is diverse.

Further breeding efforts should be made to integrate resistance to bacterial wilt with desirable agronomic traits as well as with resistances to other biotic and abiotic constraints. Any crop variety that offers only bacterial wilt resistance is unlikely to be useful in production. Special emphasis should be given to integrating resistance to bacterial wilt with resistance to late blight in potato, nematode resistance and heat tolerance in tomato, and with aflatoxin resistance in peanut. As very limited research efforts worldwide have been made for resistance to bacterial wilt in banana, it is important to initiate breeding programs in wilt hot spot regions. Because bacterial wilt of banana and plantain is largely a problem in poorer countries with limited resources, more developed countries should be encouraged to vigorously support banana breeding efforts.

The genetics of wilt resistance in different crops needs further investigation. The fundamental plant-pathogen interaction also needs further investigation in most crops. Research on molecular markers has been conducted in tomato and this useful technology should be developed for other crops as well. The recent research progress towards understanding bacterial wilt resistance and isolating resistant genes in the model plant, *Arabidopsis thaliana*, is very interesting and will hopefully eventually help us in understanding the genetics of resistance to *R. solanacearum* in agronomically important species. Finally, in the coming years it is to be hoped that more efforts will be made in genetic enhancement of bacterial wilt resistance through biotechnological approaches.

Acknowledgements

Special acknowledgements are given to Drs. J-F. Wang (AVRDC), C. Allen (USA), S. Priou (CIP), and B. Fortnum (USA), who have kindly read the paper draft and made excellent modifications. The author's attendance at the 3rd IBWS and preparation of this review were supported by the Natural Science Foundation of China (NSFC) with projects No. 3957495 (1996-1998) and 30070521(2000-2002).

Literature Cited

1. Akiew, A., and Trevorrow, P.R. 1994. Management of bacterial wilt of tobacco. Pages 179-198 in: Bacterial wilt: the disease and its causative agent, *Pseudomonas solanacearum*. A.C. Hayward and G.L. Hartman eds. CAB International.

2. Ali, M., Quadir, M.A., Okubo, H., and Fujieda, K. 1990. Resistance of eggplant, its wild relatives and their hybrids to different strains of *Pseudomonas solanacearum*. Sci. Hort. 45:1-9

3. Ano, G., Herbert, Y., Prior, P., and Messiaen, C.M. 1991. A new source of resistance to bacterial wilt of eggplant obtained from a cross: *Solanum aethiopicum* L × *Solanum melongena* L. Agronomie, 11:555-560.

4. Chaudhary, D.R., and Sharma, S.D. 2000. Screening of some brinjal cultivars against bacterial wilt and fruit borer. Agricultural Science Digest, Vol.20, No.2: 129-130.

5. Collonnier, C., Mulya, K., Fock, I., Mariska, I., Servaes, A., and Vedel, F. 2001. Source of resistance against *Ralstonia solanacearum* in fertile somatic hybrids of eggplant (*Solanum melongena L,*) with *Solanum aethiopicum* L. Plant Sci.160: 301-313.

6. Daub, M.E., and Jenns, A.E. 1989. Field and greenhouse analysis of variation for disease resistance in tobacco somaclones. Phytopathology 80:641-646.

7. Danesh, D., Aarons., S., Mcgill, G.E., and Young, N.D. 1994. Genetic dissection of oligogenic resistance to bacterial wilt in tomato. Mol. Plant-Microbe Interact. 7:464-471.

8. Duan, N., Tan, Y., Jiang, H., and Hu, D. 1993. Screening groundnut germplasm for resistance to bacterial wilt. Oil Crops China 1:22-25.

9. Fock, I., Purwito, A., Luisetti, J., Souvannavong, V., Vedel, F., Servaes, A., Ambroise, A., Kodja, H., Ducreux, G., Sihachakr, D., and Collonnier, C. 2000. Resistance to bacterial wilt in somatic hybrids between *Solanum tuberosum* and *Solanum phureja*. Plant Sci. 160:165-176.

10. French, E.R., and De Lindo, L. 1982. Resistance to *Pseudomonas solanacearum* in potato: specificity and temperature sensitivity. Phytopathology 72:1408-1412.

11. French, E.R., Anguiz, R., and Aley, P. 1998. The usefulness of potato resistance to *Ralstonia solanacearum* for the integrated control of bacterial wilt. Pages 381-385 in: Bacterial wilt disease: Molecular and ecological aspects. P. Prior, C. Allen and J. Elphinstone, eds. INRA Edition, Springer Verlag, Berlin, Germany.

12. Grimault, V., and Prior, P. 1993. Tomato bacterial wilt resistance associated with tolerance vascular tissues to *Pseudomonas solanacearum*. Plant Pathol. 42:589-594.

13. Grimault, V., Prior, P., and Anais, G. 1995. A monogenic dominant resistance of tomato to bacterial wilt in Hawaii 7996 is associated with plant colonization by *Pseudomonas solanacearum*. J. Phytopathology 143:349-352.

14. Hartman, G.L., and Elphinstone, J.G. 1994. Advances in the control of *Pseudomonas solanacearum* race 1 in major food crops. Pages 157-177 in: Bacterial wilt: the disease and its causative agent, *Pseudomonas solanacearum*. A.C. Hayward and G.L. Hartman eds. CAB International.

15. Hayward, A.C. 1986. Bacterial wilt caused by *Pseudomonas solanacearum* in Asia and Australia. Pages 15-24 in: Bacterial wilt disease in Asia and the South Pacific. G.J. Persley ed. ACIAR Proceedings no. 13. Canberra, Australian Center for International Agricultural Research.

16. Ho, G., and Yang, C., 1999. A single locus leads to resistance of *Arabidopsis thaliana* to bacterial wilt caused by *Ralstonia solanacearum* through a hypersensitive-like response. Phytopathology 89:673-678.

17. Hong, N.X., Mehan, V.K., Lieu, N.V., and Yen, N.T. 1999. Identification of groundnut genotypes resistant to bacterial wilt in Vietnam. Int. J. Pest Manag. 45: 239-243.

18. Jaynes, J.M., Nagpala, P., Destefano-Beltran, L., Huang, J.H., Kim, J.H., Denny, T., and Setiner, S. 1997. Expression of a cecropin B lytic peptide analog in transgenic tobacco confers enhanced resistance to bacterial wilt caused by *Pseudomonas solanacearum*. Plant Sci 85:43-54.

19. Jia, S.R., Qu, X.M., Feng, L.X., Tang, T.; Tang, Y.X., Liu, K., Zheng, P., Zhao, Y.L., Bai, Y.Y., and Cai, M.Y. 1998. Development of potato clones with enhanced resistance to bacterial wilt by introducing antibacterial peptide gene. Sci Ag. Sinica 31:13-18.

20. Jia, S.R., Xie, Y., Tang, T., Feng, L.X., Cao, D.S., Zhao, Y.L., Yuan, J., Bai, Y.Y., Jiang, C.X., Jaynes, J.M., and Dodds, J.D. 1993. Genetic engineering of Chinese potato cultivars by introducing antibacterial polypeptide gene. Pages 208-212 in: Biotechnology in agriculture, Proceedings of the First Asia-Pacific Conference on Agricultural Biotechnology, Beijing, China, 20-24 August 1992. Z.L. Chen, ed. Beijing.

21. Kang, Y., Xua, J., Zhang, Y., and He, L. 1989. A preliminary study on screening potato somatic variant *in vitro* for resistance to bacterial wilt. Pages 271-278 in: Plant Somaclonal Variation and Breeding. Y. Chen, W. Lu, and Q. Zheng, eds., Jiangsu Science and Technology Publishing House.

22. Krausz, J.P., and Thurston, H.D. 1975. Breakdown of resistance of *Pseudomonas solanacearum* in tomato. Phytopthology 65:1272-1274.

23. Laferriere, L., Helgeson, J.P., and Allen, C. 1999. Fertile *Solanum tuberosum* + *S. commersonii* somatic hybrids as sources of resistance

to bacterial wilt caused by *Ralstonia solanacearum*. Theoret. Appl. Gen. 98:1272-1278.

24. Liao, B., Li, W., and Sun, D. 1986. A study on inheritance of resistance to *Pseudomonas solanacearum* E.F. Smith in *Arachis hypogaea* L. Oil Crops China, 3:1-8.

25. Liao, B., Duan, N., Jiang, H., Liang, X., and Gao, G. 1998. Germplasm screening and breeding for resistance to bacterial wilt in China. Pages 75-81 in: Groundnut bacterial wilt: proceedings of the Fourth Working Group Meeting, 11-13 May 1998, Vietnam Agricultural Science Institute, Hanoi, Vietnam. S. Pande, B. Liao, N.X. Hong, C. Johansen, and C.L.L. Gowda, eds. International Crops Research Institute for the Semi-Arid Tropics, India.

26. Liao, B., Shan, Z., Lei, Y., Tan, Y., Li, D., and Duan, N. 1998. Reaction to latent infection by *Ralstonia solanacearum* in groundnut. Chinese J. Oil Crop Sci. 20:61-65.

27. Liao, B., Xu, Z., and Jiang, H. 2001. Molecular markers of resistance to bacterial wilt and their potential utilization. Chinese Journal of Oil Crop Sciences, 23:66-68.

28. Lopes, C.A., Quezado-Soares, A.M., Buso, J.A., and Melo, P.E. 1998. Breeding for resistance to bacterial wilt of potatoes in Brazil. Pages 290-293 in: Bacterial wilt disease: molecular and ecological aspects. P. Prior, C. Allen, and J. Elphinstone eds., INRA Springer.

29. Machmud, M. 1986. Bacterial wilt in Indonesia. Pages 30-34 in: Bacterial wilt disease in Asia and the South Pacific. G.J. Persley, ed. ACIAR Proceedings no. 13. Canberra, Australian Center for International Agricultural Research.

30. Mandal, A. B. 1999. Efficient somaculture system and exploitation of somaclonal variation for bacterial wilt resistance in tomato. Indian J. Hort. 56: 321-327.

31. Matsunaga, H, and Monma, S. 1999. Sources of resistance to bacterial wilt in Capsicum. J. Jap. Soc. Hort. Sci. 68: 753-761

32. Mehan,V.K., and Liao, B.S. 1994. Groundnut bacterial wilt: past, present, and future. Pages 67-88 in Groundnut bacterial wilt in Asia: proceedings of the Third Working Group meeting, 4-5 July 1994, Oil Crops Research Institute, Wuhan, China. V.K. Mehan and D. McDonald, eds. ICRISAT, India

33. Nolla, J.A.B.1931. Studies on bacterial wilt of the Solanaceae in Puerto Rico. Journal of Puerto Rico Department of Agriculture, 15:287-308.

34. Prior, P., Grimault, V., and Schmit, J. 1994. Resistance to bacterial wilt (*Pseudomonas solanacearum*) in tomato: present status and prospects. Pages 209-223 in: Bacterial wilt: the disease and its causative agent, *Pseudomonas solanacearum*. A.C. Hayward and G.L. Hartman, eds. CAB International.

35. Priou, S., Gutarra, L. and Aley, P. 1999. Highly sensitive detection of *Ralstonia solanacearum* in latently infected potato tubers by post-enrichment ELISA on nitrocellulose membrane. Bull EPPO/OEPP Bull. 29:117-125.

36. Priou, S., Salas, C., de Mendiburu, F., Aley, P. and Gutarra, L. 2001. Assessment of Latent Infection Frequency in Progeny Tubers of Advanced Potato Clones Resistant to Bacterial Wilt: A New Selection Criterion. Potato Res. 44: 359-374.

37. Quezado-Soares, A.M., and Lopes, C.A. 1995. Stability of the resistance to bacterial wilt of the sweet pepper MC4 challenged with strains of *Pseudomonas solanacearum*. Fitopatologia- Brasileira 20:638-641.

38. Rowe, P.R., Sequeira, L., and Gonzalez, L.C. 1972. Additional genes for resistance to *Pseudomonas solanacearum* in *Solanum phureja*. Phytopathology 62:1093-1094.

39. Sequeira, L., and Rowe, P.R. 1969. Selection and utilization of *Solanum phureja* clones with high resistance to different strains of *Pseudomonas solanacearum*. Am. Potato J. 46,:451-462

40. Sisson, V.A. 1999. Registration of 'Oxford 207' tobacco. Crop Science, 39: 292.

41. Thoquet, P., Olivier, J., Sperisen, C., Rogowsky, P., Laterrot, H., and Grimsley, N. 1996. Quantitative trait loci determining resistance to bacterial wilt in tomato cultivar Hawaii 7996. Mol.Plant-Microbe Interact., 9:828-836.

42. Thurston, H.D. 1976. Resistance to bacterial wilt (*Pseudomonas solanacearum*).Pages 58-62 in: Planning conference and workshop on the ecology and control of bacterial wilt caused by *Pseudomonas solanacearum*. L. Sequeira and A. Kelman, eds. Raleigh, North Carolina, NCSU.

43. Wang, J.F., and Berke, T. 1997. Source of resistance to bacterial wilt in *Capsicum annum*. Capsicum and Eggplant Newsletter 16:91-93.

44. Wang, J.F., Chen, N.C., and Li, H.M. 1998. Resistance sources to bacterial wilt in eggplant (*Solanum melongena*). Pages 284-289 in: Bacterial wilt disease: molecular and ecological aspects. P. Prior, C. Allen, and J. Elphinstone eds., INRA Springer

45. Wang, J.F., Hanson, P., and Barnes, J.A. 1998. Worldwide evaluation of an international set of resistance sources to bacterial wilt in tomato. Pages 269-275 in: Bacterial wilt disease: molecular and ecological aspects. P..Prior, C.Allen, and J.Elphinstone eds., INRA Springer.

46. Wang, J.F., Oliver, J., Thoquet, P., Mangin, B., Sauviac, L., and Grimsley, N.H. 2000. Resistance of tomato line Hawaii7996 to *Ralstonia solanacearum* Pss4 in Taiwan is controlled mainly by a major strain-specific locus. Mol. Plant-Microbe Interact. 13: 6-13.

Progress on Genetic Enhancement for Resistance to Groundnut Bacterial Wilt in China

Liao Boshou[1], Liang Xuanqiang[2], Jiang Huifang[1], Lei Yong[1],
Shan Zhihui[1], and Zhang Xinyou[3]

[1]Oil Crops Research Institute of Chinese Academy of Agricultural Sciences,
Wuhan, Hubei, 430062, China. [2]Crop Research Institute of Guangdong
Academy of Agricultural Sciences, Guangzhou, Guangdong, 510640,
China. [3]Henan Academy of Agricultural Sciences, Zhengzhou, Henan,
450002, China.

Bacterial wilt caused by *Ralstonia solanacearum* is an important constraint to groundnut (peanut) production in China, which has been among the leading countries worldwide for genetic enhancement of host-plant resistance to bacterial wilt in this crop. This paper reviews progress on genetic enhancement in China during the past decade. A total of 170 germplasm lines, distributed in all four botanical types of the cultivated groundnut, have been identified as resistant to bacterial wilt. In addition, 24 accessions of resistant *Arachis* wild species have been identified. Most resistant genotypes have showed desirable stability for resistance across regions and seasons. Germplasm accessions 89-15048 and ICG 6417 showed the highest levels of resistance without a detectable latent bacterial wilt-resistant cultivars with improved yield potential were released in China including Zhonghua 4, Zhonghua 6, Yueyou 200, Yueyou 202-35, and Quanhua 10; four cultivars were also resistant to rust. Several breeding lines with bacterial wilt resistance have been developed from the diploid species *Arachis chacoense*. Among the bacterial wilt-resistant lines derived from interspecific hybrid progenies, no obvious linkage of bacterial wilt resistance with the undesirable traits of the diploid parent was found, indicating that the resistance in the wild species might be simply inherited. In recent years, efforts were made to integrate bacterial wilt resistance with resistance to aflatoxin contamination.

Introduction

Groundnut or peanut (*Arachis hypogaea* L.) is an important oil crop as well as a cash crop in China. It is also an important source of plant protein for human consumption and livestock. By the end of the 1990s, the area planted to groundnut in China increased to about 5 million Ha, with a production of about 14 million tons. Increased groundnut production has significantly contributed to the plant oil and protein supply and to rural development in the country. For several decades, bacterial wilt caused by *R. solanacearum* has been an important constraint to groundnut production in China (9). It is considered that in recent years the groundnut fields with *R. solanacearum* infestation have increased to over 500,000 Ha, accounting for nearly 10% of the area under this crop. Incidence of bacterial wilt averaged 10 to 30% for susceptible groundnut cultivars and less than 8% for the currently grown resistant cultivars.

Extensive research efforts have been made since the 1970s at the Oil Crops Research Institute (OCRI) of the Chinese Academy of Agricultural Sciences (CAAS) and several other institutions to alleviate groundnut bacterial wilt, and effective control approaches including cultural management and use of cultivars with suitable resistance have been established. It is well known that use of genetic resistance is the most important component of any integrated management strategy. Genetic improvement for host-plant resistance has attracted much research effort during the past decade and significant progress has been made.

Germplasm Evaluation for Resistance

In China, germplasm research on the major oil crops, including groundnut, has been coordinated by the OCRI of CAAS for the past two decades. The evaluation of groundnut germplasm for resistance to bacterial wilt has been conducted continuously. Methods used to assess resistance to bacterial wilt in groundnut included screening in naturally-diseased nurseries and artificial inoculation approaches (2). Because bacterial wilt has been a serious constraint in HongAn County of Hubei Province in Central China, a field nursery has been set up there and extensively used for more than twenty years by the scientists from OCRI. In the nursery, wilt incidence of the most susceptible groundnut genotypes can be over 80%, and screening for resistance in the nursery has been very useful and reliable. For large scale screening experiments, groundnut lines were usually evaluated using single-row plots without replication in the nursery. Survival percentage of the plant populations was used to evaluate the resistance level. Genotypes that showed high survival percentage were further tested under the same natural disease pressure with three or four replications. Typical susceptible and resistant control genotypes were used to monitor disease pressure. Bacterial wilt nurseries were also established in several other provinces such as Guangdong, Guangxi and Sichuan Province. Artificial inoculation was routinely used to enhance infection rates and validate resistance properties. Infection pressure in artificial inoculation was kept close to that of natural conditions. Soaking seeds with a bacterial suspension for 30 minutes before sowing has been the most effective method for artificial infection. When the sample size was small, stem and root inoculation techniques were also used to test and confirm resistance. Multilocation tests were generally necessary to verify resistance stability.

By 2001, more than 800 newly-collected groundnut germplasm accessions were evaluated at OCRI for resistance to bacterial wilt. Fifty-three lines were identified as resistant with a population survival of over 80%. In addition to the 117 resistant genotypes identified before 1996, the total number of groundnut lines with a high level resistance to bacterial wilt was 170, among which, about 100 lines are landraces and the rest are improved lines. These lines were maintained at OCRI (Wuhan) and also at the National Gene bank in Beijing. By 2001, resistant genotypes were further positioned in all four botanic types of the cultivated groundnut: 10 were Valencia type, 53 were Spanish type, 79 were Dragon type, 23 were Virginia type, and five were other types. Besides the cultivated groundnut germplasm, 24 resistant accessions of wild *Arachis* species were identified.

Latent Infections

As in other cultivated plant species, latent infections by *R. solanacearum* in groundnut can influence growth, root system development and yield in some resistant genotypes that show no bacterial wilt symptoms (6). Reaction of groundnut to such latent infections must be considered as an important and complementary component for characterizing resistance properties. Thirty groundnut genotypes carrying resistance to bacterial wilt were artificially inoculated by soaking seeds in a bacterial suspension. The contaminated seeds were sown in sandy soil and few bacterial wilt symptoms were observed during the seedling stage. At 60 days after planting, 10 plants of each genotype were sampled and cut at root, hypocotyl and stem levels, and these segments were tested for *R. solanacearum* using ELISA. Healthy plant tissues were used as negative controls. Fewer latent infections were detected in the resistant lines that had better stability in fields across years and locations. Interestingly, groundnut genotypes with high latent colonization frequencies were more sensitive to drought stress in late growth stage, even though wilt incidence directly induced by *R. solanacearum* was low

(6). Bacterial wilt-resistant groundnut genotypes such as 89-15048, Yueyou 200, and Luhua No.3, which were less likely to be latently infected, were identified, and recommended as core parents in further breeding programs.

Mapping and Breeding for Bacterial Wilt Resistance

Since 2001, molecular diversity studies among bacterial wilt-resistant groundnut germplasm lines have been conducted at OCRI in collaboration with the International Crops Research Institute for the Semi-Arid Tropics (ICRISAT), India. Twenty-two bacterial wilt-resistant and two susceptible accessions were initially screened for molecular diversity using a Rapid Amplified Polymorphic DNA (RAPD) analysis at ICRISAT. ICG 7893, ICG 15222, and Chico were further studied for molecular diversity by Amplified Fragment Length Polymorphism (AFLP) analysis using 24 primer pairs. Some primer pairs were useful in identifying AFLP markers linked with resistance to bacterial wilt. A mapping population for marker investigation has been generated at OCRI (7).

The conventional hybridization approach was generally used in the groundnut breeding programs as the core strategy to improve resistance. In most cases, resistance to bacterial wilt in groundnut appears to be simply inherited and could be easily transferred to different varieties after a single cross (5). Selections for bacterial wilt resistance in hybrid progenies were generally made in generations F_2 through F_6, and screened in both bacterial wilt nurseries and artificial inoculations. Percentage of surviving plants was used as the resistance criterion, especially following natural field evaluation. Multilocational tests were conducted to determine stability, yield, and adaptation of selected lines.

Use of Resistant Germplasm in Breeding

In China, several resistant germplasm accessions have been used in breeding programs. Xiekangqing and Taishan Sanlirou have been most extensively used as bacterial wilt resistance donors. Improved resistant cultivars, including Ehua 5, Luhua 3, and Yueyou 92, were bred from Xiekangqing, while Zhonghua 2, and Zhonghua 4 were bred from Taishan Sanlirou. Induhuapi (a line introduced from India) has been effectively used as a resistant parent in Guangdong Province. It is interesting to note that only resistant germplasm lines belonging to *Arachis hypogaea* subsp. *fastigiata* have been successfully used as resistant donors in breeding programs. Apparently, the early maturity and tolerance to acid soil and poor soil fertility typical of Spanish or Valencia types are more desirable in agro-ecological regions where bacterial wilt is a problem. Resistant genotypes identified from *Arachis hypogaea* subsp. *hypogaea*, especially the Virginia type, are promising for increasing yield of bacterial wilt-resistant cultivars (4). However, some of their characters may inhibit integration of wilt resistance with desirable agronomic traits necessary for disease-prone areas. Large pods are usually important for high yield potential, but in most cases this trait is associated with sensitivity to calcium deficit in acid soils, a condition predominating in most regions where *R. solanacearum* causes serious groundnut losses (8). Therefore, direct use of large-podded genotypes in breeding is difficult. Efforts are currently in progress to use some of the resistant high-yielding genotypes from subsp. *hypogaea*. Genotypes with stronger resistance have been identified in the Chinese Dragon type germplasm collection, but no genotype of this type with longer growth period and spreading growth habit has been successfully used in breeding.

Recent Progress

ZHONGHUA 6

Since 1997, several improved groundnut cultivars and promising breeding lines have been developed and/or released in China. At OCRI, Zhonghua 6 was released in Hubei Province in 2000 with a high level of resistance to bacterial wilt, and improved tolerance to leaf spot and drought. In various field trials in Central China, Zhonghua 6 outyielded the currently established resistant cultivar Zhonghua 2 by 5-10%. Average bacterial wilt incidence across different years and locations was less than 5%, similar to Zhonghua 2. However, Zhonghua 6 had a better seed dormancy and very few seeds germinated before harvest even after rain, while more than 10% of Zhonghua 2 seeds germinated. With desirable pod shape, color, size, uniformity and relatively high protein content, Zhonghua 6 was thought to be suitable for confectionary processing. In a preliminary experiment, Zhonghua 6 also showed some resistance to aflatoxin production under laboratory conditions.

ZHONGHUA 4

This variety was developed at OCRI for resistance to bacterial wilt and rust, and released in Guizhou Province, two other provinces, and the central government. Zhonghua 4 had high protein content and tolerance to acid soil. This cultivar has been extensively cultivated in South and Central China. In 1998, Zhonghua 4 was recognized by the central government.

Many have been developed at OCRI, among which, 93-81 was highly resistant to bacterial wilt with tolerance to acid soil and 98-513 was resistant to bacterial wilt with improved yield. Another line, 94-305, with resistance to bacterial wilt and to rust and with high-yield potential, was selected from a cross combination between a Dragon resistant and a Spanish type susceptible genotype.

Yueyou 200, a breeding line developed at Guangdong Academy of Agricultural Sciences (GAAS) with resistance to bacterial wilt and high yield, was released as Tianfu 11. This variety was less affected by latent infection under artificial inoculation (7). Yueyou 202-35 was also developed at GAAS and released nationally in 1999 (3). It significantly outyielded local control cultivars in various yield trials and showed high resistance to rust and bacterial wilt under artificial inoculation (10.9%). Its protein (32.2%) and oil content (53.5%) was higher than in local cultivars. It was adapted to various cropping systems in South China. Yueyou 79, with desirable resistance to both bacterial wilt and rust, was developed at GAAS and released in Guangdong Province in 2000.

Groundnut cultivars with resistance to bacterial wilt have also been developed at Fujian and Hennan Province. Quanhua 10, a bacterial wilt-resistant cultivar released in Fujian Province in 1996, was rewarded by the local government in 2001 (1). Bacterial wilt-resistant cultivars have been planted to at least one million Ha since 1997 with significant impact on increasing groundnut production in the disease regions.

Interspecific Hybrids

An advanced breeding line '9102' was developed at Henan Academy of Agricultural Sciences (HAAS) and released in 2001 as an early maturing cultivar with resistance to bacterial wilt. It was developed from a cross between a Spanish-type cultivar 'Baisha 1016' and *A. chacoense*. The resistance transferred from the wild diploid species was high and stable across regions and seasons. It has high seed oil content (54%) and produced high yields in summer-sown cropping systems. Scientists from the Cash Crops Research Institute of Guangxi Academy of Agricultural Sciences, Nanning, have crossed cultivated groundnut with wild species of *Arachis* and produced many interspecific hybrid derivatives. The wild *Arachis* species involved were *A. correntina*, *A. stenosperma* and *A. cardenasii*. Up to now, seven derivatives showed over 90% survival, which is higher than the well-known bacterial wilt-resistant cultivated genotype Xiekangqing. In addition, most of the interspecific lines with resistance to bacterial wilt were also resistant to early and late leafspots.

Further Research Needs

With China's entry into World Trade Organization (WTO), groundnut production will further expand due to restructuring of agriculture and increase of market demand for plant oil and protein. Bacterial wilt will remain among the major constraints to groundnut production throughout the country. Genetic improvement for resistance will be the most important research area to further address China's bacterial wilt losses. Screening more desirable resistance resources and investigating the genetic diversity of wilt resistance in groundnut germplasm will be intensified. Yield potential and quality of wilt-resistant groundnut cultivars will be improved. Special emphasis will be given to integrating bacterial wilt resistance with resistance to aflatoxin-producing fungi.

Acknowledgements

This research was supported by the Natural Science Foundation of China (NSFC), projects No. 3957495 (1996-1998) and 30070521 (2000-2002).

Literature Cited

1. Chen, Y., and Hong, D. 1995. Breeding of a high yielding groundnut cultivar with resistance to bacterial wilt – Quanhua 10. Oil Crops China 17:44-47.
2. Duan, N.X., Tan,Y.J., Jiang, H.F., and Hu, D.H. 1993. Screening groundnut germplasm for resistance to bacterial wilt. Oil Crops China 1:22-25.
3. Liang, X., Li, S., Li, Y., Zheng, G., Li, X., and Ye, M. 1997. A new groundnut cultivar Yueyou 202-35. Oil Crops China 19:72.
4. Liao, B.S., Duan, N.X., Li, D., and Tang, G.Y. 1994. Cytoplasmic effect for resistance to bacterial wilt in Chinese dragon groundnut (Abstract). ACIAR Bacterial Wilt Newsletter 10:2.
5. Liao, B.S., Li, W.R., and Sun, D.R. 1986. A study on inheritance of resistance to *Pseudomonas solanacearum* E.F. Smith in *Arachis hypogaea* L. Oil Crops of China 3:1-8.

6. Liao, B.S., Shan, Z.H., and Lei, Y. 1998. Reaction to latent infection by *Ralstonia solanacearum* in groundnut. Chinese J. Oil Crop Sci. 20:61

7. Liao, B.S., Xu, Z.Y., and Jiang, H.F., 2001. Molecular markers of resistance to bacterial wilt in plants and their potential utilization. Chinese J. Oil Crop Sci. 23:61.

8. Mehan, V.K., Liao, B.S., Tan,Y.J., Robinson-Smith, A., McDonald, D., and Hayward, A.C. 1994. Bacterial wilt of groundnut: Information Bulletin No.35. Patancheru 502324 Andhra Pradesh, India: International Crops Research Institute for the Semi-Arid Tropics.

9. Tan, Y.J., and Liao, B.S. 1990. General aspects of groundnut bacterial wilt in China. Pages 44-47 in: Bacterial Wilt of Groundnut: Proceedings of an ACIAR/ICRISAT Collaborative Research Planning Meeting. 18-19 Mar 1990. Genting Highlands Malaysia. ACIAR Proceedings no. 31. K.J. Middleton and A.C. Hayward, eds. Canberra, Australia: Australian Centre for International Agricultural Research.

Search for Resistance to Bacterial Wilt in a Brazilian *Capsicum* Germplasm Collection

C.A. Lopes, S.I.C. Carvalho, and L.S. Boiteux

Embrapa Hortaliças, Brasília-DF, 70359-970, Brazil

Introduction

Hot and sweet peppers (*Capsicum* spp.) are important cash crops for vegetable growers in Brazil. A total of 13,000 hectares was planted to *Capsicum* species in the year 2000, with a harvest of 416,000 tons. Bacterial wilt, caused by *Ralstonia solanacearum*, is a major disease in the North region (Amazon Rain Forest), where peppers are highly appreciated but cultivated on a very small scale (2,5). In this environment, peppers have been predominantly affected by *R. solanacearum* biovar 3 with less incidence of biovar 1 isolates (3).

In Brazil, sweet peppers are traditionally cultivated in open fields in the South and Central regions, where bacterial wilt is considered a minor disease. In these areas, the importance of this disease has been neglected and its impact has been underestimated probably because the wilt symptoms have been, in many cases, erroneously attributed to *Phytophthora capsici* (the most serious pathogen in the summer season). Another reason why bacterial wilt is not observed more often in *Capsicum* spp. is that typical wilt symptoms are not always present, being sometimes restricted to plant dwarfing or to slight turgor loss limited to some branches, mainly in plants attacked by biovar 1.

In recent years, the cultivation under plastic cover of 'Lamuyo'-type *C. annuum* cultivars has dramatically increased in response to the growing demand of cosmetically-oriented consumers. Drip irrigation and black plastic mulching are employed in plastic houses, especially in the summer season, favoring bacterial wilt incidence and severity and resulting in severe yield losses to biovar 3 and biovar 1 isolates (3).

A search for sources of genetic resistance to *R. solanacearum* in hot pepper (*C. chinense*) germplasm has been initiated in Brazil (2). Additional screening work was conducted by Matos *et al.* (1) using a more diverse germplasm collection. A total of 45 *Capsicum* accessions were evaluated and three lines,. 'MC-4' ('CNPH 143'), 'MC-5' ('CNPH 144'), and 'HC-10' ('CNPH 145'), were identified as highly resistant. The *C. annuum* line 'MC-4', originating from Malaysia, was the most resistant; this genotype also had very stable resistance when challenged with a set of distinct biovar 1 and 3 strains. Interestingly, considerable variability was observed in the levels of disease regardless of the biovar employed (3). Such variability was also observed by Peter *et al.* (4) in hot pepper germplasm. The objective of this work was to estimate the resistance profile of ten peppers and a new set of lines of the Brazilian *Capsicum* collection to biovars 1 and 3.

Materials and Methods

The experiments were carried out in a greenhouse (20-40°C air temperature) in Brasília-DF, Brazil. For the virulence test, three standard genotypes 'CNPH 192' (susceptible), 'CNPH 790' (partly resistant) and 'CNPH 143' (resistant) were inoculated with 10 isolates of *R. solanacearum* obtained from pepper plants. Five isolates were classified as biovar 1 and five were classified as biovar 3.

For the screening test, 385 accessions belonging to the Brazilian *Capsicum* collection were evaluated for resistance. The lines were subdivided into four groups of approximately 90 genotypes each. These lines represented a cross-section of a large collection of 1,170 accessions maintained at Embrapa Hortaliças in Brasília-DF, Brazil. Approximately half of this collection has been characterized according to 57 morphological descriptors and also for their reaction to a set of important *Capsicum* pathogens in Brazil. The germplasm evaluated consisted of 241 accessions of *C. annuum*, 39 of *C. baccatum*, 35 of *C. chinense,* and 25 of *C. frutescens*. Plants were challenged with the isolate RS 34 (biovar 3), previously selected for its high virulence to *C. annuum* cultivars. Screening trials were conducted during the years 2000 and 2001.

For both tests, the lines were sown in styrofoam trays with 128 cells, filled with sterile substrate. When the first two pairs of true leaves were fully open, plants were removed from the cells with a gentle jet of water to preserve root integrity. They were then dipped for 1 minute in a bacterial suspension of approximately 1×10^8 CFU/ml. After inoculation, the plantlets were transplanted to 0.7 kg plastic pots, two plants per pot, with sterile substrate Plantmax® and maintained in the same greenhouse. The experimental plots contained five pots and two pots for the virulence and the screening tests, respectively, and were replicated three times in a randomized block design. Disease was assessed twice a week for three weeks using a scale from 1 to 5, where 1 indicated absence of symptoms and 5 a dead plant.

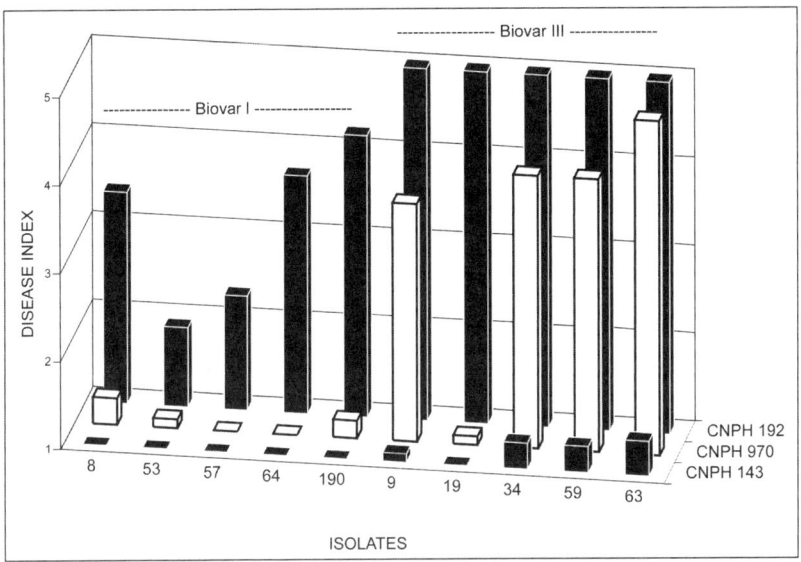

Fig. 1. Graphical representation of the reaction of three *Capsicum* genotypes ('CNPH 192', 'CNPH 970' and 'CNPH 143') challenged with ten strains of *Ralstonia solanacearum* biovars 1 and 3.

Results and Discussion

Striking differences were observed among genotypes and strains of *R. solanacearum* (Fig. 1). The line 'CNPH 143' ('MC-4') was consistently the most resistant genotype, showing only slight symptoms even when challenged with the most virulent strains. This confirms the stability of the high levels of resistance of this genotype to *R. solanacearum* strains (3). The line 'CNPH 192' had the highest disease rates.

Strains of biovar 3 were more virulent to all three genotypes than strains of biovar 1. The only exception for this trend was the isolate RS 19 (biovar 3), which incited a surprisingly low disease rate. The highest levels of virulence of biovar 3 isolates were more obvious in the line 'CNPH 970' (moderately resistant). This observation partly explains the more frequent association of pepper with biovar 3 isolates, whereas tomato plants are usually infected by biovar 1. This is very often observed in isolations from environments where both vegetable crops and both biovars are present, as in the Amazon Region. This phenomenon deserves further research, since in the previous study, conducted by Quezado-Soares and Lopes (3), this trend was not so evident.

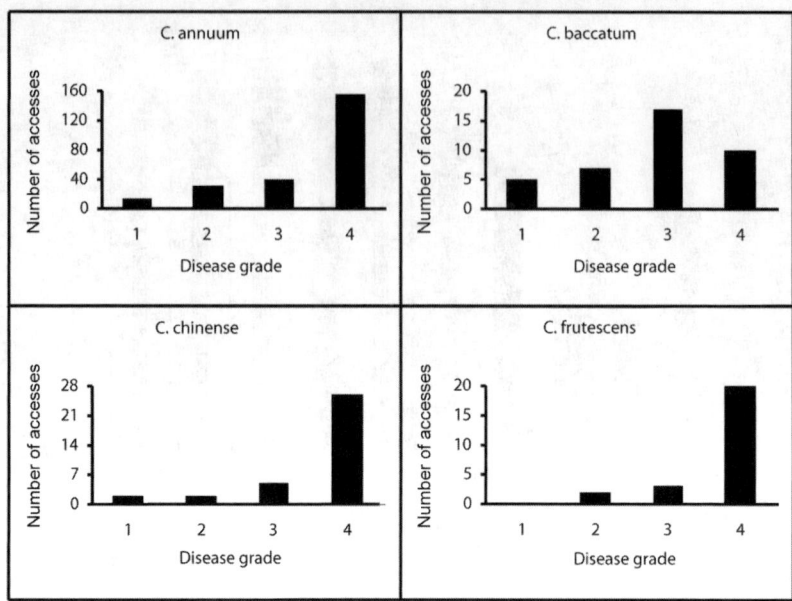

Fig. 2. Frequency distribution of genotypes within four *Capsicum* species according to their reaction to *Ralstonia solanacearum* biovar 3.

Except for the representative of *C. baccatum*, most of the genotypes were classified as highly susceptible to bacterial wilt (Fig. 2). For *C. annuum*, 13 genotypes were ranked as highly resistant, with a disease index lower than 2. Among them, the line 'MC-4' maintained its position as the most resistant genotype. This line is therefore recommended as a genitor in breeding programs aimed at developing cultivars with the resistance to the bacterial wilt disease. Studies are now underway to investigate the genetic basis of resistance to *R. solanacearum* biovar 1 and 3 in this pepper line.

Literature Cited

1. Matos, F.S.A., Lopes, C.A., and Takatsu, A. 1990. Identificação de fontes de resistência a *Pseudomonas solanacearum* em *Capsicum* spp. Horticultura Brasileira 8:22-23.
2. Cheng, S.S. 1989. The use of *Capsicum chinense* as sweet pepper cultivars and sources for gene transfer. Pages 55-62 in: Tomato and Pepper Production in the Tropics. AVRDC Publication 89-317. Tainan, Taiwan. 1989.
3. Quezado-Soares, A.M., and Lopes, C.A. 1995. Stability of the resistance to bacterial wilt of the sweet pepper 'MC-4' challenged with

strains of *Pseudomonas solanacearum*. Fitopatologia Brasileira
20:638-641.

4. Peter, K.V., Gopalakrishnan, T.R., Rajan, S., and Sadhan Kumar, P.G.
1993. Breeding for resistance to bacterial wilt in tomato, eggplant and
pepper. Pages 183-190 in: Bacterial Wilt, ACIAR Proceedings of the
International Conference, Kaohsiung, Taiwan. 1992. G.L. Hartman and
A.C. Hayward, eds.

5. Takatsu, A., and Lopes, C.A. 1997. Murcha-bacteriana em hortaliças:
avanços científicos e perspectivas de controle. Horticultura Brasileira
15: 170-177.

Solanum phureja and *S. stenotomum* Are Sources of Resistance to *Ralstonia solanacearum* for Somatic Hybrids of Potato

I. Fock[1], J. Luisetti[2], C. Collonnier[3], F. Vedel[4], G. Ducreux[5], H. Kodja[1], and D. Sihachakr[3]

[1] Laboratoire de Biologie et Physiologie Végétales, Génétique Moléculaire et Evolutive, 15 Avenue René Cassin, BP 7151, 97715 Saint Denis, La Réunion, France. [2] Laboratoire de Phytopathologie, Pôle de Protection des plantes, 7 chemin de l'IRAT, Ligne Paradis, 97410 Saint-Pierre, La Réunion, France. [3] Laboratoire de Morphogenèse Végétale Expérimentale, Bât. 360 Université Paris Sud, 91405 Orsay Cedex, France. [4] Laboratoire d'Ecologie, Systématique et Evolution, UPRESA-CNRS 8079, Bât. 360 Université Paris Sud, 91405 Orsay Cedex, France

Bacterial wilt caused by *Ralstonia solanacearum* is probably one of the most devastating plant bacterial diseases known. It affects more than 200 plant species worldwide. Under tropical conditions, broad host range race 1 strains are extremely damaging, whereas race 3 strains are responsible for wilting of potatoes and tomatoes under cool temperate conditions (4,6). Since chemicals are not effective and sanitation measures are difficult to apply, resistant or tolerant cultivars offer the best disease management strategy. But in potato, unlike tobacco or peanut, no good resistance is available and only a few tolerant cultivars are used in some countries (4). However, since the incidence of bacterial wilt depends on climatic and ecological conditions, tolerant cultivars selected under one environment may not hold up well elsewhere. Consequently, continuous development of resistant or tolerant varieties is required to improve bacterial wilt control. Some wild or related cultivated species are known to be resistant or highly tolerant, but unfortunately, crossing cultivated potato with resistant genotypes classified as Wild *Tuberosa* could lead to hybrids with some undesirable wild traits as well as a moderate level of resistance (4). Cultivated *Tuberosa Solanum phureja* and *S. stenotomum* are phylogenetically close to *S. tuberosum* and are considered to be bacterial wilt resistant. Clones of *S. phureja* have already been crossed with cultivars of *S. tuberosum* (10). Although resistance to bacterial wilt has also been identified in *S. stenotomum*

(8), this species has never been used as a source of resistance in potato breeding programs. To overcome sexual incompatibilities, somatic fusion provides an alternative for introgression of multiple resistance genes from wild *Solanum* species into *S. tuberosum* (11,12). Therefore, we performed somatic hybridization experiments between a dihaploid clone of *S. tuberosum* cultivar 'BF15' (2n=2x=24) and a diploid (2n=2x=24) clone of either of *S. phureja* or *S. stenotomum*. The nature of selected putative regenerated somatic hybrids was assessed by several analyses (2,3). In this study, somatic hybrids from *S. stenotomum* and from *S. phureja* were evaluated for resistance to strains of *R. solanacearum* originating from Reunion Is.

Materials and Methods

Six tetraploid somatic hybrids from *S. stenotomum* and six from *S. phureja* (five tetraploid and an amphiploid) were evaluated for resistance to *R. solanacearum* race 1 and race 3 strains from Reunion Is. Strains G14 (race 1, biovar 3) and PDT5 (race 3, biovar 2), were provided by CIRAD (Centre de Coopération Internationale en Recherche Agronomique pour le Développement). Root inoculation was performed by dipping freshly cut roots from 4-weeks old vitroplants for 30 min either in a 1×10^7 CFU/ml bacterial suspension (inoculated plants) or in sterile water (control plants). After inoculation, plants were kept in liquid MS medium and placed in a culture room (14 h·d–1 illumination at 55 μmol·m–2·s–1, 20°C and 60% relative humidity). Inoculations were performed on three replicates of 12 plants for each clone. Plants were observed weekly and symptoms recorded using a disease index (DI) ranging from 0 to 4: 0= no wilted leaves, 1= up to 25% wilted, 2= up to 50% wilted, 3= up to 75% wilted and 4= plants entirely wilted (2,3). Disease indices (13) were calculated as the ratio between the sum of the products of each disease index, divided by 4, and the corresponding number of plants and the total number of inoculated plants. Disease incidence was evaluated at 30 days after inoculation as percentage of wilted plants. Bacterial populations in roots and stems were also estimated. Plants sections were crushed and serially diluted and spread onto an appropriate medium (2,3).

Results

As expected, the susceptible parent *S. tuberosum* displayed high wilting rates regardless of the strain inoculated. For *S. phureja*, no wilted plant was observed and the disease index was low (0.36) following infection by the

Table 1. Disease index and disease incidence on parental lines and tetraploid somatic hybrids from *S. phureja* recorded 30 days after root inoculation with strains of *R. solanacearum*.

Genotype[1]	Disease index[2]		Disease incidence [2]	
	Race 1 strain	Race 3 strain	Race 1 strain	Race 3 strain
BF15 (parental)	0.87 b	1.00 a	94.3 a	100.0 a
BP3	0.80 b	1.00 a	30.6 bc	100.0 a
BP4	0.49 c	0.88 b	7.9 d	68.4 b
BP6	0.78 b	1.00 a	40.5 bc	100.0 a
BP9	0.08 d	0.52 c	0.0 d	2.8 d
BP15	0.43 c	1.00 a	20.5 cd	100.0 a
BP16	0.79 b	1.00 a	48.6 ab	100.0 a
S. phureja	0.36 c	0.86 b	0.0 d	50.0 b
Controls	0.0 d	0.0 d	0.0 d	0.0 d

[1] For both parents, 2n = 2x = 24. For all hybrids, 2n = 4x, except for BP9 for which 2n > 4x.

[2] Values followed by the same letter are not significantly different at *P* = 0.05

race 1 strain. Infection with the race 3 strain scored 50% disease incidence (Table 1). For *S. stenotomum*, the wilting rate was low: 0 or 30% according to the strain used (Table 2).

When inoculated with the race 1 strain, all somatic hybrids of *S. phureja* except one showed a wilting rate close to that of the wild parent species. However, when inoculated with the race 3 strain, most hybrids displayed a wilting rate of 100%, as did *S. tuberosum*. The amphiploid hybrid, BP9, showed a wilting rate and a disease index significantly lower than the wild parent (Table 1). No hybrids from *S. stenotomum* wilted when inoculated with the race 1 strain. When inoculated with the race 3 strain, based on the disease indices at day 30, no hybrids were significantly different from the wild species (Table 2). Bacterial populations recovered from roots of apparently healthy plants were higher than 1×10^6 CFU/ml regardless of strain or plant clone (Table 3). However, within stems inoculated with the race 1 strain, significant differences in population levels were recorded between *S. tuberosum*, *S. phureja*, and its hybrids (Table 3). No bacteria were recovered from stems of *S. stenotomum* and its hybrids (Table 3). Race 3 strains were detected in stems of *S. tuberosum* and *S. phureja* at high population levels ($>1 \times 10^6$ CFU/ml) whereas only a rather low bacterial population was recovered from the stems of *S. stenotomum* and hybrids tested ($<1 \times 10^4$ CFU/ml) or from stems of BP9 ($<1 \times 10^5$ CFU/ml) (Table 3).

Table 2. Disease index and disease incidence on parental lines and tetraploid somatic hybrids from *S. stenotomum* recorded 30 days after root inoculation with strains of *R. solanacearum*.

Genotype[1]	Disease index[2]		Disease incidence [2]	
	Race 1 strain	Race 3 strain	Race 1 strain	Race 3 strain
BF15 (parental)	0.98 a	1.00 a	94.3 a	100.0 a
BS2	0.04 c	0.76 b	0.0 c	16.7 c
BS31	0.10 c	0.64 b	0.0 c	16.7 c
BS33	0.11 c	0.65 b	0.0 c	16.7 c
BS37	0.10 c	0.74 b	0.0 c	30.6 b
BS42	0.09 c	0.69 b	0.0 c	27.8 b
BS44	0.04 c	0.63 b	0.0 c	13.9 c
S. stenotomum	0.10 c	0.74 b	0.0 c	30.6 b
Controls	0.0 c	0.0 c	0.0 c	0.0 c

[1] For both parents, 2n = 2x = 24. For all hybrids, 2n = 4x.
[2] Values followed by the same letter are not significantly different at $P = 0.05$.

Table 3. Populations of *R. solanacearum* within roots and stems of asymptomatic plants 30 days after root inoculation by race 1 or race 3 strains.

Genotype[1]	Race 1 strain[2]		Race 3 strain[2]	
	Root	Stem	Root	Stem
BF15	7.43 a	7.13 a	7.93 a	7.79 a
S.phureja	7.70 a	3.74 b	7.27 a	6.92 b
BP9	7.54 a	3.20 c	7.69 a	4.28 c
S.stenotomum	7.29 b	0.00 b	7.02 b	3.31 b
BS 2	6.95 c	0.00 b	6.34 c	3.32 b
BS 31	6.98 c	0.00 b	6.10 c	3.04 b

[1] For hybrids, 2n = 4x except for BP9, 2n > 4x. For both parents, 2n = 2x = 24.
[2] Expressed as log $CFU.g^{-1}$ fresh weight. Values followed by the same letter are not significantly different at $P = 0.05$.

Discussion

Susceptibility of parental lines to inoculation with *R. solanacearum* varied with the strain used. Whatever the strain, *S. tuberosum* cultivar 'BF15' was highly susceptible and all inoculated plants wilted within four weeks. Large bacterial populations were recovered from roots and stems of

BF15 (1×10^7 to 1×10^8 CFU.g^{-1} fw). Under our experimental conditions, *S. phureja* appeared tolerant of the race 1 strain as no wilt was observed, but bacterial populations were recovered from stems at low density. Nevertheless, *S. phureja* appeared moderately susceptible to the race 3 strain (50% wilt and highly colonized asyptomatic plants). The relationship between cultivar resistance/tolerance to bacterial wilt and stem bacterial populations was consistent with previous observations on tomato (9). Interestingly, among the hybrid clones of *S. phureja* tested, the amphiploid hybrid clone (BP9) (> 48 chromosomes) was as tolerant to race 1 as the wild parent but less susceptible to the race 3 strain. The wilt rating was significantly lower (2.8% *vs* 50%) in this clone than in the parent, as was the stem colonization level (4.28 versus 6.92). We speculate that this is due to the association of one copy of dihaploid potato (2x) with one copy plus a few chromosomes of the *S. phureja* genome (>2x), probably harboring the resistance genes, giving a gene dosage-effect resulting in higher tolerance in the amphiploid hybrid. The other hybrids, all tetraploids obtained from *S. phureja*, appeared as susceptible to race 1 and race 3 as was the wild parent. *S. stenotomum* and all somatic hybrids inoculated with the race 1 strain showed no disease after four weeks. Moreover, no bacterial populations were recovered from the stems. Therefore, *S. stenotomum* and its somatic hybrids were considered resistant to race 1, although high bacterial populations were found in the roots. The mechanism of resistance acting in *S. stenotomum* and its somatic hybrids may involve the diffusion of bacterial populations from roots to stems through collar and/or the capability to multiply within the stems. These results are in agreement with a report from Grimault *et al.* (5) on tomato. When inoculated with the race 3 strain, bacterial wilt developed on the wild parent and its somatic hybrids, but at a rate significantly lower than in BF15. There were no significant differences between disease indices of the wild parent and hybrids. However, *S. stenotomum* and its derivative hybrids could not be considered to be resistant to *R. solanacearum* race 3, but only tolerant, since bacterial populations were recovered from stems.

Results obtained in this study, together with those from other authors for introgression of bacterial resistance in particular (7), highlight the potential of somatic fusion as a valid way for introducing traits of resistance from wild species to cultivated potatoes. Moreover, the resistance to bacterial wilt introduced into cultivated crops like eggplant by using protoplast fusion has proved stable in field conditions (1). Nevertheless, further detailed evaluation of the somatic hybrids under field conditions is needed to confirm their potential exploitation in breeding programs for potato.

Literature Cited

1. Collonnier, C., Mulya, K., Fock, I., Mariska, I., Servaes, A., Vedel, F., Siljak-Yakovlev, S., Souvannavong, V., Ducreux, G., and Sihachakr, D. 2001. Source of resistance against *Ralstonia solanacearum* in fertile somatic hybrids of eggplant (*Solanum melongena* L.) with *Solanum aethiopicum* L. Plant Sci. 160: 301-31.
2. Fock, I., Collonnier, C., Purwito, A., Luisetti, J., Souvannagong, V., Vedel, F., Servaes, A., Ambroise, A., Kodja, H., Ducreux, G., and Sihachakr, D. 2000. Resistance to bacterial wilt in somatic hybrids between *Solanum tuberosum* and *Solanum phureja*. Plant Sci. 160: 165-176.
3. Fock, I., Collonnier, C., Luisetti, J., Purwito, A., Souvannagong, V., Vedel, F., Servaes, A., Ambroise, A., Kodja, H., Ducreux, G., and Sihachakr, D. 2001. Use of *Solanum stenotomum* for introduction of resistance to bacterial wilt in somatic hybrids of potato. Plant Physiol. Biochem. 30: 899-908.
4. French, E.R., Anguiz, R., and Aley, F.P. 1998. The usefulness of potato resistance to *Ralstonia solanacearum* for the integrated control of bacterial wilt. Pages 381-385 in: Bacterial Wilt Disease, Molecular and Ecological Aspects. P. Prior, C. Allen, and J.G. Elphinstone, eds. Springer-Verlag, Berlin.
5. Grimault, V., Gélie, B., Lemattre, M., Prior, P., and Schmit, J. 1994. Comparative histology of resistant and susceptible tomato cultivars infected by *Pseudomonas solanacearum*. Physiol. Mol. Pathol. 44: 105-123.
6. Hayward, A.C., Elphinstone, J.G., Caffier, D., Janse, J., Stefani, E., French, E.R., and Wright, A.J. 1998. Round table on bacterial wilt (brown rot) of potato. Pages 420-430 in: Bacterial Wilt Disease, Molecular and Ecological Aspects. P. Prior, C. Allen, and J.G. Elphinstone, eds. Springer-Verlag, Berlin.
7. Laferriere, L.T., Helgeson, J.P., and Allen, C. 1999. Fertile *Solanum tuberosum*+ *S. commersonii* somatic hybrids as sources of resistance to bacterial wilt caused by *Ralstonia solanacearum*. Theor. Appl. Genet. 98: 1272-1278.
8. Martin, C. 1979. Sources of resistance to *Pseudomonas solanacearum*. Pages 49-53 in: Developments in Control of Potato Bacterial Disease. Report of a Planning Conference held at CIP, Lima, Peru, June 12-15.
9. Prior, P., Bart, S., Leclercq, S., Darrasse, A., and Anais, G. 1996. Resistance to bacterial wilt in tomato as discerned by spread of *Pseudomonas* (Burkholderia) *solanacearum* in the stem tissues. Plant Pathology 45: 720-726.

10. Sequeira, L., and Rowe, P.R. 1969. Selection and utilization of *Solanum phureja* clones with high resistance to different strains of *Pseudomonas solanacearum*. Am. Potato J. 46: 451-462.
11. Serraf, I., Sihachakr, D., Ducreux, G., Brown, S.C., Allot, M., Barghi, N., and Rossignol, L. 1991. Interspecific somatic hybridization in potato by protoplast electrofusion. Plant Sci. 76: 115-126.
12. Valkonen, J.P.T., and Rokka, V.M. 1998. Combination and expression of two virus resistance mechanisms in interspecific somatic hybrids of potato. Plant Sci. 131: 85-94.
13. Winstead, N.N., and Kelman, A. 1952. Inoculation techniques for evaluating resistance to *Pseudomonas solanacearum*. Phytopathology 42: 628-634.

Assessment of Resistance to Bacterial Wilt in CIP Advanced Potato Clones

S. Priou, P. Aley, and L. Gutarra

International Potato Center (CIP), Lima, Peru

Bacterial wilt (or brown rot) caused by *Ralstonia solanacearum* (Smith) Yabuuchi *et al.* is a major constraint to potato production in most tropical and subtropical regions. At high elevations, potatoes are affected mostly by cool temperature-adapted, restricted host range strains of *R. solanacearum* (race 3/biovar 2A) that are principally transmitted through latently infected tubers. There is no high-level resistance in potato cultivars, but some are less susceptible to bacterial wilt and yield well in the presence of the pathogen. Some cultivars, such as Cruza 148 and Molinera, do not express wilt in cool conditions, but can disseminate the pathogen through progeny tubers with a high rate of latent infection. The use of the moderate levels of resistance that are available, however, can have a huge impact on ware potato production in areas where soils are highly infested if bacterial wilt-free seed can be provided (4).

In the 1990s, advanced potato clones were obtained from a 14-yr program of breeding for bacterial wilt resistance at CIP. These clones were produced after various crosses with: (i) clones derived from Colombian *S. phureja* genotypes produced at the University of Wisconsin in the 1970s, (ii) clone AVRDC-1287 derived from *S. chacoense* and *S. raphanifolium*, (iii) clone Cruza 148 of unknown origin, resistant to bacterial wilt and late blight, (iv) diploid populations derived from wild species *S. chacoense, S. sparsipilum* and the native species *S. stenotomum, S. phureja* and *S. goniocalyx*, and (v) *S. tuberosum* subsp. *tuberosum* genotypes that carry earliness, heat adaptation, resistance to late blight and/or root-knot nematode, immunity to potato virus X and Y, high yield and good agronomic characteristics (1,8). The bacterial wilt resistance of *S. phureja*-derived materials has been found to be strain-specific and sensitive to high temperatures (2, 3). However, resistance to race 3 strains is expected to be more stable than resistance to race 1 strains of *R. solanacearum* prevalent in the lowland, since strains from race 3 are a genetically homogeneous group. So far, bacterial wilt-resistant potato genotypes have been selected mostly on the absence of wilting symptoms. Very few researchers have assessed latent infection of stems or tubers, although latent infection is responsible for the spread of the disease and for overcoming resistance if infected seed tubers are planted (4).

In this paper we report a three-year evaluation of CIP advanced clones in a bacterial wilt-infested field (race 3/biovar 2A) in Peru for their resistance to wilt and tuber infection. These clones were produced from the last crosses for bacterial wilt resistance made at CIP in 1995. They have not been tested in any other country.

Materials and Methods

Among 1343 advanced clones from the last population of materials produced in 1996 at CIP's experiment station in Huancayo (3300 m altitude), 963 were selected for good agronomic traits. In October 1997, 580 clones and in November 1998, 383 clones were planted for pre-screening in a bacterial wilt -infested field at Carhuaz (2810 m), Ancash Department, Peru, with five plants each, resulting in selection of 90 genotypes resistant to bacterial wilt. These 90 clones were multiplied at Huancayo from healthy duplicates and then planted at Carhuaz again in November 1999 for a second evaluation under high disease pressure. Experimental design was 25 plants each in five replications (rows) of five plants. In February 2001, 34 of the 43 selected clones were planted for a third evaluation (because of lack of seed of the other nine), with five replications of five plants each. In 1997, 1998 and 1999, 10 miniplots of five plants each of commercial cultivars Yungay (susceptible), Revolución (susceptible), Molinera (moderately resistant), and Cruza 148 (resistant) were planted as controls and randomly distributed in the field. Molinera was not planted in 2001. Cultural practices were as recommended for commercial potato crops.

In all trials soil inoculum was enhanced one month after emergence by burying (at root level) one-eighth of a 9.0 cm diam. plate containing a 48-h agar culture of R. solanacearum CIP311 on Kelman's medium without tetrazolium chloride. Each culture piece contained approximately 3×10^9 colony-forming units (CFU). Strain CIP311 (race 3/biovar 2A) had been isolated from the same field and several sanitation precautions were taken to avoid pathogen spread. For each plant, wilt incidence was evaluated at 15-day intervals for two months using the CIP 1-5 infection scale of wilted plants (1 = 0% wilted, 2 = 1-25%, 3 = 26-50%, 4 = 51-75%, and 5 = 76-100%). The average score was recorded for the clone (e.g., the sum of scores for each plant divided by the number of plants). At harvest (about 120 days after planting), healthy yield and weight of rotted tubers (those exhibiting bacterial wilt symptoms upon slicing) were recorded.

In 1999 and 2000 all tubers of 10 plants for each of 30 and 35 clones, respectively, were graded in three size categories: 1.5-2.5 cm, 2.6-5 cm, and > 5 cm and tested individually for latent infection by *R. solanacearum* using NCM-ELISA, a post-enrichment enzyme-linked immunosorbent assay on nitrocellulose membrane (6). This is a sensitive and specific serological method developed at CIP. In 2001, tuber latent infection of 34 clones was assessed: a sample of 30 tubers per clone was tested following the sampling strategy described by Priou *et al.* (7). In 1999, enriched samples were streaked on Kelman's medium to confirm the presence of the bacterium. When ELISA was positive but the bacteria could not be isolated, DNA amplification by PCR was performed from enriched tuber extracts using primers 759 and 760 of Opina *et al.* (5).

Results

From 580 clones planted in 1997, 41 (7.1%) were selected for high resistance to bacterial wilt (no wilt). Of these, only eight remained after a second evaluation in 1999. From 383 potato clones planted in 1998, 49 (12.8%) were rated highly resistant to bacterial wilt. Severity of the disease was much higher in 1999/2000 thus, clones that had a bacterial wilt incidence up to the score of resistant cultivar Molinera were selected (2.2, i.e. 30% wilt), considering that these clones had no wilt in 1997 or 1998 evaluation trials. A total of 43 clones have been retained from 90 clones tested and only five clones (5.5%) were highly resistant to bacterial wilt (no wilt). In the 2001 trial, of the 34 planted, 21 had no wilt and four had less bacterial wilt than, or equal to the 5% wilt from Cruza 148 (Table 1). In 2001, yields were extremely low for all clones and control cultivars because the crop was planted in January 2001 instead of October-November 2000 and rain was excessive and late blight incidence was high. In harvests 1999 and 2000, most of the clones yielded well in spite of high disease pressure (many had yield ranging 1-1.5 kg per plant). However, this trait was not taken into account as a selection criterion. Molinera was reported in the 1970s as moderately resistant but high bacterial wilt incidences were observed in these trials, ranking it as susceptible.

Thirteen clones were resistant to bacterial wilt in all three evaluations (wilt score less than or equal to that of the resistant control), from which five were highly resistant (no wilt) in all trials.

Twenty-five high-yielding clones have been selected as highly to moderately resistant to bacterial wilt (the average of three evaluations being less than 6% wilt) (Table 1). However, all clones harbored tuber infection

Table 1. Wilt incidence (WI %), healthy yield (HY g/plant), percentage rotted tubers at harvest (RTH % weight) and latently infected tubers (LIT %) of advanced potato clones planted in a *Ralstonia solanacearum* (race 3/biovar 2A)-infested field in Carhuaz, Peru, selected for their high to moderate resistance to bacterial wilt in 1998-1999, 1999-2000 and 2001 crops.

N°	Clone pedigree	1998-1999				1999-2000				2001			
		WI	HY	RTH	LIT	WI	HY	RTH	LIT	WI	HY	RTH	LIT
1	(BWH87.344R x TXY.11)1	0	1048	0		0	858	3	27.0	0	246	0	3.3
2	(CRUZA-148 x C90.205)8	0	903	31		0	1268	5	36.4	0	216	1	36.7
3	(720118.1 x C90.205)21	0	1264	0	18.5	0	702	8	31.6	0	164	3	0.0
4	(720118.1 x C90.205)20	0	1378	6	19.2	0	672	0	24.7	0	188	8	8.0
5	(720118.1 x BWH87.183)3	0	860	0	19.2	0	1556	5	30.7	0	439	0.3	6.7
6	(720118.1 x C90.205)9	0	1518	0	36.1	1	1320	1	40.3	0	409	3	30.0
7	(C90.205 x 34.73)13	0	460	0		1	745	1	38.4	0	172	2	40.0
8 [a]	H89.65.44	0	680	0		1	1270	3	37.1	0	300	1	7.2
9	(BWH87.415 x DXY-7)16	0	1375	0	32.5	3	728	2	31.8	0	108	26	20.0
10	(CRUZA-148 x BWH87.344R)1	0	893	0	14.1	4	1430	5	33.6	0	326	1	10.0
11	(BWH87.230R x C90.205)1	0	1834	13	9.1	4	1420	1	31.1	0	505	1	50.0
12	(720118.1 x C90.205)17	0	750	4		5	948	3	39.8	0	327	0	6.7
13	(CRUZA-148xBWH87.344R)3	0	1136	7	29.5	6	1466	6	30.7	0	291	3	26.6
14	(28.68 x C90.205)5	0	510	0	60.0	7	700	1	18.8	5	537	10	16.7
15	(28.68 x BWH87.344R)13	0	950	5	10.4	7	1260	4	30.0	5	345	2	0.0
16 [a]	BWH87.338	0	675	0		7	1020	3	19.0	0	250	7	13.3
17	69.4	0	1840	0		8	1104	3	53.1	0	369	3	10.0
18	(CRUZA-148 x C90.205)12	0	1972	1		8	1060	4	57.0	5	135	16	64.3
19	(381064.2 x TXY-11)4	0	1444	2		10	1428	3		0	183	9	20.0
20	(BWH87.420 x C90.205)6	0	1494	4		10	809	7	50.0	0	351	2	6.7
21 [a]	SR 17.50	0	1320	0		12	564	3	24.8	0	147	5	6.7
22 [a]	392278.19	0	740	0		12	456	4	10.3	0	207	13	13.3
23	(BWH87.446R x TXY.2B)1	0	914	5		12	521	13	20.0	0	154	8	20.0
24	(C91.640 x 34.73)2	0	780	0		17	920	2		0	106	0	0.0
25	(BWH87.289 x XY-13)103	0	517	52	47.1	17	920	4	36.6	1	227	17	10.0
	Yungay (S) [b]	45.7	628	21	71.3	70	1106	34	4.7	15	222	12	6.7
	Revolucion (S)	84.2	1094	50	71.5	92	874	46	7.6	45	113	27	20.0
	Molinera (MR) [b]	54.5	870	15	27.6	33	862	27	19.5				
	Cruza 148 (R) [b]	4.0	1027	3	42.2	6	1349	12	72.8	5	352	4	36.7

[a] Clones selected from the 1997/1998 evaluation trial.

[b] S = susceptible, MR = moderately resistant, R = resistant.

(either visible at harvest or latent) in all trials, most of them at levels lower than Cruza 148. For the 30-35 clones assessed, the average tuber infection rate after harvest in 2001 (17.6%) was lower compared to the previous two years (30% in 1999 and 34% in 2000 (data not shown)). Control varieties had percentages of latently infected tubers similar to seasons 2000 and 2001 but the percentage of rotted tubers at harvest was higher.

Tubers have been graded to evaluate the effect of tuber size on latent infection levels. The size effect was not significant according to analysis of variance and Waller-Duncan's test at P=0.05. Average percentages of infected tubers among the 35 clones were 28.5, 29.3 and 30.7% in 1999, and 31.07, 33.22, and 33.17% in 2000 for tuber size of 1.5–2.5 cm, 2.6–5 cm, and > 5 cm, respectively. This result shows that infected plants produce tubers of all sizes with equal probability of being infected; thus tubers can be sampled independently of their size. This is of great concern for sampling tubers from seed lots for analysis of bacterial wilt infection.

From the 2246 tubers analyzed in 1998, 674 (30%) were positive by ELISA. The pathogen could not be isolated on Kelman's medium from 30 of these tuber extracts. The presence of *R. solanacearum* was confirmed by PCR in 27 of these 30 doubtful samples, leading to a possible cross-reaction rate of only 0.44%. However, the other reason for not confirming positive results in ELISA could be that the inoculum concentration in the extract was lower than the detectable level by plating on Kelman's medium and by post-enrichment PCR, since the sensitivity of post-enrichment NCM-ELISA is higher (2 cells/ml) than the other two techniques under our conditions (6).

Discussion

The 25 selected clones are being freed of viruses to meet international distribution standards for on-farm testing in countries where high soil bacterial wilt infestation levels limit potato cultivation. In these bacterial wilt-endemic areas, selected clones would be valuable for ware potato production but tubers should be sold right after harvest since they harbor latent infections and could rot during storage. Moreover, tubers should not be used as seed to avoid dissemination of the disease and breakdown of resistance that may occur when seed is infected, as has been reported for *phureja*-derived cultivars (4). This possibility is currently being investigated in Peru.

Susceptibility to tuber infection and to aboveground symptoms were not correlated as reported by Ciampi and Sequeira (2). Moreover, results obtained by assessing tuber infection after harvest were not consistent from one year to another; thus the latent infection potential of clones may not depend on wilt incidence but on environmental factors.

Breeding for resistance to bacterial wilt at CIP has resulted in potato clones with high to moderate levels of resistance, superior to the *phureja* x *tuberosum* hybrids. However, a high frequency of latent infection is still present in tubers at levels comparable to those observed for *S. phureja*-derived clones such as Molinera. Probably, resistance to latent infection does not occur in the genetic base of the parents used for the crosses that led to these materials. Latent infection in tubers was not a selection criterion to select original *phureja* genotypes used in the University of Wisconsin's breeding program for resistance to bacterial wilt. Neither was tuber infection a criterion in the further two decades of breeding. Therefore, the criteria formerly used in the course of selection for potato resistance to bacterial wilt should be reappraised; the sampling strategy described by Priou *et al.* (7) sets the stage for this. In the absence of better sources of higher levels of resistance, national programs should continue breeding and selecting for bacterial wilt resistance from the selected CIP advanced materials.

Literature Cited

1. Anguiz, R.J., and Mendoza, H.A. 1997. General and specific combining abilities for resistance to bacterial wilt (*Pseudomonas solanacearum* E.F. Smith) in PVX and PVY immune autotetraploid potatoes. Fitopatologia 32:71-80.
2. Ciampi, L., and Sequeira, L. 1980. Multiplication of *Pseudomonas solanacearum* in resistant potato plants and the establishment of latent infections. American Potato Journal 57: 319-329.
3. French, E.R., and de Lindo, L. 1982. Resistance to *Pseudomonas solanacearum* potato: Strain specificity and temperature sensitivity. Phytopathology 72:1408-1412.
4. French, E.R., Anguiz, R., and Aley, P. 1998. The usefulness of potato resistance to *Ralstonia solanacearum* for the integrated control of bacterial wilt. Pages 381-385 in: Bacterial wilt disease: Molecular and ecological aspects. P. Prior, C. Allen, and J. Elphinstone, eds. INRA Edition, Springer Verlag, Berlin, Germany.
5. Opina, N., Tavner, F., Hollway, G., Wang, J.F., Li, T.H., Maghirang, R., Fegan, M., Hayward, A.C., Krishnapllai, V., Hong, W.F., Holloway, B.W., and Timmis, J.N. 1997. A novel method for development of species and strain-specific DNA probes and PCR primers for identifying *Burkholderia solanacearum* (formerly *Pseudomonas solanacearum*). As. Pac. J. Mol. Biol. Biotechnol. 5:19–30.
6. Priou, S., Gutarra, L., and Aley, P. 1999. Highly sensitive detection of *Ralstonia solanacearum* in latently infected potato tubers by post-

enrichment ELISA on nitrocellulose membrane. EPPO/OEPP Bull. 29:117-125.

7. Priou, S., Salas, C., de Mendiburu, F., Aley, P., and Gutarra, L. 2001. Assessment of latent infection frequency in progeny tubers of advanced potato clones resistant to bacterial wilt: a new selection criterion. Potato Res. 44: 359-374.

8. Schmiediche, P., 1985. Breeding potatoes for resistance to bacterial wilt caused by *Pseudomonas solanacearum*. Pages 105-111 in: ACIAR Proceedings no. 13. G.J. Persley, ed. Canberra, Australia.

Screening Long Pepper (*Piper* spp.) for Resistance to Bacterial Wilt Caused by *Ralstonia solanacearum*

Maria J.B. Cavalcante[1], Carlos A. Lopes[2],
Hélia A. Mendonça[3], and Francisco J.S. Ledo[4]

[1] Embrapa Acre, Caixa Postal 321, Rio Branco 69908-970 , AC, Brazil.
[2] Embrapa Hortalicas, Caixa Postal 218, Brasilia 70359-970, Brazil.
[3] Embrapa Acre, Caixa Postal 321, Rio Branco 69908-970 , AC, Brazil.
[4] Embrapa Gado de Leite, Rua Eugênio do Nascimento, 610,
CEP 36.038-330, Juiz de Fora, MG, Brazil.

Ralstonia solanacearum is native to most Brazilian soils. It is a limiting factor for growing solanaceous crops, especially in the Amazon Region where high temperature and high humidity are present all year round (11). Confirming its high capacity to infect different hosts (4), this pathogen was recently found causing wilt in long pepper (*Piper hispidinervum*) (9). This species is a native shrubby plant of the Piperaceae family, which originated in the State of Acre. It has been commercially cultivated for extraction of a rich essential oil in safrol, used in formulations of biodegradable insecticides with low toxicity; and as a fixer of fragrances and cosmetics. Disease outbreaks in the State of Rondonia (Fig. 1) killed up to 70% of these plants and became a serious burden for the growers. Even though both biovars 1 and 3 of the pathogen are present in the Amazon, only biovar 1 has been associated with diseased long pepper plants (1). This biovar is also the only one isolated from new or unusual nonsolanaceous hosts like *Passiflora edulis* (6), *Eryngium foetidum* (8) and *Talinum triangulare* (7) found in the State of Para.

In a search for measures to control this disease, we screened progenies and populations of long pepper for resistance to bacterial wilt.

Material and Methods

The bacterial strain used as inoculum belongs to race 1, biovar I of *R. solanacearum*, according to Hayward (3). It was isolated from the stem base

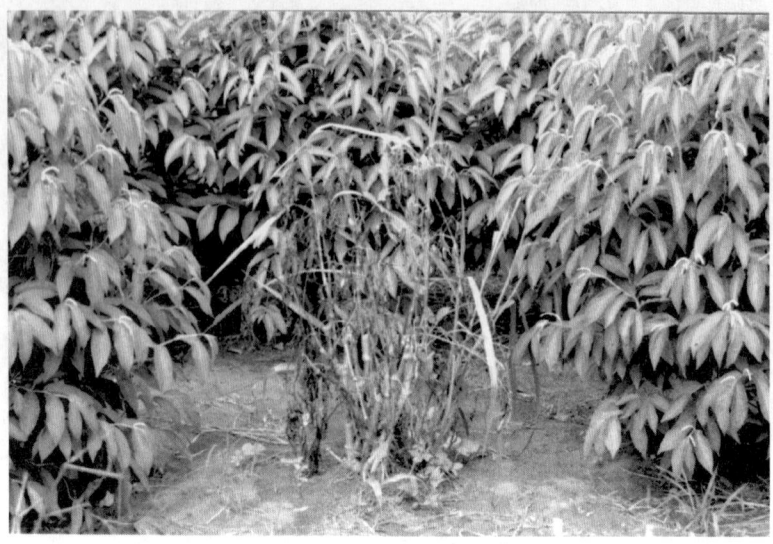

Fig. 1. Long pepper plants (*Piper hispidinervum*), infected by *Ralstonia solanacearum*.

of a wilted long pepper plant and presented typical white irregular colonies with a pink center when cultivated in TZC medium (5). Pure cultures were maintained in sterile water, and for the inoculation, they were cultivated in Kado 523 medium in a growth chamber at 28°C for 48 hours. The experimental design was randomized complete block with three replications of ten plants per plot. Twenty-five natural populations of *P. hispidinervum*, 28 open pollinated progenies of *P. hispidinervum* and 13 of *P. aduncum* were evaluated. Plants of 6-8 cm (40 days after planting) were inoculated by immersing their roots, previously pruned of the bottom third, in a bacterial suspension of 1×10^8 CFU/ml. The inoculated plants were transplanted immediately to plastic pots filled with 0.5 liter of autoclaved soil, and kept in a greenhouse (20-40°C). Disease severity was assessed 30 days after inoculation using a scale ranging from 1 to 5, where 1 = absence of symptoms; 2 = plants with 1/3 of wilted leaves; 3 = plants with 2/3 of wilted leaves; 4 = totally wilted plants and 5 = dead plants (12). The bacterial wilt index (BWI) was calculated by the formula BWI = Σ(C x P) / N, where C = grade attributed to each symptom class; P = number of plants in each symptom class and N = total number of infected plants (2).

Results and Discussion

Disease symptoms were first observed seven days after inoculation and consisted of typical wilting from top to bottom of the plants. Even though the inoculation procedure was very drastic, we observed significant differences among the progenies of *P. hispidinervum* (P <0,05) (Table 1).

Table 1. Bacterial wilt index for progenies and populations of *Piper hispidinervum* and of progenies of *P. aduncum*. Acre, 2000/2001.

	Piper hispidinervum			*Piper aduncum*	
Progenies	Mean[a]	Populations	Mean	Progenies	Mean
10	2.67 a	106	3.80 a	12	1.53 a
17	2.76 a	16	3.97 a	11	3.13 b
18	3.34 a	13	4.00 a	8	3.40 b
09	3.43 a	15	4.00 a	14	3.40 b
23	3.53 a	12	4.13 a	13	3.93 c
56	4.00 b	111	4.20 a	3	4.20 c
12	4.13 b	10	4.23 a	5	4.47 c
51	4.27 b	9	4.26 a	6	4.47 c
35	4.33 b	11	4.27 a	15	4.47 c
07	4.33 b	26	4.33 a	2	4.73 c
55	4.40 b	20	4.47 a	7	5.00 c
06	4.57 b	24	4.53 a	9	5.00 c
34	4.67 b	118	4.73 b	10	5.00 c
21	4.67 b	17	4.80 b		
33	4.67 b	115	5.00 b		
32	4.76 b	123	5.00 b		
54	4.87 b	125	5.00 b		
27	4.90 b	119	5.00 b		
52	4.93 b	122	5.00 b		
53	5.00 b	30	5.00 b		
24	5.00 b	29	5.00 b		
25	5.00 b	22	5.00 b		
01	5.00 b	114	5.00 b		
22	5.00 b	105	5.00 b		
29	5.00 b	31	5.00 b		
30	5.00 b				
26	5.00 b				
29	5.00 b				

[a] Means followed by the same letter do not differ statistically from each other for the Scott-Knott test (5%) (10).

No progeny or population of *P. hispidinervum* was completely resistant to the disease, suggesting, as for many other hosts of *R. solanacearum*, that the genetic control of the resistance is polygenic.

Significant differences in resistance were found for populations of *P. hispidinervum* and *P. aduncum* (Table 1), but high levels of resistance were again not found, except for the progeny 12 of *P. aduncum*. This is, therefore, considered an interesting source of resistance for use in breeding programs.

Additional work needs to be done to identify sources of resistance to bacterial wilt within *P. hispidinervum* genotypes, especially adjusting the screening procedures to allow the detection of intermediate levels of resistance. It is not expected that resistance alone will solve the bacterial wilt problem in long pepper, although it might contribute to an integrated approach to control the disease. The viability of using the progeny 12 of *P. aduncum* as a resistant genitor also needs further study. Finally, the pathogen's variability needs to be monitored in order to seek stable resistance.

Literature Cited

1. Cavalcante, M.J.B., and Lopes, C.A. 2000. Caracterização de isolados de *Ralstonia solanacearum* em cultivos de pimenta longa do Estado de Rondônia. Fitopatologia Brasileira. 25 (suplemento):321
2. Empig, L.T., Calub, A.G., Katgbak, M.M., and Deanon Jr., J.R. 1962. Screening tomato, eggplant and pepper varieties and strains for bacterial wilt (*Pseudomonas solanacearum*) resistance. Philippines Agriculturist 46:303-314.
3. Hayward, A.C. 1991. Biology and epidemiology of bacterial wilt caused by *Pseudomonas solanacearum*. Annu. Rev. Phytopathol. 29:65-87.
4. Hayward, A.C. 1995. The hosts of *Pseudomonas solanacearum*. Pages 39-45 in: Bacterial Wilt and its Causative Agent: *Pseudomonas solanacearum*. A.C. Hayward and G.L. Hartman, eds. CABI International.
5. Kelman, A. 1954. The relationship of pathogenicity in *Pseudomonas solanacearum* to colony appearance on tetrazolium medium. Phytopathology 44: 693.
6. Lopes, C.A., Poltronieri, L.S, Quezado-Soares, A.M., Trindade, D.R., and Albuquerque, F.C. 1999. Maracujazeiro, mais um hospedeiro de *Ralstonia solanacearum*. Summa Phytopathologica 25:26.
7. Lopes, C.A.; Poltronieri, L.S., and Poltronieri, M.C. 2001. *Talinum triangulare*, new host of *Ralstonia solanacearum* in the Brazilian

Amazon. http://ardeath.biosci.uq.edu.au/ibwc/talinum_triangulare.htm consulted on 10/05/2001.

8. Lopes, C.A, Poltronieri, L.S., and Poltronieri, M.C. 2002. Chicória, hortaliça não convencional da Amazônia, nova hospedeira de *Ralstonia solanacearum*. Horticultura Brasileira, Brasília, 20. Suplemento CD-ROM, junho 2002.

9. Lopes, C.A, Poltronieri, L.S., Trindade, D.R., and Albuquerque, F.C. 1998. *Piper hispidinervum*, a new host of bacterial wilt. Bacterial Wilt Newsletter 17:13-18.

10. Scott, A.J., and Knott, M. A. 1974. Cluster analysis method for grouping means in the analysis of variance. Biometrics, North Carolina, 30:507-512.

11. Takatsu, A., and Lopes, C.A. 1997. Murcha-bacteriana em hortaliças: avanços científicos e perspectivas de controle. Horticultura Brasileira 15: 170-177.

12. Winstead, N.N., and Kelman, A. 1952. Inoculation techniques for evaluating resistance to *Pseudomonas solanacearum*. Phytopathology 42: 628-634.

COLOR PLATES

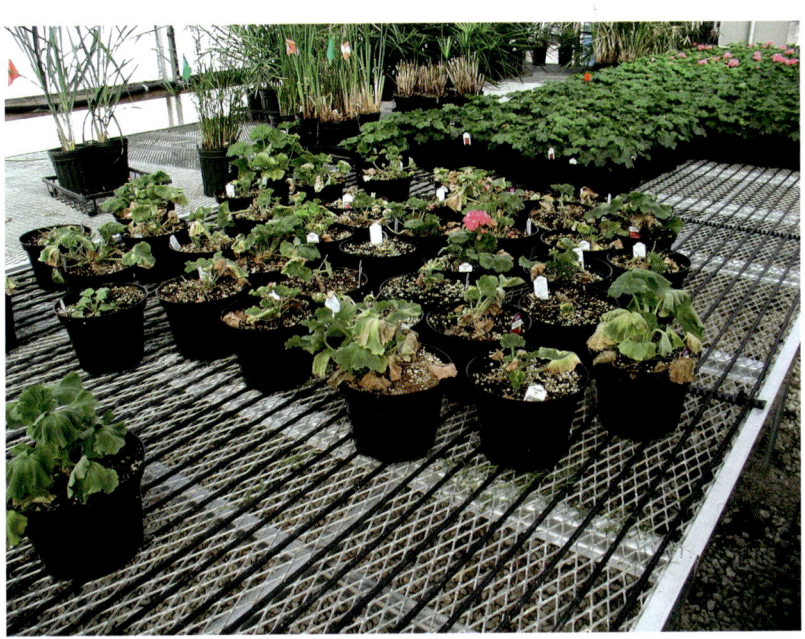

Plate 1. *Pelargonium zonale* (geranium) showing symptoms at various stages of infection by *R. solanacearum.*

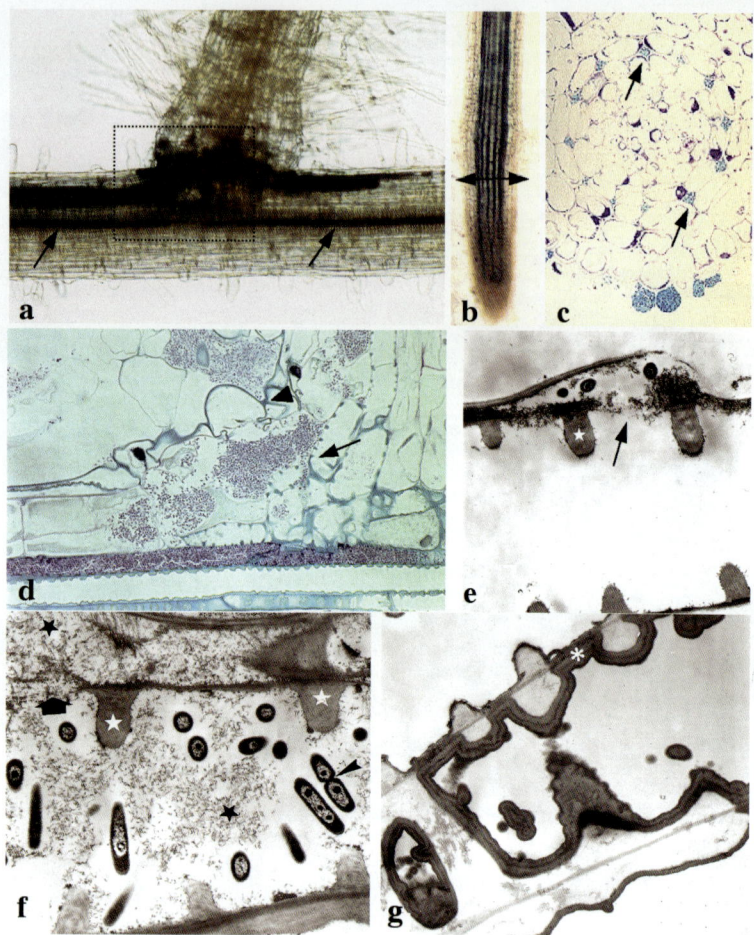

Plate 2. Root infection process of the susceptible tomato cv. Supermarmande. (a) Infected LRC and colonization of a protoxylem vessel (arrows). (b) Files of bacteria at infected root tip. (c) Cross section of infected root tip: bacteria occupy inner intercellular spaces (arrows) surrounding a central cylinder not fully differentiated. (d) Longitunal section of an infected LRC showing endodermis transgression (arrowheads) and protoxylem penetration (arrows). (e) TEM observation of bacterial degradation of pecto-cellulosic cell wall (arrow) of protoxylem between lignin encrusts (white star). (f) Bacterial colonization of xylem vessels: bacteria divides (arrowhead) within an extracellular material (black stars) and degrades pecto-cellulosic cell wall vessel (large arrow) of connecting vessel. (g) Multilamellar vascular coating (white asterisk) limit colonization.

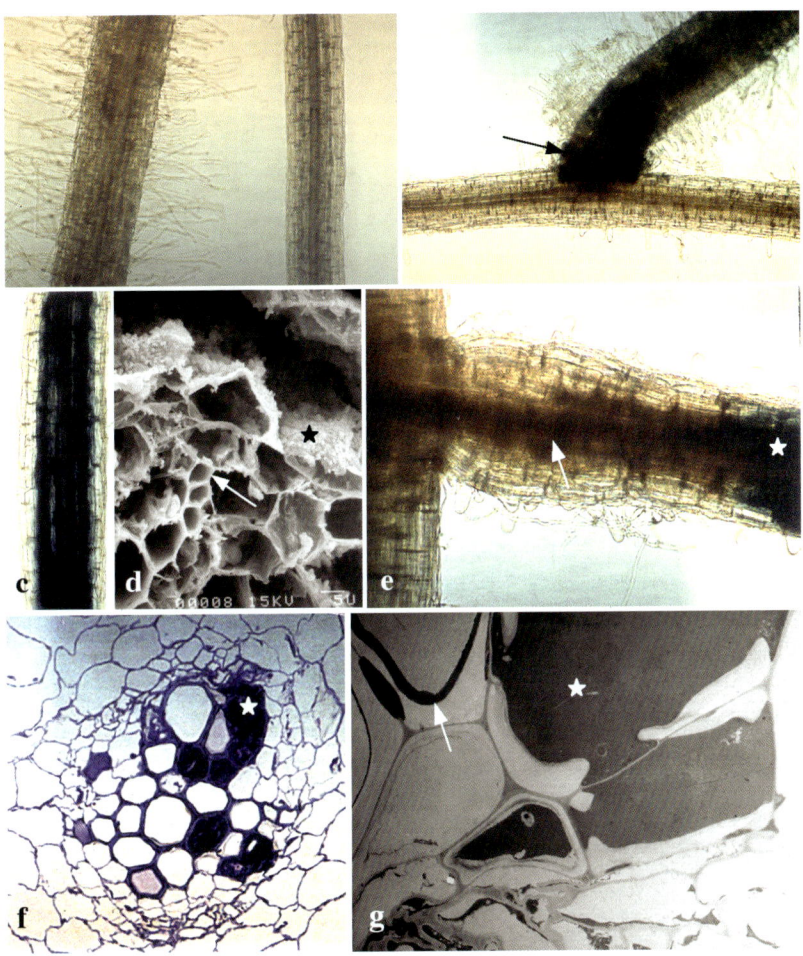

Plate 3. Root infection process of the resistant tomato cv. Hawaii 7996.
(a) Two types of lateral root: Thick and short (left), thin and long (right). (b) Crown of intercellular infection at LRC of thick and short lateral root. (c) Inner cortex infection of thin and short lateral root. (d) SEM observation of degraded inner cortex (asterisk: bacteria) without colonization of protoxylem vessel (arrow). (e) Brownish reaction in xylem vessel (arrows) correlated to cortical infection (asterisk) of thin and short lateral root. (f) Dark blue staining of phenolic compounds (white star) in brown xylem vessels observed on cross section of infected root. (g) TEM observation show electron density of phenolic compounds (white star) and vascular coating (arrow) in xylem vessels of infected root.

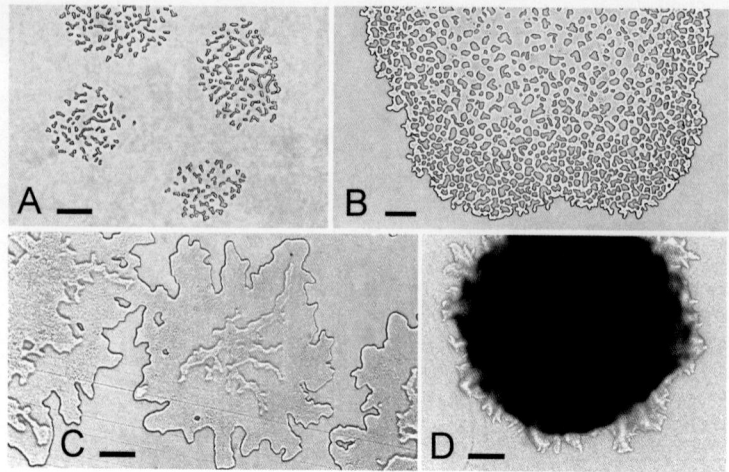

Plate 4. Micromorphology of wild-type *R. solanacearum* colonies exhibiting twitching motility on a rich medium solidified with 1.6% agar. Colonies were imaged after (A) 16 h, (B) 24 h, (C) 37 h, or (D) 44 h of incubation at 30°C. Bars = 0.1 mm.

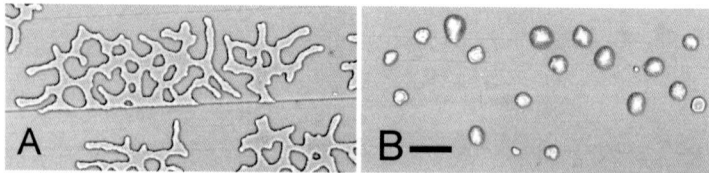

Plate 5. Micromorphology of *R. solanacearum* (A) wild-type colonies that exhibit twitching motility and (B) colonies of a *pilA* mutant that do not. Cultures were streaked on a rich medium solidified with 1.6% agar and imaged after 20 h at 30°C. Bar = 0.1 mm.

Host Resistance to *Ralstonia solanacearum*

Y. Marco, A. Trigalet, J. Vasse, J. Olivier, D.X. Feng, and L. Deslandes

Laboratoire de Biologie Moléculaire des Relations
Plantes-Microorganismes, CNRS-INRA, BP27, Auzeville,
Castanet-Tolosan, France.

Host resistance to *Ralstonia solanacearum*, a pathogen capable of infecting more than 50 botanical families (more than 200 plant species) worldwide, will doubtless continue to play an important role in the development of novel strategies to control wilt disease. Although plant materials resistant and tolerant to bacterial wilt have been known for many years, the study of the basic biology of resistance has been hindered by several obstacles linked to the nature of this important pathogen. These include: 1) the wide variability in the host-pathogen interactions, 2) the importance of environmental conditions which influence the outcomes of the interactions, and 3) the complexity of the mechanisms involved in this pathosystem, which has few gene-for-gene resistances. Although good progress has been made in the analysis of host resistance in the last few years, its molecular bases are still poorly understood. Elsewhere, this book treats several other aspects of host resistance such as breeding for resistant cultivars and biological control (see Liao, this volume). This review deals mainly with the biochemical and genetic mechanisms underlying resistance.

Inducers of Disease Resistance to *R. solanacearum*

Several lines of research have been developed around different aspects of the *Ralstonia solanacearum*-host plant interaction. Pioneering work dealt with the search for resistance inducers. Data suggested that surface components of the pathogen played a major role in the recognition between plant and bacteria. Initial studies demonstrated induction of resistance after artificial inoculations of heat-killed virulent strains or avirulent mutants of the bacteria in root, stem and leaf of host plants (3, 8, 11, 17, 22, 21, 25, 27, 28). The nature of the active determinants of the host responses has been reviewed and studies in this field showcase the complexity of factors involved in establishment of resistance. For instance, a purified lipopolysaccharide fraction (LPS) extracted from whole bacterial cells by a variety of procedures was shown to possess a high inducer activity (8). The origin of the LPS did not appear to be important since fractions purified from non-pathogenic bacteria were also active. Additionally, LPS attached to host cells in a manner similar to heat-killed bacteria; LPS could also induce ultrastructural changes in the plant cell. These data strongly suggested that the active component of heat-killed cells was the LPS fraction. These studies also demonstrated that the O-specific polysaccharide of the LPS was not required for activity.

Ultrastructural analysis of tobacco mesophyll cells in contact with virulent and avirulent strains of *R. solanacearum* identified marked differences between compatible and incompatible interactions. Virulent bacteria divided freely in the intercellular spaces of the infected plant whereas HR-inducing bacteria did not divide and were quickly surrounded by a granular and fibrillar material. It was postulated that attachment of bacteria to cell walls was associated with a recognition process between components of the outer cell walls of bacteria on the one hand and putative receptors on the host cell wall on the other hand. Sequeira and co-workers therefore tested the hypothesis that incompatible forms of *R. solanacearum* were immobilized on plant cell walls *via* a direct interaction between the LPS fraction and the lectin-like glycoproteins that are common components of plant cell walls. It was shown that virulent strains of the pathogen failed to agglutinate significantly whereas avirulent strains agglutinated rapidly after addition of lectin (24).

One of the obvious differences between virulent and spontaneous avirulent strains of the pathogen is the accumulation of extracellular polysaccharide (EPS). This polymer, which is present in low amounts or even totally absent in avirulent forms of *R. solanacearum* but abundant in the virulent ones, was hypothesised to hinder the agglutination process. Such inhibition of agglutination was indeed observed (23). Despite some inconsistencies in the data presented, this study offered a tentative model to explain differences observed between compatible and incompatible interactions. Such approaches should be re-evaluated using current tools and strategies such as novel bacterial mutants and host genetics. Indeed, recent work by Denny and co-workers (Kang, this volume) suggests that altered regulation of type-4 pili may play a role in agglutination of spontaneous mutant strains.

Genetically-engineered *hrp* mutants of *R. solanacearum* have been described as potential biocontrol agents of tomato and potato bacterial wilt (7, 26). Evidence of local resistance in tomato tissue induced by the presence of these *hrp* mutants, such as formation of tyloses and intense browning of cells in the vicinity of the invaded xylem vessels, also suggested that complex, different mechanisms are probably involved in the induced resistance, the nature of which is not yet understood (5). However, cytological studies of the infection process by non-pathogenic mutants in susceptible host plants, or by pathogenic strains in tolerant host plants underlined that an increased production of phenolic compounds is likely involved in the observed local induced resistance.

Cytological Observations of Bacterial Wilt Resistance Mechanisms

Many observations concerning resistance mechanisms have been made on tomato in the form of comparative studies of resistant and susceptible cultivars. Since the report of Grimault and Prior (9), bacterial wilt resistance in tomato has been associated with tolerance of vascular tissues to colonization by *R. solanacearum*. In the epicotyls of resistant cultivars, tyloses occlude colonized vessels and limit bacterial spread, while at the same time, in susceptible cultivars, no tyloses were observed in colonized vessels and bacterial spread was not limited (10). More recently, McGarvey *et al.* (14) have confirmed that bacterial spread was reduced in Hawaii7996, one of the most resistant tomato cultivars studied. They also observed that bacterial ingress into the taproot was 15-fold faster in the susceptible cultivar studied than in the resistant one, and further, that rates of multiplication and maximum bacterial cell densities were greater in the susceptible than in the resistant cultivar. Moreover they found that bacteria and EPS I were distributed throughout the vascular bundles and intercellular spaces of the pith in the susceptible cultivar, whereas in the resistant cultivar, bacteria and EPS I were restricted to vascular tissues. More recently, cytological observations have shown that resistance mechanisms associated with induced production of phenolic compounds can take place at the root infection level of the resistant tomato cultivar Hawaii7996 (Vasse, this volume). These mechanisms seem very similar to those developed by a susceptible tomato cultivar to limit the root infection process of non-pathogenic mutants (1,30). In both cases, activation of the secondary plant metabolic pathways for phenolic compounds appears to be essential for the control of bacterial development.

Analysis of Genes Associated with the Hypersensitive Reaction

The so-called hypersensitive reaction (HR) is a plant response which is characterised by the death of plant cells in contact with the invading microorganisms and is therefore thought to restrict the growth and ingress of the pathogen in many plant-pathogen interactions. It is generally considered as one of the most efficient possible reactions to pathogen attack, although in the case of *R. solanacearum*, no causal relationship with resistance has been yet established. The role of genes associated with this particular host re-action has been the focus of several studies which suggested strongly their importance in resistance. *Hsr203* is a tobacco gene preferentially expressed during the HR induced by an avirulent strain of the pathogen. Its promoter is rapidly, strongly and specifically activated in response to various HR-inducing bacteria including *R. solanacearum*; it does not respond to various stress conditions and is dependent on the presence of functional *hrp* (hypersensitive response and pathogenicity) genes of the pathogen (16). It was shown that HSR203 is a serine hydrolase with an esterase activity. Moreover, antisense suppression of *hsr203* in tobacco resulted in an accelerated hypersensitive response when plants were inoculated with an avirulent strain of *R. solanacearum* (29). This response was accompanied by a drastic inhibition of *in planta* bacterial growth. In addition, transgenic plants deficient in HSR203 also had increased resistance to another bacterial pathogen, *Pseudomonas syringae* pv *pisi* and to virulent and avirulent races of *Phytophthora parasitica*.

Additionally, the promoter of this gene has been used to develop genetically engineered disease resistance. For example, the *hsr203* promoter was fused to *popA*, an *R. solanacearum* gene encoding a necrosis elicitor (2). Because PopA is capable of activating the *hsr203* promoter, transgenic plants harboring this construct rapidly accumulate the bacterial elicitor at the pathogen infection sites. The outcome of induced PopA accumulation is a localized HR and a high degree of resistance to an oomycete pathogen. This kind of application, which requires a careful selection of individual transgenic plants since the induced HR may affect plant development, illustrates the potential of such strategies to engineer plants resistant to pathogens. However, it is not yet known if such transgenic plants exhibit an increased level of resistance to *R. solanacearum*.

Engineered Resistance to *R. solanacearum*

A large variety of antimicrobial proteins and peptides, purified from various sources, are known to be potent inhibitors of bacterial pathogens. A defensin from spinach (19), snakin-1, a peptide from potato (20), four proteins isolated from barley leaves and presenting homologies to non-specific lipid transfer proteins (13), two LTPs from Arabidopsis and spinach (18), a pseudothionin-St1 purified from potato (15), as well as cecropin B, a small peptide from the giant silkmoth *Hyalophora cecropia* (6), were all shown to inhibit *in vitro* growth of *R. solanacearum*. Although the mode of action of these antimicrobial compounds is still poorly understood, some of them such as wheat thionins and an LTP (LTP2) may act on membrane integrity (4). Moreover, Tn5 mutants of *R. solanacearum* were selected based on

278

their increased sensitivity to thionins. The responsible transposon insertion was in a gene that presents homology with the *rfaF* gene from *E. coli* and presumably encodes a heptosyltransferase that is involved in the synthesis of the LPS core. These mutants in fact have an altered LPS electrophoretic pattern and they died rapidly *in planta*. They also failed to produce symptoms when infiltrated into the leaves or stems of tobacco plants.

In some cases, it has been possible to engineer resistance against *R. solanacearum* by expressing these peptides or proteins in transgenic plants. For example, tobacco plants harboring constructs containing LPT2 as well as some transgenic potato lines expressing lyzozyme have an enhanced tolerance to bacterial pathogens such as *P. syringae* pv *tabaci* (13) and an increased resistance to *R. solanacearum* (A. Trigalet, pers. comm.), respectively. In contrast, tobacco plants expressing cecropin B are not resistant to *R. solanacearum*, most likely due to degradation of the protein by endogenous endoproteases (6). It is important to pursue field tests of transgenic plants expressing one or several of these potential mediators of plant resistance (see Denny, this volume).

Model Plant Systems to Understand Resistance Mechanisms to *R. solanacearum*

The finding that *Arabidopsis thaliana* is a host plant for *R. solanacearum* is very promising since resistant ecotypes have been identified. The isolation and characterization of *RRS1-R*, the first resistance gene to bacterial wilt isolated to date (for details, see Deslandes, this volume), as well as the demonstration that, depending on the *A. thaliana* ecotypes and the *R. solanacearum* strains used, different resistance mechanisms are expressed by the plant, indicates that this novel pathosystem will be of great value to decipher the signaling pathways leading to resistance. One of the greatest advantages of this model weed lies in the existence of numerous mutants affected in their response to various compounds involved in plant defense such as salicylic acid, ethylene, and jasmonic acid. It is now possible to test the influence of such compounds on disease development and resistance. Additionally, many mutants altered in their response to various pathogens are well characterized and this opens the possibility to determine if some elements of the plant response are conserved whatever the nature of the pathogen. All the studies performed so far have only led to correlations between resistance and various physiological, morphological or molecular changes occurring in the host. Development of genetic approaches is therefore essential to better understand wilt disease resistance mechanisms. Whether the results obtained in model plants will be transposable to plants of agricultural interest remains of course the main question. In this context, data presented during this meeting strongly suggest that some components of the signalling pathways leading to resistance might be conserved between tomato and Arabidopsis. Moreover, the inter-generic transfer of genes such as *RRS1-R* should bring some clues concerning the conservation of resistance mechanisms among different plant species.

Perspectives

Our knowledge of the molecular mechanisms underlying disease development and resistance is still limited but will doubtless progress rapidly using a combination of molecular, genetic, biochemical and cytological approaches. The recent sequencing of the *R. solanacearum* genome certainly will also lead to stronger interactions between microbiologists and plant molecular biologists; it is indeed obvious that a molecular dialogue takes place between the two partners in this interaction. The systematic inactivation of bacterial genes similar to genes characterized in other pathogens and known to play an important role in the infectious process should allow the identification of genes essential for the pathogen such as virulence and avirulence genes (see Genin, this volume). This in turn should lead to the search for their plant targets whose nature and function remain completely elusive to date.

Most studies of plant-pathogen interactions have focused primarily on resistance mechanisms. Disease itself, considered for a long time as a passive process during which the plant was seen as a substrate for the microorganism, was completely neglected. Recent findings, mostly in *A. thaliana*, demonstrate that active plant metabolism is necessary for the appearance of symptoms. It is now well established for instance that ethylene insensitivity greatly reduces susceptibility of various plants to different pathogens including *R. solanacearum* as reported during this meeting. It is therefore essential to develop this new field of research.

Considering approaches aimed at the isolation of pathogen inhibitors, it is quite important to understand inhibitor mode of action which remains in most cases unknown or poorly characterized. Such studies should lead to the identification of bacterial targets likely to play an important role during the interaction and possibly to development of novel strategies for wilt disease control.

Molecular mechanisms underlying biological control and resistance/tolerance caused by the infiltration of LPS and dead bacteria within the host, also remain to be elucidated although it is highly probable that SAR (systemic acquired resistance) and/or ISR (induced systemic resistance) will play an important role in theses processes.

Finally, the last few years have seen the emergence of novel and powerful approaches such as genomics and proteomics. These strategies will allow us to develop a global vision of the changes occurring during incompatible and compatible interactions. So far, while most studies have focused on resistance mechanisms, very little knowledge has been acquired on the variations in general plant metabolism and its influence on the infection process.

In conclusion, let's go back to the bench and work! There is so much to be done.

Literature Cited

1. Araud-Razou, I., Vasse, J., Montrozier, H., Etchebar, C., and Trigalet, A. 1998. Detection and visualization of the major acidic exopolysaccharide of *Ralstonia solanacearum* and its role in tomato root infection and vascular colonization. Eur. J. Plant Pathol. 104: 795-809.
2. Arlat, M., Van Gijsegem, F., Huet, J.C., Pernollet, J.C., and Boucher, C.A. 1994. PopA1, a protein which induces a hypersensitivity-like response on specific Petunia genotypes, is secreted via the *Hrp* pathway of *Pseudomonas solanacearum*. EMBO J. 113: 543-53.
3. Averre, C., and Kelman, A. (1964) Severity of bacterial wilt as influenced by ratio of virulent to avirulent cells of *Pseudomonas solanacearum* in inoculum. Phytopathology 54: 779-83.
4. Caaveiro, J.M., Molina, A., Gonzales-Manas, J.M., Rodriguez-Palenzuela, P., Garcia-Olmedo, F., and Goni, F.M. 1997. Differential effects of five types of antipathogenic plant peptides on model membranes. FEBS Lett. 410:338-42.
5. Etchebar, C., Trigalet-Demery, D., van Gijsegem, F., Vasse, J., and Trigalet, A. 1998. Xylem colonization by an HrcV⁻ mutant of *Ralstonia solanacearum* is a key factor for the efficient biological control of tomato bacterial wilt. Mol. Plant Microbe Interact. 9:869-877.
6. Florack, D., Allefs, S., Bollen, R., Bosch, D., Visser, B., and Stiekema, W. 1995. Expression of giant silkmoth cecropin B genes in tobacco. Transgenic Res. 4:132-41.
7. Frey, P., Prior, P., Marie, C., Koutoujansky, A., Trigalet-Demery, D., and Trigalet, A. 1994. Hrp6 mutants of *Pseudomonas solanacearum* as potential biocontrol agents of tomato bacterial wilt. Appl. Environ. Microbiol. 62: 473-479.
8. Graham, T., Sequeira, L., and Huang, T. 1977. Bacterial lipolysaccharides as inducers of disease resistance in tobacco. Appl. Environ. Microbiol. 34: 424-32.

9. Grimault, V., and Prior P. 1993. Bacterial wilt resistance in tomato associated with tolerance of vascular tissues to *Pseudomonas solanacearum*. Plant Pathol. 42: 589-594.

10. Grimault, V., Gélie, B., Lemattre, M., Prior, P., and Schmidt, J. (1994) Comparative histology of resistant and susceptible tomato cultivars infected by *Pseudomonas solanacearum*. Physiol. Mol. Plant Pathol. 44:105-123.

11. Lozano, J.C., and Sequeira, L. 1970. Prevention of the hypersensistive reaction in tobacco leaves by heat-killed cells of *Pseudomonas solancearum*. Phytopathology 60:875-79.

12. Molina, A., Segura, A., and Garcia-Olmedo, F. 1993 Lipid transfer proteins (nsLTPs) from barley and maize leaves are potent inhibitors of bacterial and fungal plant pathogens. FEBS Lett. 316:119-21.

13. Molina, A., and Garcia-Olmedo, F. Enhanced tolerance to bacterial pathogens caused by the transgenic expression of barley lipid transfer protein LPT2. Plant J. 12: 669-75.

14. McGarvey, J. A., Denny, T. P., and Schell, M. A. 1999. Spatio-temporal and quantitative analysis of growth and EPS I production by *Ralstonia solanacearum* in resistant and susceptible tomato cultivars. Phytopathology. 89:1233-1239.

15. Moreno, M., Segura, A., and Garcia-Olmedo, F. 1994. Pseudothionin-St1, a potato peptide active against potato pathogens. Eur. J. Biochem. 223:135-39.

16. Pontier, D., Godiard, L., Marco, Y., and Roby, D. 1994. Hsr203J, a tobacco gene whose activation is rapid, highly localized and specific for incompatible plant/pathogen interactions. Plant J. 5:507-21.

17. Rathmell, W., and Sequeira, L. 1975. Induced resistance in tobacco leaves : the role of inhibitors of bacterial growth in the intercellular fluid. Physiol. Plant Pathol. 5:65-73.

18. Segura, A., Moreno, M., and Garcia-Olmedo, F. 1993. Purification and antipathogenic activity of lipid transfer proteins (LTPs) from the leaves of Arabidopsis and spinach. FEBS Lett. 332:243-46.

19. Segura, A., Moreno, M., Molina, A., and Garcia-Olmedo, F. 1998. Novel defensin subfamily from spinach (Spinacia oleracea). FEBS Lett 435:159-62.

20. Segura, A., Moreno, M., Madueno, F., Molina, A., and Garcia-Olmedo, F. 1999. Snakin-1, a peptide from potato that is active against plant pathogens. Mol. Plant Microbe Interact. 12:16-23.

21. Sequeira, L., Aist, S., and Ainslie, V. 1972. Prevention of the hypersensitive reaction in tobacco by proteinaceous constituents of *Pseudomonas solanacearum*. Phytopathology 62:536-42.

22. Sequeira, L., and Hill, L. (1974) Induced resistance in tobacco leaves : the growth of *Pseudomonas solanacearum* in protected tissues. Physiol. Plant Pathol. 4, 447-55.
23. Sequeira, L. 1976. Specificity in the infection of plant hosts by *Pseudomonas solanacearum*. Pages 63-67 in: Proc. First International Planning Conference and Workshop on the Ecology and Control of bacterial wilt caused by *Pseudomonas solanacearum*. L. Sequiera and A. Kelman, eds. Raleigh, NC. 63-67.
24. Sequeira, L., and Graham, T.L. 1976. Agglutination of avirulent strains of *Pseudomonas solanacearum* by potato lectin. Phytopathology 66:3.
25. Sequeira, L., Gaard, G., and de Zoeten, G. 1977. Attachment of bacteria to host cell walls : its relation to mechanisms of induced resistance. Physiol. Plant Pathol. 10:43-50.
26. Smith, J., Offord, L., Kibata, G., Murimi, Z., Trigalet, A., and Saddler, G. 1998. The development of a biological control agent against *Ralstonia solanacearum* race 3 in Kenya. Pages 337-342 in: Bacterial Wilt Disease. P. Prior, C. Allen, and J. Elphinstone, eds. Springer Press, Berlin.
27. Tanaka, H. 1983. Protection of tomato and tobacco against root infection of *Pseudomonas solanacearum* by heat-killed bacteria. Ann. Phytopath. Soc. Japan 49:66-8.
28. Tanaka, H. 1985. Induced resistance in tobacco against bacterial wilt and its possible mechanism. Bull. Utsuhomiya Tobacco Expt. Station 21:1-66.
29. Tronchet, M., Ranty, B., Marco, Y., and Roby, D. 2001. HSR203 antisens suppression in tobacco accelerates development of hypersensitive cell death. Plant J. 27:115-27.
30. Vasse, J., Frey, P., and Trigalet, A. 1995. Microscopic studies of intercellular infection and protoxylem invasion of tomato roots by *Pseudomonas solanacearum*. Mol. Plant-Microbe Interact. 8:241-251.
31. Vasse, J., Génin, S., Frey, P., Boucher, C., and Brito, B. 2000. The *hrpB* and *hrpG* regulatory genes of *Ralstonia solanacearum* are required for different stages of the tomato root infection process. Mol. Plant Microbe Interact. 13:259-267.

Microscopic Studies of Root Infection in Resistant Tomato Cultivar Hawaii7996

J. Vasse, S. Danoun, and A. Trigalet

Laboratoire de Biologie Moléculaire des Relations Plantes-Microorganismes, CNRS-INRA, BP27, Castanet-Tolosan, France

Ralstonia solanacearum, a soilborne bacterium well adapted to rhizo-sphere survival and life in soil (2), can enter plant roots from artificial and natural openings (4). Root infection allows the bacteria to reach xylem ves-sels, in which bacteria develop and produce exopolysaccharide (EPS), con-tributing to wilting and death of susceptible plants. Different stages of root infection were deduced from spatio-temporal microscopic studies of inter-actions between a susceptible tomato cultivar and wild-type *R. solan-acearum* and from root infection phenotypes analysis of non-pathogenic bacterial mutants affected in either virulence factors, EPSI and cell wall de-grading enzymes, or determinant of pathogenesis, *hrp* genes (1, 8, 9). In the infection process, bacteria are confronted with the root surface, the root cortex, the endodermis and vascular tissue which represent different en-vironmental conditions. From this, two classes of mutants phenotypes can be proposed: first, bacteria are infective and infect more or less the root cor-tex but are unable to penetrate in vascular cylinder, such mutants are not invasive. Secondly, bacteria are able to reach xylem vessels but the suscep-tible tomato plants limit their development in roots and stems. In the latter case, plant-bacteria interactions are in a situation of latent infection or toler-ance. Such a situation resembles bacterial wilt resistance in tomato that Prior and co-workers (6) referred to as "any measurable plant mechanism able to overcome completely or to limit the development of a pathogen or its effects", and that "this definition emphasises the positive control of patho-gens by plant metabolism." Using grafting experiments, they thus conclude that resistance in tomato did not result from unsuccessful root infection, but is rather associated with the ability of the plant to restrict bacterial invasive-ness in the stem. Other studies on resistance have been performed following inoculation of wild-type bacteria through artificial opening of wounded roots (3, 5), even if such inoculation method rules out bacterial interactions with the root system and allows bacteria to enter straight into xylem vessels.

The objectives of this study were to analyse and compare the root infection process of a highly resistant tomato cultivar with that of a susceptible cultivar, both inoculated without root wounding by the wild-type strain of *R. solanacearum* already used as a positive control in studies of mutants root infection phenotype on tomato.

Materials and Methods

BACTERIAL STRAIN AND INOCULUM PREPARATION

The strain GMI1485 of *Ralstonia solanacearum* used in this study is a derivative of the wild-type strain GMI1000. It carries an insertion of the transposon Tn5-B20 containing a promoterless *E. coli lacZ* gene and constitutively expresses a very high level of β-galactosidase activity. GMI1485 has a wild-type pathogenic phenotype on tomato plant cultivar Supermarmande (8). Bacteria were grown in peptone broth containing kanamycin (50 mg.l^{-1}) at 28 °C for 24 h and were diluted in the plant culture medium as inoculum.

PLANT GROWTH CONDITIONS AND ROOT INOCULATION

Seeds of *Lycopersicon esculentum* cultivar Supermarmande and cultivar Hawaii7996 were surface-sterilised and germinated. Four seedlings were deposited on stainless steel mesh in large sterile test tubes with radicals in contact with the surface of 75 ml of Murashige and Skoog plant nutrient solution. The tubes were kept in a growth chamber and two leaf plantlets were inoculated with broth grown bacterial inoculum to obtain about 5x10^7 CFU/ml plant nutrient medium.

MICROSCOPIC METHODS

Light microscopy was performed on whole roots and root sections. Whole root systems of plantlets were processed 2, 4, 7 days after inoculation and then each three days over a period of 3 weeks. Roots were treated as already described (8). Briefly they were fixed with a solution of 1.25% (v/v) glutaraldehyde to inactivate endogenous plant β-galactosidase activity, rinsed and stained to reveal bacterial β-galactosidase activity using 0.1% X-Gal. After incubation overnight, whole roots were rinsed and observed by bright-field microscopy on glass slides but without cover slips to avoid pressure on samples.

Root sections were obtained from 2-3 mm root segments of interest dissected from whole roots already fixed and histochemically stained. They were successively fixed again with 2.5% (v/v) glutaraldehyde, post-fixed in 2% osmium tetroxide, dehydrated in an ethanol series, progressively embedded in Spurr resin, polymerized and sectioned. Semithin sections (1 μm thickness) were stained with a mixture of 1% (w/v) toluidine blue and 2% (w/v) methylene blue in 1 % sodium borate aqueous solution and ob-served by bright-field or differential interference contrast microscopy.

TRANSMISSION AND SCANNING ELECTRON MICROSCOPY

Ultrastructural observations were performed by transmission electron microscopy (TEM), on ultrathin sections (80 nm thickness) of the same embedded root segments already observed by light microscopy. Sections were successively stained with uranyl acetate and lead citrate. Observations were made with a TEM microscope operating at 75 kV.

Observations of samples difficult to embed due to bacteria-induced tissue degradation were performed by scanning electron microscopy (SEM). Some samples fixed and dehydrated as described above were critical-point dried with CO_2 as a transitional fluid and sputter-coated with gold-palladium. Observations were made with SEM microscope operating at 15 kV.

BIOCHEMICAL STUDIES OF PHENOLIC COMPOUNDS

Phenolic compounds were extracted from the root culture liquid medium with diethylether, pH 2, then transfered into methanolic solution. They were analyzed by RP-HPLC in a 60 min run (detection at 280 nm, flow rate of 1.5 ml.min^{-1}, linear gradient of increasing methanol from 5% to 99% with 1% phosphoric acid, RP-C18 column).

Results and Discussion

ROOT INFECTION PROCESS IN SUSCEPTIBLE TOMATOES

The fully-virulent *R. solanacearum* strain GMI1485, which expresses a *lacZ* reporter gene fusion, was used to visualize the bacterium in root tissues at various stages of infection. We focussed primarily on three stages: root surface colonization, infection of the root cortex, and invasion of the vascular tissue.

R. solanacearum preferentially colonizes intercellular grooves at the root surface of the root elongation zone, as well as intercellular spaces in lateral root cracks (LRC). All mutants already examined were able to per-form such intercellular root surface attachment (1, 8, 9).

From these sites, intercellular bacterial development into the root sig-naled the start of the cortical infection stage. At infected LRCs, multiplying bacteria formed intercellular and confluent infection pockets in the cortex of the main root. Such infections sometimes also progressed to form lines of bacteria in intercellular spaces of the inner cortex along the root endodermis along the side where a lateral root was developing (Color Plate 2a). It was easier to follow the progress of bacterial infection towards vascular tissue at LRCs than at root tips, where lines of bacteria in intercellular spaces of the inner cortex were observed all around the vascular cylinder (Color Plate 2b). Depending on the level of bacterial development, cortical cells ap-peared more or less degraded, but not the epidermis. The formation of inter-cellular lines of bacteria and the evident degradation of cortical cells indi-cated bacterial ability to progress longitudinally along the root cortex.

The endodermis, whose cells have suberized radial walls and stored phenolic compounds, is considered a physical and metabolic barrier sur-rounding the vascular cylinder. Possibly as a result, the two potential infec-tion sites are both located where the endodermal cell layer is modified due to root growth development: the endodermis is not fully differentiated in the root elongation zone and it is modified by outgrowth of lateral root meri-stems from the pericycle cell layer through the root cortex.

Crossing the endodermis is a critical step in the root infection process, and several non-pathogenic mutant strains studied previously (such as *hrp* mutants) are unable to pass through this particular cell layer (1, 8, 9). In contrast, wild-type bacteria at similar root sites quickly invade intercellular-ly and appear to pass through modified endodermal cell walls, entering the central cylinder. Once in the cylinder, the bacteria develop further, degrad-ing outer vascular parenchyma cells (Color Plate 2c). Tomato roots have two opposite clusters of vessels, each cluster containing both xylem and differentiating protoxylem, localized at two poles in the vascular cylinder. Within vessel cell walls, there is a spiral of lignin encrusting the inner sur-face. By degrading the pectin-cellulose cell wall between the lignin rein-forcement, bacteria can penetrate into these vessels (Color Plate 2d). Bac-teria multiply actively in the xylem and, by degrading the pectin pit mem-branes between vessels, they are also able to invade the metaxylem (Color Plate 2e). However, an unspecific vascular defense reaction was sometimes observed in the susceptible cultivar Supermarmande. This consisted of a continuous vascular coating of a multilamellar material resembling suberin. Vessels coated in this way never appeared colonized, suggesting that coated walls cannot be degraded by bacteria and hence limit vascular colonization, even in a susceptible cultivar (Color Plate 2f). We previously noted that xylem vessel penetration by mutant strains was generally delayed and accompanied by widespread vascular coating. A vascular hypersensitive-like response also appeared to limit bacterial development surrounding a protoxylem pole in a susceptible tomato infected by *hrpB* or *hrcV* mutant strains (9).

ROOT INFECTION PROCESS IN RESISTANT TOMATO CULTIVAR HAWAII 7996

L. esculentum cultivar Hawaii7996 had the highest level of resistance under our hydroponic conditions in growth chambers and it is reported to have a very good level of resistance in the field (7). Relative to Supermarmande, rhizogenesis in Hawaii7996 appeared to be greater. Consequently, the potential infection sites appeared to be more numerous. However, two types of secondary roots developed in Hawaii7996 during growth in Murashige and Skoog nutrient solution: some are thick and shorter, with numerous long root hairs, while others are longer and thinner without excessive numbers of root hairs (Color Plate 3a). These two types of roots reacted differently to inoculation by the wild-type bacterial strain. At the surface of the thick short roots, bacteria colonized the intercellular grooves between trichoblasts and the root tip infection is limited to the part beyond the apical meristem. No intercellular lines of bacteria developed into the root cortex. Infection of LRCs of thick roots appeared limited to an external crown of intercellular space around the root base without further infection (Color Plate 3b). We also frequently observed a brownish coloration at these LRCs suggesting oxidation of phenolic compounds proximal to these colonized intercellular spaces. Vascular colonization did not occur in thick and short roots. Resistance to root infection was never observed at such an early stage on the susceptible cultivar, whatever the non-pathogenic mutant strain studied. Infection of thin lateral roots was quite different: surface colonization was less frequent than that observed on thick and short roots, and root tip infection took place in the elongation zone behind the apical meristem. Lines of bacteria did develop in the intercellular spaces of the inner cortex. Indeed, the inner cortex was sometimes fully degraded while the outer cortex and epidermis remained free of bacteria (Color Plate 3c,d). In a few cases, we observed vascular colonization of protoxylem vessels only (not shown). At LRCs, infection developed similarly as at root tips.

ROLE OF PHENOLIC COMPOUNDS IN ROOT RESISTANCE

In both thick and thin roots of Hawaii 7996 we frequently observed a brownish reaction of xylem vessels in the vicinity of cortical infection (Color Plate 3e). Sections of such root segments revealed the presence of vascular coating and amorphous material occupying the lumen of xylem vessels. Dark blue staining by toluidine/methylene blue as well as high electron density following osmium tetroxyde fixation, suggested the polyphenolic nature of these materials (Color Plate 3f,g).

Our microscopic observations let us to hypothesize that unknown compound(s) derived from secondary metabolism of polyphenols might be responsible for the very limited root infection in the resistant cultivar Hawaii7996. Such compound(s) might originate from the root system. They could be linked to plant tissue and/or released with root exudates into the liquid nutrient medium. In preliminary experiments, we used HPLC to test for low molecular weight phenolic compounds in plant culture liquid medium containing root system exudates from each cultivar inoculated or not with wild-type bacteria. Preliminary analyses suggested that the wild–type bacteria could induce a release of phenolic compounds by the root system of the resistant cultivar. Analyses are in progress to isolate and to further characterize such compounds from root liquid medium and root tissues.

Our results demonstrate that, following inoculation without artificial root wounding, resistance mechanisms can act at different stages of root infection in tomato cultivar Hawaii7996 growing in hydroponic solution. The fact that resistance was maintained in other cultivars after inoculation by severing roots (3,5), suggests that other plant responses must also contribute to limit bacterial development at later interaction stages. It is noteworthy that mechanisms limiting the root infection process of a wild-type strain in a highly resistant cultivar resembled those deployed by the susceptible cultivar to limit root infection by non-pathogenic mutant strains. In both cases, our observations suggested that the activation of the secondary metabolism of phenolic compounds appears to contribute to the positive control of bacterial development in the plant, even if the biochemical nature of these compounds remains to be determined.

Literature Cited

1. Araud-Razou, I., Vasse, J., Montrozier, H., Etchebar, C., and Trigalet, A. 1998. Detection and visualization of the major acidic exopolysaccharide of *Ralstonia solanacearum* and its role in tomato root infection and vascular colonization. Eur. J. Plant Pathol. 104:795-809.
2. Granada, G.A., and Sequeira, L. 1983. Survival of *Pseudomonas solanacearum* in soil, rhizosphere, and plant roots. Can. J. Microbiol. 29:433-440.
3. Grimault, V., Gélie, B., Lemattre, M., Prior, P., and Schmit, J. 1994. Comparative histology of resistant and susceptible tomato cultivars infected by *Pseudomonas solanacearum*. Physiol. Mol. Plant Pathol. 44:105-123.

4. Kelman, A., and Sequeira, L. 1965. Root to root spread of *Pseudomonas solanacearum*. Phytopathology 55:304-309.
5. Nakaho, K. 1997. Distribution and multiplication of *Ralstonia solanacearum* in tomato plants resistant rootstock cultivar LS-89 and susceptible Ponderosa. Ann. Phytopathol. Soc. Japan 63:8-88.
6. Prior, P., Grimault, V., and Schmit, J. 1994. Resistance to bacterial wilt (*Pseudomonas solanacearum*) in tomato: present status and prospects. Pages 209-223 in: Bacterial wilt: the disease and its causative agent, *Pseudomonas solanacearum*. A.C. Hayward and G.L. Hartman, eds.
7. Scott, J.W., Somodi, G.L., and Jones, J. B. 1993. Testing tomato genotypes and breeding for resistance to bacterial wilt in tomato. Pages 126-131 in: Bacterial Wilt. ACIAR Proc. N°45. G.L. Hartman and A.C. Hayward, eds. Watson Ferguson, Co, Brisbane, Australia.
8. Vasse, J., Frey, P., and Trigalet, A. 1995. Microscopic studies of intercellular infection and protoxylem invasion of tomato roots by *Pseudomonas solanacearum*. Mol. Plant-Microbe Interact. 8:241-251.
9. Vasse, J., Génin, S., Frey, P., Boucher, C., and Brito, B. 2000. The *hrpB* and *hrpG* regulatory genes of *Ralstonia solanacearum* are required for different stages of the tomato root infection process. Mol. Plant-Microbe Interact. 13:259-267.

Development of Bacterial Wilt Resistant Varieties and Basis of Resistance in Eggplant (*Solanum melongena* L.)

T.R. Gopalakrishnan, P.K. Singh, K. B. Sheela, M. Asha Shankar, P.C. Jessy Kutty, and K.V. Peter

Kerala Agricultural University, Vellanikkara, Kerala, India

Kerala, the "Gods' Own Land", is located in the southwest corner of peninsular India, between the Western Ghats to the east and Arabian Sea to the west. Diverse climatic conditions prevailing in different parts of the state allows culture of an unusual variety of crops including spices, fruits, and vegetables. Bacterial wilt caused by *Ralstonia solanacearum* is common in solanaceous vegetables like tomato, eggplant and chili in the state and has also emerged as a major problem in other vegetables like bitter gourd, pumpkin, ash gourd, and others.

Bacterial wilt is the single most serious problem in the traditional brinjal (eggplant)-growing tracts in the state. In the local cultivars grown in Kerala, the disease incidence ranges from 15 to 60 per cent and it can be as high as 100 per cent in high yielding varieties (2). Bacterial wilt also assumes serious proportions elsewhere in India, especially in the central and Deccan plateau of Karnataka, Western Maharashtra, Madhya Pradesh, Orissa, the eastern plains of Assam, West Bengal, and Bihar.

Chemical control of the disease is impractical because the pathogen is soilborne, so concerted efforts were made at Kerala Agricultural University to develop bacterial wilt-resistant varieties. This paper deals with the development of different bacterial wilt resistant varieties and the basis of resistance in eggplant.

Materials and Methods

This study was undertaken in Kerala, a hot spot for bacterial wilt incidence. High temperature, high rainfall and prevalence of laterite and acidic soil conditions combine to make the region quite conducive to the multiplication of *Ralstonia solanacearum*. Race 1 and race 3 strains of the pathogen have been isolated from Kerala soils. Resistance breeding was based on *S. melongena* line SM-6, the only brinjal accession identified as resistant in preliminary screening studies during 1979. SM-6 was highly segregating, grouping into 11 phenotypic classes based on fruit color, shape and presence or absence of thorns on the stem. The eleven groups were subjected to four methods of selection, namely, mass, line, single plant, and single seed descent method for four cycles. Single plant selections of line SM 6-6 alone were subjected to rigorous selection for two more cycles.

SCREENING AND ARTIFICIAL INOCULATION

Screening for wilt resistance was conducted in a wilt disease nursery where the previous crop had failed due to bacterial wilt disease. Artificial inoculation of the wilt pathogen was done as per Winstead and Kelman (6) by injecting bacterial ooze collected from freshly wilted plants into the axils of third or fourth fully opened leaves at 15 and 30 days after planting. Bacterial wilt was confirmed by the ooze test and degree of wilt was quantified or grouped as per Mew and Ho (5).

INHERITANCE STUDIES

The bacterial wilt resistant selection, SM 6-7 (Surya), was utilized further for understanding the genetic, biochemical and anatomical basis of resistance to wilt. Surya was crossed to the susceptible variety, Pusa Kranti to develop F_1, F_2, BC_1 and BC_2 generations. All the generations were raised during September-December, 1996 under artificial inoculation.

Anatomical studies. The transverse section of the roots of the resistant variety Surya and the susceptible variety Pusa Kranti were observed microscopically to study the anatomical basis of wilt resistance.

BIOCHEMICAL STUDIES

Alcoholic extracts of the roots of 60 days old plants of the resistant Surya and the susceptible Pusa Kranti were taken for estimation of total phenol by Folin-Ciocalteau method and O.D phenol by Arnow's method as suggested by Mahadevan and Sridhar (4).

Results and Discussion

DEVELOPMENT OF WILT-RESISTANT VARIETIES

Out of the twenty-six brinjal varieties/cultivars screened for resistance to bacterial wilt in the wilt disease nursery at Kerala Agricultural University,

Table 1. Performance of eleven phenotypic groups of *S. melongena* line SM 6 for yield and bacterial wilt resistance.

| Group* | Yield/plant (kg) | | Wilt (%) |
	Range	Mean	
SM 6-1	0.60-1.35	0.88	18.49
SM 6-2	0.83-3.01	1.68	16.94
SM 6-3	0.55-1.10	0.74	6.30
SM 6-4	0.59-1.35	0.91	16.40
SM 6-5	0.75-1.46	1.08	7.01
SM 6-6	0.10-1.38	1.24	14.33
SM 6-7	0.50-1.40	0.87	5.42
SM 6-8	0.50-0.83	0.61	1.80
SM 6-9	0.55-0.90	0.66	3.00
SM 6-10	0.35-1.08	0.67	2.57
SM 6-11	0.60-1.55	1.15	7.75
Mean		0.95	9.01
CD		1.82	

*Phenotypic Group Charcteristics:

SM 6-1 Thorned, long purple

SM 6-2 Thornless, long purple

SM 6-3 Thorned, long green

SM 6-4 Thornless, long green

SM 6-5 Thorned, long white

SM 6-6 Thornless, long white

SM 6-7 Thornless, oval purple

SM 6-8 Thorned, oblong green

SM 6-9 Thornless, oblong green

SM 6-10 Thorned, oblong white

SM 6-11 Thornless, oblong white

in 1979, twenty were completely killed by wilt by the early flowering stage. Line SM-6, the single resistant accession, exhibited considerable variation for fruit and plant characters. SM-6 was partitioned into 11 phenotypic groups based on color (purple, white, green) and fruit shape (long, oval and round) and by the presence or absence of thorns on the stem and leaves. In the selected phenotypic groups, disease incidence varied from 1.8% in SM 6-8 to 18.49% in SM 6-1 under artificial inoculation. However, the average yield of the 11 groups was only 0.95 kg/plant (Table 1).

"Surya" The 11 phenotypic groups were subjected to four methods of selection over four cycles, which increased the mean yield by 40.85%. In SM 6-7 a yield increase of 20.2% was achieved by resorting to single plant selection (Table 2), ultimately yielding 1.19 kg / plant. SM 6-7 attained perfect homogeneity for its purple oval fruits and thornless stem by the fourth cycle (Table 2). Based on its high resistance and good productivity (40.5 t/ha), the 16th State Seed Sub-Committee Meeting on Crop Standards

Table 2. Performance as % wilt incidence and (yield/plant in kg) of SM 6-7 (eventually "Surya") in different cycles of selection.

Selection Cycle	Mass	Line	Single plant	Single seed descent
C1	0.0 (0.88)	0.0 (0.64)	0.0 (0.99)	0.0 (0.63)
C2	3.3 (1.14)	0.0 (0.81)	0.0 (1.05)	0.0 (0.77)
C3	8.3 (0.92)	6.7 (0.86)	10.0 (0.98)	10.0 (0.70)
C4	0.0 (1.03)	3.3 (0.87)	0.0 (1.19)	6.7 (0.82)

released line SM 6-7 under the name "Surya" for commercial cultivation. It was also identified nationally by the 12th AICVIP Workshop held at Hyderabad, India during 6-7th February, 1992. To test the specificity of resistance, the Kerala Agricultural University has collaborated with USDA laboratory, BARC–W, USA where Goth and co-workers (3), observed that Surya (SM 6-7) had high resistance to the most virulent isolates of *R. solanacearum*. Surya has thornless stems and green leaves with a violet tinge. It bears small to medium sized violet oval fruits with an average length of 9.45 cm and girth of 3.85 cm.

"*Swetha*" The single plant selection of SM 6-6 was not stable even after four cycles (yield :1.42 kg/plant). This line was further subjected to rigorous single plant selection for two more cycles and attained a yield level of 3.86 kg/plant. The resulting wilt-resistant, white, long-fruited eggplant, SM 6-6 with a productivity as high as 73 t/ha was identified at the national level by the working group meeting of AICVIP held from 15-18th March 1996 at Varanasi, UP. The 18th State Seed Sub-Committee Meeting on Crop Standards held on the 17th of September, 1996 recommended this selection for release under the name "Swetha" for large scale cultivation in the wilt-prone region of the state. Swetha is characterized by thornless stems with a bushy and compact growth habit. The leaves have a peculiar semi-erect

Table 3. Performance as % wilt incidence and (yield/plant in kg) of *S. melongena* line SM 6-6 (eventually "Swetha") in different selection cycles.

Selection Cycle	Mass	Line	Single plant	Single seed descent
C1	10.0 (0.83)	3.3 (0.69)	3.3 (0.96)	0.0 (0.59)
C2	6.7 (0.97)	3.3 (0.74)	3.3 (1.06)	0.0 (0.76)
C3	33.3 (1.03)	10.0 (0.81)	20.0 (1.17)	18.3 (0.85)
C4	13.3 (1.39)	0.0 (0.96)	5.0 (1.42)	10.0 (0.91)
C5	-	-	0.0 (1.64)	-
C6	-	-	0.0 (3.86)	-

orientation. Small to medium long white fruits with an average length of 13.85 cm and a weight of 63.6 gm have excellent cooking quality.

"Haritha" During this rigorous selection on line SM-6 and its descendants, germplasm collection continued and 320 collections were screened for wilt resistance. SM-141, a light green-fruited line found to be resistant to wilt, was also subjected to rigorous single plant selection for high productivity and uniformity in plant and fruit characters. The results are furnished in Table 4. After the fifth cycle of single plant selection, SM 141 reached a yield level of 6.4 kg/plant. Based on its bacterial wilt resistance, high yield and specific consumer preference, line SM 141 was recommended by the 19th State Seed Committee on Crop Standards held on 15-6-98 for disease endemic areas and this line was released as a cultivar under the name "Haritha". Haritha is a long duration, spreading variety with white flowers, light green, soft, cylindrical fruits. This high-yielding variety (68.8 t/Ha) is ideal for ratooning. Table 5 gives an overall comparison of the three open pollinated varieties. Haritha is a long duration variety with large cylindrical fruits having light green color and excellent cooking quality.

Table 4. Improvement of *S. melongena* line SM-141 (eventually "Haritha") yield through selection.

Selection cycles	Year	Yield/plant (kg)	Wilt incidence (%)
C 1	1988	0.90	0
C 2	1989	1.27	0
C 3	1992	2.39	0
C 4	1993	3.85	0
C 5	1995	6.40	0

Table 5. Comparative performance of Surya, Swetha, and Haritha with susceptible cultivar Pusa Kranti.

Character	Surya	Swetha	Haritha	Pusa Kranti
Plant height (cm)	83.20	111.50	155.63	97.90
Plant spread (cm)	113.20	107.00	154.43	61.65
Days to flower	22.50	29.70	40.50	32.80
Days to 1st harvest	43.50	47.20	57.40	50.40
Fruit length (cm)	9.45	13.85	16.60	12.90
Fruit girth (cm)	3.85	2.95	4.07	4.35
Av. fruit weight (g)	62.40	63.60	128.27	68.50
No. of fruits/plant	66.60	117.20	113.50	7.30
Yield/plant (kg)	3.06	3.86	6.40	0.38
Productivity (t/Ha)	40.50	73.00	68.80	1.80
Wilt incidence (%)	0.00	0.00	0.00	100.00

"Neelima." An F_1 hybrid Surya X SM 116, was highly wilt-resistant and productive. This line been recommended for the state of Kerala and released as a cultivar under the name Neelima. The plants are spreading and thornless with violet flowers and glossy violet fruits with an average length of 12.0 cm and and weight of 176 g. The potential productivity is as high as 101.33 t/Ha.

INHERITANCE STUDIES AND HETEROSIS BREEDING

Earlier studies on the inheritance of bacterial wilt resistance found a monogenic and incomplete dominance of susceptibility over resistance. In the present investigation, six hybrids developed by crossing resistant parents were totally free from bacterial wilt (Table 6). However, in three hybrids the percentage of wilt ranged from 4-18% as one of the parents involved in the hybridization program exhibited 6 to 18% wilt. These results suggest that resistance to wilt is recessive. Unfortunately, a more detailed

Table 6. Mean bacterial wilt incidence values in 11 parents and nine F_1 hybrids November 1995-June 1996

Sl. No.	Genotype	Wilt (%)	Disease Reaction
	PARENTS		
1	Surya	0	R
2	Composite2	18	R
3	SM 116 Annapurna	0	R
4	Arka Keshav	0	R
5	SM 71	0	R
6	Swetha	0	R
7	Haritha	0	R
8	SM 63	0	R
9	WCG (S)	12	R
10	TGR	0	R
	F_1 HYBRIDS		
1	Surya x Composite2	6	R
2	Surya x SM 116 (Neelima)	0	R
3	Surya x Annapurna	0	R
4	ArkaKeshav x Composite2	18	R
5	Arka Keshav x SM 71		R
6	Swetha x SM 71	0	R
7	Swetha x SM 63	0	R
8	Haritha x WCG (S)	4	R
9	Haritha x TGR	0	R
10		0	R

evaluation, involving large F_2, BC_1 and BC_2 populations along with parents and the F_1, was terminated without results due to complications caused by the fungal pathogen *Fusarium* and termites.

ANATOMICAL STUDIES

In anatomical studies, we observed large sized and loosely arranged cortical cells in the roots of the susceptible variety Pusa Kranti. In contrast, the cortical cells of the resistant line Surya were small and compactly arranged. This correlative observation suggested that pathogenic bacteria may enter easily through the loosely arranged cortical cells of the susceptible variety. In the resistant variety, the compactly arranged cortical cells could provide a shield against the entry of bacteria into the roots from the soil. Secondary xylem and phloem vessels were damaged in the roots of the susceptible variety, as a result of bacterial invasion. During disintegration of xylem, phloem vessels and the connected tissues, phenolic compounds are released. These later oxidize to quinones, giving a black discoloration in the xylem and phloem vessels of susceptible varieties. We speculate that damage and subsequent obliteration of physiologically active secondary xylem results in the blocking of water and nutrient flow to the stem and leaves, and ultimately leads to wilting of the plants. Our observations suggest that the damage of physiologically active secondary phloem may contribute to the blocking of photosynthates to the roots, resulting in the cessation of root production.

BIOCHEMICAL STUDIES

The roots of resistant variety Surya had a high total phenol content (0.36%) and O.D phenol (0.02%) compared to the roots of the susceptible variety, Pusa Kranti (0.22% and 0.001% respectively) (Table 7). Geetha (1) also reported a high content of OD phenol in the roots of wilt-resistant eggplant varieties. The correlation between high content of phenols and resistance suggests that phenols may be one mechanism that impedes pathogen entry and further multiplication in the roots of resistant varieties.

Table 7. Total phenol and O.D phenol contents in the roots of wilt-resistant and susceptible varieties

Varieties	Resistance reaction	Total phenol (%)	OD phenol (%)
Swetha	R	0.38	0.022
Surya	R	0.36	0.021
Pusa Kranti	S	0.22	0.001

Conclusions

Operating since 1979, a breeding program for resistance to bacterial wilt at Kerala Agricultural University, India, has resulted in the development of three agronomically distinct wilt-resistant varieties, namely, Surya (oval purple fruits) , Swetha (long white fruits) and Haritha (long, light green fruits) as well as an F_1 hybrid, Neelima. Inheritance studies demonstrated that susceptibility to bacterial wilt was dominant over resistance. In the roots of resistant varieties, the outer cortical cells are small sized and tightly packed, possibly acting as a shield to prevent pathogen entry. In contrast, loose and large cells in the outer cortex of the susceptible varieties may facilitate easy entry of pathogen. High phenolic content in the roots of resistant varieties may also prevent the entry and further multiplication of bacteria in the resistant varieties.

Literature Cited

1. Geetha, P.T. 1989. Heterosis and genetic analysis involving isogenic lines in brinjal resistant to bacterial wilt. MSc. (Hort) Thesis, Kerala Agricultural University, Thrissur.
2. Gopimani, R., and George, M.K. 1989. Screening brinjal varieties for wilt resistance. Agricul. Res. J. Kerala.17: 7-10.
3. Goth, R.W., Peter, K.V., and Webb, R.R. 1983. Bacterial wilt: *Pseudomonas solanacearum* resistance in pepper and eggplant. Phytopathology 73: 808.
4. Mahadevan, A., and Sridhar, R. 1982. Methods in Physiological Plant Pathology, 2nd Edn. Sivakasi Publications, Indira Nagar, Madras.
5. Mew, T.W. and Ho, W.C., 1977. Effect of soil temperature on resistance of tomato cultivars to bacterial wilt. Phytopathology 67:907-911
6. Winstead, N.N., and Kelman, A. 1952. Inoculation techniques for evaluation of resistance to *Pseudomonas solanacearum* Phytopathology. 42: 628-634.

QTL Mapping for Bacterial Wilt Resistance in Hawaii 7996 Using AFLP, RGA, and SSR Markers

Conrado H. Balatero[1], Desiree M. Hautea[1], Josefina O. Narciso[1], and Peter M. Hanson[2]

[1] Institute of Plant Breeding, College of Agriculture, University of the Philippines Los Baños, 4031 College, Laguna, Philippines; [2] Plant Breeder, Asian Vegetable Research and Development Center, Shanhua, Tainan, Taiwan, People's Republic of China

Bacterial wilt, caused by the soilborne pathogen *Ralstonia solanacearum*, continues to be a major production constraint in tropical and subtropical environments, particularly during the rainy season. There is no effective chemical control, hence, breeding for resistant varieties is still considered the most practical and economical control measure.

Bacterial wilt resistance, however, is a complex trait. Inheritance studies for resistance to bacterial wilt indicated both simple inheritance patterns of major genes for resistance (1,8), and quantitative (polygenic) inheritance (6,12,13). The environment and strains of *R. solanacearum* also influence resistance expression. These factors make breeding for resistance using conventional selection based on phenotypic resistance expression a relatively difficult task.

Rapid advances in DNA marker technologies, however, have provided new tools in plant breeding. DNA markers can generate high-density molecular maps that locate more precisely genes affecting either simple or complex traits (10,16). If DNA markers are strongly linked to a trait of interest, then molecular marker-assisted selection can greatly improve breeders' efficiency.

In tomato, molecular mapping of bacterial wilt resistance genes led to the identification of molecular markers linked to quantitative trait loci (QTL) controlling bacterial wilt resistance (6,12,13,15). Although important QTL were identified in the two F_2 mapping populations, the level of marker saturation was low for efficient marker-aided selection or map-based cloning of resistance genes. Most of the linked markers are also RFLP markers and are therefore too costly and laborious to use in routine marker-assisted breeding. Furthermore, the F_2 or F_3 mapping populations used in previous studies did not allow extensive evaluation of effects of environment (location or growing conditions) or of different pathogen strains. The use of recombinant inbred lines (RIL), as in this study, can overcome these limitations, since RIL can serve as a permanent mapping resource that will enable replicated tests in multiple environments using different pathogen strains.

This paper describes the results of our molecular mapping work for bacterial wilt resistance using F_6 recombinant inbred lines of Hawaii 7996 x WVa700 mapping population.

Phenotyping F_6 RILs of Hawaii 7996 x WVa700 for Bacterial Wilt Resistance

EVALUATION OF PARENTAL LINES AND F_6 RILS
AGAINST TWO VIRULENT *R. SOLANACEARUM* STRAINS

A total of 189 F_6 RILs generated by single seed descent from the original 200 F_2 mapping population used earlier by Thoquet et al (12), were evaluated for resistance to two highly virulent *R. solanacearum* strains (Tm-22 and Tm-151). The F_6 RILs, together with the parental lines Hawaii 7996 and WVa700, were transplanted 7-10 days from sowing onto small plastic cups (7.62 cm in diameter) filled with steam-sterilized soil mix. Plants were artificially inoculated about one month after sowing by drenching individual plants with 25 ml of bacterial suspension at $1X10^6$ CFU/mL. Plant response to bacterial infection was determined weekly based on three resistance parameters: wilt disease index score, proportion of plants showing wilt symptoms, and percent survival. Each plant was indexed on a scale of 0 to 5 as follows: 0 – no symptom; 1 – 1 leaf wilted (partial or complete); 2 – 2 to 3 leaves wilted (partial or complete); 3 – more than 3 leaves to about of 2/3 of leaves wilted; 4 – more than 2/3 or all leaves are wilted (apex is still erect), and 5 – whole plant wilted (collapsed).

PHENOTYPIC DISTRIBUTION OF RESISTANCE IN THE F_6 RILS

The phenotypic distribution (as wilt index score) was almost normally distributed, but with a skew towards resistance in terms of percent survival. The resistant parent Hawaii 7996 showed a high resistant reaction (low mean wilt index score and high percent survival) compared to the susceptible parent WVa700.

The response of F_6 RILs to strain Tm-151 did not follow a normal distribution but was skewed towards susceptibility. Wilt symptoms developed very rapidly such that only 6.3% of the WVa70 plants survived one week after inoculation. The resistant parent Hawaii 7996, on the other hand, was highly resistant to strain Tm-151 with 93.8% of the plant surviving four weeks after inoculation.

Greenhouse tests also found a strain-specific response. Some of the F_6 RILs that were rated highly resistant against strain Tm-22 succumbed to strain Tm-151 and vice-versa. This observation indicates the importance of genotype x pathogen strain interaction, a type of interaction that needs to be carefully addressed by plant breeders in breeding for bacterial wilt resistant tomato lines. It should be noted that none of the previous studies on QTL mapping for bacterial wilt resistance (6,12,13,15) examined in detail genotype x strain interaction.

QTL Mapping for Bacterial Wilt Resistance

SEARCH FOR NEW PCR-BASED DNA MARKERS
IN HAWAII 7996 X WVA700 MAPPING POPULATION

DNA from the parental lines and F_6 RILs were extracted using both a medium-scale (4) and microprep method (7). Extracted DNA was further purified using 25:24:1 phenol:chloroform:octanol. The parental lines Hawaii 7996 and WVa700 and few randomly selected F_6 RILs were initially screened for marker polymorphism using AFLP, RGA and SSR markers. For amplified fragment length polymorphism (AFLP), 64 *EcoR1/MseI* selective primer pairs based on the AFLP Analysis System I (GIBCO-BRL Life Technologies) were screened for polymorphism. Restriction digestion of genomic DNA, ligation of adapter sequences, preamplification and selective amplification were based on the protocol of Vos *et al.* (14) with minor modifications.

For resistance gene analog (RGA) markers, a total of 19 RGA primers were evaluated for polymorphism in the resistant and susceptible tomato parental lines. PCR amplification was carried out following the protocol of Chen *et al.* (5) with minor modifications. For simple sequence repeat (SSR) or microsatellites, we evaluated 28 primers provided by Drs. P. Arens and B. Vosman of the DLO-Center for Plant Breeding and Reproduction Research (CPRO-DLO), Wangeningen, The Netherlands (now Plant Research International). PCR amplification conditions and polyacrylamide gel electrophoresis (PAGE) were as described (3). Bands were detected using a non-radioactive silver staining method (2).

Segregation of markers was tested using chi-square analysis. The software MAPMAKER V2.0 for Macintosh (9) was used to construct the linkage map. QTL-marker associations were determined using both single-

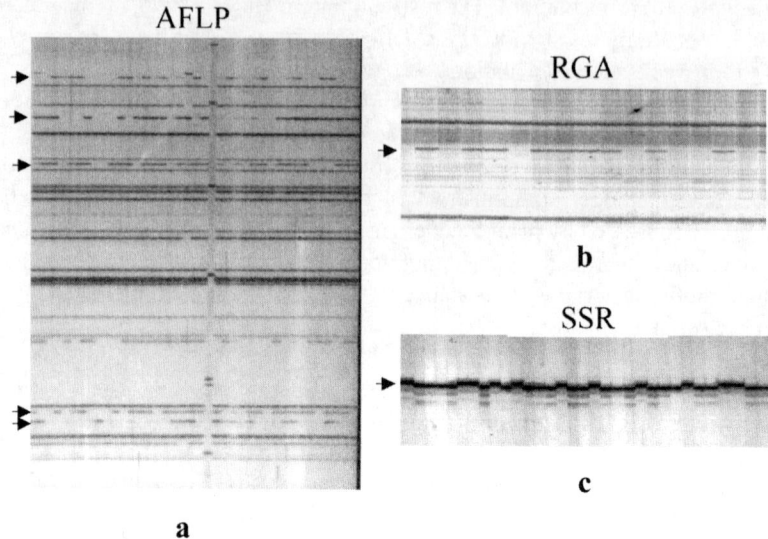

Fig. 1. Segregation of AFLP (a), RGA (b) and SSR (c) markers in the Hawaii 7996 x WVa700 F_6 recombinant inbred lines. Arrows indicate polymorphic markers

marker analysis and composite interval mapping using the QTL Cartographer Version 1.2 software (Statistical Genetics, North Carolina State University, 2001).

A highly reproducible and high-resolution non-radioactive detection of AFLP, RGA and SSR bands was obtained (Fig. 1). A linkage map consisting of 12 linkage groups and a total of 80 markers (72 AFLP, 7 RGA and 1 SSR) was earlier constructed using MAPMAKER Version 2.0 software (3). The total map length covered by the 12 linkage groups is 378.1 cM, or about 1/3 of the total map length for tomato covered by RFLP-based markers (11).

DNA MARKERS ASSOCIATED WITH BACTERIAL WILT RESISTANCE QTL

Based on single marker analysis, 7 markers (6 AFLP and 1 RGA) were tentatively associated with resistance to both Tm-22 and Tm-151 strains of *R. solanacearum* for three resistance parameters – wilt score, percent survival, and proportion of plants with wilt symptoms. The variance explained ranged from 4.8% to 32.6%. The markers were clustered in at least two genomic regions in linkage group B (Fig. 2a). The AFLP markers were derived from four primer pairs (af02, af16, af20, and af37) while the RGA primers were based on the conserved leucine-rich repeats (LRR) of the cloned

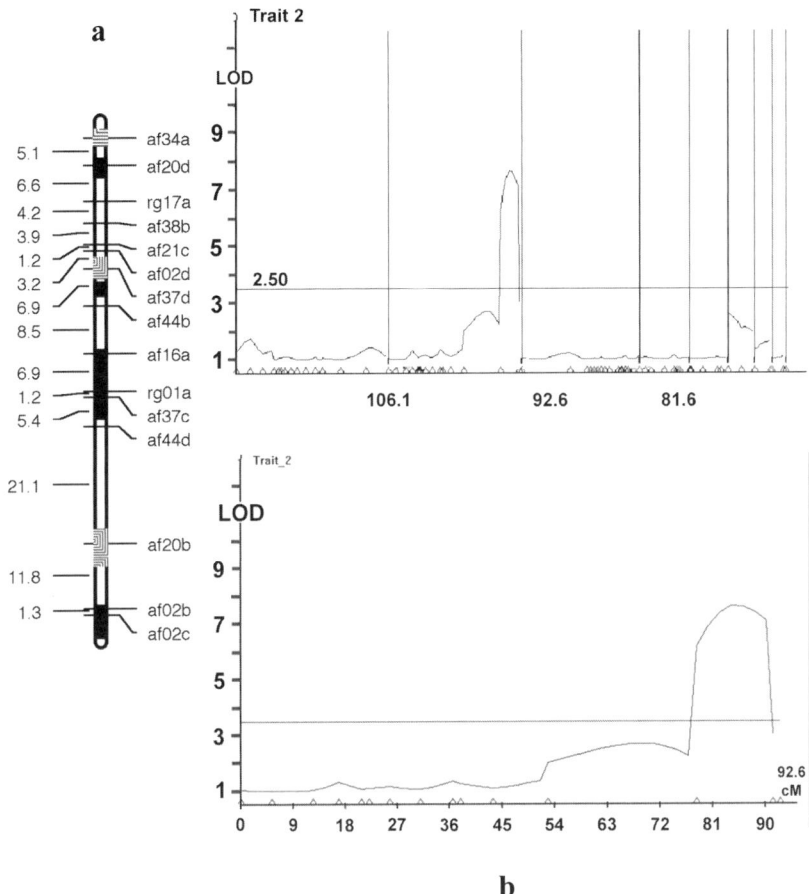

Fig. 2. QTL analysis showing **a**) putative AFLP and RGA markers associated with bacterial wilt resistance based on single marker analysis (solid black regions are associated with both strains Tm-22 and Tm-151; striped regions are specific to strain Tm-22), and **b**) composite interval mapping results showing genomic region in linkage group B with very strong association to bacterial wilt resistance QTL (LOD>5) based on mean wilt index scores.

Xa21 gene, which confers resistance to *Xanthomonas oryzae* in rice (3). Composite interval mapping (CIM) analysis indicated one major bacterial wilt resistance QTL (LOD>5.0) in Hawaii 7996 strongly linked to a co-dominant AFLP marker (af02b/af02c) (Fig. 2b). A minor QTL was also detected in another linkage group (data not shown). Strain-specific marker-QTL associations were also observed. Two minor strain-specific QTL against strain Tm-151 were observed; however, the contribution of the other resistance QTL came from the susceptible parent WVa700, which is an *L. pimpinellifolium* line.

Acknowledgements

We acknowledge financial support from the International Foundation for Science (IFS), PCASTRD-DOST of the Philippines, University of the Philippines Los Baños, and the Asian Pacific Economic Conference (APEC). We also thank Dr. Nigel Grimsley of CNRS-INRA (France) for sharing the Hawaii 7996 x WVa700 mapping population, Dr. H. Leung of IRRI, Philippines for sharing resistance gene analog (RGA) primers, Dr. Ben Vosman of CPRO-DLO (now Plant Research International), The Netherlands for sharing tomato SSR primers and Ms. J.T. Bituin, Ms. R.L. Tiongco, Ms. M. Latiza, Ms. R.B. Franke, and Mr. C.S. Caspillo for technical assistance.

Literature Cited

1. Acosta, J.C., Gilbert, J.C., and Quinon, V.L. 1994. Heritability of bacterial wilt resistance in tomato. Proc. Am. Soc. Hortic. Sci. 84:455-462.
2. Balatero, C.H., Galvez, H.F., Padlan, C.P., Segovia ,S.E., and Hautea, D.M. 1999. Optimization of non-radioactive AFLP protocol for genome analysis of important Philippine crops. Phil. J. Crop Sci. 24:66.
3. Balatero, C.H., Hautea, D.M., Narciso, J.O., Hanson, P.M., Bituin, J.T., and Tiongco, R.L. 2001. Identification of AFLP and RGA markers associated with bacterial wilt resistance QTL derived from wild tomato *Lycopersicon pimpenillifolium*. Pages 225-243 in: SOLANACEAE V. Advances in Taxonomy and Utilization. R.G. Van der Berg, G.W.M. Barendse, G.M. van der Weerden, and C. Marani, eds. Nijmegen University Press. The Netherlands.
4. Bernatzky, R., and Tanksley, S.D. 1986. Genetics of actin related sequences in tomato. Theor. Appl. Genet. 72:314-321.
5. Chen, X.M. Line, R.F., and Leung, H. 1998. Genome scanning for resistance-gene analogs in rice, barley, and wheat by high-resolution electrophoresis. Theor. Appl. Genet. 97:345-355.
6. Danesh, D., Aarons, S., McGill, G.E., and Young, N.D. 1994. Genetic dissection of oligogenic resistance to bacterial wilt in tomato. Mol. Plant-Microbe Interact. 7:464-471.

7. Fulton, T.M, Chunwongse, J., and Tanksley, S.D. 1995. Microprep protocol for extraction of DNA from tomato and other herbaceous plants. Plant Mol. Biol. Rep. 13:207-209.

8. Grimault, V., Prior, P., and Anais, G. 1995. A monogenic dominant resistance of tomato bacterial wilt in Hawaii 7996 is associated with plant colonization by *Pseudomonas solanacearum*. J. Phytopath. 143:349-352.

9. Lander, E.S., Green, P., Abrahamson, J., Barlow, A., Daly, M.J., Lincoln S.E., and Newburg, L. 1987. Mapmaker: an interactive computer package for constructing primary genetic linkage maps of experimental and natural populations. Genomics 1:174-181.

10. Paterson, A.H., Tanksley, S.D., and Sorrells, M.E. 1991. DNA markers in plant improvement. Advances in Agronomy 46:39-90.

11. Tanksley, S.D., Ganal, M., Prince J.P., Devicente, M.C, Bonierbale, M.W., Broun, P., Fulton, T.M., Giovanonni, J.J., Grandillo, S., Martin, G.B., Messequer, R., Miller, J.C., Miller, L., Paterson, A.H., Pineda, O., Roder, M., Wing, R.A., Wu, W., and Young, N.D. 1992. High density molecular linkage maps of the tomato and potato genomes: biological inferences and practical applications. Genetics 132:1141-1160.

12. Thoquet, P., Olivier, J., Sperisen, C., Rogowsky, P., Laterrot, H., and Grimsley, N. 1996a. Quantitative trait loci determining resistance to bacterial wilt in tomato cultivar Hawaii 7996. Mol. Plant-Microbe Interactions 9:826-836.

13. Thoquet, P., Olivier, J., Sperisen, C., Rogowsky, P., Prior, P., Anais, G., Mangin, B., Bazin, B., Nazer, R., and Grimsley, N. 1996b. Polygenic resistance of tomato plants to bacterial wilt in the French West Indies. Mol. Plant-Microbe Interactions 9:837-842.

14. Vos, P., Rogers, R., Bleeker, M., Reijans, M., Lee, T., Hornes, M., Frijters, A., Pot, J., Peleman, J., Kuiper, M., and Zabeau, M. 1995. AFLP: a new technique for DNA fingerprinting. Nucleic Acids Research 23:4407-4414.

15. Wang, J.F., Oliver, J., Thoquet, P., Mangin, B., Sauviac, L., and Grimsley, N.H. 2000. Resistance of tomato line Hawaii 7996 to *Ralstonia solanacearum* Pss4 in Taiwan is controlled mainly by a major strain-specific locus. Mol. Plant-Microbe Int. 13:6-13.

16. Young, N.D. 1996. QTL mapping and quantitative disease resistance in plants. Annual Rev. Phytopathol. 34:479-501.

Genetic Basis of Resistance to Bacterial Wilt in *Arabidopsis thaliana*

L. Deslandes, D. X. Feng, J. Hirsch, L. Godiard, J. Olivier, N. Grimsley, H. Zhu, S. Legay, and Y. Marco

Laboratoire de Biologie Moléculaire des Relations Plantes-Microorganismes, CNRS-INRA, BP27, Castanet-Tolosan, France

The establishment of a pathosystem between the model crucifer *Arabidopsis thaliana* and *Ralstonia solanacearum* has allowed the study of plant genetic determinants associated with resistance to this important pathogen. Two interactions have been studied. In one case, it was shown that resistance to a French isolate of the pathogen was conferred by three QTLs. The study of a second interaction between ecotypes Col-5 and Nd-1 and a tropical strain GMI1000, using a classical genetic study and positional cloning, led to the isolation of an R gene, RRS1-R (Resistance to *Ralstonia solanacearum*). This gene, which confers resistance to several isolates of *R. solanacearum*, encodes a deduced protein with a novel modular structural organization. This novel class of R genes is characterized. Additionally, in order to understand the molecular mechanisms involved in the establishment of resistance and disease development, we initiated transcriptome analysis of resistant and susceptible plants challenged with strain GMI1000. Preliminary results indicate that around 5% of the plant genes are affected during disease resistance.

Introduction

Bacterial wilt caused by the phytopathogenic bacterium *Ralstonia solanacearum* is one of the most important plant diseases worldwide (5). This pathogen has a large range of hosts with more than 200 species including approximately 50 families of mono- and dicotyledons. Among these are many species of agronomic importance, such as potatoes, tomatoes, peanuts, and bananas. Recently detected in Europe, this disease is endemic in all the tropical and subtropical areas. This bacterial pathogen is soilborne and therefore methods to control the disease have limited effects. The most effective method is the use of resistant crop varieties, which can be effective in one environment but are often overcome by virulent pathogen isolates when environmental conditions or local strain populations are different. Studies of the genetic basis of resistance to *R. solanacearum* in tomato found complex resistance mechanisms such as polygenic resistance (7).

In order to simplify the study of the genetic basis of this resistance, a new pathosystem between the model crucifer *Arabidopsis thaliana* and *R. solanacearum* has been established (2). The genetic variability of *A. thaliana* allowed the identification of ecotypes resistant and susceptible to different strains of the pathogen. Results indicate that the pathosystem offers a great variability and is particularly well suited for identification and isolation of host R genes against this pathogen.

Results

POLYGENIC RESISTANCE OF *A. THALIANA* TO A EUROPEAN STRAIN
OF *R. SOLANACEARUM*

Outbreaks of bacterial wilt have been reported on solanaceous crops (especially potato) in Europe. Several strains isolated in Europe were virulent to varying extents on different ecotypes of the crucifer. One strain, 14.25, isolated in France could induce disease on ecotype La-er but did not induce symptoma on another ecotype, Col-0. Both bacterial multiplication and development of disease symptoms in *A. thaliana* were dependent upon functional *hrp* genes. Using recombinant inbred lines, it was shown that three loci govern resistance carried by ecotype Col-0. Temporal analysis of the data demonstrated that the LOD value of these three QTLs, which are located on chromosome 2 and 5, reached a maximum at a late stage after inoculation.

MONOGENIC RESISTANCE OF *A. THALIANA* TO *R. SOLANACEARUM*
STRAIN GMI1000

Isolation of RRS1-S and RRS1-R by positional cloning. Resistance to *R. solanacearum* strain GMI1000, normally virulent on tomato, segregated as a simply inherited recessive trait in a genetic cross between *A. thaliana* accessions Col-5 (susceptible) and Nd-1 (resistant). The Col-5 *RRS1* locus was previously localized between RFLP markers *mi61* and *mi83*. The positional cloning of this locus was performed and allowed to position the *RRS1* locus on an 18 kb cosmid called B1 whose nucleotide sequence was determined and which contained two *R*-gene-like open reading frames (ORF1 and ORF2) and a third unrelated gene (ORF3). The development of

310

two additional CAPS markers (an amplified PCR fragment whose digestion by a restriction enzyme distinguishes the 2 parental alleles), 1b and 2b, corresponding to ORF1 and ORF3 respectively, defined a mapping interval that contained only ORF2. We concluded that ORF2, which is 6.3 kb long and contains 6 introns, is the *RRS1-S* gene.

Deduced primary structures of RRS1-R and RRS1-S, which correspond to the alleles present in susceptible Col-5 and resistant Nd-1 plants, respectively. The deduced protein corresponding to ORF2 has a modular organization. Motifs common to the TIR-NBS-LRR class of resistance gene products are present in the NH_2-terminus of RRS1-S. Its C-terminal region contains a potential nuclear localization signal and a WRKY domain, a 60 amino acid conserved motif characteristic of transcription factors identified only in plants and involved in many biological processes (3).

A cosmid, H, carrying the allele associated with resistance, *RRS1-R*, was isolated by screening a Nd-1 cosmid library using the *RRS1-S* gene as a probe. Its nucleotide sequence indicated a high level of identity (98%) between the sequences of the two alleles. This level of conservation (98%) extends through 1.1 kb of the potential promoter region 5' to the gene although the two genes differ in the position of a stop codon that leads to a protein truncated by 90 amino acids in *RRS1-S*, the Col-5 allele (Fig.1).

Analysis of the derived amino acid sequences of the RRS1 proteins revealed the presence of several domains found in many resistance proteins of the TIR-NBS-LRR subclass. The consensus leucine rich repeats (LRR) of RRS1 proteins consists of 6 imperfect 23 amino acids motifs. All the domains are extremely well conserved among the 2 RRS1 proteins and structure-function analysis of RRS1-R and RRS1-S should clarify the importance of the various minor amino acid differences detected between the two proteins on RRS1-R function.

RRS1-R represents therefore the first R protein containing a conserved WRKY domain, which suggests that it has a regulatory role in the expression of the signalling pathways leading to resistance or susceptibility. This potential role in transcriptional activation is also indicated by the presence

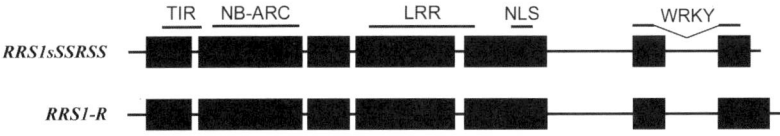

Fig. 1. Structural gene organization of the *RRS1* genes. Exons are shown as rectangles and motif similarities at the amino acid levels are indicated above the figure.

of a putative nuclear localization signal which suggests that this protein is targeted to the nucleus. Interestingly, some *avr* gene products such as AvrBs3 have been shown to be nuclear localized (1,8) indicating that a direct or indirect interaction between products of some *avr* genes and those of the corresponding *R* genes may occur in the plant nucleus.

RRS1-R confers resistance to strain GMI1000 of R. solanacearum. In order to confirm the function of *RRS1-R* and *RRS1-S*, constructs were introduced into both parental accessions. Nd-1 plants containing either a cosmid containing the *RRS1-S* gene and the 2 ORFs previously mentioned (119 independent transformants), or a 9.3 kb genomic fragment containing only the *RRS1-S* gene and its flanking regions (24 independent transformants) did not develop wilt disease. This indicated that *RRS1-S* is not in itself a susceptibility gene capable of suppressing the resistance phenotype of Nd-1.

Susceptible Col-5 plants were transformed with either the cosmid containing *RRS1-R*, or a 9.3 kb genomic clone corresponding to the *RRS1-R* gene and its flanking regions. All of the transgenic lines (19 independent for each construct) were resistant and failed to develop wilt symptoms upon inoculation with strain GMI1000. Col-5 plants transformed with constructs containing a truncated *RRS1-R* gene remained fully susceptible. These data demonstrated that *RRS1-R* is an *R* gene.

RRS1-R restricts pathogen growth in infected plants and confers broad spectrum resistance to R. solanacearum. The growth of the pathogen within control plants and a selected transgenic line, CH1.2, homozygous for both *RRS1-R* and *RRS1-S*, was estimated. Bacterial multiplication in Col-5 plants containing the *RRS1-R* transgene was comparable with that obtained in Nd-1 resistant plants, and lower by more than five orders of magnitude than that in susceptible Col-5 plants. Therefore, the *RRS1-R* gene behaves as a dominant resistance gene capable of limiting bacterial growth in a Col-5 genetic background.

Col-5 transgenic plants carrying the resistance allele *RRS1-R* were also inoculated with four strains of the pathogen that induce differential responses on accessions Nd-1 and Col-5 (2). Transgenic Col-5 plants were shown to respond in a similar way to Nd-1 plants and were fully resistant to strains AW1, GA4, GT4, and 0170 isolated from different host plants in various geographic areas. *RRS1-R*, therefore, provides resistance to several different strains of *R. solanacearum* strains.

RRS1-R-mediated resistance is dependent upon salicylic acid and NDR1. Most *A. thaliana R* genes characterized so far require salicylic acid and the defense signalling pathway genes *NDR1* or *EDS1* (4). We determined that salicylic acid plays a role in *RRS1-R*-mediated resistance since Nd-1 plants containing salicylate hydroxylase, which converts salicylic acid into inactive catechol, developed wilt symptoms. Resistance was also abolished when Nd-1 plants were crossed into the *ndr1/ndr1* mutant background and

RRS1-R/RRS1-R ndr1/ndr1 offspring selected. In both cases however, complete wilting of the plant occurred four to seven days after the death of susceptible Col-5 plants, implying that other signalling components must also play a role in *RRS1*-mediated resistance.

<small>TRANSCRIPTOME ANALYSIS OF RESISTANT AND SUSCEPTIBLE *ARABIDOPSIS THALIANA* PLANTS CHALLENGED WITH STRAIN GMI1000 OF *R. SOLANACEARUM*</small>

RRS1-R is a gene which confers resistance to several *R. solanacearum* strains isolated from different plant species. So far, no other R protein exhibiting such a structural organization has been described and the existence of a WRKY domain in both the resistant and susceptible forms of RRS1 indicate that this protein probably plays an important role in the activation of signaling pathways leading to resistance. Besides, *RRS1*-mediated resistance is not accompanied by the development of an HR. Microarray technology applied to this pathosystem will likely bring novel data on the pathways controlled by this unusual *R* gene and on the transcriptional changes associated with resistance and wilt disease development. Little is indeed known about the molecular mechanisms leading to this type of plant disease. We have ongoing analysis of the early and late events accompanying the natural interaction between *R. solanacearum* and the susceptible and resistant ecotypes, Col-5 and Nd-1 respectively. In addition, mutant lines including Col-5 transgenic plants which have been made resistant by the introduction of the resistant allele, *RRS1-R*, will be used in this study. Another interesting point will be the comparison of pathways controlled by *RRS1-R* in two different genetic backgrounds (Col-0/*RRS1-R* and Nd-1).

This study was initiated using microarrays containing around 9000 *A. thaliana* genes and using cDNA prepared from mRNA populations from Nd-1 and Col-5 plants inoculated with strain GMI1000. Preliminary results indicate that approximately 5% of the genes are affected during the infectious process. Our long-term goal is the isolation and characterization of genes whose expression is controlled by *RRS1-R,* as well as genes playing an important role during disease development.

Conclusions

In summary, the pathosystem *A. thaliana*/*R. solanacearum* constitutes a powerful tool for the identification of genetic determinants governing resistance to *R. solanacearum*. Our results demonstrate that depending on the bacterial strains and plant ecotypes used, resistance can be either polygenic or monogenic and that tools developed using Arabidopsis may lead to the isolation of novel *R* genes. This is exemplified by the positional cloning of the *RRS1-R* gene, which is the first *R* gene against *R. solanacearum* isolated so far. RRS1-R is also the first TIR-NBS-LRR resistance protein that contains a putative transcriptional activation domain. Potentially, their modular structure suggests that RRS1-S and RRS1-R proteins have a dual function: the NH_2-terminus may bind a pathogen-derived signal *via* the LRR motifs known to mediate protein-protein interactions. This recognition event may lead to the activation of the C-terminus WRKY transcriptional factor domain. This, in turn, would activate a signaling cascade, or directly activate defense-related genes, leading to the plant resistance response. Additionally, the strong similarity between the RRS1 proteins strengthens the possibility that they may compete for some essential component(s) involved in the pathogen perception or in signal transduction pathways. In this case, RRS1-R function may be affected or inhibited as the DNA binding sites are occupied by RRS1-S. In addition, minor differences in the NH_2-terminal region of RRS1 proteins may also modify their respective affinities, either for an *Avr*- or a pathogen-derived factor, or for a plant protein.

Transcriptome analysis of resistant and susceptible plants and of various mutants should bring some insight on the signalling pathways leading to resistance or susceptibility as well as on the mode of action of the *RRS1-R* gene and its potential targets. Our long-term goal is the intergeneric transfer of key genes such as *RRS1-R* in plants of agronomical importance such as potato and tomato.

Literature Cited

1. Bonas, U., and Van Der Ackerveken, G. 1997. Recognition of bacterial avirulence proteins occurs inside the plant cell: a general phenomenon in resistance to bacterial diseases Plant J. 12:1-7.
2. Deslandes, L., Pileur, F., Liaubet, L., Camut, S., Can, C., Williams, K., Holub, E., Beynon, J., Arlat, M., and Marco Y., 1998. Genetic characterization of RRS1, a recessive locus in *Arabidopsis thaliana* that confers resistance to the bacterial soilborne pathogen *Ralstonia solanacearum*. Molecular. Plant-Microbe Interact. 11, 659-667.
3. Eulgem, T., Rushton, P. J., Robatzek, S., and Somssich, I. 2000. The WRKY superfamily of plant transcription factors Trends Plant Sci. 5:199-206.
4. Glazebrook, J. 1999. Genes controlling expression of defense reponses in Arabidopis Curr. Opin. Plant Biol. 2:280-286.
5. Hayward, A.C. 1999. Biology and epidemiology of bacterial wilt caused by *Pseudomonas solanacearum* Annu. Rev. Phytopathol. 29:65-87.

6. Thoquet, P., Olivier, J., Sperisen, C., Rogowsky, P., Laterrot, H., and Grimsley, N. 1996. Quantitative trait loci determining resistance to tomato bacterial wilt in tomato cultivar Hawaii 7996. Mol. Plant-Microbe Interact. 9:826-836.

7. Thoquet, P., Olivier, J., Sperisen, C., Rogowsky, P., Prior, P., Anaïs, G., Mangin, G., Bazin, B., Nazer, R., and Grimsley, N. 1996. Polygenic resistance of tomato plants to bacterial wilt in the French West Indies Mol. Plant-Microbe Interact. 9:837-842.

8. Yang, P., Wang, Z., Fan, B., Chen, C., and Chen, Z. 1999. A pathogen- and salicylic acid-induced WRKY DNA binding activity recognizes the elicitor response element of the tabacco class I chitinase gene promotor. Plant J. 18:141-149

Roles of the Hrp-Secreted PopA Protein in *Ralstonia solanacearum* Interactions with Plants

F. Van Gijsegem[1], E. Farcy[2], J. Zethof[3], L. Zolobowska[3], and T. Gerats[3,4]

[1] University of Gent, Ledeganckstraat 35, B-9000 Gent, Belgium and Laboratoire de Biologie Moléculaire des Relations Plantes-Microorganismes, INRA-CNRS, BP27, F-31326 Castanet Tolosan Cedex, France; [2] Station de Génétique et d'Amélioration des Plantes, INRA, Dijon, France; [3] VIB Department of Plant Genetics, University of Gent, Ledeganckstraat 35, B-9000 Gent, Belgium; Gerats; [4] Present address: Dept Exp Botany, Univ of Nijmegen, Toernooiveld 1, 6525 ED Nijmegen, The Netherlands

In the interactions between pathogens and their hosts, the molecular cross talk that modulates gene expression in both partners is of crucial importance for the establishment of the disease and for disease resistance. Protein secretion systems play a pivotal role in this dialogue. In particular, the type III secretion systems encoded by the *hrp* genes in most Gram-negative bacterial plant pathogens, are essential both for expression of the disease in susceptible plants and for elicitation of resistance in resistant or non-host plants (reviewed in 4).

In *R. solanacearum*, three proteins are known to be secreted by the Hrp pathway and many other candidates arose from the analysis of the complete genome sequence (Genin, this volume). One of these *R. solanacearum* Hrp-secreted proteins, PopA, is able to elicit a necrotic reaction mimicking the hypersensitive reaction (HR) on certain plants. In all plant species tested so far, reactivity to PopA is associated with resistance to bacterial wilt. In *Petunia*, most lines are reactive to PopA. Pathogenicity tests performed on 2 reactive lines and on the few *Petunia* lines not reactive to PopA also disclosed an association between reactivity and disease resistance (1). This prompted us to analyse both plant responses activated by PopA inoculation and the involvement of PopA reactivity in resistance to bacterial wilt.

Early *Petunia* Responses to PopA

To identify plant genes whose expression is modulated upon treatment with PopA, a transcript profiling analysis was undertaken. A modified cDNA-AFLP procedure generating only one amplified fragment per plant gene was used (reviewed in 3). Leaves of reactive *Petunia* plants were infiltrated with either a PopA-containing bacterial supernatant, the supernatant of an *hrp⁻* mutant or bacterial growth medium alone. At different times after treatment, total plant RNA was isolated, reverse-transcribed into cDNAs and submitted to AFLP analysis. Within the first hour after infiltration, the expression of many genes was already affected by the different treatments. Compared to untreated leaves, numerous genes are activated or, more rarely, repressed in all three treatments by the stress of infiltration. In contrast, only a few genes appeared to be differentially modulated by the supernatant of the *hrp⁻* mutant as compared to the mock inoculation, indicating that active signals present in supernatants are mostly delivered via the type III Hrp system.

Several AFLP fragments corresponding to genes whose expression is activated or repressed specifically by a PopA-containing bacterial supernatant have also been identified. These fragments were sequenced and searches in databases revealed some interesting homologies (see Table 1). Various PopA-modulated AFLP fragments encode proteins showing similarities with the Gag-Pol polyprotein or reverse transcriptase of diverse plant retrotransposons. This indicates that, as was shown in tobacco by using fungal elicitors (7), gene expression of several transposons is activated in the early steps of the defense gene activation pathways in *Petunia*. Another PopA-modulated AFLP fragment exhibits similarities with a family of proteins shown to be implicated in defense pathways, the cystein protease inhibitor family, the more similar protein being the tomato cystatin.

Table 1. Homologies of some cDNA-AFLP fragments modulated by PopA action (E-score given at the protein level)

Fragment	Size	E-score	Homologies
TP3-3	179 bp	10^{-13}	Retroviral protein
TP3-4	165 bp	10^{-11}	Retroviral protein
TP9-9	107 bp	10^{-5}	*Arabidopsis* β-gal like protein
TP12-4	335 bp	10^{-7}	Cystein protease inhibitor *(L. esculentum* cystatin)
TP12-6	120 bp	10^{-4}	*Arabidopsis* putative protein phosphatase
TP13-6	427 bp	10^{-4}	*Arabidopsis* GTP-binding nuclear protein
TP3-12	145 bp	10^{-70}	ABC transporter
TP13-7	424 bp	10^{-12}	*E. coli* MalT

Proteins of this family were shown to be activated in various plants after wounding, herbivory, or attacks by fungi or viruses (reviewed in 5).

Finally, amongst the fragments that were found to be specifically modulated upon infiltration with a PopA-containing supernatant, were several encoding products similar to proteins like phosphatases, GTP-binding proteins, transporters or regulators, which could be involved in signal transduction cascades (Table 1).

Involvement of PopA Recognition in Disease Resistance

The association between reactivity to PopA and resistance to bacterial wilt observed in different plants as well as the genotype-dependence of PopA reactivity found in *Petunia* (1) led us to examine the involvement of PopA recognition in disease resistance in more detail. For that, the genetic determinism of PopA reactivity was analysed and *Petunia* near-isogenic lines differing in the chromosomal region carrying the reactivity locus were constructed.

REACTIVITY TO POPA BEHAVES AS A DOMINANT MONOGENIC TRAIT
LOCATED ON CHROMOSOME IV IN *PETUNIA*

Analysis of an F1 progeny from a cross between a reactive and a non-reactive *Petunia* line showed that both reactivity to PopA and resistance to bacterial wilt are dominant traits. Segregation studies in backcrosses revealed a 1:1 segregation for PopA reactivity indicating that this character is monogenic. AFLP analysis of one BC1 backcross population coupled with the segregation analysis of phenotypic markers allowed us to map the reactivity locus on chromosome IV. The parent lines used in this study are highly polymorpic (~20 polymorphic markers per primer combination) but unfortunately the region encompassing the reactivity locus is not. So, even though 600 AFLP primer combinations were tested, we could identify only one marker closely linked to the reactivity locus (linked at ~1 centimorgan).

REACTIVITY TO POPA IS LINKED TO RESISTANCE
TO BACTERIAL WILT IN *PETUNIA*

To analyze the linkage between reactivity to PopA and resistance to bacterial wilt, near-isogenic lines were constructed by introgressing the PopA reactivity locus into the non-reactive Tr66 line. Loss of the genetic material from the reactive parent was confirmed by AFLP at the BC4 level. This allowed us to choose for the subsequent crosses a plant lacking all markers (out of 100) specific to the reactive parent except for PopA reactivity and the marker closely linked to it. Plants from both a homozygous reactive and a homozygous non-reactive near-isogenic line were soil-infected with *R. solanacearum*. The reactive plants presented only minor symptoms while the non-reactive plants almost all wilted showing that reactivity to PopA is associated with resistance to bacterial wilt.

This result indicates at least a strong linkage between reactivity to PopA and resistance. However, due to the scarcity of recombination events occurring in chromosome IV in the tested cross, no predictions about the size of the region introgressed from the reactive parental line can be made.

MUTAGENESIS OF THE REACTIVITY GENE IN *PETUNIA*

To address the involvement of PopA recognition in disease resistance more closely, mutants impaired in reactivity to PopA and, ideally, cloning of the reactivity gene are needed. To tackle that, we undertook a mutagenesis of a reactive *Petunia* line by using the high copy number *Petunia* endogenous transposon d*Tph1*. This mobile element can transpose at high frequency in some highly mutable *Petunia* lines giving a frequency of mutation that might be as high as 10^{-4} (8). Since the highly mutable line W138 is reactive to PopA, it was crossed with the non-reactive Tr66 line and about 10,000 F1 plants were screened for reactivity. About 100 non-reactive mutant candidates were picked out of this first screening, and their progenies are currently being retested for reactivity. To date, progeny analysis has confirmed the mutation and its heritability for three mutants. All three mutants unfortunately also lost the marker closely linked to the reactivity locus, indicating that these mutations are not caused by a simple insertion of a transposon copy into the reactivity gene but are due to more profound chromosomal rearrangements or maybe even chromosome replacement.

Conclusions

Expression profiling analysis revealed that several *Petunia* genes are modulated very early after infiltration of a PopA-containing supernatant. Among them, the identification of a cystatin homolog can be correlated with the fact that, in transgenic tobacco lines carrying the *popA* gene under the control of a pathogen-inducible promoter, local accumulation of PopA can turn a compatible fungal interaction into an incompatible interaction. This strongly indicates that PopA can mediate the elicitation of plant defense mechanisms sufficiently to restrain fungal pathogens (2).

In most plant species resistance/tolerance to bacterial wilt is polygenic. The only example of resistance determined by a single gene was recently reported *in Arabidopsis thaliana* for the RRS1-R recessive gene (6,

Deslandes *et al.*, this volume). Analysis of our near-isogenic lines showed that in *Petunia*, resistance to bacterial wilt segregates as a dominant single locus. We are currently comparing the *R. solanacearum* infection process in susceptible and resistant *Petunia* lines to determine if resistance might also have an effect on latent infection. The near-isogenic lines exhibiting susceptibility/resistance to bacterial wilt were constructed by selecting for the introgression of the reactivity to PopA, revealing a linkage between reactivity to PopA and resistance. Failure to isolate a non-rearranged non-reactive mutant did not allow us however to assess directly the involvement of PopA recognition in resistance.

Literature Cited

1. Arlat, M., Van Gijsegem, F., Huet, J.C., Pernollet, J.C., and Boucher, C.A. 1994. PopA1, a protein which induces a hypersensitivity-like response on specific *Petunia* genotypes, is secreted vie the Hrp pathway of *Pseudomonas solanacearum*. EMBO J. 13: 543-553.
2. Belbahri, L., Boucher, C., Candresse, T., Nicole, M., Ricci, P., and Keller, H. 2001. A local accumulation of the *Ralstonia solanacearum* PopA protein in transgenic tobacco renders a compatible plant-pathogen interaction incompatible. Plant J. 28: 419-430.
3. Breyne, P., and Zabeau, M. 2001. Genome-wide expression analysis of plant cell cycle modulated genes. Curr. Opinion Plant Biol. 4: 136-142.
4. Cornelis, G.R., and Van Gijsegem, F. 2000. Assembly and function of type III secretory systems. Annu. Rev. Microbiol. 54: 735-774.
5. De Bruxelles, G.L., and Roberts, M.R. 2001. Signals regulating multiple responses to wounding and herbivores. Crit. Rev. Plant Sci. 20: 487-521.
6. Deslandes, L., Olivier, J., Theulières, F., Hirsch, J., Feng, D.X., Bittner-Eddy, P., Beynon, J., and Marco, Y. 2002. Resistance to *Ralstonia solanacearum* in *Arabidopsis thaliana* is conferred by the recessive *RRS1-R* gene, a member of a novel family of resistance genes. Proc. Natl. Acad. Sci. USA 99: 2404-2409.
7. Grandbastien, M.A. 1998. Activation of plant retrotransposons under stress conditions. Trends Plant Sci. 3: 181-187.
8. Maes, T., De Keukeleire, P., and Gerats, T. 1999. Plant tagnology. Trends Plant Sci. 4: 90-96.

A Short History of the Biochemical and Genetic Research on *Ralstonia solanacearum* Pathogenesis

Timothy P. Denny

Department of Plant Pathology, University of Georgia,
Athens, GA 30602-7274, USA

Just over 100 years ago Erwin Frink Smith provided convincing evidence that several bacteria, including what is now called *Ralstonia solanacearum*, are plant pathogens. Since then, many outstanding scientists have studied this important pathogen and have generated a body of research that epitomizes the development of phytobacteriology as a discipline. Up until the early 1950's, most research focused on cataloging the pathogen's distribution and host range, investigating symptomatology, etiology and epidemiology, and developing control practices. In 1953 Arthur Kelman summarized this early research in a monograph (8), a landmark publication that is still useful today. At about the same time, a few researchers began studying the biochemical and genetic mechanisms of *R. solanacearum* pathogenesis. This chapter provides a brief history of this latter era, which I have divided into three parts: the Physiology/Biochemistry Phase (early 1950s to early 1980s), the Genetics Phase (early 1980s to the present) and the imminent Genomics Phase. I hope that readers will gain a general appreciation of how this field has developed, our current status, and where research may be heading in the near future. To save space, citations are limited to the most important review articles and to selected recent publications.

The Physiology/Biochemistry Phase

This approximately 30-year period began with Arthur Kelman's program on the involvement of extracellular polysaccharide (EPS) and plant cell wall-degrading enzymes in disease. It is less commonly known that he isolated the type strain (K60), which has used in so many studies, from a wilting tomato plant in his back yard in Raleigh, North Carolina. Although never losing his passion for *R. solanacearum*, in the early 1960s Kelman graciously made way for Luis Sequeira, who investigated diverse aspects of host-pathogen biology over the next 20 plus years. Two underappreciated legacies of their programs are (i) the many graduate students that went on to distinguished careers and (ii) a large, irreplaceable collection of *R. solanacearum* strains. Other researchers contributed during this phase, but none as consistently or as influentially as these two pioneers.

During this phase many fundamental observations were made and important hypotheses developed about virulence factors and the mechanisms of pathogenesis and wilt induction. This progress occurred despite the relatively limited knowledge concerning plant and bacterial biology. Researchers also had to rely heavily on correlative data, because the experimental methods necessary to critically test hypotheses about the role of potential virulence factors were unavailable. Nevertheless, each time I review this literature I am impressed by how many of the conclusions have been proven correct, and how much those of us who worked primarily during the Genetics Phase built on this foundation. More details concerning this phase are available in several reviews (3, 7, 12).

EXTRACELLULAR POLYSACCHARIDE

EPS was among the first potential *R. solanacearum* virulence factors to be studied. Okabe reported in the 1940's that virulent cultures had mucoid colonies, whereas spontaneous nonmucoid (butyrous) colonies were avirulent. Kelman made a similar observation, and introduced the use of 2,3,5-triphenyltetrazolium chloride (TZC) as a media additive to make the nonmucoid colonies more noticeable. Husain and Kelman found that crude EPS from a broth culture of strain K60 caused tomato cuttings to wilt, as did xylem fluid from infected plants. They also isolated the spontaneous EPS⁻ avirulent mutant, strain B1, and found that its culture supernatant lacked wilt-inducing activity. These authors correctly concluded that wilt is primarily due to a vascular dysfunction caused by copious amounts of EPS produced by the pathogen.

The first biochemical characterization of the wilt-inducing EPS in 1959 found that galactosamine was the predominant sugar. Unfortunately, the inherent difficulties in analyzing complex polysaccharides delayed more precise studies, and it was more than three decades before Orgambide *et al.* reported that the high molecular mass acidic exopolysaccharide made by GMI1000 in culture, now referred to as EPS1 (or EPS I), has a trimeric repeating unit of *N*-acetylgalactosamine, 2-*N*-acetyl-2-doxy-L-galacturonic acid, and 2-*N*-acetyl-4-*N*-(3-hydroxybutanoyl)-2,4,6-trideoxy-D-glucose. Subsequent assays with a EPS1-specific monoclonal antibody showed that diverse *R. solanacearum* strains produce EPS1, or a very similar polysaccharide, in culture and *in planta*. EPS1 normally occurs in association with a mixture of other polysaccharides and noncarbohydrate materials.

PLANT CELL WALL-DEGRADING ENZYMES

Because *R. solanacearum* degrades tissues of herbaceous annuals in the later stages of pathogenesis, Kelman and his students also studied the involvement of the pathogen's extracellular enzymes that could attack plant cell walls. They reported that culture supernatants of K60, although lacking pectate lyase activity, have pectin methylesterase (Pme) and polygalacturonase (Pgl) activities, which could degrade pectin to galacturonic acid. An endoglucanase (Egl; originally referred to as Cx 'cellulase') that releases primarily cellobiose from carboxymethylcellulose also was detected in culture. Cultures of strain B2, a weakly virulent, spontaneous mutant, had more Pgl activity but less Pme and Egl activities than K60, an early indication that more than just EPS1 production is affected in such mutants. The conclusion from these studies, again correct, was that extracellular plant cell wall-degrading enzymes are not involved directly in wilting, but could aid bacterial movement through tissues. The involvement of different proteases and lipases remains poorly studied to this day.

PLANT GROWTH REGULATORS

The leaf epinasty and adventitious root initials seen on tomato plants infected by *R. solanacearum* suggested that there is an auxin imbalance. Serious work on Indole-3-acetic acid (IAA) began with the observation that levels of IAA are higher in infected banana and tobacco plants than in healthy plants and that both K60 and B1 produce IAA in culture. However, the amount of IAA made by *R. solanacearum* in culture is low compared to *Pseudomonas syringae* pathovars that cause hyperplastic symptoms. Although tomato cuttings placed in a solution of IAA and scopoletin (which inhibits destruction of IAA by plant IAA oxidase) at concentrations like those found in plants resulted in disease-like symptoms, experiments with radiolabeled IAA precursors showed that most of the IAA accumulating in infected tobacco plants is of plant origin. Thus, IAA production by *R. solanacearum* does not appear to be a virulence factor, but it remains unclear whether IAA accumulation in tobacco contributes to pathogenesis or disease.

Several research groups examined the possible involvement of ethylene made by *R. solanacearum* in pathogenesis. Although K60 and several other *R. solanacearum* strains produce ethylene in culture, the rates are at least 200-fold less than by some *P. syringae* strains (14), and do not correlate with virulence of the strains on tomato. In addition, most of the ethylene recovered from infected plants probably is made by host tissues. So, as with IAA, ethylene production by *R. solanacearum* does not appear to contribute to virulence.

SPONTANEOUS NONMUCOID MUTANTS

Although spontaneous nonmucoid mutants generally are avirulent, because they are pleiotropic, they could not be used to prove the role of EPS1 in wilt. For example, strain B1, which for many years was the paradigm for all such mutants, makes less Egl, more IAA and Pgl, and is more motile than its K60 parent. An intriguing difference between these two strains is that only B1 elicits a hypersensitive response (HR) when infiltrated into tobacco leaves, where it is rapidly bound to mesophyll cell walls and then enveloped by a pellicle. For over a decade, Sequeira and his coworkers compared K60 and B1 hoping to identify surface components that are responsible for these differences in host response.

The most obvious potential surface components are pili (also called fimbriae) and lipopolysaccharide (LPS) O-antigen side chains. Electron micrographs revealed that K60 cells have few pili whereas some B1 cells are heavily piliated. Unlike K60, B1 cells are aggregated by a hydroxy-proline rich glycoprotein isolated from potato, and also bind more readily to human erythrocytes and tobacco cell walls than do K60 cells. These results suggested that pili-mediated cellular interactions might promote the HR-eliciting ability of B1. However, attempts to prove this hypothesis failed when there was uncertainty regarding the source of purified pili and non-piliated mutants could not be created (but, see Kang *et al.* in this volume).

Early work on LPS also was encouraging, because B1 and some other spontaneous mutants that induced a HR lacked the O-antigen side chain. Mutants were generated that specifically lacked the O-antigen, but contrary to expectations, they did not elicit a HR. Thus, after many years of effort, the biochemical basis of HR-elicitation by B1 remained unknown, and in 1985 Sequeira concluded that "a correlative approach to the problem of HR induction.... is not practical" and that a more direct, genetic approach is necessary (12). Based on my experience with B1 and other spontaneous mutants (see below), I suspect that B1 has a very unusual mutation or, more likely, has suffered additional mutations during storage, and that even now an attempt to understand its unusual abilities probably would fail.

The Genetics Phase

During the 1970s, there was increasing interest in the genetics of phyto-pathogenic bacteria (see Ref. 4 for a thorough review), but progress was hampered by the lack of generally applicable methods to create and characterize mutants and to clone desired genes. Typical of these early years was David Coplin's report in 1974 of chemical mutagenesis to create tryptophan auxotrophs of K60 and the rejection of his manuscript describing natural transformation of K60 with *R. solanacearum* genomic DNA. This decade also saw the earliest work by Christian Boucher and coworkers, who reported in the late 1970s that *R. solanacearum* strains can exchange genetic information, that some strains will accept the RP4 plasmid by conjugation, and that bacteriophage Mu could insert into the genome.

THE HRP PROTEIN SECRETION SYSTEM

The Genetics Phase really began in the early 1980s when Boucher and associates developed a robust transposon mutagenesis procedure for *R. solanacearum*. In 1985, they were among the first in the field of phytobacteriology to identify avirulent transposon mutants that, although not recognized at the time, had insertions in the *hrp* gene cluster that is required for the HR on nonhosts and pathogenesis on hosts. Despite being unable to cause wilt symptoms, *hrp* mutants still invade unwounded tomato roots and spread into the lower stem, albeit at bacterial densities at least 1000-fold lower than the wild type. Recent microscopic observations show that *hrp* mutants also survive less well in stem tissues than do the wild type, suggesting that Hrp-related functions may suppress a resistance response.

A cadre of French researchers has devoted most of the last 15 years to characterizing the *hrp* gene cluster in strain GMI1000, first defining it physically (e.g., mapping genes, delineating transcriptional units, and sequencing DNA) and then investigating its function. Remaining steadily in the vanguard of this research area, they helped establish that *hrp* genes encode a type III protein secretion system similar to that previously identified in some human pathogens, and that *R. solanacearum* requires a Hrp pilus for protein secretion but not for binding to plant cells. GMI1000 secretes at least five potential effector proteins (Pop proteins A, B, C, F1 and F2), and strains that elicit a HR in tobacco also, presumably, secrete AvrA protein. PopA protein elicits a HR-like response when infiltrated into tobacco and some petunia cultivars, whereas PopB and PopC have protein sequence motifs that suggest they are designed to function after introduction into plant cells. However, none of these proteins is required for normal pathogenesis on tomato.

Much has also been learned about how *hrp* genes in GMI1000 are regulated. As in most other phytopathogens, most of the transcriptional units (i.e., 1, 2, 3, 4 and 7) in this gene cluster are repressed in rich media and induced by minimal medium. Unlike fluorescent pseudomonads, *R.*

solanacearum uses an AraB-type transcriptional regulator (HrpB) to control expression of other *hrp* transcriptional units. Recently, the French have pieced together the regulatory cascade upstream of HrpB (PrhA → PrhR + PrhI → *PrhJ* → *hrpG* → *hrpB*) that induces expression of HrpB 15 to 20-fold in response to physical contact with plant cell walls (2). Although intriguing and, so far, unique among phytobacteria, the significance of *hrp* gene regulation in response to plant cells is still unclear. First, all of the regulatory studies have been done in growth media or in cell-suspension cultures rather than in plants. Second, it is only the expression of transcriptional unit 1 (which contains *hrpB*), and not the downstream transcriptional units (2, 3 or 4), that is consistently and significantly increased after plant cell contact. Third, a GMI1000 *prhA* mutant is fully virulent on tomato, hypoaggressive on *Arabidopsis thaliana*, and elicits a delayed and partial HR on tobacco. Several reviews cover aspects of this work, and that in the following sections, in more detail (1, 5, 6, 7, 11).

EXTRACELLULAR VIRULENCE FACTORS

Joining the Genetics Phase a bit later than the French, Mark Schell and I at University of Georgia and later Caitilyn Allen at the University of Wisconsin, used random and targeted mutagenesis of strains AW1 and K60 to test critically whether the putative *R. solanacearum* virulence factors identified during the Biochemistry/Physiology Phase contribute to wilting of tomato plants. The earliest studies focused on the endoglucanase (Egl) and endo-polygalacturonase (PglA, also called PehA), which are the enzymes most likely to attack components of plant cell walls, and found that individually they contribute slightly to virulence. More recently, Allen and her students have shown that PehB, one of the two exo-poly-galacturonases, also contributes slightly to virulence, but that pectin methylesterase is dispensable. Although double mutants (e.g. *egl pglA*, *pehA pehB*) are less virulent than the single mutants, they still cause considerable disease. The role of the combined exoenzymes in virulence is unknown, but inactivation of the type II protein secretion system, which eliminates secretion but not production of the exoenzymes, results in an almost avirulent strain. However, since an unknown number of additional proteins also are secreted by the type II system, the basis of this reduced virulence remains unclear.

The other obvious target for elimination was EPS1. My students used random transposon mutagenesis to find the large *eps* operon, which encodes up to 16 proteins for biosynthesis of EPS1, and a single gene nearby that, for unknown reasons, interferes with EPS1 production, but not *eps* gene expression, on rich media. We originally referred to the *eps* mutants as EPS deficient, because on rich media containing TZC their colonies look different from spontaneous EPS⁻ mutants; this is, however, not due to differences in EPS1 production. These results proved that EPS1 is more important than the individual exoenzymes for AW1 to cause wilt symptoms, and similar work with K60 confirmed this conclusion. A third, complex locus originally thought to be involved in EPS production actually primarily encodes LPS biosynthesis and was later renamed the *ops* locus. The *opsG* locus has at least two genes (*rfbA* and *rfbC*) that encode enzymes required for rhamnose biosynthesis (C. Cheng Kao, personal communication). Inspection of the GMI1000 genomic DNA sequence reveals that most of the other *ops* genes encode enzymes for biosynthesis of the LPS core.

PHENOTYPE CONVERSION

While screening AW1 transposon mutants for loss of EPS, we found colonies that looked identical to spontaneous avirulent mutants and had the same pleiotropic phenotype (loss of EPS, reduced Egl and increased Pgl activities). Genetic tests proved that one of two small loci had been mutated, which meant that the changes in multiple traits were due to simple mutations rather than to a large deletion or multiple mutations as was previously supposed. To indicate that much more than just virulence was affected by mutations in these loci, I proposed that the phenomenon be called phenotype conversion and that the mutants (induced or spontaneous) be designated as phenotype conversion-types. Thus, the first locus studied, which encodes a LysR-type transcriptional regulator, was designated as *phcA* for phenotype conversion. The second locus studied contains the *phcBSR* operon. Phenotype conversion is now a widely accepted term, and I suggest that it only be used when there are changes in *phcA* sequence or PhcA function.

The discovery of the PhcA transcriptional regulator initiated more than 10 years of research at Georgia into PhcA-mediated regulation of *R. solanacearum* genes (10, 11). Many PhcA-regulated genes have been identified, but the total number of genes in the PhcA regulon is unknown. PhcA can act as an activator or a repressor of transcription, and thereby controls expression of traits either positively (e.g., EPS, Egl, Pme, acylhomoserine lactone-mediated quorum sensing) or negatively (e.g., PglA, flagellar motility, siderophore biosynthesis, twitching motility). PhcA may bind directly to a gene's promoter or act indirectly via a downstream signal cascade. The function of PhcA is itself regulated, at least in part, by the Phc confinement-sensing system encoded by *phcBSR*, which both produces and senses the unique autoinducer, 3-hydroxy palmitic acid methylester (3-OH PAME). Thus, when cells do not sense confinement (e.g., at low cell density in liquid culture or in microscopic colonies on agar media) the absence of functional PhcA allows PhcA-repressed genes to be expressed. Confinement sensing results in the generation of functional PhcA, which activates expression of positively regulated genes. The complexity of the Phc confinement-sensing system has thwarted our attempts to understand it completely. For example, we do not know why addition of 3-OH PAME to low-density cultures (< 5 x 10^6 cells per ml) does not cause immediate expression of PhcA-activated genes. It may be that *R. solanacearum* also requires an intracellular signal, possibly related to cellular metabolic status, before it will respond to 3-OH PAME.

Our image of *R. solanacearum* changed drastically with the realization that spontaneous phenotype conversion-type mutants are the result of a genetic error that locks *R. solanacearum* into one of two phenotypic states (but, see Poussier *et al.* in this volume), and that 'wild-type' colonies on agar media are only mucoid because the cells are at high density. Extrapolating what occurs in culture would suggest that there is an *R. solanacearum* 'life-cycle' where cells alternate between low and high cell-density phenotypes. It may be that the low-density form is adapted for survival in soil, whereas the high cell-density form is better at multiplying in plants.

INVASION AND SYSTEMIC COLONIZATION OF TOMATO PLANTS

One prediction of the life cycle model is that, unless *R. solanacearum* multiplies extensively in the rhizosphere, roots will be invaded and initially colonized by bacteria with the low-density phenotype. This hypothesis was supported when inoculation of unwounded tomato roots with mutants specifically lacking EPS1 or Egl showed that loss of these traits had almost no effect on the earliest stages of pathogenesis. However, EPS1 was found to contribute to the subsequent systemic bacterial colonization of stems. Similarly, a mutant lacking the type II protein secretion system is almost unable to colonize roots of tomato plants grown in peat or pine bark-based growth media, and a mutant lacking flagella invades unwounded roots much less frequently than does the wild type (13). Invasion of hydroponically-grown tomato plants is slightly different, since an EPS⁻ mutant invades secondary root axils, but is almost unable to colonize the vascular cylinder. Inoculation of a severed petiole, which it thought to test primarily for the ability of a strain to systemically colonize plants, showed that flagella are unessential *in planta* (13), whereas type-4 pili are important (see Kang *et al.* in this volume). Further work is needed to determine exactly how each of these factors or secretion systems aids invasion and/or colonization.

As bacteria systemically colonize susceptible tissues they again should fluctuate between the two phenotypes, because recently invaded tissues will have low-density pathogen populations while higher pathogen populations will develop in parts of the plant that were invaded earlier. This pattern was observed when quantitative immunofluorescence was used to measure *eps* expression in individual AW1 cells that had been recovered from tomato plant stems at different stages of colonization. Additional experiments to study gene expression *in situ* using a reporter system based on production of green or red fluorescent proteins are ongoing in my laboratory.

The Genomics Phase

The recent publication of the complete GMI1000 DNA sequence (6, 9, Genin *et al.*, this volume) ushered in the newest research phase. Now, anyone with an internet connection can immediately access data that previously would have required months of laboratory work. For example, it became trivial to determine that, in addition to the *hrp* gene cluster, many of the known virulence genes are located on the megaplasmid. The initial annotation also revealed a number of additional genes that, based on knowledge from other bacteria, might be important during pathogenesis.

How will knowing the genomic sequence of *R. solanacearum*, and an increasing number of other bacteria, help our research on the mechanisms of pathogenesis? The most straightforward way to use the DNA database will be as a guide to identify potentially important genes and/or to efficiently create mutants necessary to test whether the attributes in question contribute to virulence. This approach was applied successfully using the incomplete genomic sequence, and it greatly accelerated the research on flagella and type-4 pili. Similarly, if one has cloned promoters that are preferentially expressed *in planta* using a technique like *in vivo* expression technology (IVET), as Darby Brown and Caitilyn Allen are trying to do, then sequence data will simplify studying the attendant gene.

Rather than just providing shortcuts in existing procedures, the real potential in having the genomic sequence is that it makes possible novel approaches to study bacterial gene content and gene expression on a large scale. For instance, minute spots of DNA from every GMI1000 open reading frame (ORF) can be applied to nylon membranes (macroarrays) or glass slides (microarrays), which can then be hybridized either to genomic DNA or to cDNA libraries produced from bacterial mRNA. Genomic DNA probes prepared from other *R. solanacearum* strains, such as those with different host ranges, will reveal the ORFs in GMI1000 that are absent in those strains. This approach could be particularly instructive for *R. solanacearum*, because the high genetic diversity within the species may reflect an unusual degree of genomic plasticity. cDNA probes are useful for determining which genes are controlled by global-acting transcriptional regulators like PhcA or whose expression changes when bacteria are exposed to a new environment.

One negative aspect of DNA arrays is that they are, at least initially, quite expensive to make and to use. In contrast, genes that are coordinately controlled due to similarities in their promoter sequences can be found quickly and inexpensively using computer-aided DNA sequence analysis. The French group has used this approach to identify over 50 potential Hrp-secreted effector proteins based on their probable regulation by HrpB and the presence of encoded amino acid motifs typical of eukaryotic proteins (see Genin *et al.* in this volume). Bioinformatics approaches also can be used for genome-wide comparison of any sequenced bacteria. Comparing the genomes of bacteria that are closely related but inhabit different environmental niches, should separate the less interesting house-keeping genes from the more interesting niche-specific genes. Of course, this approach will be particularly informative once additional strains of *R. solanacearum* are sequenced. Bioinformatics also is essential for proteomics research, where one examines the proteins produced and works backwards to the genes encoding them. This approach is necessary, because sequence analysis alone is still insufficient to predict which ORFs actually encode proteins and when they might be expressed.

The Challenge of Applied Research

A relatively small number of researchers have been responsible for most of the biochemical and genetic research on *R. solanacearum*. I believe that this is appropriate, because compared to scientists that study epidemiology, develop disease management practices, or produce and certify clean seed, those studying basic aspects of pathogenesis have done little to help growers produce a healthier crop or improve their profit margin. However, this goal is much closer than it was a decade ago, and within the next decade we could begin to see tangible benefits of applied biochemical and genetic research.

A potentially serious constraint to applying our knowledge is that most strategies will require releasing transgenic plants. Presently, there is opposition in the United States and Western Europe to the introduction of genetically modified crops. There are some legitimate concerns about releasing genetically modified plants, such as the escape of transgenes into populations of wild species, but many people oppose genetically modified crops for non-scientific reasons. It will be difficult to convince such people, who are accustomed to plentiful, inexpensive food supplies and know little or nothing about agriculture, that the benefit of genetically modified crops may outweigh the potential risks. In developing countries, on the other hand, where agriculture is more personal and only minimal mechanical, chemical or genetic inputs are available, genetically modified varieties with enhanced disease resistance may be more readily accepted. For example, a potato resistant to *R. solanacearum* might be very popular in parts of Africa and South America.

Nevertheless, creating genetically modified crops resistant to *R. solanacearum* for use in developing countries will be difficult. First, because such varieties are unlikely to be profitable, agricultural biotechnology companies probably will not be interested in them. This leaves the public sector to take the initiative and bear the cost, which will be substantial, because one must add to the expense of the necessary research the price of leasing the many patented molecular genetic techniques that are needed to produce genetically modified plants for commercial purposes. Second, even when technically and fiscally possible, genetically modified crops must be agronomically and culturally acceptable where they are to be introduced. Therefore, throughout the process of cultivar development, scientists must work with the intended local growers and eventual consumers to ensure that the final genetically modified variety will be a success. I see the introduction of genetically modified crops as an equal or greater challenge than the scientific research need to produce them, but one that I hope we are capable of meeting.

Literature Cited

1. Boucher, C.A., Gough, C.L., and Arlat, M. 1992. Molecular genetics of pathogenicity determinants of *Pseudomonas solanacearum* with special emphasis on *hrp* genes. Annu. Rev. Phytopathol. 30:443-461.
2. Brito, B., Aldon, D., Barberis, P., Boucher, C., and Genin, S. 2002. A signal transfer system through three compartments transduces the plant cell contact-dependent signal controlling *Ralstonia solanacearum hrp* genes. Mol. Plant-Microbe Interact. 15:109-119.
3. Buddenhagen, I., and Kelman, A. 1964. Biological and physiological aspects of bacterial wilt caused by *Pseudomonas solanacearum*. Annu. Rev. Phytopathol. 2:203-230.
4. Chatterjee, A.K., and Vidaver, A.K. 1986. Advances in plant pathology, Vol. 4. Genetics of pathogenicity factors: application to phytopathogenic bacteria. Academic Press, New York.
5. Denny, T.P. 2000. *Ralstonia solanacearum*--a plant pathogen in touch with its host. Trends Microbiol. 8:486-489.
6. Genin, S., and Boucher, C. 2002. *Ralstonia solanacearum*: secrets of a major pathogen unveiled by analysis of its genome. Mol. Plant. Pathol. 3:111-118.
7. Hayward, A.C. 1995. *Pseudomonas solanacearum*. Pages 139-151 in: Pathogenesis and host specificity in plant diseases: histopathological,

biochemical, genetic and molecular bases. vol. I. Prokaryotes. U.S. Singh, R.P. Singh, and K. Kohmoto, eds. Elsevier Science, Inc., Tarrytown, N.Y.

8. Kelman, A. 1953. The bacterial wilt caused by *Pseudomonas solanacearum*. N.C. Agric. Exp. Sta. Tech. Bull. 99.

9. Salanoubat, M.; Genin, S., Artiguenave, F., Gouzy, J., Mangenot, S., Arlat, M., *et al.* The genome sequence of the wide host-range plant pathogen *Ralstonia solanacearum*. Nature 415:497-502.

10. Schell, M.A. 1996. To be or not to be: how *Pseudomonas solanacearum* decides whether or not to express virulence genes. Eur. J. Plant Pathol. 102:459-469.

11. Schell, M.A. 2000. Control of virulence and pathogenicity genes of *Ralstonia solanacearum* by an elaborate sensory array. Annu. Rev. Phytopathol. 38:263-292.

12. Sequeira, L. 1985. Surface components involved in bacterial pathogen-plant host recognition. J. Cell. Sci. Suppl. 2:301-316.

13. Tans-Kersten, J., Huang, H.Y., and Allen, C. 2001. *Ralstonia solanacearum* needs motility for invasive virulence on tomato. J. Bacteriol. 183:3597-3605.

14. Weingart, H., Volksch, B., and Ullrich, M.S. 1999. Comparison of ethylene production by *Pseudomonas syringae* and *Ralstonia solanacearum*. Phytopathology 89:360-365.

The *Ralstonia solanacearum* Complete Genome Sequence: Outputs and Prospects

S. Genin[1], M. Salanoubat[2], C.J. Gouzy[1], A. Moisan[3], T. Schiex[3], S. Cunnac[1], M. Lavie[1], C. Zischek[1], P. Barberis, and C. Boucher[1]

[1] Laboratoire de Biologie Moléculaire des Interactions Plantes-Microorganismes, INRA-CNRS, BP 27,31326 Castanet-Tolosan, France; [2] Genoscope and CNRS UMR-8030, 2 rue Gaston Crémieux, CP5706, 91057 Evry Cedex, France; [3] Laboratoire de Biométrie et Intelligence Artificielle, INRA-CNRS, BP 27, 31326 Castanet-Tolosan, France

The complete DNA sequence of an organism can now be determined, thereby offering a comprehensive view of all the genes present and permitting prediction of many of its biochemical functions. Even though this methodology has been recently applied to eukaryotic organisms including humans and the model plant *Arabidopsis*, a larger number of complete genome sequences have been determined for diverse prokaryotes. Due to the relative simplicity of their genomes (haploids with a total genome size usually below 8 million base pairs) rapid progress has been achieved. In our effort to unravel the molecular determinants of pathogenicity in *Ralstonia solanacearum* we undertook such an approach in order to develop a comprehensive view of the bacterial functions which play a role in the control of this plant-bacteria interaction. In collaboration with the French genome sequencing center Genoscope we have recently completed the sequencing and annotation of the race 1 strain GMI1000 which Bernard Digat isolated in French Guyana from a wilted tomato plant and which we have used to intensively analyze the molecular determinants that govern pathogenicity. In this report we will summarize the major features of this genome and illustrate how this information can be used as a starting point for further investigations concerning the molecular basis of pathogenicity. More extensive information can be obtained from a recent paper (10).

General Organization of the Genome

A BIPARTITE GENOME

Establishment of the complete genome sequence was done using a shot gun sequencing strategy. The principle of this strategy is illustrated schematically in Fig. 1. In the first step the DNA molecules are randomly fragmented into small pieces and the DNA sequence of each fragment is established. In the second step, partial overlaps between pieces of DNA sequences are used to coherently reassemble the different fragments according to their relative position in the genome, thereby reconstituting the complete genome sequence. The total length of the DNA fragments that were sequenced represented approximately 9 times the total length of the genome, offering sufficient sequence redundancy to accurately reassemble the total sequence into two contigs of 3,716,413 bp and 2,094,509 bp. In addition, fragments were found that overlapped with the two ends of each contig, establishing the circularity of the two DNA molecules. This genomic organization into two DNA molecules and the size of these molecules is in agreement with the two bands obtained from pulsed field electrophoresis of total of unfragmented DNA extracted from strain GMI1000. This work also establishes the average Guanine+Cytosine (G+C) value close to 67%,

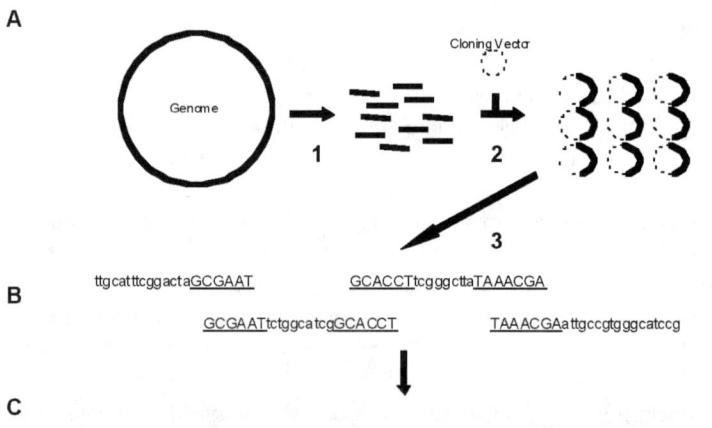

Fig. 1. Schematic representation of the "shotgun sequencing strategy": random DNA fragments from the genome are cloned in a plasmid (A), The sequence of each insert is established (B) and overlaps between individual sequences are used to reassemble the complete genome sequence (C).

336

which is in good agreement with values previously published on the basis of DNA melting temperature analysis (9). Altogether, this length of sequence offers a coding capacity for over 5100 proteins.

Analysis of gene distribution between the two molecules shows that the larger replicon probably encodes all of the genes absolutely essential to sustain life. These include all of the genes required for purine and pyrimidine biosynthesis, and all other absolutely essential genes encoding ribosomal proteins, 3 complete rDNA loci, and 55 identified tRNAs allowing recognition of all possible codons. In addition, the large molecule harbors all of the genes required for DNA replication and cell division. This molecule is therefore probably sufficient to support life of the bacterium and therefore is assumed to be the bacterial chromosome.

Since analysis of the DNA sequence establishes that *hrp* (host response and pathogenicity) genes are located on the smaller molecule, this molecule must correspond to the megaplasmid previously identified in strain GMI1000 (1). However, genes governing amino acid and cofactor biosynthesis are distributed on both replicons. In addition, several chromosomal genes have been duplicated on the megaplasmid, including a complete copy of a rDNA locus with 2 tRNA genes, a gene coding for the alpha subunit of DNA polymerase III, and a gene for the protein elongation factor G. This suggests that the two molecules have co-evolved for a long time in this bacterium and that a process of redistribution of genetic information between the chromosome and the megaplasmid might be in progress.

Mosaic Structure of the Genome

Because of the degeneracy of the genetic code (the incorporation of one particular amino acid within a protein can often be encoded by two or more codons or triplets of three successive bases within a gene) each organism has been able to evolve its own coding preference. The codon usage of an organism, defined as the frequency with which each possible alternative codon is used, is generally considered characteristic for that organism. During the process of genome annotation we found that the codon usage for 7% of *R. solanacearum* genes differs significantly from the standard codon usage for the rest of the genome. Regions in which the codon usage significantly differs from the average *R. solanacearum* codon usage were designated ACURs for Alternative Codon Usage Regions. They are found in 91 distinct loci between 3 to over 20 kb long and having a base composition ranging from 50% to 70% G+C. Most ACURs differ significantly from the average 67% G+C value calculated for the entire genome. Furthermore, ACURs have a tendency to form clusters and are most often found in the vicinity of phages, insertion sequences or other genetic elements such as those encoding Rhs and Vgr proteins generally associated with genetically

337

unstable loci (13). This is an indication that ACURs might have been acquired relatively recently through horizontal gene transfers. In addition these regions may be involved in processes of duplication/evolution which contribute to genetic variability by catalyzing acquisition, loss, or alteration of genetic material. Such genome plasticity is also exemplified by the presence in the genome of a perfect tandem duplication of a 31 kb region flanked by insertion sequences and by the previously described occurrence of genomic deletions in strain GMI1000 (2). Such flexibility of the genome might also be a source of the large genomic diversity observed within *R. solanacearum*, manifested at the biological level in the pathogen's wide host range.

R. solanacearum Has Over 200 Candidate Pathogenicity Genes

In the process of genome annotation (*i.e.* identification of the potential genes and prediction of their corresponding functions), we paid particular attention to potential pathogenicity genes, initially by searching for homologies with proteins known to play a role in pathogenicity in other bacteria-host interactions. Since we had previously established the key role in pathogenicity of the type III protein secretion system (TTSS) encoded by the *hrp* genes (4) we looked for candidate proteins that might be translocated through this system, such as those with sequence homology with other TTSS effectors; proteins having structural features characteristic of proteins from eukaryotes; and regulatory elements in the gene promoters that suggest that transcription of the corresponding genes might be co-regulated with *hrp* genes.

R.SOLANACEARUM ENCODES MANY POTENTIAL ATTACHMENT FACTORS

The *R. solanacearum* genome contains an unusually large number of genes encoding outer-membrane proteins or components of bacterial appendages (pili, fimbriae) potentially involved in attachment of the bacterium to (plant) surfaces. These include genes for type IV pili and for a new type of pilus similar to the Tad pilus of *Actinobacillus actinomycetemcomitans* which is involved in tight adherence to surfaces (8). Interestingly, there are multiple copies of the structural genes for these two types of pili/fimbriae (5 and 8 respectively). In addition, strain GMI1000 caries 28 genes encoding proteins related to various adhesins and hemagglutinins such as the filamentous hemagglutinin (FhaB) of *Bordetella pertussis*, and the HMW1A/ HMW2A adhesins of *Haemophilus influenzae* (7). Among the bacteria which have been entirely sequenced, *R. solanacearum* carries the most hemagglutinin-related proteins, a characteristic that may be correlated with its ability to colonize a wide-range of host plants as well as other environments including soil.

TYPE III TRANLOCATED EFFECTOR PROTEINS

Twenty-nine ORFs (open reading frames) encoding proteins having partial or global homology with Avr proteins found in other plant patho-genic bacteria have been identified in strain GMI1000. These include 3 homologs of the YopJ/AvrRxv proteins, one AvrBs3-related protein (other-wise found only in *Xanthomonas* strains to date) and several avirulence pro-teins from *P. syringae* [AvrE, AvrPpiA1, AvrPpiC2, AvrPphD, AvrPphE, AvrPphF (orf2)]. *R. solanacearum* also carries sequences homologous to genes located in the vicinity of the *hrp* gene clusters of *P. syringae* and *Erwinia amylovora*. Moreover, based on structural features, we have iden-tified several ORFs predicted to encode different repetitive motifs (Leucine Rich Repeats, Ankyrin repeats, and Pirin-like proteins) which may be trans-located into plant cells. Additional candidates with features characteristic of proteins from eukaryotes include an EF-hand Ca^{++} binding protein, serine/threonine protein kinases, and a tyrosine phosphatase.

Figure 2 shows that genes for such candidate effectors are distributed on the two replicons where they have a tendency to form clusters, certain of which have the characteristics of pathogenicity islands (6). Interestingly

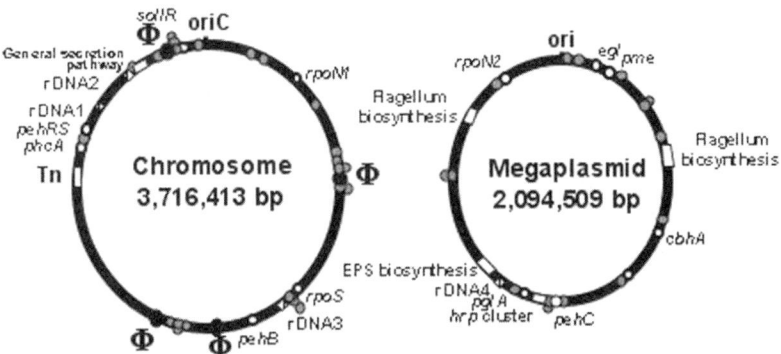

Fig. 2. Structural organization of the *R. solanacearum* genome: the two replicons are represented by circles. Localization of the predicted origins of replication (ori), of the major prophage loci (Φ), of a conjugative transposon (Tn) and and of various additional genes are represented on the maps. The 4 rDNA loci are represented by hatched circles. Dotted circles localize structural genes for candidate type III secreted effector proteins, and additional known pathogenicity determinants are represented by open circles.

enough, certain of the candidate effectors are members of multigenic protein families. For example, three genes encoding proteins related to the YopJ/AvrRxv family (12) are present in strain GMI1000, one of which is probably inactivated by a copy of the insertion sequence (ISRso13). Similarly, at least two families of leucine rich repeat proteins (LRR) have been identified based on the conservation of consensus LRR motifs and five members of a new protein family called AWR (10) have been identified.

ADDITIONAL PATHOGENICITY GENE CANDIDATES

Apart from attachment factors and type III effectors, over 30 additional candidate pathogenicity factors have been identified. These include genes governing production of plant hormones and plant signalling molecules (salicylic acid degradation, ethylene synthesis and degradation, auxin synthesis), resistance to oxidative stress (SOD and hydrogen peroxide reductase), plant cell wall degrading enzymes and synthesis of hemolysins or other RTX toxins.

Conclusions and Future Prospects

It is already clear that knowledge of the complete genome sequence of bacterial pathogens has tremendous potential for advancing our understanding of plant-pathogen interactions. Based on the criteria that are presented in this paper, about 200 candidate pathogenicity genes, including about 50 potential type III-secreted effectors, have been identified. Functional analysis in progress has already established that a large proportion of the candidate TTSS effector proteins actually belongs to the *hrpB* regulon. In addition two of these candidate effectors behave as avirulence proteins towards specific *Petunia* and *Arabidopsis thaliana* genotypes (our own unpublished data) and some of them have a significant effect on aggressiveness of the bacterium towards its hosts.

The development of DNA chips representative of the complete genome is presently under development in our laboratory. These micro arrays will be used to identify additional pathogenicity genes based on transcriptome analysis using various regulatory mutants affected in virulence (see references 3 and 11 for a review).

The complete sequence of the genome and the development of microarrays also offer new means to investigate the genetic diversity within strains of *R. solanacearum* and will hopefully lead to the identification of new genes governing host range and specificity. If such genes can be identified, diagnostic tests for their presence or absence will help determine the pathological potential of individual isolates and will support epidemiological studies.

Because they allow the analysis of the physiology of the organism under diverse environmental conditions, the development of transcriptome analysis through DNA microarrays should also be a valuable tool for analysis of the mechanisms involved in the survival of the bacterium in the environment in the absence of compatible host plants.

Literature Cited

1. Boucher, C., Martinel, A., Barberis, P., Alloing, G., and Zischek, C. 1986. Virulence genes are carried by a megaplasmid of the plant pathogen *Pseudomonas solanacearum*. Mol. Gen. Genet. 205: 270-275.
2. Boucher, C., Barberis, P., and Arlat, M. 1988. Acridine orange selects for deletion of *hrp* genes in all races of *Pseudomonas solanacearum*. Mol. Plant-Microbe Interact. 1: 282-288.
3. Brito, B., Aldon, D., Barberis, P., Boucher, C., and Genin, S. 2002. A signal transfer system through three compartments transduces the plant cell contact-dependent signal controlling *Ralstonia solanacearum hrp* genes. Mol. Plant-Microbe Interact. 15: 109-119.
4. Cornelis, G.R., and Van Gijsegem, F. 2000. Assembly and function of type III secretory systems. Annu. Rev. Microbiol. 54: 735-774.
5. Heidelberg, J.F. *et al.* 2000. DNA sequence of both chromosomes of the cholera pathogen *Vibrio cholerae*. Nature 406: 477-483.
6. Hentschel, U., and Hacker, J. 2001. Pathogenicity islands: the tip of the iceberg. Microbes Infect. 3: 545-548.
7. Jacob-Dubuisson, F., Locht, C., and Antoine, R. 2001. Two-partner secretion in Gram-negative bacteria : a thrifty, specific pathway for large virulence proteins. Mol. Microbiol. 40: 306-313.
8. Kachlany, S.C., Planet, P.J., DeSalle, R., Fine, D.H., and Figurski, D.H. 2001. Genes for tight adherence of *Actinobacillus actinomycetem-comitans*: from plaque to plague to pond scum. Trends Microbiol. 9: 429-437.
9. Palleroni, N.J., Kunisawa, R., Contopoulou, R., and Doudoroff, M. 1973. Nucleic acid homologies in the genus *Pseudomonas*. Int. J. Syst. Bacteriol. 23: 333-339.
10. Salanoubat, M. *et al.* 2002. Genome sequence of the plant pathogen *Ralstonia solanacearum.* Nature 415: 497-502.
11. Schell, M. 2000. Control of virulence and pathogenicity genes of *Ralstonia solanacearum* by an elaborate sensory network. Annu. Rev. Phytopathol. 38: 263-292.

12. Staskawicz, B.J., Mudgett, M.B., Dangl, J.L., and Galan, J.E. 2001. Common and contrasting themes of plant and animal diseases. Science 292: 2285-2289.
13. Wang, Y.D., Zhao, S., and Hill, C.W. 1998. Rhs elements comprise three subfamilies which diverged prior to acquisition by *Escherichia coli*. J. Bacteriol. 180: 4102-4110.

Genes Involved in Early Bacterial Wilt Pathogenesis

Caitilyn Allen, Julie Tans-Kersten, and Enid González

Department of Plant Pathology, University of Wisconsin-Madison, Madison, WI 53706 USA

Ralstonia solanacearum confronts a series of challenges during its life cycle as a plant pathogen and saprophyte. It must survive and compete effectively in the soil, a challenging and diverse environment. To make the transition to the pathogenic phase with its attendant explosive population growth, the bacterium must locate and approach a host rhizosphere, and, once there, it must find a wound or natural opening through which to enter the plant. Inside the root cortex, the pathogen must multiply using the available nutrients, and find the developing protoxylem vessels that lead to its optimal habitat inside the plant. The xylem vessels themselves pose particular challenges. The xylem fluid is not a nutritionally rich environment; the internal pressure is high, and rapid transpirational flow can scatter bacteria, impeding their aggregation and attachment to vessel walls. If the plant recognizes it, the invading bacterium may be killed by inducible antimicrobial defenses. Pit membranes and pit parenchyma cells block passage between adjacent xylem vessels, impeding bacterial spread. Infected vessels are often obstructed by tyloses, gels, and the bacterium's own extracellular polysaccharide (EPS). If the pathogen does multiply successfully, the resulting collapse and death of its plant host creates an environment thick with phenolics and other toxic byproducts of lysed cells. The desiccated dying plant puts the bacteria under water stress. *R. solanacearum* must find a way to escape from the dying plant and re-enter the saprophytic life. As a saprophyte, *R. solanacearum* must also adapt to life in waterways and be able to multiply and thrive in a variety of latent hosts without triggering plant defenses or disease symptoms.

Accumulating genetic evidence suggests that *R. solanacearum* adapts to these different environmental challenges by expressing specific sets of genes during each of its different life phases. An interlocking regulatory cascade that we are only beginning to understand controls expression of these various gene suites (11). Bacterial cell density is a key regulatory signal. When *R. solanacearum* reaches high population densities in culture (possibly corresponding to growth in the confined spaces inside plants), the PhcA global regulator is induced by intracellular accumulation of a novel diffusible quorum sensing signal, 3-OH-PAME (Denny, this volume). Often acting indirectly, PhcA activates transcription of several virulence factors, most notably EPS. This level of gene expression is believed to correspond to the full-blown pathogenesis observed when bacteria reach *in planta* population densities greater than 10^8 CFU/gm.

However, PhcA also represses expression of another regulator, PehSR. This two-component regulator positively controls expression of the bacterium's three extracellular polygalacturonases (PGs), type-4 pili-mediated twitching motility, and flagellar swimming motility (2, 12; Kang, this volume). All of these traits contribute quantitatively to virulence, and none are indispensable for pathogenesis. A *pehSR* mutant strain is quite reduced in virulence, but it still causes symptoms on about 20% of inoculated tomatoes in our assay. Our working model is that these PehSR-dependent traits are expressed at low bacterial population densities, corresponding to saprophytic life and early plant invasion and colonization. They are thus called the early virulence genes.

Degradation of Plant Pectins

EXO-PG PEHC IS CO-TRANSCRIBED WITH A GALACTURONATE TRANSPORTER

R. solanacearum strain K60 produces three extracellular PGs, which hydrolytically cleave the pectic polymers that make up the plant primary cell wall and middle lamella. An endo-PG, PehA (PglA), degrades the polymer internally at random, rapidly macerating plant tissue and releasing large polygalacturonate (PGA) oligomers. PehB, in contrast, cleaves digalacturonate residues from the non-reducing ends of PGA. Virulence assays with site-directed mutants demonstrate that each of these PGs contribute significantly to virulence, with PehA playing a larger role (6). In particular, PehA and PehB help the bacterium colonize host plants (7). We searched the *R. solanacearum* strain GMI1000 genome sequence (10) for sequences resembling known PGs in order to identify and clone *pehC*, which encodes the last of the three PGs. This gene, interestingly located near one end of the *hrp*-type 3 secretion system gene cluster, encodes a 70.35 kDa exo-PG that releases monogalacturonate (galUA) from pectin. Immediately (75 bp) downstream of the *pehC* stop codon is a gene encoding a protein 56% identical to ExuT, a galacturonate transporter found in *E. coli* and in the soft rot pathogen *Erwinia chrysanthemi* (5). A polar insertion in *pehC* resulted in a mutant that was both unable to release galUA from PGA (a *pehC* mutant phenotype) and unable to grow on galUA as a sole carbon source (suggesting loss of transporter function). In contrast, a non-polar insertion in the same location destroyed PehC function but did not affect growth on galUA. These data demonstrate that *pehC* and *exuT* are co-transcribed from a single promoter in an operon.

PEHC DOES NOT CONTRIBUTE TO BACTERIAL WILT VIRULENCE

Strain K60-409, a non-polar *pehC* mutant, was as virulent on tomato as its wild-type parent in both a naturalistic soil-soak virulence assay and in a cut-petiole inoculation assay that introduced bacteria directly into the xylem vessels. We therefore concluded that this exo-PG does not contribute measurably to virulence; the virulence of a triple mutant lacking all three PGs remains to be determined, but we predict that it will not differ from that of a PehA/PehB double mutant. If PehC is not a virulence factor, what then is the biological role of this abundantly-produced extracellular enzyme that specifically degrades a component of plant cell walls?

PECTIC SUBSTANCES AREN'T A SIGNIFICANT NUTRIENT SOURCE *IN PLANTA*

A gentamycin resistance gene insertion in the *exuT* open reading frame produced a mutant strain, K60-T09, which could not grow on galUA or PGA as a sole carbon source, though it still produced all three extracellular PGs. This mutant, which can macerate plant tissue like its parent strain but can no longer uptake and metabolize pectin degradation products, offered the opportunity to test the long-standing hypothesis that PGs contribute to pathogen success in the plant by releasing a valuable nutrient source from plant pectins. However, we found *exuT* mutant K60-T09 was as virulent as its parent strain, effectively refuting the hypothesis that *R. solanacearum* depends on host pectins as an energy source during pathogenesis. These results suggest that the ability to degrade pectic substances down into monomers and metabolize them as an energy source most likely contributes to bacterial fitness during the final stages of pathogenesis or during saprophytic life away from a living host, possibly in the soil.

Regulation of Swimming Motility *in Planta*: A Puzzle

FLAGELLAR MOTILITY IS REQUIRED FOR PLANT INVASION

R. solanacearum has swimming motility conferred by 1 to 6 polar flagella. The ability to move through the environment offers obvious advantages to a soil-borne pathogen that must find and invade host plant roots. We previously demonstrated that a site-directed mutant lacking FliC, the protein that makes up the flagellar filament, is nonmotile, aflagellate, and significantly reduced in virulence in a soil soak assay that required the bacteria to actively locate and invade tomato roots from the soil. However, when this nonmotile mutant was applied directly to cut tomato petioles, it was as virulent as the wild-type parent strain (12). We concluded that pathogen motility contributes to virulence early in bacterial wilt disease development, during host location, invasion and colonization. A future priority is to identify the signal(s) that turn off motility during growth in the host plant.

R. SOLANACEARUM IS NONMOTILE IN THE PLANT

In culture, *R. solanacearum* motility is regulated in response to cell density via the quorum sensing-responsive global virulence gene regulator PhcA. Around 65% of cells are motile at 10^8 CFU/ml, with lower levels of motility at both lower and higher cell densities (3). However, when we measured the motility of bacteria in xylem fluid taken directly from infected tomato stems, we did not observe any motile cells until cell densities reached 10^9 CFU/ml xylem fluid, and even only 5% of the population was motile (12). This result is consistent with the observation that nonmotile mutants are fully virulent when introduced directly into the xylem, but it also suggests that this trait is regulated differently *in planta* than in culture.

MOTILITY IS REGULATED BY PHCA, PEHSR, FLHDC, AND OTHER FACTORS

In enterics, bacterial swimming motility, a complex and expensive trait requiring an estimated 50 gene products, is regulated in a three-level cascade. At the top of this cascade is the master regulator of motility, FlhDC, which is a heterotetrameric transcriptional activator (8). The *R. solanacearum* genome contains homologues of the genes involved in this regulatory cascade, and in order to better understand regulation of motility in this species, we created site-directed *flhDC* mutant K702. K702 was nonmotile, as expected, and was quantitatively reduced in virulence to the same degree as the *fliC* mutant. To better understand the position of *flhDC* in the *R. solanacearum* motility regulon, we inserted the *flhDC* promoter region immediately upstream of a promoterless gus (*uidA*) gene in the broad host range plasmid pLAFR3 and used this reporter gene construct to measure *flhDC* expression under various conditions.

Mutants lacking the PehSR two-component regulator are non-motile, so it was not surprising that there was no detectable *flhDC::gus* expression in a *pehSR* mutant background. This result confirmed that PehSR modulates expression of motility via the transcription of *flhDC*. But in culture at least, *flhDC* expression was not proportional to *pehSR* expression; while expression of a *pehR::gus* fusion decreases steadily as cell density increases, *flhDC* expression increases with cell density. Previously we found that *pehSR* expression increases around 12-fold in a *phcA* mutant background, indicating that PhcA represses expression of *pehSR* at higher cell densities in culture (2). One might therefore predict that a *phcA* mutant would have increased *flhDC* activity at higher cell densities. However, to our surprise, expression of *flhDC::gus* was the same in a *phcA* mutant background as it was in the wild-type parent strain. Thus, our data suggest that *flhDC* does not respond to overexpression of *pehSR*, possibly because of an intervening regulator. These results with regulator::reporter gene fusions are supported by our direct observation that a *phcA* mutant of strain K60 has the same motility phenotype on soft agar plates as the wild-type strain.

We also measured *flhDC::gus* expression in *R. solanacearum* cells extracted from infected tomato plants. Since the bacteria are essentially nonmotile in the plant, we expected that *flhDC* would not be expressed in the plant. However, *flhDC::gus* activity per cell was in fact about 10-fold higher in bacteria growing *in planta* than in those growing in culture. There are several possible explanations for this unexpected finding. Perhaps FlhDC's activity indicates that *R. solanacearum* is paralyzed in the xylem vessel, secreting and assembling flagella but not rotating them. This scenario seems unlikely given that the flagellum is complex and costly to synthesize, and that some evidence suggests that flagellin may trigger plant recognition and defense responses (4). Several bacterial animal pathogens are nonmotile inside the host, and in one system expression of motility in the host destroys virulence, suggesting that motility can be actively disadvantageous to pathogens (1). Alternatively, *flhDC* may be upregulated in the plant because it controls other functions needed during pathogenesis. In addition to motility, in other species FlhDC also regulates secretion through the flagellar basal body, as well as stationary phase and cell division functions (9, 13). In either case, it appears that an intervening regulatory mechanism, either transcriptional or post-transcriptional, prevents the increased *flhDC* expression from inducing motility in planta. Further research is needed to identify the signal or condition in the plant that down-regulates bacterial motility downstream of FlhDC.

Conclusions

Plant pathologists understandably focus on the pathogen traits that are directly responsible for symptoms and economic losses. In the case of *R. solanacearum*, attention has centered on the period of explosive growth in the plant xylem vessel that coincides with plant wilting and death. However, accumulating data are gradually forcing us to develop a broader per-

347

spective on the life of *R. solanacearum*, one that includes its ability to escape a dying plant, survive between hosts, and initiate pathogenesis. These abilities are mediated by interlocking sets of regulons that turn on expression of traits needed in each of the bacterium's several different habitats – and turn off traits that are unnecessary or disadvantageous. Our findings concerning this bacterium's pectin metabolic pathway and its regulation of swimming motility reveal a set of traits that contribute to bacterial fitness in the early stages of pathogenesis or during saprophytic life. We need to develop methods to better measure and understand this obscure but epidemiologically important part of the life cycle.

Literature Cited

1. Akerley, B.J., Cotter, P.A., and Miller, J.F. 1995. Ectopic expression of the flagellar regulon alters development of the *Bordetella*-host interaction. Cell 80:611-620.
2. Allen, C., Gay, J., and Simon-Buela, L. 1997. A regulatory locus, *pehSR*, controls polygalacturonase production and other virulence functions in *Ralstonia solanacearum*. Mol. Plant-Microbe Interact. 10:1054-1064.
3. Clough, S.J., Flavier, A.B., Schell, M.A., and Denny, T.P. 1997. Differential expression of virulence genes and motility in *Ralstonia* (*Pseudomonas*) *solanacearum* during exponential growth. Appl. Environ. Microbiol. 63:844-850.
4. Felix, G., Duran, J.D., Volko, S., and Boller, T. 1999. Plants have a sensitive perception system for the most conserved domain of bacterial flagellin. Plant J. 18:265-276.
5. Haseloff, B.J., Freeman, T.L., Valmeekam, V., Melkus, M. W., Oner, F., Valachovic, M. S., and Francisco, M. J. S. 1998. The *exuT* gene of *Erwinia chrysanthem* EC16: nucleotide sequence, expression, localization, and relevance of the gene product. Mol. Plant-Microbe Interact. 11:270-6.
6. Huang, Q., and Allen, C. 1997. An *exo*-poly-a-D-galacturonosidase, PehB, is required for wildtype virulence in *Ralstonia solanacearum*. J. Bacteriol. 179:7369-7378.
7. Huang, Q., and Allen, C. 2000. Polygalacturonases are required for rapid colonization and full virulence of *Ralstonia solanacearum* on tomato plants. Physiol. Mol. Plant Pathol. 57:77083.
8. MacNab, R.M. 1996. Flagella and motility. Pages 123-145 in: *Escherichia coli* and *Salmonella*: Cellular and Molecular Biology, 2nd ed, vol. I. F.C. Niedhardt, ed. ASM Press, Washington D.C.

9. Prub, B.M., and Matsumura, P. 1996. A regulator of the flagellar regulon of *Escherichia coli*, flhD, also affects cell division. J. Bacteriol. 178:668-674.

10. Salanoubat, M., Genin, S., Artiguenave, F., Gouzy, J., Mangenot, S., Arlat, M., *et al.* 2002. Genome sequence of the plant pathogen *Ralstonia solanacearum*. Nature 415:497-502.

11. Schell, M.A. 2000. Control of virulence and pathogenicity genes of *Ralstonia solanacearum* by an elaborate sensory array. Annu. Rev. Phytopathol. 38:263-292.

12. Tans-Kersten, J., Huang, H., and Allen, C. 2001. *Ralstonia solanacearum* needs motility for invasive virulence on tomato. J. Bacteriol. 183:3597-3605.

13. Young, G., Schmiel, D., and Miller, V.L. 1999. A new pathway for the secretion of virulence factors by bacteria: the flagellar export apparatus functions as a protein secretion system. Proc. Nat'l Acad. Sci USA 96:6456-6461.

Phase Reversion from Phenotype Conversion Mutants to Wild Type May Be Induced in *Ralstonia solanacearum* by a Susceptible Host Plant

S. Poussier, D. Trigalet-Demery, S. Barthet, P. Thoquet, M. Arlat, and A. Trigalet

Laboratoire de Biologie Moléculaire des Relations Plantes-Microorganismes, INRA/CNRS, UMR 215, BP 27, 31326 Castanet-Tolosan, Cedex, France

The phenotype conversion phenomenon in *Ralstonia solanacearum* has long been identified (11) and abundant information is now available about its occurrence and molecular mechanism. Briefly, the wild-type strain undergoes loss of pathogenicity associated with changes in colony morphology (10, 11), motility (5,12) and pathogenicity traits such as impaired exopolysaccharide production (6,10,11), decreased endoglucanase production (13) and increased polygalacturonase production (1,10,15). These pathogenicity determinants are governed by a complex regulatory network under the control of the *phc*A gene, a LysR-type transcriptional global regulator gene (4,14). A working hypothesis states that the phenotype conversion form is a survival state of the pathogen in natural settings, and that some environmental factors induce a reverse shift from phenotype conversion to wild-type. (7).

To address this latter speculation we first generated a series of spontaneous phenotype conversion mutant strains from the GMI1000 wild type strain, or from GMI1557, a constitutive beta-glucuronidase (gus)-expressing derivative of GMI1000 (8). We then screened for appearance of the wild-type form in stem or in the rhizosphere of tomato plants that had been inoculated by the phenotype conversion mutant strains. Finally, we assessed the potential ability of susceptible tomato root extracts to induce the reverse shift from phenotype conversion back to wild-type.

Isolation and Phenotypic Characterization
of Phenotype Conversion Mutants

Wild-type strain GMI1000 of *Ralstonia solanacearum* (a race 1/biovar 3 strain) and its GMI1557 derivative both form ovoid to irregular-shaped smooth colonies with a pink centre when grown on BGT rich medium (peptone 1%, yeast extract 0.1%, glucose 0.5%, triphenyltetrazolium chloride 50mg.l^{-1}, 1.5% agar). Spontaneous phenotype conversion mutant strains were obtained from the two latter strains, according to the Hruschka and Kelman's procedure (1973) at a frequency of 1 in 20, and developed on the same medium as small, round, dark red colonies often surrounded by a translucent halo. The halo was best observed under oblique transmitted light. 116 independent phenotype conversion mutant strains were isolated on the basis of their colony morphology, and their reduced endoglucanase and increased polygalacturonase activities relative to the parent strain.

All phenotype conversion mutant strains were non-pathogenic on the susceptible tomato cv. Supermarmande. Immunofluorescence labelling with EPS-specific monoclonal antibodies (2) showed that all of these phenotype conversion mutant strains were EPS-impaired (EPS^i) or even totally EPS$^-$ when compared to those of the parent strain. They were all stable and retained their phenotype conversion phenotypic traits when cultivated on rich medium, i.e. no conversion from phenotype conversion to wild-type was ever observed even though an average of 50,000 individual colonies were examined over a 2-week period of observation for each phenotype conversion mutant strain, and over subculturing for months.

Characterization of Indels Within the *phc*A Gene

The nucleotide sequence of *phc*A from strain AW1 (GenBank # L19269) was used to design two primers, TGGTACGACAACGAGTGG (phca1) and AAGGAACCCTGCCCGCAC (phca2) to amplify DNA sequences of the *phc*A gene from parent strains and from their related phenotype conversion mutants strains. Agarose gel electrophoresis showed that specific PCR products amplified from parent strains and from 13 phenotype conversion mutant strains clearly differed in size, suggesting that an insertion or a deletion occurred in the *phc*A gene of these 13 phenotype conversion mutant strains. *Alw*1 digestion of the PCR products from the remaining 103 phenotype conversion mutant strains and from parent strains generated six subfragments and revealed changes in mobility in 8 additional phenotype conversion mutant strains. To sum up, differences in mobility in agarose gels identified significant rearrangements in the *phc*A gene in 21 out of the 116 phenotype conversion mutant strains. PCR products corresponding to these 21 *phc*A genes were then cloned and sequenced.

Nucleotide sequence analysis revealed that a 64 bp DNA stretch between nucleotide position 843 and 906 in the *phc*A gene of the pathogenic GMI1557 (GenBank # AF239238) was duplicated in tandem in phenotype conversion mutant strain 9-4c (GenBank accession number AF 239239). In phenotype conversion mutant strain 9-3 an 884 bp additional sequence was inserted at nucleotide 527 of the GMI1559 *phc*A gene. The latter insertion belongs to the IS5 family and IS1031 subfamily; it was named ISRso1 and registered in IS Finder (http::/www.is.biotoul.fr) and in NCBI (Genbank # AF239240).

Nucleotide sequences analyses of the *phc*A genes of 19 phenotype conversion mutant strains originating from GMI1000 led to identification of six distinct deletions ranging from 2 bp to 215 bp in various locations. Two duplications (7 bp and 28 bp) and one single bp change (A to C) occured in the last three phenotype conversion mutant strains. Five phenotype conversion mutant strains harbor the ISRso1 at the unique location 527, as formerly identified in phenotype conversion mutant strain 9-3. Four insertions belonging to the IS3 family were identified in the vicinity of the start codon, as well as one IS4 nearby the stop codon.

Plant-Induced Shift from Phenotype Conversion to Wild-Type in Susceptible Tomato Plants

When inoculated with each of 116 phenotype conversion mutants strains, susceptible tomato plants cultivated in peat pots remained symptomless 21 days after inoculation, whereas inoculation with the pathogenic GMI1000 or GMI1557 strains led to total wilting within 15 days post-inoculation. Phenotype conversion mutant strains were isolated from epicotyls of symptomless plants at densities around 10^5CFU/g dry weight of stem tissue. Unexpectedly, wild-type-like revertants were also isolated at lower densities of an average of 10^3CFU/g dry weight from the same symptomless plants inoculated with some of the phenotype conversion mutant strains under study. Isolation and colony counting from inoculated plants was carried out using the Spiral Plater on rich medium in 14 cm diameter Petri dishes. This method allowed a single specific colony type to be quickly identified among thousands of colonies prior to confluent growth.

An average of 8% of wild-type revertants were identified among approximately 60,000 individual colonies independent experiments from symptomless plants inoculated with phenotype conversion mutant strain 9-4c (64 bp duplication in tandem). Wild-type revertants from phenotype conversion mutant strain 9-3 (with an IS5 insertion) were also isolated at frequencies

353

about 3 x 10^{-3}, which means that we identified only 2 wild-type-revertants out of 130,000 individual phenotype conversion colonies examined. Wild-type revertants were also isolated following inoculation with phenotype conversion mutant strain 99 (with an IS5 insertion) or with the phenotype conversion mutant strain 13 (with an IS3 insertion), both at frequencies about 5 x 10^{-3}.

Plant-Induced Shift from Phenotype Conversion to Wild-Type in Axenically-Grown Plants

To rule out the possibility of an accidental contamination by the wild-type parental strain we conducted additional experiments with tomato grown in axenic conditions. Briefly, tomato seeds were surface sterilised, and allowed to germinate on BG (rich) medium. Germinated seeds were deposited onto 0.8% agar containing Musrashige and Skoog medium in sterile test tubes or in Magenta boxes. Tomato plants at the two-leaf stage were inoculated with a calibrated suspension of a phenotype conversion mutant strain. Sterile water was used to rinse the soft culture medium at 18 days post inoculation before screening for potential wild-type-revertants by plating on rich medium.

To obtain tomato root extracts (TRE), 10 sterile 5 cm long root systems taken from Magenta boxes were soaked in 5 ml of sterile water and sterile-filtered through 0,45μ and 0,22μ membranes successively. Aliquots of freshly prepared TRE were poured onto individual 14 cm diameter rich medium-containing Petri dishes and allowed to dry in a laminar sterile flow cabinet. The rich medium complemented with TRE was used to check for presence of potential wild-type-revertants by the Spiral Plater method.

Wild-type revertants were detected in both the rinsings of the culture medium at 18 dpi, and on rich medium complemented with TRE, from the above-mentioned phenotype conversion mutants, namely 9-4C (64 bp duplication) at frequencies about 4 x 10^{-3}, 9-3 and 99 (IS5 insertion) and 13 (IS3 insertion) at frequencies about 5 x 10^{-4}. No wild-type revertants were ever observed from the four phenotype conversion mutant strains after inoculation of Musrashige and Skoog medium alone or medium only complemented with glucose and incubated for 18 days before plating on BG rich medium in the absence of any TRE. About 130,000 individual colonies were checked for each of the four phenotype conversion mutant strains of interest, which indicates that either these phenotype conversion do not spontaneously revert to wild-type in the absence of TRE, or that spontaneous reversions occurred at frequencies lower than 3 x 10^{-5}. These data strongly suggest that a soluble plant factor induces the shift from phenotype conversion to wild-type at a distance from the root.

All of these four types of wild-type revertants were pathogenic on the susceptible tomato cv Supermarmande and exhibited the phenotypic traits associated with wild-type, such as EPS, endoglucanase and polygalac-turonase production comparable to those of parental strains. DNA sequence analysis of the wild-type revertants will be presented elsewhere. Interest-ingly, the four "tomato-reversible" phenotype conversion mutant strains retained their phenotype conversion phenotypes in the presence of root ex-tracts from Spring Barley cv. Cork and of Celery cv. Géant doré, both of which are non-host plants for *R. solanacearum.*

Conclusion and Prospects

Our data indicate that a variety of DNA rearrangements in the *phc*A gene can be responsible for the phenotype conversion phenotype, and that a com-plete phase variation cycle can occur in *R. solanacearum* from the patho-genic GMI1000 or GMI1557 strains (ON) to nonpathogenic phenotype con-version mutants strains (OFF), and from some phenotype conversion mu-tant strains to reverse pathogenic strains (ON again). Our data suggest a route by which pathogenicity can be switched ON in a non-pathogenic phenotype conversion variant by a soluble inducer at a distance from the root system of a susceptible host plant. In addition preliminary results strongly suggest that some susceptible crops can specifically induce the

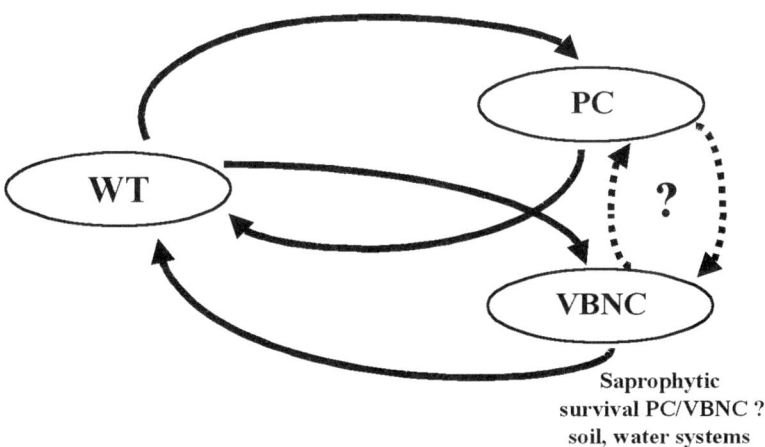

Fig. 1. Working model of reversible conversion from non pathogenic phenotype conversion to pathogenic wild-type and/or from nonculturable VBNC to wild-type.

reversion from phenotype conversion to wild-type while non-host plants do not. Further studies are still needed to identify the chemical nature of the tomato root inducer.

These results as a whole support the speculative hypothesis originally presented by Denny *et al* (1994). In the meantime the discovery of the VBNC in *R. solanacearum* (9,16) will probably boost a revival of interest in the different survival forms of the pathogen in natural settings. Notably, the potential link (Figure 1) which could exist between the phenotype conversion form and VBNC form of biovar 2 strain 1609 is under study in by a collaborative European group. A practical issue from the studies of pathogen survival in naturally-infested fields would be to explore the role of rotation crops and/or of agricultural pratices in inducing potential shifts from pathogenic to non pathogenic forms of *R. solanacearum*. Such studies could lead to recommendations of specific agricultural pratices or use of selected rotation crops by farmers in order to eradicate the pathogenic form from survival niches, avoid regrowth from VBNC, or to minimize phenotype conversion to wild-type.

Literature Cited

1. Allen, C., Huang, Y., and Sequeira, L. 1991. Cloning of genes affecting polygalacturonases production in *Pseudomonas solanacearum* Mol. Plant-Microbe Interact. 4:147-154.
2. Araud-Razou, I., Vasse, J., Montrozier, H., Etchebar, C., and Trigalet, A. 1998. Detection and vizualization of the major acidic eopolysaccharide of *Ralstonia solanacearum* and its role in tomato root infection and vascular colonization. Eur. J. Plant Pathol.104:795-809.
3. Boucher, C., Barberis, P., Trigalet, A., and Demery, D. 1985. Transposon mutagenesis of *Pseudomonas solanacearum*: isolation of Tn5-induced avirulent mutants. J. Gen. Microbiol. 131:2449-2457.
4. Brumbley, S., Carney, B., and Denny, T. 1993. Phenotype conversion in *Pseudomonas solanacearum* due to spontaneous inactivation of PhcA, a putative LysR transcriptional regulator. J. Bact. 175:5477-5487.
5. Clough, S., Flavier, A., Schell, M., and Denny, T. 1997. Differential expression of virulence genes in motility in *Ralstonia* (*Pseudomonas*) *solanacearum* during exponential growth. Appl. Environ. Microbiol. 63:844-850.
6. Denny, T., Makini, F., and Brumbley, S. 1988. Characterization of *Pseudomonas solanacearum* Tn5 mutants deficient in extracellular polysaccharide. Mol. Plant-Microbe Interact. 1:215-223.

7. Denny, T., Brumbley, S., Carney, F., Clough, S., and Schell, M. 1994. Phenotype conversion of *Pseudomonas solanacearum*: its molecular basis and potential function. Pages 137-143 in: Bacterial Wilt: the disease and its causative agent *Pseudomonas solanacearum*. A.C. Hayward and G.L. Hartman, eds. CAB International, Wallingford, UK.

8. Etchebar, C., Trigalet-Demery, D., van Gijsegem, F., Vasse, J., and Trigalet, A. 1998. Xylem colonization by an HrcV- mutant of *Ralstonia solanacearum* is a key factor for the efficient biological control of tomato bacterial wilt. Mol. Plant-Microbe Interact. 9:869-877.

9. Grey, B., and Steck, T. 2001. The viable but nonculturable state of *Ralstonia solanacearum* may be involved in long-term survival and plant infection. Appl. Environ. Microbiol. 67:3866-3872.

10. Husain, A., and Kelman, A. 1958. Relation to slime production to mechanism of wilting and pathogenicity of *Pseudomonas solanacearum*. Phytopathology 48:155-165.

11. Kelman, A. 1954. The relationship of pathogenicity in *Pseudomonas solanacearum* to colony appearance on a tetrazolium medium. Phytopathology 44:693-695.

12. Kelman, A., and Hruschka, J. 1973. The role of motility and aerotaxis in the selective increase of avirulent bacteria in still broth culture of *Pseudomonas solanacearum* J. Gen. Microbiol. 76:1787-188.

13. Schell, M. 1987. Purification and characterization of an excreted endoglucanase from *Pseudomonas solanacearum*. Appl. Environ. Microbiol. 53:2237-2241.

14. Schell, M. 1996. To be or not to be: how *Pseudomonas solanacearum* decides whether or not to express virulence genes. Eur. J. Plant Pathol. 102:459-469.

15. Schell, M., Roberts, D., and Denny, T. 1988. Analysis of the *Pseudomonas solanacearum* polygalacturonase encoded by *pgl*A and its involvement in pathogenicity. J. Bact. 170:4501-4508.

16. Van Elsas, J., Kastelein, P., de Vries, P., and van Overbeek, L. 2001. Effects of ecological factors on the survival and physiology of *Ralstonia solanacearum* bv. 2 in irrigation water. Can. J. Microbiol. 47:842-854.

Insertions in the Avirulence Gene *AvrA* Alter the Virulence of *Ralstonia solanacearum* on *Nicotiana tabacum*

A.E. Robertson[1], B.A. Fortnum[2], W.P. Wechter[1],
T.P. Denny,[3] and D.A. Kluepfel[1]

[1] Department of Plant Pathology and Physiology, Clemson University, 120 Long Hall, Clemson SC 29634-0377. [2] Department of Plant Pathology and Physiology, Pee Dee Research and Education Centre, 2200 Pocket Rd, Florence, SC 29506-9706. [3] Department of Plant Pathology, University of Georgia, Plant Science Building, Athens, GA 30602-7274

Bacterial wilt is a major disease of tobacco in both North and South Carolina, but it rarely occurs on tobacco in Georgia and Florida, although it is common on tomato in tobacco-growing counties there (5,7). We examined the genetic diversity of *R. solanacearum* in the southeastern U.S. using rep-PCR (9). Neighbor-joining tree analysis showed that South Carolina isolates segregated from Georgia, North Carolina and Florida isolates (9). To further investigate this apparent diversity, the avirulence gene *avrA* was cloned and sequenced from selected *R. solanacearum* isolates from the Carolinas and Georgia. Avirulence genes determine race specificity of a pathogen by limiting the range of host cultivars or host species and genera that the pathogenic strain may attack. Therefore loss or inactivation of an avirulence gene often extends the host range of a pathogen to include plants that were previously resistant because they contained the corresponding resistance gene. Here we describe characteristics of *avrA* in the *R. solanacearum* populations of the southeastern U.S. and their correlation with the differences in bacterial wilt incidence between the Carolinas and Georgia/ Florida.

Materials and Methods

Bacterial strains and media. Eighty-eight isolates of *R. solanacearum*, collected from soil and wilted tomato and tobacco plants in the southeastern U.S., were grown on CPG, TTC media (6) or in one-tenth BG broth at 28°C (2).

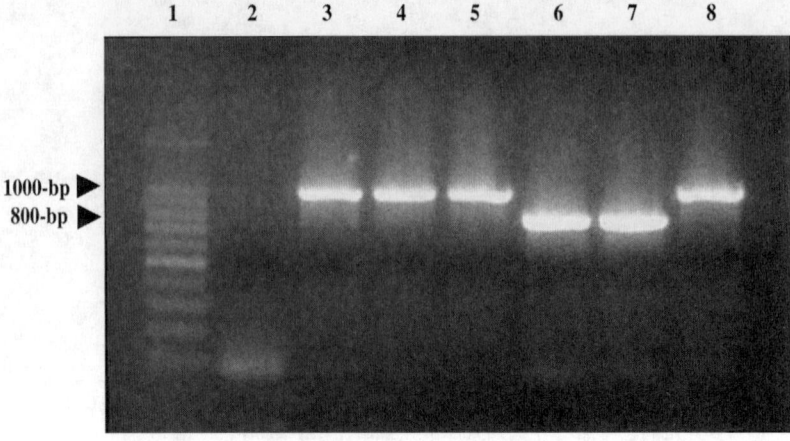

Fig. 1. Amplification of *avrA* from isolates of *Ralstonia solanacearum* from the southeastern U.S. (lane 1 = 100 bp size marker; lane 2 = water control, lane 3 = NC116 , lane 4 = SC06; lane 5 = SC10 ; lane 6 = AW1; lane 7 = K74 ; lane 8 = GA102)

Hypersensitivity and Pathogenicity tests. Leaf infiltration hypersensitivity assays with *R. solanacearum* isolates and transconjugants were performed on fully expanded leaves of tobacco cv. 'K326'(2). Reactions were scored daily for up to four days after inoculation. The pathogenicity of *R. solanacearum* isolates was tested on tomato cv. 'Marion' and tobacco cv. 'K326'. A soil drench method was used to inoculate the seedlings. Wilting symptoms were assessed every three days from seven days after inoculation for a total of 21 days.

Recombinant DNA techniques. Standard methods were used for *R. solanacearum* genomic DNA isolation, plasmid DNA isolation, Southern blotting and hybridization, sequencing, and triparental matings (11). DNA primers were designed to amplify the 5' and 3' ends of *avrA*, and to amplify either end of the 180-bp insertion sequence, IS180-bp.

Results

A radiolabelled copy of the cloned 804 bp *avrA* gene hybridized to a 6-kb *Eco*RI DNA fragment in all *R. solanacearum* strains tested. PCR amplification of *avrA* from each isolate resulted in either a 804-bp fragment or a 984-bp fragment (Figure 1). All isolates that elicited a HR on tobacco, that is necrosis by 16-24 h after inoculation, contained the 804 bp wild-type allele. However, in all HR-negative isolates the *avrA* allele was 984 bp long. Pathogenicity assays on tobacco and tomato revealed a perfect correlation between HR and pathogenicity on tobacco. In all cases, the HR-positive isolates were pathogenic on tomato but avirulent on tobacco, while HR-negative isolates wilted both tomato and tobacco.

MUTANT *AVRA* ALLELES CONTAIN INSERTIONS

The mutant 984 bp *avrA* allele from HR-negative isolates SC06, NC116, and GA102 was cloned, sequenced and compared to the wildtype *avrA* allele from strain AW1 (HR-positive). Two DNA insertions were discovered. A 155-bp insertion was found in GA102, between nucleotides 541 and 542 in the *avrA* gene; this insertion had no homology to any other sequence in the GeneBank database. In SC06 and NC116, a 180-bp insertion was found between nucleotides 455 and 456. A BLASTn search of the GeneBank database revealed a greater than 99% homology to a 171-bp fragment within the 722-bp intergenic region upstream of the *phcA* gene in *R. solanacearum* AW1 (1). Southern blot analysis of *Eco*RI-digested genomic DNA from each of a selection of *R. solanacearum* isolates showed that sequences homologous to this 180-bp insertion were present in multiple copies throughout the genome; it was named IS180. Both of these insertions have characteristics of mobile genetic elements: they are flanked by terminal indirect repeats and have a direct repeat of the insertion site sequence.

EFFECT OF IS180 ON HR AND PATHOGENICITY ON TOBACCO

A plasmid-borne copy of *avrA* was introduced into four strains that are pathogenic on tobacco: SC06, NC116, GA102 and NC25. In each case, the resulting transconjugants all elicited a HR on tobacco and no longer caused wilt symptoms on tobacco. Therefore, *avrA* functioning *in trans* could restrict the host range of these four strains.

Discussion

The incidence of bacterial wilt of tobacco in the southeastern U.S. varies considerably between the Carolinas and Georgia and Florida. Kelman and Person reported in 1961 that Georgia strains of *R. solanacearum* have low virulence on tobacco and that bacterial wilt on tomato does not necessarily indicate a hazard for tobacco or peanut production in that state (7). Our detection of three different *avrA* alleles in 88 strains collected from the southeastern U.S. may explain this phenomenon. Strains with the 804 bp wild-type *avrA* allele were HR-positive on tobacco, whereas strains with either of the modified alleles, 959 or 984 bp, caused only a chlorosis of the infiltrated tobacco tissue 48-96h after inoculation, which eventually developed into necrosis. In addition, strains with either of the modified alleles, 959 or 984 bp, were pathogenic on tobacco. Moreover, strains containing the modified alleles were more prevalent in the Carolinas than in Georgia and Florida and these data correlate well with the observed disease incidence.

Under controlled environmental conditions, all HR-positive isolates were pathogenic on tomato but were avirulent on tobacco, whereas HR-negative isolates wilted both tomato and tobacco. In a study of *R. solanacearum* strains from the French West Indies, most strains developed a typical HR on tobacco; however, they were also pathogenic on tobacco (8). Therefore the characteristics of our strains, HR-positive/pathogenic negative on tobacco, may be unique to the southeastern U.S., but this remains to be verified. Jackson *et al.* showed that *virPphA* in *P. syringae* pv. *phaseolicola* acted as a virulence determinant on bean but as an *avr* gene in soybean (3). Similarly, insertions in the *avrA* locus allow *R. solanacearum* to evade the recognition and defense response of tobacco while remaining pathogenic on tomato. This is not the first report of a DNA insertion in an *avr* gene which expanded a host range. For example, a 104 bp DNA insertion was found in the *avrPphE* gene of *P. syringae* pv. *phaseolicola* race 8, which resulted in virulence on bean cultivars carrying the resistance gene *R2* (12). Kearney *et al.* found an insertion sequence, IS476, in the *avr*Bs1 locus in spontaneous mutants of *X. campestris* pv. *vesicatoria* race 2 that were virulent on normally resistant cultivars of pepper (4).

Bacterial wilt-resistant tobacco cultivars developed for one location may not be resistant to *R. solanacearum* strains found in another location (8) presumably because of differences in environmental conditions and *R. solanacearum* genetic diversity. Here we demonstrate that one specific gene, the *avrA* gene, may play a major role in determining the incidence of bacterial wilt throughout the southeastern U.S. and that insertions in an avirulence gene extend the host range of selected *R. solanacearum* isolates to tobacco.

Analysis of the *R. solanacearum* genome has revealed multiple *avr* genes related to those described in other bacteria (10). Investigation of these loci will aid our understanding of host range and perhaps other ecological parameters such as survival, colonization and competition. Improved understanding of *avr-R* interactions between *R. solanacearum* and susceptible and resistant hosts will provide new insights into *R. solanacearum* pathogenesis and lead to new practical strategies for managing bacterial wilt on tobacco and other crops.

Literature Cited

1. Brumbley, S.M., and Denny, T.P. 1990. Cloning of wild-type *Pseudomonas solanacearum phcA*, a gene that when mutated alters expression of multiple traits that contribute to virulence. J. Bacteriol. 172:5677-5685.
2. Carney, B.F., and Denny, T.P. 1990. A cloned avirulence gene from *Pseudomonas solanacearum* determines incompatability on *Nicotiana tabacum* at the host species level. J. Bacteriol. 172:4836-4843.
3. Jackson, R.W., Athanassopoulos, E., Tsiamis, G., Mansfield, J., Sesma, A., Arnold, D., Gibbon, M.J., Murillo, J., Taylor, C.B., and Vivian, A. 1999. Identification of a pathogenicity island which contains genes for virulence and avirulence on a large native plasmid in the bean pathogen *Pseudomonas syringae* pv phaseolicola. PNAS USA 96:10875-10880.
4. Kearney, B., Ronald, P.C., Dhalbeck, D., and Staskawicz, B. 1990. Characterization of IS476 and its role in bacterial spot disease of tomato and pepper. J. Bacteriol. 172:143-148.
5. Kelman, A. 1953. The bacterial wilt caused by *Pseudomonas solanacearum*, Technical Bulletin, North Carolina Agricultural Experiment Station. Raleigh, North Carolina.
6. Kelman, A. 1954. The relationship of pathogenicity of *Pseudomonas solanacearum* to colony appearance in a tetrazolium medium. Phytopathology 44:693-695.
7. Kelman, A., and Person, L.H. 1961. Strains of *Pseudomonas solanacearum* differing in pathogenicity to tobacco and peanut. Phytopathology 51:158-161.
8. Prior, P., and Steva, H. 1990. Characteristics of strains of *Pseudomonas solanacearum* from the French West Indies. Plant Disease 74: 13-17.
9. Robertson, A.E., Fortnum, B.A., Wood, T., and Kluepfel, D. 2001. Diversity of *Ralstonia solanacearum* in the Southeastern United States. Beiträge zur Tabakforschung International/International Contributions to Tobacco Research 19:319-327.
10. Salanoubat, M., Genin, S., Artiguenave, F., Gouzy, J., Mangenot, S., Arlat, M., *et al.* 2002. Genome sequence of the plant pathogen *Ralstonia solanacearum*. Nature 415: 497-502.
11. Sambrook, J., Fritsch, E.F., and Maniatis, T. 1989. Molecular Cloning: A Laboratory Manual. 2nd Ed. Cold Spring Harbor Laboratory Press. Cold Spring Harbor, NY:
12. Stevens, C., Bennett, M.A., Athanassopoulos, E., Tsiamis, G., Taylor, J.D., and Mansfield, J. W. 1998. Sequence variations in alleles of the avirulence gene avrPphE.R2 from *Pseudomonas syringae* pv. *phaseolicola* lead to loss of recognition of the AvrPphE protein within bean cells and again in cultivar-specific virulence. Mol. Microbiol. 29:165-177.

Ralstonia solanacearum Requires Type-4 Pili for Twitching Motility, Adherence, Natural Transformation, and Virulence

Yaowei Kang[1], Huanli Liu[1], Stéphane Genin[3], Mark A. Schell[1, 2], and Timothy P. Denny[1]

Departments of Plant Pathology[1] and Microbiology,[2] University of Georgia, Athens, GA 30602-7274, USA, and Laboratoire de Biologie Moléculaire des Relations Plantes-Microorganismes, INRA-CNRS, Toulouse, France[3]

Everyone who has taken a bacteriology course knows that many bacteria propel themselves rapidly through liquid media using rotating flagella. It is less widely known that bacteria have other means of locomotion that are independent of flagella, one of which is the relatively slow migration of bacteria over a solid surface, known as twitching motility (4). Although originally named for the jerky, intermittent movement of individual cells that is sometimes observed, twitching motility can result in continuous and coordinated cell movements. A model organism for investigating twitching motility is *Pseudomonas aeruginosa*, whose very active movement results in microscopic colonies having thin, ragged margins with protruding 'spearheads' and groups of cells, called 'rafts', that separate from the colony (9). Macroscopically, twitching motility can result in colonies that enlarge to cover much of the agar surface of a Petri dish.

Both genetic and biophysical data show that twitching motility requires polar, retractile type-4 pili (Tfp) (11). Tfp are flexible filaments, about 6 nm in diameter and up to several micrometers long, composed of many subunits of a single pilin protein monomer. In *P. aeruginosa* over 30 additional proteins are required for assembly, display and function of Tfp (3). Sophisticated microscopic techniques have provided direct evidence that retraction of Tfp, probably by filament disassembly, generates sufficient force to move bacterial cells (5). Tfp also can be important for adhesion, autoaggregation, biofilm formation, horizontal gene transfer, and virulence (8). The gliding motility exhibited by *Myxococcus xanthus* also requires functional Tfp (11).

While developing *R. solanacearum* strains that express green fluorescent protein we observed that microscopic colonies resembled those of twitching motility-positive *P. aeruginosa* strains PAO1 and PAK. We summarize here our results showing that *R. solanacearum* exhibits twitching motility mediated by Tfp and that piliation plays an important role in the interaction of this pathogen with its surroundings (6, 7).

Micromorphology of Colonies Exhibiting Twitching Motility

When isolated colonies of *R. solanacearum* strain AW1 develop on a rich medium containing 1.6% agar they exhibit a remarkable set of micro-morphologies (Color Plate 4). Colonies begin as a small cluster of cells, but after about 15 hours at 30°C they split into rafts that migrate away from one an-other (Color Plate 4a). These rafts often develop multiple irregularly-shaped 'tendrils' that join at their tips, sometimes making a colony that is transiently reticulated (Color Plate 4b). The rafts may instead expand and join at multiple points to give a large, thin colony with multiple spearheads at its margin (Color Plate 4c). Cell density then begins to increase starting near the center of the colony, usually resulting in one or more distinct tiers of bacteria. Up to this point (about 24 to 30 hours), colonies of a wild-type, an extracellular polysaccharide (EPS)-negative mutant, and a *phcA* mutant (a phenotype conversion-type) are indistinguishable. Subsequently, in wild-type colonies twitching motility slows and then stops while cell density and EPS production increase (Color Plate 4d). By the time plates are usually examined at about 48 hours, most or all evidence of twitching motility is obscured. In contrast, colonies of a *phcA* mutant remain relatively thin (they are translucent when triphenyl tetrazolium chloride is not added to the medium) and continue to enlarge for several more days, reaching diameters more than three times larger than that of wild-type colonies.

Colony development of strains K60 and GMI1000 were very similar to that described for AW1. It should be noted that the twitching motility of all of these strains was much less than that of *P. aeruginosa* cultured at the same time. To determine if twitching motility is a characteristic trait of *R. solanacearum*, we examined a selected group of 32 strains from around the world isolated over many years from diseased plants of the major suscep-tible host species. Twenty-five strains exhibited twitching motility similar to AW1, seven strains (six of which were race 3) exhibited lesser motility, and two strains were nonmotile. We believe that the nonmotile strains are probably mutants and that twitching motility is a characteristic of *R. solanacearum* as a species.

Twitching Motility Requires Functional Type-4 Pili

Examination of the GMI1000 genomic DNA sequence revealed a large number of open reading frames (ORFs) that are predicted to encode proteins like those essential for Tfp biogenesis in *P. aeruginosa*. Because there were multiple ORFs that might encode the pilin protein, we initially focused on the putative PilQ and PilT proteins, which should be the highly conserved outer membrane secretin through which the pilus projects, and the cytoplasmic ATPase that energizes retraction of Tfp, respectively. The putative *pilQ* and *pilT* genes were site-specifically inactivated in the genomes of AW1 and K60, and as expected the resulting mutants no longer exhibited twitching motility (Color Plate 5). Although young colonies of the mutants were smaller and more domed than wild-type colonies, these differences were completely (for *pilQ*) or mostly (for *pilT*) eliminated by the time colones were 2 days old. The mutants multiplied normally, produced wild-type amounts of EPS and two enzymes (endoglucanase and endopolygalacturonase), and elicited a normal HR defense response when infiltrated into nonhost tobacco leaves. Thus, neither type II nor type III protein secretion systems were affected by the apparent loss of functional Tfp.

To visualize *R. solanacearum* Tfp and to identify the pilin protein required multiple steps. Because *R. solanacearum* makes polar Hrp pili (10) that could be mistaken for Tfp in electron micrographs, we created an AW1 *hrpY* mutant, which cannot make the Hrp pilin protein, and a AW1 *hrpY pilQ* double mutant that should make neither Hrp pili nor Tfp. Electron micrographs revealed that *hrpY* cells from 1-day old colonies had polar pili, whereas no pili were observed on *hrpY pilQ* cells. Polyacrylamide gel electrophoresis of proteins sheared from the surface of wild-type cells and those lacking one or both types of polar pili (*hrpY*, *pilQ*, and *hrpY pilQ* mutants) showed that production of Tfp correlated with the presence of a 17-kDa protein. After determining the amino acid sequence of an internal fragment of this protein, we ascertained that it was similar to the internal sequence of many type-4 pilins found in the NCBI protein database and thus was likely to be the *R. solanacearum* type-4 pilin.

The ORF for the presumed type-4 pilin was found in the GMI1000 chromosome and its gene designated as *pilA*. A very similar gene is present immediately upstream, and was designated as *plpA* (pilin-like protein A). These two genes appear to be transcribed independently from promoters with a RpoN (sigma[54]) transcription factor binding motif, which was not unexpected, since in *P. aeruginosa* transcription of *pilA* is RpoN-dependent. The putative PilA and PlpA proteins resemble typical type-4A prepilins in every way, except for possibly a longer leader peptide. Inactivation of *pilA* in AW1, K60 and GMI1000 resulted in mutants that lacked the 17-kDa pilin protein and did not exhibit twitching motility. Complementation of the

AW1 mutant with a cloned wild-type copy of *pilA* restored twitching motility. In contrast, inactivation of *plpA* in GMI1000 had no effect on twitching motility. Therefore, we concluded that PilA is the type-4 pilin and PlpA is a pseudopilin.

Tfp are Important for Adherence, Transformation and Virulence

We compared wild-type AW1 to its *pilA* mutant to test whether Tfp promote adherence, as is the case with some other bacteria. In unshaken broth cultures, only AW1 cells formed large three-dimensional aggregates. Similarly, when a strip of clear polyvinyl chloride plastic was inserted into these cultures at the start of incubation, AW1 produced a reticulate biofilm on the plastic surface, whereas the *pilA* mutant formed only scattered clumps of cells. The ability to adhere to each other and to inert surfaces might help *R. solanacearum* to survive in the soil. Aldon *et al.* (1) observed that GMI1000 adheres to suspension-cultured plant cells primarily by one pole and that absence of Hrp pili did not affect this adherence. We similarly observed preferential polar attachment of AW1 bacteria to suspension-cultured tobacco cells and to tomato roots, and found that adherence of the *pilA* mutant was unoriented.

The *pilA* mutant wilted tomato plants more slowly than wild-type AW1 regardless of whether a soil drench was used to inoculate unwounded roots or the inoculum was applied to the stub of a severed petiole. The difference in virulence between the wild type and *pilA* mutant was distinctly less on young, succulent plants (3 weeks from transplanting) than on older, more woody plants (5 weeks old). Because the *pilA* mutant was less virulent even when introduced directly into the xylem of cut petioles, it appears that Tfp have a role inside plants in addition to any that they might have for invasion of roots. Additional experiments will be required to determine if the reduced virulence of the *pilA* mutant was due to altered adherence to plant cells or to a lack of twitching motility, either of which might retard colonization of roots or tissues.

We also found that Tfp are part of the natural transformation in *R. solanacearum*, as they are in many other bacteria. For example, a suicide plasmid that can site-specifically integrate into the *R. solanacearum* genome naturally transformed AW1 but not its *pilA* mutant. However, when the plasmid DNA was introduced into cells by electroporation, an equal number of transformants were recovered for the wild type and the *pilA* mutant.

Twitching Motility Is Indirectly Regulated by the Phc Confinement-Sensing System

As noted above, twitching motility does not stop as early in colonies of a *phcA* mutant as it does in wild-type colonies. Mutations in other known regulatory genes in AW1 (*vsrAD*, *vsrBC*, *xpsR*, *rpoS*, *solR*, *solI*) and GMI1000 (*prhA*, *prhI*, *prhJ*, *hrpG*, *hrpB*), had no effect on twitching motility. These results might be explained by the Phc confinement-sensing system, which is responsible for positively and negatively regulating a variety of genes as *R. solanacearum* cell density increases. In this case, as PhcA becomes fully active in maturing wild-type colonies it appears to down regulate Tfp biogenesis or activity. This hypothesis was supported by our finding that transcription of a *pilA*::*lacZ* reporter fusion in AW1 decreased nine-fold as cell density of a broth culture increased from 3×10^8 CFU/ml to 6.4×10^9 CFU/ml. In contrast, expression of an *esp*::*lacZ* fusion, which is positively regulated by PhcA, increased about 100-fold.

In *P. aeruginosa* expression of *pilA* is positively regulated by PilR and RNA-polymerase holoenzyme containing sigma[54]. Based on its similarity to PilR, Allen *et al.* (2) suggested that in *R. solanacearum* the PehR response regulator might similarly regulate expression of *pilA*. Our finding that *pilA* appears to have a sigma[54]-dependent promoter strengthens this hypothesis. As predicted, inactivating *pehR* in an AW1 *pilA*::*lacZ* strain decreased expression of the reporter fusion 10-fold. Significantly, transcription of *pehR* (and thus *pilA*) is negatively regulated by functional PhcA (2). Therefore, we propose that in young, developing colonies the absence of functional PhcA allows PehR to promote transcription of *pilA*, resulting in Tfp biogenesis and twitching motility. When cells sense confinement (due in part to accumulation of the 3-OH PAME autoinducer) PhcA becomes functional and represses transcription of *pehR* and *pilA*, thereby reducing Tfp biogenesis and twitching motility. Why *R. solanacearum* regulates production of Tfp in this way is still under investigation.

Literature Cited

1. Aldon, D., Brito, B., Boucher, C., and Genin, S. 2000. A bacterial sensor of plant cell contact controls the transcriptional induction of *Ralstonia solanacearum* pathogenicity genes. EMBO J. 19:2304-2314.
2. Allen, C., Gay, J., and Simon-Buela, L. 1997. A regulatory locus, *pehSR*, controls polygalacturonase production and other virulence functions in *Ralstonia solanacearum*. Mol. Plant-Microbe Interact. 10:1054-1064.

3. Alm, R.A., and Mattick, J.S. 1997. Genes involved in the biogenesis and function of type-4 fimbriae in *Pseudomonas aeruginosa*. Gene 192:89-98.
4. Henrichsen, J. 1983. Twitching motility. Annu. Rev. Micro. 37:81-93.
5. Kaiser, D. 2000. Bacterial motility: how do pili pull? Curr. Biol. 10:R777-R780.
6. Kang, Y., Liu, H., Genin, S., Schell, M.A., and Denny, T.P. 2002. *Ralstonia solanacearum* requires type-4 pili to adhere to multiple surfaces and for natural transformation and virulence. Mol. Microbiol., in press.
7. Liu, H., Kang, Y., Genin, S., Schell, M.A., and Denny, T.P. 2001. Twitching motility of *Ralstonia solanacearum* requires a type IV pilus system. Microbiology-UK 147:3215-3229.
8. Manning, P.A., and Meyer, T.F. 1997. Type-4 pili: biogenesis, adhesins, protein export and DNA import. Gene 192:1-198.
9. Semmler, A.B.T., Whitchurch, C.B., and Mattick, J.S. 1999. A re-examination of twitching motility in *Pseudomonas aeruginosa*. Microbiology-UK 145:2863-2873.
10. van Gijsegem, F., Vasse, J., Camus, J.C., Marenda, M., and Boucher, C. 2000. *Ralstonia solanacearum* produces Hrp-dependent pili that are required for PopA secretion but not for attachment of bacteria to plant cells. Mol. Microbiol. 36:249-260.
11. Wall, D., and Kaiser, D. 1999. Type IV pili and cell motility. Mol. Microbiol. 32:1-10.

Understanding the Molecular Basis of Bacterial Wilt Disease: A View from the Inside Out

Darby Brown and Caitilyn Allen

Department of Plant Pathology, University of Wisconsin-Madison, Madison, WI 53706 USA

The ability of a bacterium to cause disease is determined by complex interactions among many different gene products, each contributing to the bacterium's ability to persist and multiply within the host and/or in the environment. Much work has been done to identify and elucidate the functions of *Ralstonia solanacearum* virulence factors during plant pathogenesis. Specifically, we know that the global regulator PhcA regulates expression of many virulence factors in response to changes in bacterial cell density (12). Additionally, a separate host-contact-induced regulatory pathway mediated through PrhA and HrpB controls the expression of the type III secretion system and its presumptive secreted virulence factors, whose identities and functions are only beginning to be explored (2). While it is apparent that these two regulatory pathways play a crucial role in the development of bacterial wilt disease, we do not know the identity of every gene product regulated by PhcA and PrhA/HrpB. Moreover, it is likely that many functions necessary for virulence are not controlled by either of the two known regulatory cascades. Thus, our understanding of the molecular basis of bacterial wilt disease is incomplete and limited, and our existing knowledge and expectations tend to constrain our search for additional virulence genes. Fresh approaches are needed to identify all the traits that function together to bring about one of the world's most destructive plant diseases.

The lack of a comprehensive understanding of the physiological and genetic factors involved in *R. solanacearum* pathogenesis may be due in part to the approaches used to identify these genes. Most of the research to identify *R. solanacearum* virulence factors has involved screening mutants for loss of virulence. The non-pathogenic mutant is then isolated and the corresponding gene is identified through complementation experiments. Loss-of-function analyses fail to detect genes with subtle phenotypes, and are especially problematic since successful pathogenesis relies on the presence and interaction of many gene products; most with redundant and/or additive functions. However, standard plant virulence assays often fail to detect loss of additive or redundant virulence factors. Therefore, we decided to develop an alternative approach that does not rely on loss of function and/or lack of pathogen virulence.

The IVET Approach

This technique, known as an _in vivo_ expression technology (IVET) screen, is designed to specifically identify bacterial genes necessary for successful growth _in planta_ and pathogenesis (reviewed in 4,5,8). IVET uses the host itself as a selective medium that supports only the growth of strains containing plant-induced promoters. Briefly, a library of potential promoter-containing DNA fragments are cloned upstream of a promoterless copy of a gene that is absolutely required for the pathogen to grow in the host. The promoter-trapping plasmid containing the library is introduced into a pathogen strain that carries a deletion in this absolutely required gene, so that growth and/or pathogenesis can occur only if genetic complementation occurs. Additionally, a reporter gene (usually, _gfp_, _lacZ_ or _uidA_) is present on the vector to allow for detection of promoter activity both in

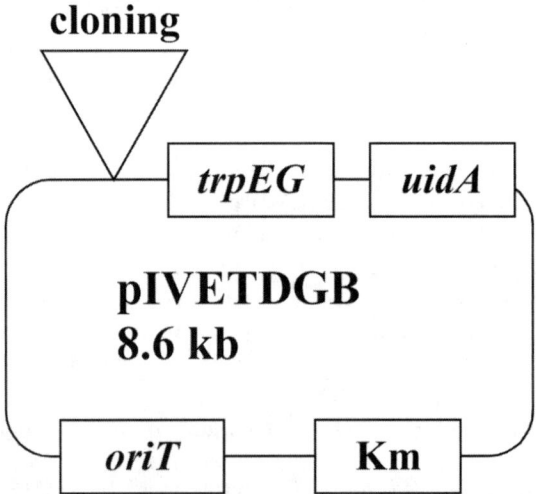

Fig. 1. Integrative promoter-trapping vector pIVETDGB, derived from pVO155 (11). Random chromosonal fragments ranging from 1-5 kb are cloned into the polylinker to create transcriptional fusions to the promoterless _trpEG_ and _uidA_ genes. pIVETDGB is 8.6 Kb and cannot replicate in _R. solanacearum_.

and out of the host-plant. The promoter-trapping vector is usually derived from a plasmid that does not replicate in the bacterial host, so that the vector must integrate into the bacterial chromosome by homologous recombination. To screen for host-active promoters, the strains containing the integrated vector are pooled and then inoculated into the host. After a given time period, the complemented bacteria, which were able to multiply *in planta*, are retrieved from the host and screened for constitutive promoter activity using the second reporter gene described above. Once strains containing specifically host-induced promoters are identified, the sequence of the corresponding gene is obtained and the identity and function of the gene and its product are determined.

Our IVET screen makes use of an integrative, promoter-trapping vector, pIVETDGB (Figure 1), to select for host-induced promoters that can drive the expression of a promoterless tryptophan biosynthetic gene (*trpEG*). The important features of pIVETDGB include the *ori*T, which allows pIVETDGB to be introduced into an *R. solanacearum trpEG* deletion mutant by triparental conjugation. Additionally, a kanamycin resistance gene allows the initial selection of integrants as well as facilitating extraction of bacteria from the plant tissue after the screening step. The promoterless *trpEG* locus was cloned upstream of the promoterless *uid*A (gus) reporter gene. The promoterless *uidA* gene allows an output screen for the undesired constitutive promoters (those that are active under both *in planta* and free-living conditions).

We will conduct an initial IVET screen by pooling several hundred integrants and inoculating them directly into susceptible tomato seedlings via the cut petiole. Preliminary experiments indicate that with this inoculation method, 1000 bacteria are enough to reliably kill a tomato; thus, pools containing 100 or more strains can be applied to a single plant. After 72-96 hours, the bacteria will be isolated from the plant tissue and screened on plates containing X-gluc to differentiate between genes that are presumably plant-induced and those that are constitutively expressed. This screen is based on the assumption that bacteria that are recovered from the host plant were able to multiply effectively in the host, and that this multiplication was driven by an active promoter cloned upstream of the promoterless *trpEG* locus. Sequencing primers on either side of the promoter library-cloning site, together with the use of recently completed *R. solanacearum* genome sequence (11), will allow rapid identification of active promoter sequences.

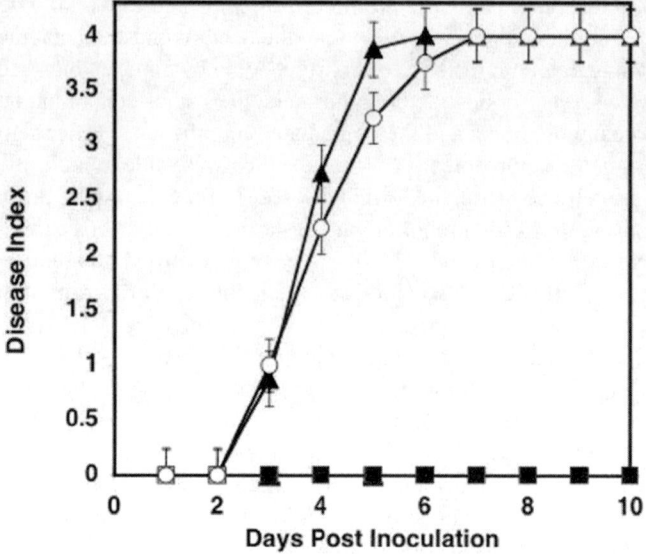

Fig. 2. Virulence of various IVET strains: 20 day-old tomato seedlings were petiole-inoculated with 2000 CFU/petiole. Plants were rated daily for disease symptoms. Triangles: K60 (wild-type strain); Circles: K909/ pIVET::PtrpEG (IVET + a 550 bp *trpEG* promoter region cloned upstream of *trpEG*); Squares: K909 (Δ*trpEG*). Each point represents the mean of three independent assays; each assay contained eight plants for each treatment.

Tryptophan Biosynthesis is Necessary for Growth and Virulence

TrpE and TrpG are the large and small subunits of anthranilate synthase, respectively. Anthranilate synthase is the enzyme that catalyzes the first dedicated step in the biosynthesis of the essential amino acid tryptophan (10). We specifically deleted the *trpEG* locus of *R. solanacearum* strain K60 and replaced it with a gentamycin resistance gene cassette. This Δ*trpEG* mutant, called K909, is unable to grow in tobacco or tomato plants and is completely avirulent on tomato (Figure 2). This result demonstrates that *R. solanacearum* must be able to synthesize tryptophan to cause disease, suggesting that this amino acid is a limiting factor for bacterial multiplication in the xylem tissue.

The growth and virulence defect of strain K909 can be restored to wild-type levels by the integration of a construct containing the *trpEG* promoter cloned upstream of the promoterless *trpEG* locus in pIVETDGB (Figure 2). Moreover, the promoters of *pilA*, *flhDC*, and *hrpB*, which are known to be expressed *in planta*, can also rescue the avirulent phenotype of K909 if they are cloned upstream of the promoterless *trpEG* locus in pIVETDGB. In contrast, if the *pilA* promoter or the *trpEG* promoter are cloned in the opposite orientation with respect to the *trpEG* ORF, the resulting construct cannot rescue the avirulent phenotype of K909. Taken together, these control data suggest that our IVET screen should effectively identify plant-induced promoters in a library of random chromosomal fragments cloned into pIVETDGB upstream of the promoterless *trpEG* locus and integrated into the chromosome of K909. The resulting information should prove useful for understanding the identity, function and interactions of additional *R. solanacearum* virulence factors.

Expected Outcomes and Limitations

IVET has successfully identified host-induced genes in many microbes, including such plant-associated bacteria as *Xanthomonas campestris, Rhizobium meliloti, Pseudomonas putida, Pseudomonas syringae,* and *Pseudomonas fluorescen*s *(*1,3,6,7,9*)*. Interestingly, many of the genes identified to date by IVET in these organisms have unknown functions. Other host-induced genes identified by this approach include those involved in general bacterial metabolism, secretion, stress response, and regulation, as well as previously known virulence genes, which provide a useful internal control. Not surprisingly, these lists of host-induced genes indicate that successful pathogenesis, symbiosis, or root colonization relies on many genes acting in concert to obtain required nutrients, evade defense responses, survive drastic environmental changes, colonize the rhizosphere, and control populations of competing microbes in the soil. Although the initial temptation may be to study single potential virulence genes tagged by an IVET screen, a thoughtful global examination of all host-induced genes has the potential to define precisely the biochemical environment experienced by the bacterium growing in or near a host plant.

While IVET can successfully find host-induced genes using the host as the selective medium, there are a few drawbacks to this approach. First, the strength of the IVET screen relies on the stringency of the screen through the host, and this stringency depends in part on the relative strength of the promoters and their level of activity within the host environment. We may fail to identify some promoters that are active in the host because they are not strong enough to drive the expression of the *trpEG* locus, or because the promoters may be only transiently expressed. To identify those promoters that are transiently active, a modified IVET screen called RIVET has been developed (13). However, our control experiments indicate that even the promoter of a relatively weakly-expressed regulatory gene like *flhDC* (which encodes a transcriptional activator of the motility regulon) can drive sufficient expression of *trpEG* to restore virulence and growth to *trpEG* mutant strain K909.

Additionally, the library of putative promoter fragments must be complete, giving a 99% probability that the active promoter is within 1000 bp of the fusion junction (i.e. the cloned fragment and the reporter gene). The number of clones necessary to achieve this high coverage is about 70,000. Therefore, pooling bacterial strains for plant inoculation is essential to efficiently handle large numbers. However, because the strains are pooled, strains with very active promoters may out-compete those with less active promoters, and so the population of bacteria obtained from the plant may be biased towards the strains with the most active promoters. Other techniques, such as microarray technology, can also be used to identify host-induced genes. Microarrays have the further advantage of identifying genes that are down-regulated in the host, while IVET strictly identifies genes that are up-regulated in the host. A complementary microarray approach to find *R. solanacearum* genes for which expression is altered in the plant is currently underway (J. Elphinstone and S. Simpson, pers. comm.).

Finally, by introducing pooled integrants directly into tomato xylem vessels via cut petioles we are unlikely to identify pathogen genes that are only induced in the first stages of wilt disease development, during root invasion and early colonization. A different screening method must be designed to find this set of genes.

Although some limitations exist, there are many advantages to using IVET. In addition to the identification of *R. solanacearum* genes that are induced in the host-plant under *in vivo* conditions, the IVET vector also can be used to monitor the relative activity level of various promoters under different conditions without the need for additional molecular manipulations because the *uidA* gene is present in the vector and is thus expressed whenever the promoter of interest is active. Additionally, there are many other applications (some realized, some yet to be realized) of the IVET system. For example, comparing the specific gene expression profiles between bacteria multiplying in resistant and susceptible plant cultivars may provide insight into the biochemical nature of plant resistance. IVET also may be used to find genes necessary for soil survival, and genes upregulated during latent infection of tolerant or weed hosts. Using IVET in different strains of the pathogen may provide insight into the unique host-interaction genes found among the highly heterogeneous strains that make up the *R. solanacearum* species complex. Overall, we expect that IVET will not only help us to identify additional specific *R. solanacearum* virulence genes, but that this approach will also improve our global understanding of what it takes to be a successful plant pathogen.

Literature Cited

1. Boch, J., Joardar V., Gao, L., Robertson, T.L., Lim, M., and Kunkel, B. 2002. Identification of *Pseudomonas syringae* pv. *tomato* genes induced during infection of *Arabidopsis thaliana*. Mol. Micro. 44: 73-88.

2. Brito, B., Aldon, D., Barberis, P., Boucher C., and Genin, S. 2002. A signal transfer system through three compartments transduces the plant cell contact-dependent signal controlling *Ralstonia solanacearum hrp* genes. Molec. Plant Micro. Interac. 15: 109-119.

3. Lee, S., and Cooksey, D.A. 2000. Genes expressed in *Pseudomonas putida* during colonization of a plant-pathogenic fungus. Appl. Environ. Micro. 66:2764-2772.

4. Mahan, M.J., Heithoff, D.M., Sinsheimer, R.L., and Low, D.A. 2000. Assessment of bacterial pathogenesis by analysis of gene expression in the host. Annu. Rev. Genet. 34: 139-164.

5. Merrell, D.S., and Camilli, A. 2000. Detection and analysis of gene expression during infection by *in vivo* expression technology. Phil. Trans. R. Soc. Lond. B. 355:587-599.

6. Oke, V., and Long, S.R. 1999. Bacterial genes induced within the nodule during the *Rhizobium*-legume symbiosis. Mol. Micro. 33:837-849.

7. Osbourne, A.E., Barber, C.E., and Daniels, M.J. 1987. Identification of plant-induced genes of the bacterial pathogen *Xanthomonas campestris pathovar campestris* using a promoter-probe plasmid. Embo J. 6: 23-28.

8. Rainey, P.B., and Preston, G.M.. 2000. *In vivo* expression technology strategies: valuable tools for biotechnology. Curr. Opin. Biotech. 11:440-444.

9. Rainey, P.B. 1999. Adaptation of *Pseudomonas fluorescens* to the plant rhizosphere. Environ. Micro. 1:243-257.

10. Romero, R.M., Roberts, M.F., and Phillipson, J.D. 1995. Anthranilate synthase in microorganisms and plants. Phytochemistry. 39: 263-276.

11. Salanoubat, M.S., Genin, S., Artiguenave, F., Gouzy, J., Mangenot, S., Arlat, M., *et al.* 2002. Genome sequence of the plant pathogen *Ralstonia solanacearum*. Nature 415:497-502.

12. Schell, M.A. 2000. Control of virulence and pathogenicity genes of *Ralstonia solanacearum* by an elaborate sensory array. Annu. Rev. Phytopathol. 38:263-292.

13. Slauch, J.M. and Camilli, A. 2000. IVET and RIVET: use of gene fusions to identify bacterial virulence factors specifically induced in host tissues. Methods Enzymol. 326: 73-96.

Bacterial Wilt Diseases of Banana: Evolution and Ecology

M. Fegan

Cooperative Research Centre for Tropical Plant Protection,
Department of Microbiology and Parasitology, The University
of Queensland, St. Lucia, Queensland, Australia

Bacterial wilt diseases continue to be major limiting factors to cultivation of banana. Three diseases, moko, bugtok (also known as tibaglon and tapurok),and blood disease, have been described as being caused by *R. solanacearum* or the closely related blood disease bacterium (BDB). Moko disease was first recognized in Trinidad in the 1890s (17) and the disease is now known to be endemic in Central and South America and is also present in the southern Philippines. Bugtok disease is only known in the Philippines and was first reported in the mid-1960s (16) although it has probably been present in the Philippines since the early 1950's (19). Blood disease is restricted to Indonesia and was first recognised in the islands close to Sulawesi in 1906.

For a detailed description of the diseases, see reviews by Stover (20), Jeger *et al.* (13) and Thwaites *et al.* (22). Here I will discuss the evolutionary relationships among the causal agents of the diseases and their relationship to the epidemiology and ecology of bacterial wilts of *Musa*.

Diseases Caused by *R. solanacearum*

EVOLUTIONARY RELATIONSHIPS AMONG MOKO DISEASE-CAUSING STRAINS IN CENTRAL AND SOUTH AMERICA

The first analysis of the evolutionary relationships of *R. solanacearum* race 2 strains was that of Cook *et al.* (6) using restriction fragment length polymorphism (RFLP). *R. solanacearum* race 2 strains were found to belong to three multi-locus genotypes (MLGs), MLG 24, MLG 25 and MLG 28. These groupings were found to correlate with the geographic origin of the strains; MLG 24, Central America; MLG 25 Columbia and Peru; MLG 28, Venezuela. This grouping of *R. solanacearum* race 2 strains into the three MLGs is mirrored in the new phylotyping scheme proposed by Fcgan and Prior (this volume). In this scheme all race 2 strains belong to phylo-type II; all MLG 24 strains cluster together in sequevar 3; all MLG 25 strains cluster together in sequevar 4, and all MLG 28 strains cluster in sequevar 6. However, the genetic diversity of race 2 strains may be greater than these three multi-locus groups. Granada (11) indicates that there are more MLGs of *R. solanacearum* race 2 strains and Prior and Fegan (this volume) have also identified strains causing moko disease that do not belong to MLG 24, 25 or 28.

Prior to the subdivision of *R. solanacearum* race 2 strains into MLGs, strains of *R. solanacearum* causing moko disease were classified by their pathogenic and cultural characteristics (see Table 5.1 in Thwaites *et al.* (22) and Table 1).This nomenclature for subdivision of *R. solanacearum* race 2 strains is still in use today. However, this means of subdividing moko dis-ease-causing strains does not match the genetic grouping of strains (Table 1). Strains identified as "SFR" (small fluidal round colony form, insect transmitted) are found in MLGs 25 and 28. The strains identified as "D" (causing leaf distortion and slow wilting of banana) belong to MLGs 24 and 25. In contrast, the strains designated as "B" (large elliptical colony form, rapid wilt of banana, not commonly insect transmitted) are present in

Table 1. Characteristics of strains of race 2 adapted from Thwaites *et al.* (22), French and Sequeira (9) and Fegan and Prior (this volume)

Strain Type[a]	Distribution[a,b]	Characteristics[a]	Ecology[a]	MLG[b,c]
SFR (Small fluidal round)	Central America, Venezuela, Colombia, Caribbean	Small fluidal round, slight formazan pigment	Highly pathogenic Insect transmission high, soil trans-mission low	25, 28
B (banana rapid wilt)	Central and South America, The Philippines	Large elliptical colonies, slight formazan pigment	Highly pathogenic Insect transmission low, soil trans-mission high	24
D (Distortion)	Costa Rica, Surinam, Guyana	As for B above	Low pathogenicity for banana/ plan-tain / heliconia	24, 25
H	Costa Rica	As for B above	Pathogenic for plan-tain but not banana	24

[a] From Thwaites *et al* (22).
[b] From Fegan and Prior (this volume).
[c] From Cook and Sequeira (5).

MLG 24 only, as are the strains classified as "H" (slightly pathogenic on plantain but not pathogenic to banana). The phylogenetic work of Prior and Fegan (this volume) showed that isolates of MLGs 24 and 25 are closely related to each other. MLG 28, by contrast, is relatively distantly related to MLGs 24 and 25. Given that strains classified as SFR are present in MLGs 25 and 28 it is conceivable that these strains may have differing properties including survival in soil and host range. As yet no work addressing the potential differences in strains representing each MLG has been undertaken. Strains belonging to MLG 28 have been isolated from naturally infected tomato (Prior and Fegan, this volume). There is an urgent need to confirm this important finding.

MOKO AND BUGTOK DISEASES: ARE THEY ONE AND THE SAME?

The symptoms of insect transmitted moko disease on the cooking banana variety bluggoe (ABB) and bugtok disease on the cooking banana varieties Saba or Cardaba (ABB or BBB) are very similar. In both bugtok and insect transmitted moko disease of bluggoe the symptoms are first seen in the flower buds or peduncles which become blackened and wrinkled. The bacterium spreads to the fruit and causes a rot. In insect transmitted moko disease of bluggoe, systemic invasion of the rhizome is typically incomplete and the disease is essentially one of the fruit raceme (3); the same is true of bugtok disease (14). However, there are differences in the symptomatology of these two diseases later in the infection.

Eden-Green (8) first proposed that strains causing moko and bugtok diseases in the Philippines were indistinguishable; the information confirming this hypothesis is summarised below. Both moko and bugtok disease-causing strains of *R. solanacearum* from the Philippines cluster with the moko disease-causing isolates belonging to MLG 24 (sequevar 3) (Prior and Fegan, this volume). Molecular fingerprinting studies have demonstrated that bugtok disease-causing strains and moko disease-causing strains from the Philippines share the same fingerprinting patterns. Using the same molecular typing techniques these Philippine bugtok and moko disease-causing strains are most closely related to moko disease-causing strains from Honduras (15); Bagsic-Opulencia, Raymundo and Fegan, unpublished data). Therefore, bugtok and moko disease are caused by the same *R. solanacearum* strains in the Philippines and are most closely related to MLG 24, "B" strains from Honduras. As bugtok disease has been known in the Philippines since the early 1950s (19), moko disease was probably introduced into the Philippines from Honduras at that time, contrary to the widely accepted view that it was introduced in the late 1960s (4). It is unlikely that moko disease originated in the Philippines and was then introduced into Central and South America, because the genetic diversity of the pathogen is greatest in Central and South America and the genetic diversity of a pathogen is generally accepted to be greatest where the organism originates.

As the symptoms of bugtok disease of cooking banana in the Philippines are extremely similar to the insect transmitted moko disease of cooking banana in South America and both moko and bugtok diseases in the Philippines are caused by the same strains of R. *solanacearum*, I suggest that the diseases are one and the same. The slight differences in symptomatology later in the disease are probably due to differences in the banana genotype and the interaction of the pathogen with this varying host genotype. Bluggoe is considered an ABB genotype plantain whereas Saba and Cadaba are BBB genotype plantains, although this requires confirmation (1).

As mentioned above the insect transmitted bugtok disease-causing strains belong to MLG 24. Therefore all genetic groups of R. *solanacearum* race 2 (MLGs 24, 25 and 28), given the correct conditions, contain strains that are insect transmitted. Although it seems to be commonly accepted that the B-type strains of MLG 24 are transmitted only via root-to root contact these strains have been described by Stover as oozing from diseased peduncle cushions and can therefore be insect transmitted (20). Insect transmission of the B strain is more common on bluggoe (ABB) than it is on banana (AAA) (20). It seems that insect transmission of moko disease (including bugtok) is commonly associated with bananas of the ABB (or in the case of 'Saba' and 'Cardaba' in the Philippines BBB) genotype. It is interesting to postulate that insect transmission of R. *solanacearum* race 2 strains is more a consequence of the interaction of the host and the bacterium than just a property of the strain infecting the plant. If this is the case, then the classification of insect transmitted strains of R. *solanacearum* race 2 as 'SFR' strains is flawed and actually confuses the issue of the relative virulence of strains by subdividing them based upon phenotypic traits which, as pointed out by French and Sequeira (9), are not stable.

Given that the "insect transmitted" and "soil transmitted" phenotypes of R. *solanacearum* race 2 strains have the same genetic background this has potential implications for the control measures used for these supposedly different variants of R. *solanacearum* race 2. For the "insect transmitted" variant a 6 month fallow period is recommended and for the "soil transmitted" variant a 12 month fallow period. If there is no discernible difference in the genotype of these organisms then the fallow period for "insect transmitted" strains may need to be extended. At the very least more work needs to be done on the strains from each of the three genetic groups to identify any difference in their survival in the field.

Blood Disease: Convergent Evolution?

The literature addressing blood disease or the BDB is not large. Most reviews on the disease still quote the work of Gäumann (10) from the 1920s when describing the pathology of the disease and the host range of the pathogen. Research addressing such questions as host range/alternative hosts, disease ecology, and even pathogen biology are sadly lacking.

The BDB is phenotypically and genotypically distinct from the *R. solanacearum* strains that cause moko disease. The BDB is a member of phylotype IV (Fegan and Prior, this volume) and is closely related to other members of the *R. solanacearum* complex from Indonesia, whereas the strains of *R. solanacearum* race 2 belong to phylotype II. *R. solanacearum* race 2 moko disease causing strains and the BDB are two different organisms causing similar diseases (7). It has been reported that *Musa balbisiana* (BB) and *Pelipita* (ABB) which have some resistance to moko disease are susceptible to the BDB (18), confirming that the organisms causing these diseases are different. However, there still seems confusion in the literature as to the exact nature of these organisms and misnaming of the BDB as *R. solanacearum* could lead to confusion with *R. solanacearum* race 2 strains. The symptomatology of blood disease is almost exactly the same as insect transmitted moko disease; in fact the symptoms are so similar that Wardlaw (23) concluded that the two diseases are caused by the same organism. As originally proposed by Eden-Green in 1994 (8) until the BDB is formally described it is vitally important that it should be known as "the BDB" or "BDB" to avoid any confusion which may lead to incorrect naming of the organism in legislation.

Because of the similarity of symptoms of blood disease and moko disease and the close evolutionary relationship between the two causative organisms it seems that similar diseases have evolved in two different continents (21). Questions as to the similarities of the genetic basis for the two diseases should be answered in order to understand the evolution of pathogenicity.

Recently blood disease has spread rapidly across the Indonesian archipelago and is now present from West Java to Irian Jaya (Supriadi, this volume). This disease was confined to Sulawesi from its discovery in 1916 until 1987, probably due to a quarantine order on the movement of bananas from Sulawesi from the time the disease was discovered. However, blood disease is now known throughout Indonesia. The reasons for this rapid movement of the disease are not known. Possibly since the quarantine was broken on Sulawesi in 1987 (8) and the bacterium became established in Java it has spread naturally throughout the Indonesian archipelago due to a lack of effective quarantine. It is also possible that a more pathogenic variant of the BDB has emerged. Research is urgently required to help answer these questions.

Future Prospects

We still know very little about the ecology of *R. solanacearum* race 2 in its natural environment. Are there reservoirs of these organisms yet to be discovered? Some observations suggest the presence of weed hosts for strains of *R. solanacearum* that cause wilting of banana (2) but what is the importance of this finding with respect to persistence of strains in soil and transmission to banana? Are there any other 'new' hosts of *R. solanacearum* race 2 strains? The work of Prior and Fegan (this volume) indicates that other hosts such as pothos and anthurium may harbor these organisms. Hunt (12) also indicates the potential for *Dieffenbachia* and tannia to be hosts. All of these plants are aroids (Araceae). Are aroids, many of which originate from South America, natural hosts of *R. solanacearum* race 2?

Within MLG 24 strains there appear to be strains with varying pathogenicity. Strains are reported to vary from severe wilting of banana to those causing only disease in plantain but not banana (9). These results need to be examined in the light of the genetic evidence and if these strains are in fact different, we should further investigate the genetic mechanisms of pathogenicity of these strains.

With the development of diagnostic tests for the different genotypes of *R. solanacearum* that cause moko disease (Prior and Fegan, this volume) we may now be in a position to answer some of these questions about ecology and pathogenicity. It is hoped that future research into the pathogens causing moko disease will fill the many gaps in our knowledge of a subject on which little has been published since the 1970s.

We know little about the epidemiology and ecology of the BDB. How widespread is the pathogen in naturally occurring *Heliconia* and *Musa* spp.? Are there any other alternate hosts such as weeds? How long does the pathogen survive in soil? Does the pathogen associate with the root systems of non-host plants? It is obvious that in-depth studies on the epidemiology of the disease need to be carried out. The observations of Gäumann in the early 1900's that the bacterium can infect a plant via the stigma of the female flower need to be confirmed as this will affect control measures for the disease.

Molecular diagnostic tests specific for this organism need to be developed to accurately resolve the ecological and epidemiological questions posed above as well as for the accurate identification of diseased material. The BDB is now known to be as close to Australia as Irian Jaya and as close to Singapore and Malaysia as the Kempar district of Riau Province in Sumatra (18). The rapid spread of this disease across Indonesia should serve as a warning to all countries in South East Asia.

Literature Cited

1. Anonymous. 1999. Workshop on banana cultivar names in and synonyms in Southeast Asia. Infomusa 8:37-39.
2. Berg, L.A. 1971. Weed hosts of *Pseudomonas solanacearum* (SFR strain) causing banana bacterial wilt. Phytopathology 61:1314-15.
3. Buddenhagen, I., and Kelman, A. 1964. Biological and physiological aspects of bacterial wilt caused by *Pseudomonas solanacearum*. Annu. Rev. Phytopathol. 2:203-230.
4. Buddenhagen, I.W. 1986. Bacterial wilt revisited. Pages 126-143 in: Bacterial wilt disease in Asia and the South Pacific: proceedings of a workshop, PCARRD, Los Banos, Philippines, 8-10 October 1985, edited by G. Persley. ACIAR Press, Canberra.
5. Cook, D., and Sequeira, L. 1994. Strain differentiation of *Pseudomonas solanacearum* by molecular genetic methods. Pages 77-93 in: Bacterial Wilt: the Disease and its Causative Agent, *Pseudomonas solanacearum*, A.C. Hayward and G.L. Hartman, eds. CAB International, Wallingford, UK.
6. Cook, D., Barlow, E., and Sequeira, L. 1989. Genetic diversity of *Pseudomonas solanacearum*: detection of restriction fragment polymorphisms with DNA probes that specify virulence and hypersensitive response. Mol. Plant-Microbe Interact. 2:113-121.
7. Cook, D., Barlow, E., and Sequeira, L. 1991. DNA probes as tools for the study of host-pathogen evolution: The example of *Pseudomonas solanacearum*. Pages 103-108 in: Advances in Molecular Genetics of Plant-Microbe Interactions. H. Hennecke and D.P.S. Verma, eds. Kluywer Academic Publishers, Dordrecht.
8. Eden-Green, S.J. 1994. Diversity of *Pseudomonas solanacearum* and related bacteria in South East Asia: new direction for moko disease. Pages 25-24 in: Bacterial wilt: the disease and its causative organism, *Pseudomonas solanacearum*, A.C. Hayward and G.L. Hartman, eds. CAB International, Wallingford, UK.
9. French, E.R., and Sequeira, L. 1970. Strains of *Pseudomonas solanacearum* from Central and South America: a comparative study. Phytopathology 70:506-512.
10. Gäumann, E. 1921. Onderzoekingen over de bloedziekte der bananen op Celebes I. Mededeelingen van het Instituut voor Plantenziekten No. 48.

11. Granada, G., Howell, M, and Cook, D. 1993. Genotypic variation in Columbian isolates of *Pseudomonas solanacearum* race 2 determined by RFLP analysis. Phytopathology 83:1404.

12. Hunt, P. 1987. Current Strategies for moko control in Grenada: technical and logistical constraints. Pages 121-129 in: Proceedings of the Conference on Improving citrus and banana production in the Caribbean through phytosanitation. St. Lucia West Indies 2-5 December 1986. CTA/CARDI, Wageningen.

13. Jeger, M.J., Eden-Green, S.J., Thresh, J.M., Johanson, A., Waller, J.M., and Brown, A.E.. 1995. Pages 3117-3381 in: Banana diseases. In Bananas and Plantains. S. Gowen, ed. London: Chapman and Hall.

14. Molina, G.C. 1996. Integrated management of 'Tibaglon,' a bacterial fruit rot disease of cooking bananas under farmer's field. Philippine Phytopathol. 32:83-91.

15. Raymundo, A.K., Aves-Ilagan, Y, and T.P. Denny, T.P. 1998. Analysis of genetic variation of a population of banana infecting strains of *Ralstonia solanacearum*. Pages 56-60 in: Bacterial Wilt Disease: Molecular and Ecological Aspects. P. Prior, C. Allen, and J. Elphinstone, eds. Springer Publishing, Berlin.

16. Roperos, N.I. 1965. Note on the occurrence of a new disease of cooking banana in the Philippines. Coffee Cacao J. 8:135-136.

17. Rorer, J.B. 1911. A bacterial disease of bananas and plantains. Phytopathology 1:45-49.

18. Setyobudi, L., and Hermanto, C. 1999. Rehabilitation of cooking banana farms: base line status of banana disease bacterium distribution in Sumatera. Pages 117-120 in: Advancing Banana and Plantain R & D in Asia and the Pacific: Proceedings of the 9th INIBAP-ASPNET Regional Advisory Committee meeting held at South China Agricultural University, Guangzhou, China - 2-5 November 1999, A.B. Molina and V.N. Roa, eds. INIBAP, Los Banos.

19. Soguilon, C.E., Magnaye, L.V., and Natural, M.P. 1994. Bugtok disease of cooking bananas: 1. Etiology and diagnostic symptoms. Philippine Phytopathol. 30:26-34.

20. Stover, R.H. 1972. Banana, Plantain and Abaca diseases. Commonwealth Mycological Institute Surrey, England.

21. Stover, R.H., and Espinoza, A. 1992. Blood disease of bananas in Sulawesi. Fruits 47:611-613.

22. Thwaites, R., Eden-Green, S.J., and Black, R. 2000. Diseases caused by bacteria. Pages 213-239 in: Diseases of Banana, Abaca and Enset. D.R. Jones, ed. CABI Publishing, Wallingford UK.

23. Wardlaw, C.W. 1972. Banana diseases, 2nd Ed.. Longman, London.

Comparative Genome Plasticity of Tomato and Banana Strains of *Ralstonia solanacearum* in the Philippines

A.K. Raymundo[1], M.E. Orlina[1], W.A. Lavina[1], and N.L. Opina

[1] Institute of Biological Sciences and [2] Institute of Plant Breeding, University of the Philippines Los Baños, College, Laguna, Philippines

Ralstonia solanacearum causes bacterial wilt, the most widespread and destructive disease of solanaceous crops and bananas in the warm temperate and tropical areas of the world. In the Philippines it causes tremendous losses of bananas and solanaceous crops, especially tomato (11). Use of resistant varieties, quarantine and sanitation are the best strategies to reduce yield losses.

R. solanacearum is a pathogen of great diversity. This diversity causes problems, especially in breeding for resistance, where strain diversity likely explains the difficulty of breeding universally resistant lines. Tomato-infecting strains in particular have high genetic diversity (4, 6). In contrast, banana bugtok and moko strains are almost genetically homogeneous (8), based on hybridization with seven probes and PCR experiments using rep primers in 94 banana strains of *R. solanacearum* collected in 1989-92. No differences in fingerprints were observed except when repetitive elements were used as probe (9) and in Rep-PCR where there was a second haplotype which was not exclusive to either moko or bugtok strains (8).

We compared the genomic plasticity of the banana and tomato strains. Although earlier results suggested that the banana strains are highly homogeneous and the tomato strains highly diverse, new sets of isolates were obtained to confirm the result. Plant samples showing symptoms of bacterial wilt were collected from the southern region of the Philippines (2), using standard isolation procedures and pathogenicity testing. (2, 8). Genomic DNA isolation and PCR using REP and RAPD primers were as described (3, 6). DNA fingerprint banding patterns were compared by aligning the bands and scoring for the presence (1) or absence (0) of a band along a lane. Cluster analysis was used to generate a dendrogram showing the relationships among the strains (8).

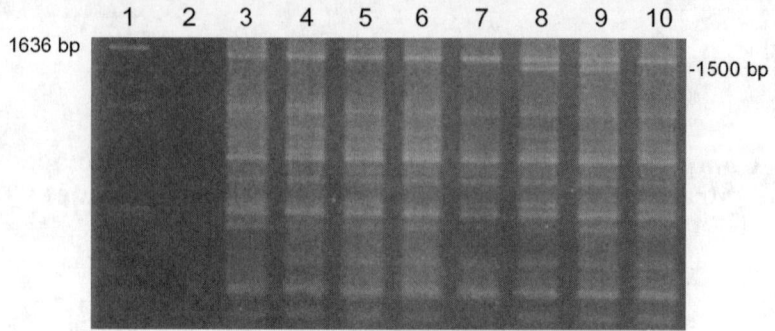

Fig. 1. Rep-PCR banding patterns of new isolates of Philippine banana infecting strains of *Ralstonia solanacearum* collected 1995-2000. Lane 1: 1 Kb Ladder; Lane 2: negative control (no template); Lane 3: positive control (Bu24W, bugtok isolate); Lane 4: BuTK4; Lane 5: BuTK3; Lane 6: BuTK5; Lane 7: BuTK6; Lane 8: BOFA 1; Lane 9: BOFA 2; Lane 10: BAMP 12. (Lanes 4-10 are all bugtok isolates)

Banana Isolates

In 1995 – 2000, we isolated a total of 81 new isolates of *R. solanacearum* from *Musa* plant samples showing symptoms of bacterial wilt or fruit hardening from the southern part of the Philippines (2). All of the isolates induced wilting on yellow plum tomato plants 5 to 12 days after inoculation (DAI). They were all confirmed to be *R. solancaearum* by PCR using the species-specific primer set 759/760 (7). The DNA of all the isolates were also amplified using the Philippine banana strain specific primer M114 (2) except the isolate from the plant abaca (*Musa textiles*) (2).

Among the three rep-PCR primers, REP was used in the study because only this primer set detected polymorphism among local banana strains (2). Of the 81 isolates, 73 were found to have genetic profiles similar to that of the reference strains Bu24W and MoD6 (2) while seven possessed an extra band at about 1500 bp (Fig. 1). These seven strains, which were isolated from the Cardaba variety of banana, came from BPI, Bago Oshiro, Davao. This result confirms the very low variability of the banana strains, which are considered almost monomorphic. The isolate from *Musa textiles* (abaca) produced using a REP primer genetic fingerprint that was completely distinct from the banana isolates of *R. solanacearum*.

Tomato Strains

There was a very high degree of diversity in the 53 tomato strains gathered from different parts of the Philippines from 1975-1995 and analyzed by PCR using RAPD Operon primers OPD-11, 13 and 18. At a similarity level of 50%, there were 17 clusters (Fig. 2). With a few exceptions, most of the isolates belonged to biovar 3. While geographic clustering of strains could be discerned, the Bukidnon strains were classified into seven clusters and the Laguna isolates into five clusters, underlining the highly diverse nature of the tomato strains.

To study the effect of host genotype on the variability of the tomato strains, ten *R. solanacearum* strains were inoculated to seven tomato cultivars with varying levels of resistance. These strains had different degrees of virulence. Four strains, T151, T280, T290 and T523, were considered more virulent based on their ability to cause a greater number of wilted plants among resistant cultivars. One month after inoculation, the pathogen was reisolated from the wilted plants. DNA from three isolates obtained from each of five plants belonging to the seven varieties for each of the four more virulent strains was extracted and subjected to REP-PCR. No changes in fingerprints were observed among the reisolated strains from the susceptible varieties. Only those reisolated from plants inoculated with strains T280 and T523 from moderately resistant and resistant cultivars showed variability. The rest of the study, however, focused on the most virulent strain, T523.

DNA fingerprinting using REP-PCR of strain T523 produced 31 bands ranging from 0.2 Kb to over 6 Kb in size from most of the reisolates. However, a mutant strain isolated from a moderately resistant variety (L-180) had an extra 0.3 Kb and a missing 0.7 Kb fragment.

To determine if there was any change in virulence, T523 (the wild type strain), T523-726 (a reisolate from L-180, a moderately resistant plant, which has the same fingerprint as the wild type and T523-731 (the mutant isolate) were inoculated individually to the same set of tomato cultivars used in the initial test. Wilting was observed in the susceptible plants (Yellow Plum and L-390) four days after inoculation (DAI) with the mutant isolate T523-731. At 10 DAI, it also caused wilting of 92% and 100 % of the resistant cultivars C 108 and 508, respectively. An average of 68% wilting was obtained for all resistant cultivars and 74% for moderately resistant cultivars. In contrast, the wild type strain T523 and the other isolates T523-726 wilted susceptible plants 7 DAI. The isolates elicited 8.33 - 16.6% wilting of lines C 108 and 508, respectively. The wild type strain and T 523-726 wilted 3% and 4% of the resistant cultivars, respectively, one month after inoculation. The genomic fingerprints of the reisolates were determined by REP-PCR. The haplotype of all isolates obtained from sus-

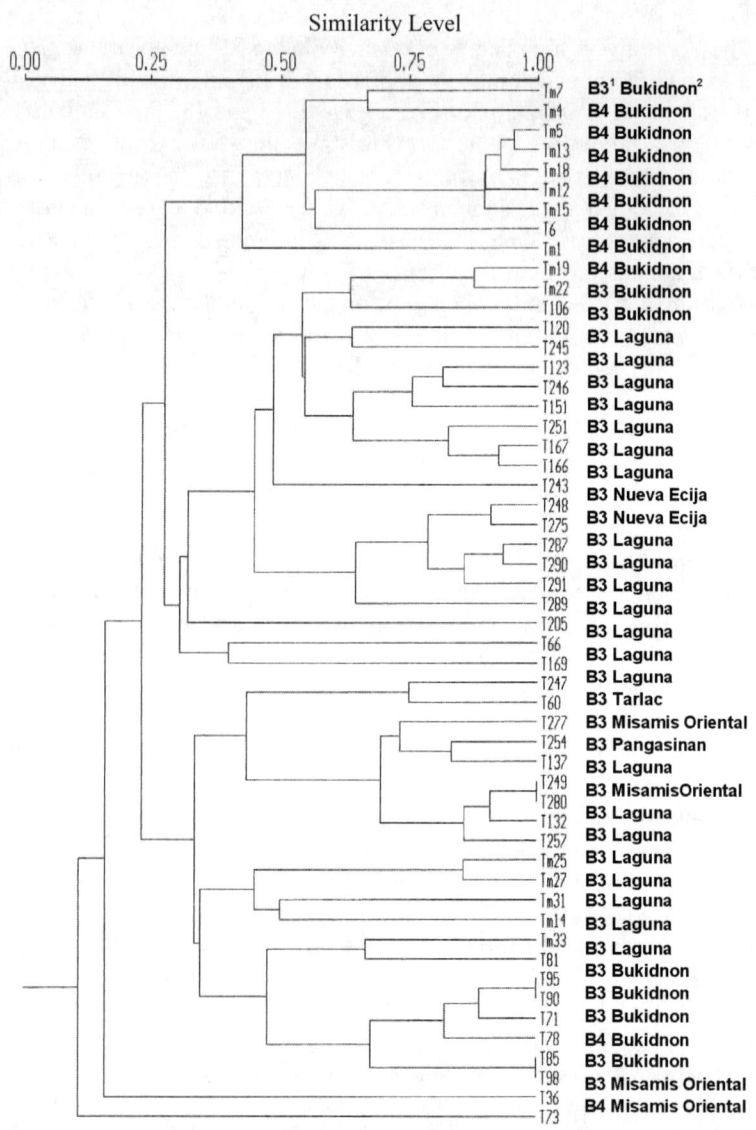

Similarity Level

0.00	0.25	0.50	0.75	1.00

Strain	Description
Tm7	B3[1] Bukidnon[2]
Tm4	B4 Bukidnon
Tm5	B4 Bukidnon
Tm13	B4 Bukidnon
Tm18	B4 Bukidnon
Tm12	B4 Bukidnon
Tm15	B4 Bukidnon
T6	B4 Bukidnon
Tm1	B4 Bukidnon
Tm19	B4 Bukidnon
Tm22	B3 Bukidnon
T106	B3 Bukidnon
T120	B3 Laguna
T245	B3 Laguna
T123	B3 Laguna
T246	B3 Laguna
T151	B3 Laguna
T251	B3 Laguna
T167	B3 Laguna
T166	B3 Laguna
T243	B3 Nueva Ecija
T248	B3 Nueva Ecija
T275	B3 Laguna
T287	B3 Laguna
T290	B3 Laguna
T291	B3 Laguna
T289	B3 Laguna
T205	B3 Laguna
T66	B3 Laguna
T169	B3 Laguna
T247	B3 Laguna
T60	B3 Tarlac
T277	B3 Misamis Oriental
T254	B3 Pangasinan
T137	B3 Laguna
T249	B3 MisamisOriental
T280	B3 Laguna
T132	B3 Laguna
T257	B3 Laguna
Tm25	B3 Laguna
Tm27	B3 Laguna
Tm31	B3 Laguna
Tm14	B3 Laguna
Tm33	B3 Laguna
T81	B3 Bukidnon
T95	B3 Bukidnon
T90	B3 Bukidnon
T71	B4 Bukidnon
T78	B3 Bukidnon
T85	B3 Misamis Oriental
T98	B4 Misamis Oriental
T36	
T73	

Fig. 2. Dendrogram derived by UPGMA (Unweighted Pair Group Method Arithmetic Mean) showing the similarity among tomato strains of *R. solanacearum* based on RAPD PCR. [1]Biovar and [2]Place of Collection.

ceptible cultivars remained the same. In contrast, changes in the DNA fingerprints of isolates from moderately resistant and resistant plants were observed.

DNA was extracted from three reisolates/plant/variety collected. Three to six percent of the T523-731 reisolates from the moderately resistant Improved Pope and L-180 shifted back to the parent or the wild type haplotype. Four haplotypes were observed on the reisolates from the second virulence test in contrast to two haplotypes after the first virulence test. Some reisolates of the mutant T523-731 from Hawaii 7996, which were observed to exhibit another haplotype, are characterized by an additional band (0.2 Kb).

In order to be successful, pathogens need mechanisms for entry into and movement within the plant, acquiring nutrients, escape from plant defense reactions, and finally, egress of reproductive structures from the host and dissemination (5). It is most probable, therefore, that after strain T523 had passed through the resistant tomato cultivars, genes for preexisting virulence factors expressed in a minor component of the population conferred a selective advantage. Thus the substrain T523-731 may have existed in the population at a low level and host selection increased frequency of these more virulent members of the population when they were inoculated to plants grown on a larger scale with particular resistance genes. This appears to be a case of a gene-for-gene interaction, based on correlated studies of the host and the parasite and where the expression of a gene for resistance is conditioned by a corresponding gene for virulence in the parasite (1). The virulence of the reisolate T523-731was apparently conditioned by genes for resistance in the host, as evidenced by the enhanced virulence of the reisolates of this strain obtained from moderately resistant and resistant cultivars.

This increased virulence of *R .solanacearum* strain T523 and the apparent increase in its genetic variability suggest that it was able to adapt to the pressure exerted by the resistant host. The resistance gene(s) in the cultivars C108, 508 and Hawaii 7996 became ineffective, apparently due to the response of the *R. solanacearum* strains to the selective pressure exerted by the resistant cultivars.

Our data confirm the low and high genome plasticity of the banana and the tomato strains, respectively. We found that the low plasticity of the banana strains may have been due to the limited host species on which these strains thrive and the absence of resistance genes to bacterial wilt in edible bananas (8,10). In contrast, there are resistance genes in tomato, and our results suggest the host genotype plays a key role in the development of variability of the organism.

Literature Cited

1. Flor, H. 1971. Current status of the gene-for-gene concept. Annu. Rev. Phytopathol. 9:275-296.
2. Ilagan, Y.A., Raymundo, A.K., Lavina, W.A., and Natural, M.P. 2003. Genetic homogeneity of the Philippine banana strains of *Ralstonia solanacearum* (Smith) Yabuuchi *et al.* in the Philippines. Philipp. Agric. Scientist. 86:394-402.
3. Ilagan, Y.A., Raymundo, A.K., Lavina, W.A., and Denny, T.P. 2003. Development of a polymerase chain reaction-based technique for the detection of Philippine banana strains of *Ralstonia solanacearum.* Philipp. Agric. Scientist. 86: 385-393.
4. Jaunet, T., and Wang. J.F. 1997. Population structure of *Ralstonia solanacearum* in a disease nursery in Taiwan. Pages 82-88 in: Bacterial Wilt Disease: Molecular and Ecological Aspects. P. Prior, C. Allen, and J. Elphinstone, eds. Springer-Verlag, Berlin.
5. Keen, N. 1999. Plant disease resistance: progress in basic understanding and practical application. Adv. Bot. Res. 30: 291-328.
6. Opina, N.L., Villa, J.E., and Raymundo, A.K. 2000. Genetics and agressiveness diversity of *Ralstonia solanaceraum* affecting tomato in the Philippines. Proceedings of the 31st annual Scientific Conference of the Pest Management Council of the Philippines. May 3-6, 2000, Baguio City.
7. Opina, N.L., Tavner, F., Holloway, G., Wang, J.F., Li, T.H., Maghirang, R., Fegan, M., Hayward, A.C., Krishnapillai, V., Hong, W.F., Holloway, B.W., and Timmis, J.M. 1997. A novel method for development of species and strain-specific DNA probes and PCR primers for identifying *Burkholderia solanacearum*). Asia Pac. J. Mol. Biol. Biotech. 5: 19-30.
8. Raymundo, A.K., Ilagan, Y.A., and Denny, T.P. 1998. Analysis of genetic variation of a population of banana-infecting strains of *Ralstonia solanacearum.* Pages 56-60 in: Bacterial Wilt Disease: Molecular and Ecological Aspects. P. Prior, C. Allen, and J. Elphinstone, eds.. Springer, Berlin.
9. Raymundo, A.K., and Ilagan, Y.A. 1999. Cloning of a repetitive element which distinguishes banana strains of *Ralstonia solanacearum* in the Philippines. Philipp. Agric. Scientist 82: 338-350.
10. Sequiera, L. 1998. Bacterial wilt: the missing element in international banana improvement programs. Pages 4-15 in: Bacterial Wilt Disease: Molecular and Ecological Aspects. P. Prior, C. Allen and J. Elphinstone, eds. Springer, Berlin.

11. Soguilon, C.E., Magnaye, L.V., and Natural, M.P. 1994. "Bugtok" disease of cooking bananas: etiology and diagnostic symptoms. Philippine Phytopathol. 30:26-34.

Present Status of Blood Disease in Indonesia

Supriadi

Research Institute for Spice and Medicinal Crops,
Jalan Tentara Pelajar No. 3, Bogor 16111 Indonesia

Since 1921, blood disease of banana in Indonesia was confined to Sulawesi (Celebes) and the neighboring Salayar Island. It was the subject of a quarantine order that restricted the export of banana fruits and vegetation from that region. No record was found after this first outbreak until it appeared in Jonggol, West Java in 1987. In 2001, the disease was found in Lombok and Sumbawa Islands, West Nusa Tenggara, new endemic islands outside Sulawesi, Java and Bali. The disease has also occurred in the provinces of Lampung and North and West Sumatra. Unconfirmed data also report the disease in West Kalimantan, Ambon and Timika Irian Jaya. It is not known whether this rapid spread is from one source or from different sources of origin. Artificial inoculation revealed that the pathogen, the blood disease bacterium (BDB) has a very narrow host range, limited to the banana plant. Most local varieties belonging to cooking (ABB group) and dessert (AAA group), are susceptible. Few banana varieties showed tolerance in the field, but these should be evaluated for further use in breeding improvement. Almost all isolates of BDB carry temperate phages that can be used to distinguish them from *R. solanacearum* race 2. Several male flower-visiting insects including the families of Cloropidae, Drosophilidae, Flatypezidae, Culicidae, Muscidae, Antomyiidae, Sarcopangidae (Diptera), Coleophoridae (Lepidoptera), Blattidae (Blattaria), and Apidae (Hymenoptera) are able to carry the pathogen, and these are strongly suspected as vectors. Artificial feeding of some insects demonstrated that the bacterium was carried in the mouth but did not persist in the abdomen or thorax. Although it has rapidly distributed almost all over Indonesia, very little effort has been made to stop the disease from spreading. International assistance is urgently required. There is now a great risk that some islands in East Nusa Tenggara, which are known to be areas of banana culture, and which are connected to Sumbawa Island by busy public transportation, will become infested by BDB.

Introduction

Gäumann first used "blood disease" for a bacterial disease on banana confined to South Sulawesi and the neighboring Salayar Island in 1920. The disease was the subject of a quarantine order that restricted the export of banana fruits and plant materials from that region since 1921. The pathogen was named *Pseudomonas celebensis* (9). Since this finding, there has been no report of the disease. The description of the pathogen did not meet the requirements for inclusion in the Approved List of bacterial names (14); accordingly, the name *P. celebensis* is no longer valid and has disappeared from the literature. In this paper, the pathogen is called BDB (blood disease bacterium).

Blood disease on banana in Indonesia has attracted international interest since the findings of Eden-Green *et al.* (5) confirmed that the disease had occurred in Jonggol, near Jakarta, the capital city of Indonesia. These authors suggested reinstatement of the *P. celebenses* name for the causal agent of blood disease of banana.

ECONOMIC IMPORTANCE

The banana plant is one of the most popular economic plants in Indonesia. The plant grows almost everywhere, and banana is the main cheap source of vitamins and carbohydrate for a majority of Indonesian people. In 1999, the banana production area was estimated 70,560 Ha, with total production of 3,376,661 tons. The national loss of banana production due to the disease was estimated around 36% in 1991 (15). In 1993, reports of losses from several districts in Lampung showed that about 963,380 plants died in Lampung Selatan, and 1,101,000 plants in Lampung Utara. Cahyaniati *et al.* (2) estimated the actual loss from Lampung Province was about 64%. For example, before the outbreak of the disease some farmers in Pekat District Sumbawa could harvest 100-banana bunches/Ha every week. After the outbreak, these farmers got nothing. Damage of banana plants in Lombok and Sumbawa was very serious because the commonly-planted variety Pisang Kapok (ABB type) was highly susceptible.

Symptoms and Causal Agent

DISEASE SYMPTOMS

Symptoms of blood disease are similar to those of Moko disease on banana in Central and South America, and also to Bugtok or Tapurok disease in the Philippines, which is caused by *Ralstonia solanacearum* race 2 (banana race) (7). Externally, the midribs and petioles of the oldest leaves become flaccid, and petioles collapse near the junction with the pseudo-stem. Younger leaves become bright yellow, then necrotic and dry. Fruit bunches may appear outwardly normal, even when all of the leaves are dis-colored, but a few split, blackened or prematurely ripened fruits may be present. Male flower buds are shriveled. Finally the diseased plant dies.

Internally, brown vascular streaking is seen throughout the plant extend-ing into the roots. In mature plants, this is concentrated in the fruit stem and extends into the fruits, which are internally discolored and contain dry cavities or pockets of reddish-brown mucoid or gelatinous tissue. Charac-teristically, all of the fruits show internal symptoms. A white to reddish-brown 'blood-like' bacterial ooze exudes slowly from cut vascular bundles.

CAUSAL AGENT

Based on the cultural characteristics of the bacterium on agar media such as sucrose peptone, and on its pathogenicity, blood disease on bananas is caused by a plant pathogenic bacterium whether it is called *R. solan-acearum* race 2, *P. celebensis,* or BDB. The colonies of BDB on media containing tetrazolium chloride are small, mucoid or slightly viscid with red centers and well-defined white margins (5,7,28). Pathogenicity studies in-dicated that BDB wilted banana but not solanaceacous plants (7,13,26, 27). Pathogenicity of BDB also differed from other closely related plant patho-gens such as *P. syzygii*, the cause of Sumatra disease of clove (7,8) as well as from other *R. solanacearum* non-banana races from Indonesia (26, 27).

BDB, however, is closely related serologically to *R. solanacearum* and *P. syzygii* (6,17,27). Fatty acid and protein profiles of BDB are also related to those of *R. solanacearum* (21,28). Based on the nucleotide sequences of 16S rRNA BDB is placed in the same group as *R. solanacearum* race 2 and *P. syzygii* (3,19,30).

PHAGE TYPING

We have explored the potential use of lysogenic phage to distinguish BDB from other closely related plant pathogens such as *R. solanacearum* and *P. syzygii* (25,29). We found that 53 of 59 (95%) BDB isolates from Sulawesi and Java during 1988-1995 were lysogenic on indicator strains. Further tests of the BDB isolated from several new outbreaks of diseased bananas in Java, Lombok and Sumbawa during 1995-2001, supported pre-vious findings. In total, 81 BDB isolates have been tested for lysogeny

Table 1. Frequency of lysogeny among isolates of BDB, *Ralstonia solanacearum,* and *Pseudomonas syzygii* (some data from 25,29).

Isolate types	Host	Country	Number tested	Number lysogeny
R. solanacearum race 1, 3, 4	non banana	Indonesia	55	10 (18.2%)
BDB	banana	Indonesia	81	78 (96.3%)
R. solanacearum race 1, 3, 4, 5	non banana	Other countries	40	10 (25%)
R. solanacearum race 2	banana	Other countries	16	0 (0%)
P. syzygii	clove	Indonesia	5	0 (0%)

(Table 1). In this respect BDB differs from *R. solanacearum* race 2 which causes Moko disease in Central and South America, and also from the closely related *P. syzygii* It seems that the lysogeny property is a specific bacteriological character of BDB which can be used to support identification and differentiation amongst very closely related bacteria. Practically, the lysogeny test is very simple and can be performed in the laboratory with basic equipment.

Epidemiology

DISEASE DISTRIBUTION

During 1987-1990, several scientists in various locations in Indonesia conducted disease observations independently. In Sulawesi, the disease was actively spreading through South, North and Central Sulawesi (5,20). Since the first finding in Jonggol, near Jakarta in 1987 by Eden-Green *et al.* (5), the disease has been found in various location in West Java (10, 18,27). In Yogyakarta, Central Java, the disease was also observed (1), whereas from East Java the disease was reported as well (23,13,16). In Sumatra, blood disease was recognized in 1993 in Lampung (2,4), Medan North Sumatra (Sitepu, pers. comm.), and Solok West Sumatra (I. Jatnika, pers. comm.). Outside Sumatra and Java, the disease was confirmed in 1994/ 1995 in Bali (22), Lombok and Sumbawa Islands in 1998/1999 (24). A recent visit by the author to Sumbawa has confirmed the disease has appeared in that island. BDB has also killed banana plants in Ambon, Maluku (Leiwakabessy, pers.com). Unconfirmed reports also indicated that the disease has appeared on banana plants in Timika Irian Jaya. The most recent

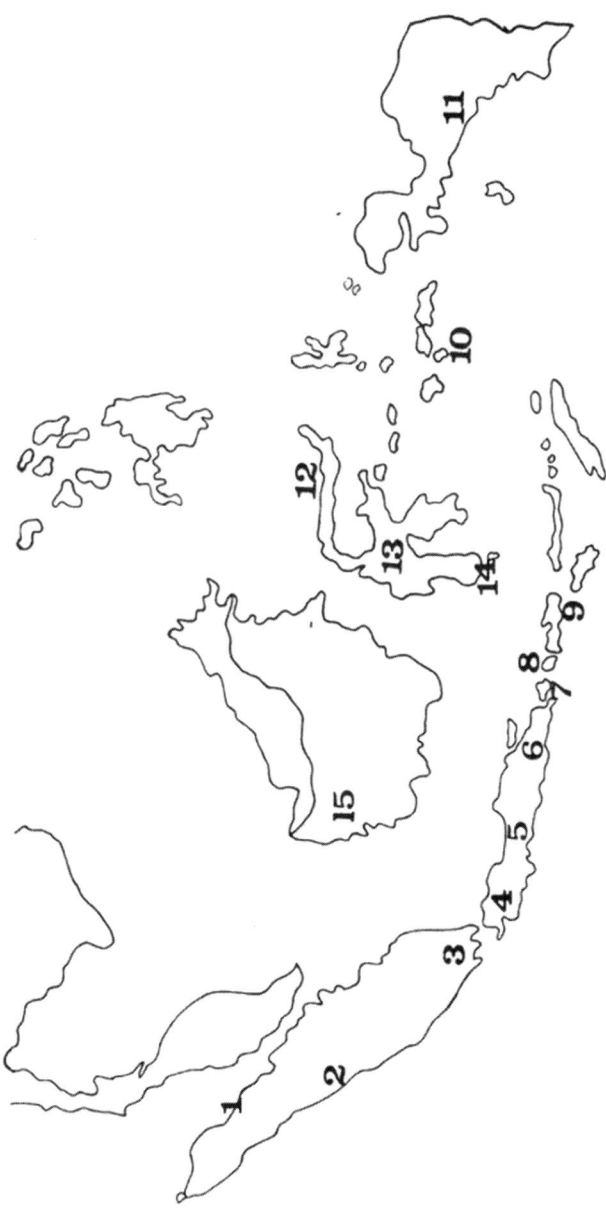

Fig. 1. Distribution of blood disease of banana in Indonesia. 1:Medan, North Sumatra, 2: Solok, West Sumatra, 3: Lampung (1997), 4: West Java (1987), 5: Central Java (1997), 6: East Java (1997), 7: Bali (1994), 8: Lombok (1999), 9: Sumbawa (1999), 10: Ambon, 11: Timika, Irian Jaya, 12: North Sulawesi (1920), 13: Central Sulawesi (1920), 14: South Sulawesi (1920) 15: Kalimantan.

information on blood disease distribution in Indonesia is presented in Figure 1.

Eden-Green (8) has estimated the spread of blood disease at a speed of 100km/year, and suggested that it threatens all banana plants in Indonesia. Since there is no significant activity to stop the disease, it appears that the disease is progressively spreading eastwards from the 'first appearance' in Jonggol, near Jakarta alongside the north coastline of Java to Bali, Lombok and Sumbawa, and westwards following the direction of Lampung and Solok in Sumatra. Disease origins may come from various independent sources such as from Sulawesi to Kalimantan, Ambon, and Irian Jaya.

HOST PLANTS

Pathogenicity tests of BDB isolates show that the pathogen has a very narrow host range, i.e. banana and *Heliconia* sp. Various plants such as tomato, eggplant, ginger, black nightshade (*Solanum torvum*) and a weed (*Phylanthus niruri*) artificially inoculated with BDB cultures showed negative symptoms. This is further evidence that BDB differs from *R. solanacearum* causing Moko disease, which has several alternate hosts excluding banana.

RESISTANCE SCREENING

Intensive screening and field trials of large numbers of banana varieties in Indonesia has been conducted by Hanudin *et al.* (10) in Bogor with artificial inoculation, and Sudana *et al.* (22) based on a field trial in Bali. They showed that most of local banana varieties are susceptible to BDB.

However, there are several local varieties, which show less susceptibility or tolerance (22) (Table 2). Further study is required to confirm whether those tolerant lines are only escapes from infection or if they have some degree of resistance which can be used for breeding improvement of

Table 2. Preliminary results: Banana varieties tested for resistance to BDB (10,22)

Susceptible banana ('Pisang') varieties	Tolerant varieties
Ambon Lumut, Ambon Jepang, Ambon Putih, Ampyang, Badak, Bangkahulu, Barangan, Emas, Embe, Jambe, Jimbluk, Kepok (Saba), Lilin, Nangka, Raja Sere, Seribu, Siman, Sogit, Siam, Tanduk	Batu (Klutuk), Bancan, Bunting, Bojong, Dak Nangka, Kayu, Ketip, Marga, Kepet, Muli, Papan, Rempeneng, Susu Ketan, Susu, Plepeden, Telu (Telur), Udang

bananas. Clarification of genetic variation amongst local variety names is also necessary.

Potential insect vectors of BDB have been studied by Maryam *et al.* (12) and Leiwkabessy (11). Maryam *et al.* showed that following artificial membrane feeding, an unidentified flower-visiting insect (Diptera, Drosopholilidae) was able to acquire the pathogen in the mouth, but the pathogen did not persist in the abdomen or thorax. Leiwkabessy isolated BDB from macerated tissues and washed surfaces of several male-flower-visiting insects belonging to the family Cloropidae, Drosophilidae, Flatypezidae, Culicidae, Muscidae, Antomyiidae, Sarcopangidae (Diptera), Coleophoridae (Lepidoptera), Blattidae (Blattaria), and Apidae (Hymenoptera) collected from diseased banana plants in Lampung. The isolated bacterium was pathogenic to banana seedlings. Undoubtedly, the role of insects as vector or carrier of BDB may explain the spread of the disease throughout Indonesia. The role of banana traders, however, is also important. For example, according to local farmers in Lombok and Sumbawa islands, traders directly harvest banana bunches from fields possibly using tools which may have been contaminated from other banana plants. Disease spread within fields is probably due to tools used in traditional practices by farmers such as cutting old banana leaves or unwanted shoots.

Control Strategies

Blood disease is actively spreading throughout Indonesia and is becoming a major threat for banana production. Diseased plants and their shoots should be totally eradicated to eliminate the sources of the inoculum. To speed up the process, the plants may be treated with herbicide. Meanwhile, rehabilitation, especially for isolated islands, has to be planned using disease-free planting materials generated via tissue culture. Tight monitoring of the disease outbreaks requires close coordination between government officials and local farmers.

Searching for resistant genes in local varieties of bananas followed by their utilization for breeding improvement needs to be deepened. The role of insects as vectors, and monitoring of vectors in healthy regions need to be seriously studied. International assistance is required to assist research to stop further spread of the disease, and to evaluate strategies to control it.

Acknowledgements

I wish to thank the INIBAP (International Network for Improvement of Banana and Plantain) and the Agency for Agriculture Research and Development of Indonesia for sponsorship to attend the Symposium, and to Dr. Karden Mulya for fruitful discussion.

Literature Cited

1. Arwiyanto, T. 1988. Identifikasi penyebab penyakit baketerial pada tanaman pisang di Yogyakarta. Proceedings of the 8th Indonesian Phytopathology Society, Jakarta 29-31 October 1985: 46-47.
2. Cahyaniati, C., Mortensen, N., and Mathur, S.B. 1997. Bacterial Wilt of Banana in Indonesia. Technical Bulletin. Directorate Plant Protection. Directorate General of Food Crops and Horticulture.
3. Cook, D., Barlow, E., and Sequeira, L. 1991. DNA probes as tools for the study of host-pathogen evolution: The example of *Pseudomonas solanacearum*. Pages 103-108 in: Advances in Molecular Genetics of Plant-Microbe Interactions. H. Henneke and D. Verma, eds. Kluwer Academic Publishing, The Netherlands.
4. Dikin, A., Kornahen, F., and Hermawan. 1977. Perbedaan isolate bakteri penyebab penyakit layu pisang di Lampung dan Jawa Barat. Proceedings of the XIII Indonesian Phytopathological Society, Mataram 27-29 September 1995: 407-410.
5. Eden-Green, S.J., Supriadi, and Hartati, S.Y. 1988. Characteristics of *Pseudomonas celebensis*, the cause of blood disease of bananas in Indonesia. Proceedings of the 5th International Congress of Plant Pathology, August 20-27, Kyoto, Japan: 389 (abstr).
6. Eden-Green, S.J., Supriadi, Hasnam, N., and Hunt, P. 1988. Serological relationship between the xylem-limited bacteria causing Sumatra disease in Indonesia and *Pseudomonas solanacearum*. Pages 357-363 in: Proceedings of the 6th International Conference on Plant Pathogenic Bacteria, Maryland USA 1985. E. Civerolo, A. Collmer, R.E. Davis, and A. Gillaspie, eds. Martinus Nijhoff, Dordrecht.
7. Eden-Green, S.J., and Sastraatmadja, H. 1990. Blood disease bacterium present in Java. FAO Bulletin 38: 49-90.
8. Eden-Green, S.J. 1994. Diversity of *Pseudomonas solanacearum* and related bacteria in Southeast Asia: New directions for Moko disease. Pages 25-34 in Bacterial Wilt: The Disease and Its Causative Agent, *Pseudomonas solanacearum*. A.C. Hayward and G.L. Hartman, eds. CAB International, Wallingford, Oxon UK.

9. Gäumann, E. 1921. Ondezoekingen over de bloedziekte der banananen op Celebes I (Investigations on the blood-disease like of banana in Celebes I). Mededeelingen Van Het Instituut Voor Planten Ziekten 50.

10. Hanudin, B. Tjahjono, and Sugiharso. 1993. Uji resistensi varietas pisang terhadap bakteri layu. Jurnal Hortikultura 3: 37-42.

11. Leiwakabessy, C. 1999. Potensi beberapa jenis serangga dalam penyebaran penyakit layu bakteri *Ralstonia* (*Pseudomonas*) *solanacearum* Yabuuchi et al pada pisang di Lampung. Master of Science Thesis, Bogor Agriculture University. 64 pages.

12. Maryam, A., Rasta, T., Handayani, W., and Sihombing, D. 1997. Akuisisi dan persistensi bakteri layu pada tanaman pisang oleh seranga. National Seminar of the Indonesian Entomology Society, Bogor 8 January 1997: 154-161.

13. Masnilah, R., Yuliani, A., Tjahjani, A., and Trisusilowati, E.B. 2001. Karakterisasi bakteri penyebab penyakit layu pada pisang di daerah Jember. Proceedings of the XVI Indonesian Phytopathological Society, Bogor 22-24 August 2001.

14. Moffett, M.L., and Dye, D.W. 1983. Valid names of plant pathogenic bacteria. Pages 299-315 in: Plant Bacterial Diseases: A diagnostic guide. P.C. Fachy and G.J. Persley, eds. Academic Press, Australia.

15. Muharam, A. and Subijanto. 1991. Status of banana diseases in Indonesia. Pages 44-49 in: Banana Diseases in Asia and the Pacific. Proceedings of a technical Meeting on Diseases Affecting Banana and Plantain in Asia and the Pacific. Brisbane, Australia, 15-18 April 1991. R.V. Valmayar, B.E. Umali, and C.P. Bejosano, eds. INIBAP.

16. Mulyadi, and Hernusa, T. 2001. Intensitas penyakit darah pada tanaman pisang disebabkan oleh bakteri *Pseudomonas solanacearum* di Kabupaten Bondowoso. Proceedings of the XVI Indonesian Phytopathological Society, Bogor 22-24 August 2001.

17. Robinson-Smith, A., Jones, P., Elphinstone, J.G., and Forde, S.M.D. 1995. Production of antibodies to *Pseudomonas solanacearum*, the causative agent of bacterial wilt. Food and Agricul. Immun. J. 7: 67-79.

18. Satari, U., and Sumaraw, I.O. 1990. Penyakit layu bakteri pada pisang di daerah Bogor dan sekitarnya. Jurnal Fitopatologi Indonesia 3: 53-55.

19. Seal, S.E., Jackson, L.A., Young, J.P.W., and Daniels, M. 1993. Differentiation of *Pseudomonas solanacearum*, *Pseudomonas syzygii*, *Pseudomonas pickettii* and blood disease bacterium by partial 16S rRNA sequencing: construction of oligonucleotide primers for sensitive detection by polymerase chain reaction. J. Gen. Microbiol. 139: 1587-1594.

20. Stover, R.H., and Espinoza, A. 1992. Blood disease of bananas in Sulawesi. Fruits 47: 611-613.
21. Stead, D.E. 1992. Grouping of plant-pathogenic and some other *Pseudomonas* spp. by using cellular fatty acid profiles. Int. J. System. Bacteriol. 42: 281-295.
22. Sudana, I.M., Suprapto, D.N., Arya, N., and Sukanaya, W. 1999. Usaha pengendalian penyakit layu pada pisang di Bali. Proceedings of the XV Indonesian Phytopathological Society, Purwokerto 16-18 September 1999: 404-410.
23. Sumardiyono, C., Subandiyah, S., Sulandari, S., and Martoredjo, T. 1997. Peningkatan ketahanan terhadap penyakit layu bakteri (*Pseudomonas solanacearum*) pisang dengan radiasi kultur jaringan. Proceedings of the XIV Indonesian Phytopathological Society, Palembang 27-29 October 1997.
24. Supeno, B. 2001. Isolasi dan identifikasi penyakit darah pisang di Lombok . Proceedings of the XVI Indonesian Phytopathological Society, Bogor 22-24 August 2001.
25. Supriadi. 1994. Studies on the characteristics of *Pseudomonas solanacearum* and related species from Indonesia, and the potential use of bacteriophage and bacteriocin for biological control of bacterial wilt disease. PhD Thesis, Wye College, University of London.
26. Supriadi. 1999. Karakterisasi kultur dan patogenisitas isolat *Pseudomonas celebensis* penyebab penyakit darah pada tanaman pisang. Jurnal Hortikultura 9:129-136.
27. Supriadi, Elphinstone, J.G., Eden-Green, S.J., and Hartati, S.Y. 1995. Physiological, serological and pathological variation amongst isolates of *Pseudomonas solanacearum* from ginger and other hosts in Indonesia. Industrial Crop Research Journal 1(2): 88-98.
28. Supriadi, Elphinstone, J.G., Hennessy, J., and Robinson, A. 1997. Analysis of whole protein profiles of isolates of *Pseudomonas solanacearum* and related species from Indonesia by SDS-page. Jurnal Penelitian Tanaman Industri 3: 6-12.
29. Supriadi, Elphinstone, J.G., Eden-Green, S.J., and Mansfield, J.M. 1997. Bacteriopage typing of *Ralstonia solanacearum*, *Pseudomonas syzygii*, and blood disease bacterium of banana. Hayati 4: 72-77.
30. Taghavi, M., Hayward, A.C., Sly, L.I., and Fegan, M. 1996. Analysis of the phylogenetic relationships of strains of *Burkholderia solanacearum*, *Pseudomonas syzygii*, and the blood disease bacterium of banana based on 16S rRNA gene sequence. Int. J. System. Bacteriol. 46: 10-15.

Diversity and Molecular Detection of *Ralstonia solanacearum* Race 2 Strains by Multiplex PCR

P. Prior[1] and M. Fegan[2]

[1] INRA, Unité de Pathologie Végétale, Domaine St Maurice, BP 94, 84143, Montfavet, France. [2] Cooperative Research Centre for Tropical Plant Protection, Department of Microbiology and Parasitology, The University of Queensland, St. Lucia, Queensland, Australia

R. solanacearum strains infecting *Musa* spp (known as race 2 strains) pose a major threat to dessert and cooking banana (plantain) production worldwide (10). Unravelling the phylogenetic relationships among these strains is essential for quarantine purposes and scientifically promising for investigation of the basis of host specificity. *R. solanacearum* is a very heterogeneous species (7) and even within race 2 strains, there is variation at both the phenotypic and genotypic level (3,6).

French and Sequeira (6) defined five groups or ecotypes within strains of *R. solanacearum* race 2 causing bacterial wilt on banana, plantain and *Heliconia* sp. in Central and South Americas. These groups are: type A (Amazon basin), SFR (small, fluidal, round), B (banana), D (distortion), and H (heliconia). Strains within each group differ in virulence, some are pathogenic on both banana and plantain (A, SFR, B, and D types) and others are only pathogenic to plantain but not to banana (H). The groupings were also based on the major mode of transmission of strains by insects (SFR) (1) or soilborne (B-type). Moreover, some groups consist of highly aggressive strains (SFR, A, B) and others of less aggressive strains (D-type). All the ecotypes are naturally pathogenic on *Musa* spp. and tested pathogenic to tomato and other solanaceous hosts if bacteria were directly injected into the stem. However, they have never been isolated from a naturally wilted solanaceous plant in the field.

Based upon RFLP analysis Cook and Sequeira (2) found that all *R. solanacearum* race 2 strains cluster into three multi-locus genotypes (MLGs), defined as MLGs 24, 25 & 28. A hierarchical classification scheme based on phylogenetic analysis of 16S-23S intergenic spacer region (ITS) and endoglucanase (*egl*) gene sequences has also been described (Fegan and Prior, this volume). In this scheme *R. solanacearum* race 2 strains have been found to belong to Phylotype II, sequevars 3, 4 and 6. In this study the phylogenetic position of *R. solanacearum* race 2 strains within the phylotyping scheme of Fegan and Prior (this volume) is confirmed. Furthermore, the phylogenetic position of strains, determined by *egl* sequence analysis, was used to as a basis to choose strains for a subtractive hybridization approach to identify *R. solanacearum* race 2-specific DNA fragments. These specific genomic DNA fragments have been used to develop PCR-based molecular tests for *R. solanacearum* race 2.

Phylogenetic Position of *R. solanacearum* Race 2 Strains in the Phylotyping Scheme

The endoglucanase gene of 31 strains of *R. solanacearum* isolated from *Musa* sp. or *Heliconia* sp. and 25 *R. solanacearum*-species complex strains from other hosts was sequenced and phylogenetically analysed using the methods described by Fegan *et al.* (5) (Table 1). All strains sequenced fell

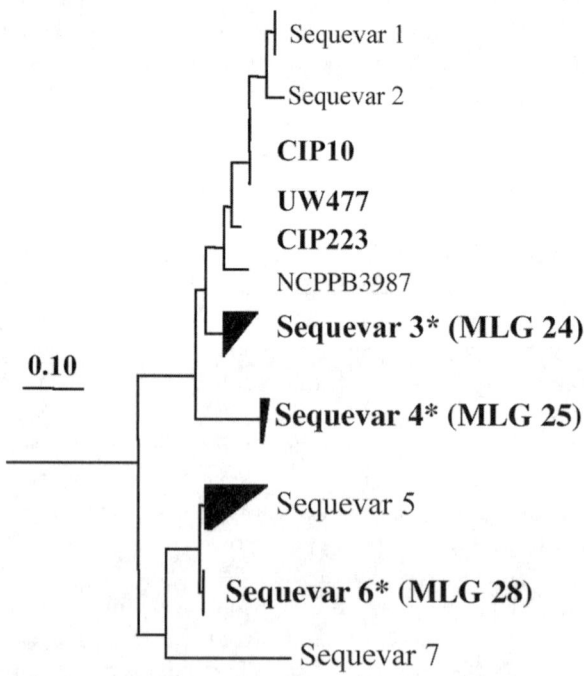

Fig. 1. Phylogenetic tree of phylotype II based upon partial endoglucanase gene sequences. The asterisk indicates the sequevars to which *R. solanacearum* race 2 strains belong.

into three sequence variants equivalent to sequevars 3, 4 and 6 described by Fegan and Prior (this volume) (Fig. 1).

All strains previously identified to be MLG24 (2) fell within sequevar 3 (Table 1). Strains in this sequevar were isolated from Costa Rica, Honduras and Panama from the hosts banana, plantain and *Heliconia* sp. A strain of *R. solanacearum* isolated from peanut in Indonesia (CIP418; Table 1) was unexpectedly found to belong to sequevar 3 (MLG 24). Further work on the pathogenicity of this strain found it to be pathogenic on banana (P. Prior, unpublished). As moko disease is not known to be present in Indonesia this important finding needs to be confirmed. However, the possibility that this strain has become mislabelled has to be considered. All strains of sequevar 3 were also found to belong to biotype 3 (Table 1) as described by Fegan and Prior (this volume)

All strains previously identified as belonging to MLG25 (2) fell in sequevar 4. Strains in this sequevar were isolated from Peru, Columbia, Costa Rica, Martinique and Florida, USA from the host plants banana, plantain, *Heliconia* sp., pothos *(Epipremnum aureum)* and *Anthurium*. Strains isolated from bacterial wilt-infected *Anthurium* from Martinique in the French West Indies and from pothos in Florida were found to cluster with *R. solanacearum* strains belonging to sequevar 4. The strains from *Anthurium* were non-pathogenic on banana (Prior, pers comm.).

However, the strains from pothos are described as causing wilt of banana (8,9). The pathogenic potential of these strains for banana needs to be confirmed. At the very least this extends the known host range of sequevar 4 (MLG 25) strains to include pothos and *Anthurium*. All strains of sequevar 4 were also found to belong to biotype 4 (Table 1) as described by Fegan and Prior (this volume), with the exception of strain UW170 which typed as biotype 3. This organism gave inconsistent PCR results as well (see below).

Strains belonging to sequevars 3 (MLG24) and 4 (MLG25) are closely related and form a branch together with sequevars 1 and 2, which contain potato disease-causing strains belonging to race 3/biovar 2. All strains previously identified as belonging to MLG28 (2) fell in Sequevar 6. Strains in this sequevar were isolated from Honduras, Venezuela, Hawaii and Australia (where the disease has since been eradicated) from the hosts banana, plantain and *Heliconia* sp. Sequevar 6 (MLG 28) clusters closely with sequevar 5 strains (Fig. 1). The strains in sequevar 5 are pathogenic on solanaceous hosts such as eggplant and tomato but not on *Musa* spp. and are found in central Africa and the Caribbean. Sequevar 6 is phylogenetically distinct from strains of sequevars 3 (MLG 24) and 4 (MLG 25) in which the other moko disease causing strains are found. Hence the *R. solanacearum* race 2 strains are polyphyletic, which indicates a separate evolutionary origin for the two groups of strains. All strains of sequevar 6 were also found to belong to biotype 6 (Table 1) as described by Fegan and Prior (this volume).

During the course of this study use of the primer pairs specific for sequevars 3, 4 and 6 (MLG 24, 25 and 28) to identify strains of *R. solanacearum* in Brazil by collaborating scientists at INPA (Instituto Nacional de Pesquisas da Amazônia) revealed a tomato plant naturally infected with a sequevar 6 (MLG 28) strain. This expands the known host range of this organism and is the first description of tomato as a natural host of *R. solanacearum* race 2/biovar 1.

R. solanacearum race 2 PCR Tests

To develop PCR-based diagnostic tests for *R. solanacearum* race 2 sequevars 3, 4 and 6, we used a subtractive hybridization approach. Central to this approach is the assumption that the phylogenetic relationship of strains revealed by analysis of the *egl* gene reflects the organismal (total genome) phylogeny. Therefore comparison of genomic sequences between closely related strains is likely to reveal unique DNA regions. Using the phlogenetic data from the *egl* sequences, strains were chosen to be "tester" (genome containing the sequences of interest – an *R. solanacearum* race 2 strain) and "driver" (the reference sample – a closely related non-banana pathogenic strain). Tester and driver DNAs were hybridized, and the hybrid sequences removed. Consequently, the remaining unhybridized DNAs represented tester-specific sequences. The Clontech PCR-Select™ Bacterial Genome Subtraction Kit was used, as per the manufacturers' instructions, to generate the subtracted genomic DNA fragments. Subtracted genomic DNA fragments were cloned using the Advantage™ PCR Cloning Kit from Clontech Laboratories Inc. (Palo Alto, CA USA). The specificity of subtracted genomic DNA fragments was assessed by dot-blot hybridization.

To find sequences specific to sequevar 6 (MLG28) strains, we used tester strain UW21 (sequevar 6), a strain pathogenic on banana from Honduras and driver strain CIP301 (sequevar 5), a broad host range strain from potato, isolated in Peru, that is not pathogenic on banana. Similarly, to find sequences specific to sequevar 4 (MLG 25), the moko strain CFBP1419 from Costa Rica was subtracted against driver strain Ant307 isolated from *Anthurium* in the French West Indies (FWI). From each subtraction experiment about 50 fragments with sizes ranging from 50bp to 2Kb were cloned and their specificity established. Subtracted fragments of interest were sequenced and based on these results, PCR primers were designed with the aid of OLIGO Version 6 primer design software (Molecular Biology Insights, Inc. CO, USA) (Table 1) and tested for specificity. Four primer

Table 1. List of strains used in this study, including PCR and biotype results.

Strain No[1]	Origin/Host	Other No[1]	Bv[2]	Phylo[3]	MLG[4]	Primer pair[5] 35	20	06	28	Bt[6]
UW20	Honduras/Banana		1/SFR	II / 6	28	-	-	-	+	6
UW21	Honduras/Banana	R371, CIP21	1/SFR	II / 6	28	-	-	-	+	6
UW181	Venezuela/Plantain	K261	1	II / 6	28	-	-	-	+	6
DAR64836	Australia/*Musa* sp		1	II / 6	28	-	-	-	+	6
A3907	Hawaii/Heliconia		1	II / 6	ND	-	-	-	+	6
A3909	Hawaii/Heliconia		1	II / 6	ND	-	-	-	+	6
A3911	Hawaii/Heliconia		1	II / 6	ND	-	-	-	+	6
UW 127	Peru/Plantain	CIP4	1/A	II / 4	25	+	+	+	-	4
UW129	Peru/Plantain		1/A	II / 4	25	+	+	+	-	4
UW131	Peru/Plantain		1/A	II / 4	ND	+	+	+	-	4
UW160	Peru/Plantain	R282	1/A	II / 4	25	+	+	+	-	4
UW162	Peru/Plantain	JT 648	1/A	II / 4	25	+	+	+	-	4
UW163	Peru/Plantain		1/A	II / 4	ND	+	+	+	-	4
CFBP1419	Costa Rica/*Musa* sp	K163, JS847	1	II / 4	ND	+	+	+	-	4
CIP20	Peru/Plantain	UW156,S249	1	II / 4	25	-	+	+	-	4
UW70	Colombia/Plantain	CIP70	1/SFR	II / 4	25	-	+	+	-	4
UW179	Colombia/Plantain	R368, CIP30	1/SFR	II / 4	ND	-	+	+	-	4
UW175	Colombia/Plantain		1/SFR	II / 4	25	-	+	+	-	4
CFBP2144	Colombia/Plantain	IW1509	1/SFR	II / 4	ND	-	+	+	-	4
CFBP1412	Colombia/Plantain	NCPPB2314	1/SFR	II / 4	ND	-	+	+	-	4
R368	Colombia/Plantain	UW179	1/SFR	II / 4	ND	-	+	+	-	4
P515	USA/Pothos		1	II / 4	ND	-	+	+	-	4
P548	USA/Pothos		1	II / 4	ND	-	+	+	-	4
ANT307	FWI/ Anthurium		1	II / 4	ND	-	+	-	-	4
ANT11212	FWI/Anthurium		1	II / 4	ND	-	+	-	-	4
UW170	Colombia/Heliconia	PD1453	1/D	II / 4	ND	-	-	-	-	3
UW09	Costa Rica/ Heliconia	JT644	1	II / 3	24	+	-	-	-	3
UW11	Costa Rica/ Heliconia		1/D	II / 3	ND	+	-	-	-	3
UW135	Honduras/Banana	CIP7, S228	1/B	II / 3	24	+	-	-	-	3
UW138	Costa Rica/Plantain		1/H	II / 3	24	+	-	-	-	3
UW166	Costa Rica/Plantain	CIP27	1/B	II / 3	ND	+	-	-	-	3
UW167	Costa Rica/Banana	R283, CIP125	1/B	II / 3	24	+	-	-	-	3
CFBP1183	Costa Rica/ Heliconia	JS793	1/D	II / 3	ND	+	-	-	-	3
CFBP1409	Honduras/*Musa* sp	K135, JS77	1	II / 3	ND	+	-	-	-	3
CFBP1482	Panama/*Musa* sp	K168, JS730	1	II / 3	ND	+	-	-	-	3

Table 1 (continued). List of strains used in this study, including PCR and biotype results.

Strain No.[1]	Origin/Host	Other No.[1]	Bv[2]	Phylo[3]	MLG[4]	Primer Pair[5] 35	20	06	28	Bt[6]
CIP418	Indonesia/Peanut	MOH6	1	II / 3	ND	+	-	-	-	3
CFBP2957	FWI/Tomato	MT5	1	II / 5	ND	-	-	-	-	5
CIP301[DI]	Peru/Potato	R311	1	II / 5	3	-	-	-	-	5
CIP239	Brazil/Potato	R306	1	II / 5	38	-	-	-	-	5
CFBP3858	Netherlands/Potato	JS907	2	II / 1	ND	-	-	-	-	1
CIP 117	Nigeria/Potato	UW453	2	II / 1	34	-	-	-	-	1
CIP309	Colombia/Potato	UW80, S206	2	II / 1	27	-	-	-	-	1
CIP10	Peru/Potato	UW477, R569	2T	II / 2	29	-	-	-	-	2
ICMP7969	Kenya/Potato		1	II / 7	ND	-	-	-	-	7
K60	USA/Tomato	UW25	1	II / 7	1	-	-	-	-	7
JT528	Reunion Is./Potato		1	III / 19	ND	-	-	-	-	10
CFBP3059	Burkina Faso/Eggplant	JCG.AU28	1	III / 23	ND	-	-	-	-	10
J25	Kenya/Potato		2T	III / 22	ND	-	-	-	-	9
GMI1000	French Guyana/Tomato		3	I / 12	ND	-	-	-	-	8
CFBP765	Japan/Tomato	JS771	4	I / ND	ND	-	-	-	-	8
R288	China/*Morus alba*	JT659	5	I / 18	ND	-	-	-	-	8
PSI07	Indonesia/Tomato		2	IV / 8	ND	-	-	-	-	11
ACH732	Australia/Tomato	UW433	2	IV / 9	ND	-	-	-	-	11
R24	Indonesia/Clove	*P. syzygii*	NA	IV / 10	ND	+	-	-	-	NA

[1] UW; University of Wisconsin USA; R, Rothamsted Experimental Station UK; CFBP, Collection Française des Bactéries Phytopathogènes, France; CIP, International Potato Center, Peru; ACH, A.C. Hayward, University of Queensland, Australia.

[2] Biovar and ecotypes of *Musa* sp strains of *R. solanacearum* (5) where known, NA – not applicable.

[3] Phylotype/Sequevar as defined by Fegan and Prior (this volume); ND – not determined.

[4] MLG – Multi-locus genotype – as defined by Cook and Sequeira (2), ND – not determined.

[5] PCR primer pairs, 20 – Mus20-F/Mus20-R; 35 – Mus35-F/Mus35-R; 06 – Mus06-F/Mus06-R; 28 – SI28-F/SI28-R (see Table 1) + indicates an amplicon was produced, - indicates that an amplicon was not produced.

[6] Biotype after Fegan and Prior (4), NA – not applicable.

pairs were eventually chosen for testing on an extended set of *R. solan-acearum* strains (Table 2).

The primer pair Mus20-F/Mus20-R specifically amplified all strains from sequevar 4 (MLG 25), with the exception of strain UW170 (Table 2). The reason for this has yet to be confirmed. Primer pair SI28-F/SI28-R specifically amplified the seven strains belonging to sequevar 6 (MLG 28) (Table 2). The Mus35-F/Mus35-R primer pair amplified all 10 strains of sequevar 3 (MLG 24), some sequevar 4 (MLG 25) strains and the *P. syzygii* strain R24. All but one (the ecotype of this strain has not been determined) of the sequevar 4 (MLG 25) strains which amplified with the Mus35-F/Mus35-R primer pair were of the A-ecotype (5) (Table 1); the signifi-cance of this is unknown. The cross-reactivity of the primer pair with *P. syzygii* is not considered a problem as *P. syzygii* is a pathogen of clove but not any of the hosts known to be infected by *R. solanacearum* race 2 strains. *P. syzygii* is also easily separated from *R. solanacearum* race 2 strains by using the phylotype PCR described by Fegan and Prior (this volume) as it belongs to phylotype IV and *R. solanacearum* race 2 strains all belong to phylotype II. However this result requires further clarification to establish if any other members of phylotype IV cross react with this pri-mer pair.

The primer pair designed to target the subtracted fragment Mus06 (Mus6-F/Mus6-R) specifically amplified sequevar 4 (MLG 25) strains of. *R. solanacearum* that were known to be pathogenic on *Musa* sp. This pri-mer pair failed to produce the expected amplicon from the sequevar 4 (MLG25) strains ANT307 and ANT11212 (Table 1, Fig. 2) isolated from *Anthurium,* which are not pathogenic on banana. However, the primer pair

Table 2. Musa-specific primers designed from the subtracted sequences specific to the phylotype II sequevars 3, 4 and 6 and used in a multiplex PCR.

Primer	Sequence (5' to 3')	Product size	Specificity
Mus20-F	CGGGTGGCTGAGACGAATATC	351bp	Sequevar 4
Mus20-R	GCCTTGTCCAGAATCCGAATG		
Mus35-F	GCAGTAAAGAAACCCGGTGTT		Sequevar 3, som
Mus35-R	TCTGGCGAAAGACGGGATGG	400bp	Sequevar 4 and *P. syzygii*
Mus06-F	GCTGGCATTGCTCCCGCTCAC		Sequevar 4
Mus06-R	TCGCTTCCGCCAAGACGC	167bp	pathogenic on *Musa* sp.
Si28-F	CGTTCTCCTTGTCAGCGATGG	220bp	Sequevar 6
Si28-R	CCCGTGTGACCCCGATAG C		

did amplify the sequevar 4 (MLG 25) strains P515 and P548 recently isolated from pothos in Florida, which are pathogenic on banana (7) (Table 1). This sugests that this primer pair may amplify a genomic DNA fragment associated with pathogenicity in sequevar 4 (MLG 25) strains. This finding requires confirmation.

From the four PCRs described above a multiplex PCR was developed (Fig. 2 and Appendix 1). This PCR incorporated all primer pairs in a single reaction to allow rapid identification of the sequevar to which an *R. solanacearum* strain belongs. All sequevar 6 (MLG 28) strains produced a single amplification product of 220bp due to amplification by the Si28-F/Si28-R primer pair (Fig. 2 lanes 2-4). All sequevar 4 (MLG 25) strains produce an amplification product of 351bp and may also produce 167bp and 400bp products due to amplification with Mus06-F/Mus06-R and/or Mus35-F/ Mus35-R respectively as described above (Fig. 2 lanes 5-9). All sequevar 3 (MLG 24) strains produced only a single amplification product of 400bp due to amplification by the Mus35-F/Mus35-R primer pair (Fig. 2 lanes 10-13). Although the Mus35-F/Mus35-R primer pair also amplifies certain strains belonging to sequevar 4 (MLG 25) (for example Fig. 2 lanes 5 and 6) these sequevar 4 (MLG 25) strains will also produce a second amplicon of 351bp thus allowing sequevar 3 (MLG 24) to be distinguished. Thus, using this multiplex PCR all strains belonging to sequevars 3, 4 and 6 can be conclusively identified.

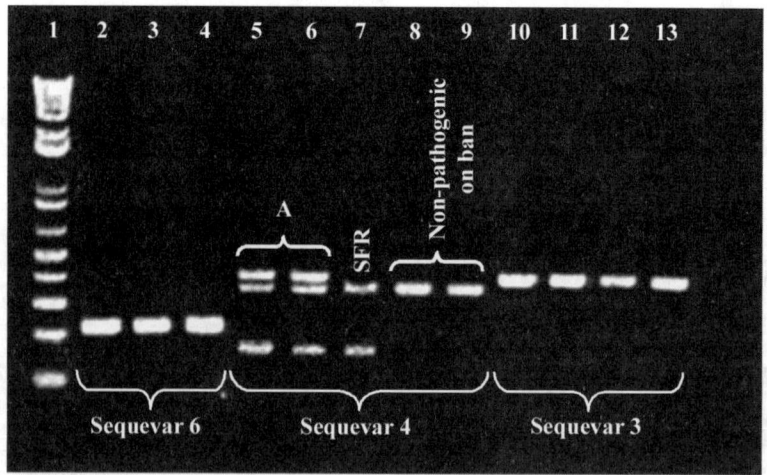

Fig. 2. Sample multiplex PCR gel. Lane 1 contains a 1kb plus DNA ladder from Invitrogen. Lanes 2, 3 and 4 contain sequevar 6 (MLG 28) strains UW20, UW21 and UW182 respectively. Lanes 5 – 9 contain sequevar 4 (MLG 25) strains UW127, UW131, UW179, UW70, ANT307 and ANT11212. Lanes 10 – 13 contain the strains UW09, UW11. UW135 and UW138.

This multiplex-PCR test must be validated further using a greater number of isolates including more recently isolated strains of *R. solanacearum*. However, this PCR has already been useful in improving our understanding of the phylogenetic relationships within this group of *R. solanacearum* strains and may also prove useful in epidemiological studies and for quarantine purposes. It is anticipated that validation of this multiplex-PCR in an epidemiological survey may allow identification of isolates that would otherwise escape diagnosis. A negative result from this PCR for an *R. solanacearum* strain of phylotype II isolated from *Musa* spp. should be taken as strong indication of emerging or unsuspected strains which will add to the global phylogenetic scheme. This molecular test should be accompanied by tests assessing pathogenicity on banana to allow the complete phenotypic and genetic description of isolates.

The *egl* gene phylogeny-based phylotyping scheme (Fegan and Prior, this volume) used to choose strains for the subtractive hybridization approach resulted in the identification of sequevar-specific genomic DNA fragments. The success of this approach validates the phylogenetic relationships identified by the *egl* gene based phylogeny and a similar approach may be employed to identify areas of the genome specific for other important groups within the *R. solanacearum* species complex.

Literature Cited

1. Buddenhagen, I.W., and Elsasser, T.A. 1962. An insect-spread bacterial wilt epiphytotic of bluggoe banana. Nature 194:164-165.
2. Cook, D., and Sequeira, L. 1994. Strain differentiation of *Pseudomonas solanacearum* by molecular genetic methods. Pages 77-94 in: Bacterial wilt: the disease and its causative agent, *Pseudomonas solanacearum*, A.C. Hayward and G.L. Hartman, eds. CAB International, Wallingford, UK.
3. Cook, D., Barlow, E., and Sequeira, L. 1989. Genetic diversity of *Pseudomonas solanacearum*: detection of restriction fragment polymorphisms with DNA probes that specify virulence and hypersensitive response. Mol. Plant-Microbe Interact. 2:113-121.
4. Fegan, M., Taghavi, M., Sly, L.I., and Hayward, A.C. 1998. Phylogeny, diversity and molecular diagnostics of *Ralstonia solanacearum*. Pages 19-33 in: Bacterial Wilt Disease: Molecular and Ecological Aspects, edited by P. Prior, C. Allen, and J. Elphinstone, eds. Springer, Berlin.
5. French, E.R., and Sequeira, L.. 1970. Strains of *Pseudomonas solanacearum* from Central and South America: a comparative study. Phytopathology 70:506-512.

6. Hayward, A.C. 1994. Systematics and phylogeny of *Pseudomonas solanacearum* and related bacteria. Pages 123-136 in: Bacterial wilt: the disease and its causative agent, *Pseudomonas solanacearum*, A.C. Hayward and G.L. Hartman, eds. CAB International, Wallingford.
7. Norman, D.J., and Yuen, J.M.F. 1998. A distinct pathotype of *Ralstonia (Pseudomonas) solanacearum* race 1, biovar 1 entering Florida in pothos (*Epipremnum aureum*) cuttings. Can. J. Plant Pathol. 20:171-175.
8. Norman, D.J, and Yuen, J.M.F. 1998. First report of *Ralstonia (Pseudomonas) solanacearum* infecting pot anthurium production in Florida. Plant Dis. 83:300.
9. Sequeira, L. 1998. Bacterial wilt: the missing element in international banana improvement programs. Pages 6-14 in: Bacterial Wilt Disease; Molecular and Ecological Aspects. P. Prior, C. Allen, and J. Elphinstone, eds. Springer, Berlin.

Appendix

MULTIPLEX PCR METHOD

Reactions were carried out in a total volume of 25 µl containing 1x PCR buffer (supplied by the manufacturer of the polymerase) 1.5 mM $MgCl_2$, 0.2 mM of each dNTP, 2U of *Taq* Polymerase (Biotech International, Perth WA, Australia), 6 pmoles of each primer (Table 2). Reactions were heated to 96°C for 5 min and then cycled through 30 cycles of 94°C for 15s, 59°C for 30s and 72°C for 30s, followed by a final extension period of 10 min at 72°C. Samples (5 µl) of reaction mixtures were examined by electrophoresis through 2% agarose gels and bands were revealed by staining in 0.5 µg/ml ethidium bromide.

Bacterial Wilt Disease Complex of Banana in Indonesia

Siti Subandiyah[1], Siwi Indarti[1], Tri Harjaka[1], Sri N.H. Utami[2], Christanti Sumardiyono[1], and Mulyadi[1]

[1]Dept. of Entomology and Plant Pathology, [2]Dept. of Soil Science, Faculty of Agriculture, Gadjah Mada University Yogyakarta 55281, Indonesia

Banana is cultivated in Indonesia with little or no input and attention and grows anywhere in the yards surrounding the houses, in the villages, and in the fields. However, banana and plantain are quite important commodities as fresh or cooking fruits for dessert, substitute food, or snacks and they are consumed continuously. The high economic value of the plant led to the development of *in vitro* propagation of banana in Indonesia and therefore, some extensive banana plantations have been established with more intensive cultivation and a formal banana industry is developing.

The rapid spread of blood disease since the 1980s in most islands of the country reduced banana production markedly. The disease was endemic at first only in South Sulawesi and Selayar island in the 1920s (5) and was confined there for about 60 years. However, in the early 1980s the disease was found in some spots in Yogyakarta with low severity and little damage (1). Another incident was reported in Bogor and as a result the bacterial pathogen *Pseudomonas celebensis* was described (4); following this, the pathogen spread explosively through the islands of the country causing quite severe damage. Transportation among the islands has been going on in Indonesia for hundreds of years; therefore, distribution of banana materials apparently occurred without increasing the incidence of the disease until the 1980s.

Global warming due to the greenhouse effect, with burning of forests which occurred in most islands of Indonesia, may have caused an increase in the aggressiveness of the blood disease bacterium (BDB) and of the insect vectors associated with the disease. However, there is no proof since BDB isolates from the past do not exist and cannot be compared with those from the present. Molecular analysis suggests that BDB is closely related to *Ralstonia solanacearum* within a distinct group belonging to Phylotype IV, found only in Indonesia (Fegan and Prior, this volume).

The epidemiology of blood disease is quite similar to that of Moko disease, except that BDB is only infectious on banana but not on *Heliconia* spp. nor on solanaceous plants. However, different species of Heliconia may have different responses to BDB and it has been reported that the bacterium can infect *Helionia*. BDB is transmitted both through the soil and running water and by insect vectors. A wide distribution of common insects visits banana inflorescences (14). Many inflorescence-visiting insects from different families were reported to carry BDB (15, 16).

This paper discusses the association of blood disease with banana insect pests or pollinating insects and nematodes in the endemic areas of Yogyakarta province. The infestation of insect pests and nematodes weakens the host plant so it becomes more susceptible to BDB, and the insect pests or nematode also have the potential to vector the bacterial pathogen. Therefore, the bacterial wilt disease complex demands integrated disease control that may include sanitation, pest and nematode control, resistant cultivars or induced resistance mechanism as the components for integrated pest management.

Materials and Methods

FIELD LOCATION

Three districts in Yogyakarta province with 13 endemic areas of BDB were observed using the method of Stratified Random Sampling from September to December 2001. The distance between endemic areas in each district was about 5–10 km. The altitudes ranged from a few metres to about 130 m above sea level. Banana plantations belonged to local farmers with more than 20 banana clusters in each locality. Cultural practice was conducted traditionally with little or no input of fertilizer or pesticide. There were no seedlings sown from *in vitro* propagation used as planting materials. The plants were self propagated or farmers propagated from their own banana plantation for new plantings. Farmers apply simple cultural practices some-times by cutting the old leaves, suckers, and male inflorescences, removing the decaying pseudostems and cleaning the yard.

FIELD OBSERVATIONS

Field observations were conducted for disease intensity, insect pest infestation, inflorescence-visiting insects, nematodes, soil type and soil pH. Disease intensity was measured by calculating the percentage of infected banana clusters in one location. The only insect pests studied were major pests (11) that may relate to BDB infection or transmission. Common pollinating insects visiting the inflorescence were observed and identified. Nematodes were observed in the root and the rhizosphere by collecting roots and the soil samples, which were extracted in the laboratory in order to calculate the population density and nematode identification. Soil samples were also collected for pH analysis and soil texture.

BDB IDENTIFICATION

Wilting banana samples found in the field were collected and brought to the laboratory for BDB isolation and quick identification to confirm that the plant samples were infected by BDB. Bacterial isolation was conducted from the fruits, peduncles, true stem, or corm and plated on CPG medium (13). Suspected bacterial colonies were checked for Gram reaction using 3% KOH and used for tobacco hypersensitivity tests. When the bacteria were Gram-negative and the tobacco hypersensitivity test was positive, the plant sample was confirmed as BDB infection. Two BDB isolates were sent for further confirmation by Dr. Mark Fegan at the University of Queensland.

When BDB detection was negative, we referred back to the recorded field symptoms to check for likely *Fusarium* infection. Fusarium infection in the field usually resulted in discoloration of vascular bundles in the pseudostem in contrast with BDB where these were in the true stem. Furthermore, *Fusarium* infection frequently causes longitudinal breakdown of the infected pseudostem and it does not cause any rotting or ripening of immature fruits, which is quite different from BDB symptoms (18). The samples of wilt were also tested for *Fusarium* using PDA isolation medium to identify the fungal colonies. In the field, usually cv. Kepok (ABB) was the most susceptible to BDB, whereas *Fusarium* more commonly attacked Ambon (AAB) and closely related cultivars.

INSECT IDENTIFICATION

Insect pest identification was mainly for major insect pests associated with the larvae or the adult attacking leaves, stem, or inflorescence/fruits. Leaves damaged by insects were observed for the typical damage appearing on the leaves and the presence of the larvae on the leaves or the adult insect in the environment. Stem damage was observed by cutting or sectioning the pseudostem and the true stem or corm both longitudinally and transversely and looking for larvae and adult insects in the infested stem. Damage on the inflorescence and fruit was observed closely and examined for the insect attacking the plant. Insect samples were collected and identified in the laboratory. (2,14).

Pollinating insects visiting the inflorescence were observed early in the morning, in the afternoon, and early in the evening. The insects were collected using an insect catching screen and brought to the laboratory for further identification (2,14).

SOIL ANALYSIS

Soil samples were obtained from the rhizosphere of BDB-infected banana and from healthy plants, and from the area surrounding the banana plantation. The samples were taken to the laboratory for pH and soil texture analysis. Soil pH and soil texture were observed using the method of Tan (25). Soil taxonomy was determined using keys to soil taxonomy (19, 24).

Results and Discussion

Table 1 shows that higher BDB intensity is associated with insect pests or nematode infestation. Two species of insect pests were related to high intensities of BDB. They were *Erionata thrax* (Lepidoptera) and *Cosmopolites sordidus*, whereas *Nacoleia octasema* was found only in few samples. Infestation of *E. thrax* associated with high densities of leaf rolling symptoms was found in the districts of Kotamadya and Sleman. The larvae in the rolling leaves became butterflies that must feed on banana inflorescences; therefore they have potential to spread BDB. *E. thrax* infestation was correlated with high incidence of BDB whenever there was pathogen inoculum and susceptible host plants.

The other lepidopteran found in BDB endemic areas was *N. octasema*. The pest was found only in a few BDB infected fruits with some larvae and scabby fruits. The moths lay eggs near the bracts of an emerging inflorescence. The larvae feed on the inflorescence and young fruits, causing wounds that may increase the susceptibility of the host plant to BDB infection. The pest life cycle is completed in a single inflorescence until the moth is ready to lay eggs on other inflorescences; therefore, this insect may have less potential for spreading BDB. High BDB intensities (30%) in Wonosari 2 (Table 1) and the infestation of *N. octasema* seemed to be more correlated with the high population density of *Pratylenchus* sp. nematodes.

True stem or corn borer *C. sordidus* has been reported in combination with nematode infestation on banana (8,21,22). The damage to roots caused by parasitic nematodes weakens the infected plant and makes it more susceptible to other pathogens or insect pests. Jumjunidang *et al.*(12) reported that the increase of banana root damage by parasitic nematodes was correlated with the increase of damage by *C. sordidus* in West Sumatra

Table 1. Banana Bacterial Wilt Disease Complex in Yogyakarta Province[a]

Locality	BDB (%)	Insect Pest Occurrence	Pratylenchus density[b]	Fusarium wilt	Soil Type and pH
Yogya city1	80	Erionata	1334.78	no	Entisol, sandy, 6.86
Yogya city 2	30	Erionata	27	no	Entisol, sandy, 7.14
Yogya city 3	25	Erionata	0	no	Entisol, sandy loamy, 7.33
Banana germplasm	10	Erionata	333.33	no	Entisol, loamy, 5.71
Sundak1	50	Cosmopolites	16.67	no	Entisol, loamy, 6.59
Sundak 2	40	Cosmopolites	90.25	yes	Inceptisol, clay-loamy, 5.87
Tunjungsari 1	0	Cosmopolites	42.20	yes	Inceptisol, clay-loamy, 6.59
Tunjungsari 2	0	Cosmopolites and Nacolea	7.95	yes	Inceptisol, clay-loamy, 7.53
Tepus 1	0	Cosmopolites	0	yes	Inceptisol, clay-loamy, 7.33
Tepus 2	0	Cosmopolites	12.0	yes	Inceptisol, clay-loamy, 6.52
Wonosari 1	70	none	831.42	no	Vertisol, clay, 7.12
Wonosari 2	30	Nacolea	1009.27	no	Vertisol, clay, 7.45
Wonosari 3	0	none	116.67	no	Vertisol, clay, 6.62

[a] Data observed from September – December 2001.
[b] Population density of *Pratylenchus* per 10 g banana roots.

Furthermore, in this study we found that the infestation of *C. sordidus* was also correlated with high BDB incidence (Table 1). The BDB infected banana samples were found to have many larvae of *C. sordidus* in the true stems and even in the peduncles. The insect pest is not very active and moves >25 m in six months, and the weevils rarely fly (6); therefore, the infestation by this pest may increase the susceptibility of the host plant to BDB rather than leading to long-distance disease transmission. In addition, plantain (ABB) was reported to be the most susceptible to *C. sordidus* (3,6) and also to BDB (10,24).

Several insects visiting banana inflorescences may be pollinating insects. The butterfly of *Erionata thrax* was found quite frequently as an inflorescence visitor in the morning and late in the afternoon. Other Dipteran and Hymenopteran insects were found in almost all areas and we identified *Apis trigona* as the most common insect visiting banana inflorescence in Yogyakarta.

Several genera of nematodes were found attacking banana in the BDB endemic areas, including *Pratylenchus* sp., *Meloidogyne* sp., *Haplolaimus* sp., *Rhadopholus* sp.. However, *Pratylenchus* sp. was the most common and was found in almost all samples with population densities ranging from 16.67 – 1334.78 nematodes per 10 gram of root sample. Higher population densities of *Pratylenchus* sp. showed higher intensities of BDB in Yogya city 1, Wonosari 1, and Wonosari 2 (Table 1). *Pratylenchus* sp. is a migratory endoparasite that causes wounds and root damage and actively moves from one root to others (7). Therefore, this nematode may increase the susceptibility of the host plant and transmit the bacterial pathogen as well.

The distribution of BDB in relation to soil pH suggested that BDB occurred at the soil pHs ranging from 5.71 to 7.45. BDB was also found in soil types with sandy to clay loams classified as Entisol, Inceptisol and Vertisol, the most common soil types found in Yogyakarta (24). Further research on the survival of BDB in different soil pH and soil texture should be conducted.

The incidence of BDB in Yogyakarta province seemed to be associated with a complex infestation of insect pests and nematodes. Fusarium wilt was also found and sometimes was in the same location as BDB (Table 1). Therefore, integrated control is needed for the disease management. Insect pest control to prevent infestation by pests that weaken banana plants, create entry wounds for the bacterium, and may spread BDB is quite important for effective management of BDB.

Acknowledgements

The authors would like to thank ACIAR especially Dr. Paul Ferrar for his effort to gain the travel grant and Gadjah Mada University for the research grant. Our appreciation also to the scientific committee of 3rd IBWS in White River, RSA, especially Prof. C. Allen and Dr. P. Prior. Our gratitude to Dr. A.C. Hayward for good discussion in preparing this manuscript.

Literature Cited

1. Arwiyanto, T. 1985. Identifikasi penyakit bakterial pada tanaman pisang di Yogyakarta. Pages 46-47 in: Proc. 8th Conf. of the Indonesian Plant Pathology Soc. Jakarta 29-31 Oct. 1985.
2. Borror, D.J. 1992. Pengenalan Pelajaran Serangga. Gadjah Mada University Press.
3. Desmawati, A., Hasyim, and Harlion. 1997. Intensitas kerusakan hama penggerek bonggol pisang padaberbagai kelompok genom pisang. In: Proc. 5th Con. of Indonesian Entomology Soc. Bandung 24-26 Juni 1997.
4. Eden Green, S.J., Supriadi, and Hartati, S.Y. 1988. Characterization of *Pseudomonas celebensis*, the cause of blood disease of bananas in Indonesia. Page 349 (abstract) in: Proc. 5th Int. Con. Plant Pathology. Kyoto, 20-27 August.
5. Gäumann, E. 1921. Ondezoekingen over de bloedziekte der banananen op Celebes I. Mededeelingen Van Het Inst. Voor Planten Ziekten 50.
6. Gold, C.S., and Messianen, S. 2001. The banana weevils *Cosmopolites sordidus*. Musa Pest Fact Sheet No. INIBAP.
7. Gowen, S., and Quenerheve, P. 1990. Nematode parasite of banana, plantains, and abaca. Pages 431-460 in: Plant parasitic nematodes in subtropical and tropical agriculture. CAB. Int. Inst. of Parasitology.
8. Hadisoeganda, W.W. 1994. Status of nematode problems affecting banana in Indonesia. Pages 63-73 in: Banana nematodes and weevil borers in Asia and the Pacific. INIBAP.
9. Hanudin, Tjahjono, B., and Sugiharso. 1993. Uji resistensi varietas pisang terhadap bakteri layu. J. Hortikultura. 3:37-42.
10. Hardoo, A., and Golden, I.M. 1989. A key and diagnostic Compendium to the species of the genus Pratylenchus Filipjew. J. Nematol. 21:202-218.
11. Hasyim, A., Harlion, Desmawati, and Junjunidang. 1996. Hama-hama penting pada pertanaman pisang. In:Buku Komoditas Pisang. Badan Litbang Pertanian. Puslitbang Hortikultura. Research Inst. For Horticulture, Solok.
12. Jumjunidang, Hasyim, A., Desmawati, Harlion, and Sumargono, A. 1998. Distribusi geografis nematoda parasit akar pisang dan hubungannya dengan hama penggerek bonggol *Cosmopolites sordidus* Germ. Di Sumatra Barat. J. Hortikultura 8:1095-1101.
13. Kelman, A. 1953. The bacterial wilt caused by *Pseudomonas solanacearum*. NC Agric. Exp. Stn. Tech. Bull. 99, Raleigh N.C.
14. Klashoven, L.G.E. 1981. Pest of Crops in Indonesia. P.A. Van der Laan ed. PT. Ichtisar Baru, Jakarta.

15. Leiwakabessy, C. 1999. Potensi beberapa jenis serangga dalam penyebaran penyakit layu bakteri *Ralstonia (Pseudomonas) solanacearum* Yabuuchi *et al* pada pisang di Lampung. Master Thesis. Bogor Agriculture University.
16. Maryam, A.B.N., Rasta, T., Handayani, W., and Sihombing, D. 1997. Akuisisi dan persistensi bakteri layu pada tanaman pisang oleh serangga. Pages 154-161 in: Proc. of National Seminar of Indonesian Entomology Soc. Bogor 8 Jan. 1997.
17. Moi, W.F. 1968. Pictorial key to genera of plant parasitic nematodes. Art Craft, Ithaca. NY.
18. Semangun, H. 2000. Penyakit-penyakit Tanaman Hortikultura di Indonesia. 2nd ed. Gadjah Mada University Press. Yogyakarta
19. Soil Survey Staff. 1999. Keys to Soil Taxonomy. SMSS Technical Monograph No. 6.
20. Southey, J.F. 1985. Laboratory methods for work with plant and soil nematodes. Her Majesty's Stationary Office. London.
21. Spijer, P.R., Budenberge, W.J., and Sikora, R.A. 1993. Relationship between nematodes, weevils, banana and plantain cultivars and damage. Ann. Appl. Biol 123:517-525.
22. Spijer, P.R., Gold, C.S., Karamura, E.B., and Kshaija, I.N. 1994. Banana weevils and nematode distribution pattern in Highland banana system in Uganda. Preliminary results from diagnostic survey. Pages 285-289 in: African Crop Sci. Proc. I.
23. Subandiyah, S., Nursilaturahmu, Nugrahaningsih, A.E., and Sumardiyono, C. 2001. The antagonism and induced resistance by fluorescent pseudomods against the banana blood disease pathogen *Ralstonia solanacearum*. Page 257 in: 13th Biennial Plant Pathology Conference Handbook, Cairns 24-27 September 2001. Australian Plant Pathologicial Society.
24. Sutanto, R., Maas, A., Ranst, E.V., Stoops, G., and Eswaran, H. 1994. Pedological excursion areas around Yogyakarta and Central Java, Indonesia. ITC-Gent. Pub. Series No. 6.
25. Tan, Him H. 1996. Soil samplings, preparations and analyses. Marcell Dekker, Inc. NY.

Bacterial Wilt of *Heliconia* in Pernambuco, Brazil: First Report and Detection by PCR in Soil and Rhizomes

S.M.P. Assis[1], I.S. Oliveira[2], V.N. Covello[2], K.G. Rehn[3], and R.L.R. Mariano[2]

[1] Botânica/Depto. Biologia,[2] Fitossanidade/Depto. Agronomia/ UFRPE, 52171-900, Recife-PE. [3]Departamento de Bioquímica/ CCB/UFPE, 50670-901, Recife-PE

The genus *Heliconia* belongs to the family Heliconiaceae and, along with the family Musaceae, is included in the Zingiberales. The inflorescences of *Heliconia* species are very popular in Brazil because of their exuberance and durability. However, crop expansion, which demands importing and commercializing rhizomes, risk pathogen and pest dissemination. Bacterial wilt caused by *Ralstonia solanacearum* is the only bacterial disease of *Heliconia* species around the world.

Race 2 of *R. solanacearum* infects triploid bananas and heliconias, and is found in Hawaii, Costa Rica, Mexico, Guatemala, Honduras, Colombia, Venezuela, Peru, Brazil, Suriname, the Guyanas, Trinidad, Grenada, India and the Philippines (3, 19). In Brazil, *R. solanacearum* race 2 is widespread on bananas in the states of Amapá, Amazonas, Pará and Rondônia (18). In the Northeast, centers of disease were detected in the states of Paraíba, Ceará, Sergipe and Alagoas (20).

Heliconia species can be asymptomatically infected by race 2 (7). *Heliconia* spp. can also host isolates not pathogenic to banana or giving only atypical symptoms, but causing tomato wilt and apparently belonging to race 1. An association of *R. solanacearum* with heliconia wilt does therefore not necessarily mean that the isolate in question can infect banana. Thus, various pathogenicity tests and observation of all symptoms are necessary to establish the proper race identity (3).

In heliconias, bacterial wilt has been reported in Costa Rica in *Heliconia latispatha, H. caribaea, H. acuminata, H. imbricata* (3,15) and *H. bihai* (15), in Hawaii (USA) in *H. psittacorum* and *H. rostrata* (4) and in Colombia in *H. latispatha* (5). In Brazil this is also the only bacterial disease in *Heliconia* spp., reported in the states of Pernambuco (1) and Amazonas (Dr. Bernard Boher, pers. comm.).

423

First Report of *Ralstonia solanacearum* in Heliconia in Pernambuco and Brazil

In March of 1999, in the State of Pernambuco, Brazil, tropical flower plantations were visited and different species of *Heliconia* were collected showing symptoms similar to those observed in the Moko disease of banana. Adult plants showed wilting, yellowing and leaf necrosis. These symptoms started in central leaves and were followed by xylem collapse. The center of the pseudostem was discolored and a transverse section revealed bacterial ooze. These symptoms agree with those described in Hawaii by Sewake and Uchida (16). However, the upper part of the pseudostem and plants in the initial stages of disease did not always show discoloration or bacterial ooze. Unfolding new leaves in new shoots showed distortion, yellowing and necrosis, which impaired their development. These symptoms frequently preceded rot, collapse and plant death. Infected plants were observed in *H. bihai*, *H. caribaea*, *H. humilis*, *H. nickeriensis* (*H. psittacorum* x *H. marginata*) *H. psittacorum* cv. Lady Di, cv. Red Opol, cv. Sassy, cv. Strawberries, *H. psittacorum* x *H. spathocircinata* cv. Golden Torch, *Heliconia rauliniana* (*H. marginata* x *H. bihai*), *H. stricta* and *H. wagneriana*.

Bacterial isolates obtained from infected rhizomes of *Heliconia* spp. presented the same morphological and biochemical features as those described by Yabuuchi *et al.* (25) for *R. solanacearum* and for biovar 2 according to Hayward (6). The hypersensitivity reactions were positive in tobacco leaves. In pathogenicity tests, the characteristic symptoms of bacterial wilt were observed 20 to 30 days after inoculation in heliconia and banana cv. Pacovan but no disease appeared in tomato cv. Santa Clara. Amplification by PCR using the primers OLI1 and Y2 from a diagnostic region of *R. solanacearum* 16S rRNA (14) produced a band with a molecular weight of approximately 300 bp,. The pathogen was therefore identified as *R. solanacearum*, race 2, biovar 1.

Bacterial wilt in heliconias has seriously affected the commercialization of rhizomes and the establishment of new plantations in Pernambuco, Brazil. Bacterial wilt of heliconia was found in five out of seven commercial plantations of tropical flowers, a high prevalence (71%). In the species of *Heliconia* with obvious symptoms, disease incidence varied from 2 to 10%. All contaminated sites were visited over a period of two years and in spite of an initially low disease incidence in some areas, the majority suffered appreciable yield losses. This can be attributed to the ability of the pathogen to survive in the soil for many years, and to the high virulence of the isolates of *R. solanacearum* present in these areas. During the rainy season, several species of *Heliconia* showed 50% mortality. Mortality diminished considerably in the dry period, when the irrigation was kept at a minimum level and the pathogen was thereby eradicated in four of the five flower plantations. A new crop planted after a 6-12 month fallow was disease-free. According to Ferreira (3), in conditions favorable to symptom development such as high temperature and humidity, heliconia wilt becomes irreversible and leads to plant death. On the other hand, even under favorable conditions latent infection may occur, or the infected plants have only yellowing and stunting.

In Brazil bacterial wilt of heliconias occurred at nearly the same time in many plantations and in different *Heliconia* species, those recently imported and in those already cultivated. This pattern suggests an epidemiology of inadvertent pathogen dissemination in Pernambuco and Brazil by the import of rhizomes, probably with latent infections. The same mode of introduction occurred in Australia after the import of *Heliconia* rhizomes from Hawaii, and a quarantine strategy was successfully implemented to eradicate the disease (7).

Thus, the vigorous exchange of infected germplasm, plantlets and rhizomes, at short or long distances, was a major factor for the dissemination of *R. solanacearum* in heliconia and in bananas. In addition, the pathogen is easily spread across soil and surface water by root contact, by mechanical transmission in cultural practices such as pruning and harvesting, by nematodes and humans (9). In heliconia cultivation, crop harvesting favors the pathogen dissemination, not only by means of the inoculum present on the knife but also by the inoculum from soil, because the inflorescence is harvested near the ground.

High soil humidity (8), a common condition in the culture of heliconias, which are frequently irrigated, actively promotes survival and dissemination of *R. solanacearum*. Moreover, the dense foliage in a heliconia plantation creates a humid microclimate and the crop is frequently cultivated at the edges of water streams. This last fact is probably responsible for the frequent pathogen spread inside flower farms and among different host species. According to Buddenhagen and Kelman (2), dry periods reduce the viability of the pathogen and diminish the intensity of the disease. Otherwise, the long-term soil survival of *R. solanacearum* is due to the presence of weed hosts and volunteer plants, which contribute as alternative sources of inoculum for the maintenance of high population levels of the bacteria in the soil (8). In the specific case of heliconia culture, pruning and harvesting always generates a large amount of crop residue. This is used as mulch and together with the weed hosts contributes further to bacterial survival.

Detection of *Ralstonia solanacearum* by PCR in Soil and Rhizomes

Five soil samples from the state of Pernambuco, Brazil, were used for DNA extraction, all with a pH around 6.5. Two of these samples were collected from the rhizosphere of wilted heliconias in production areas. Two samples came from maize plantations, where *R. solanacearum* had been observed in tomato two years before. These four samples represented naturally infested soils. The fifth sample, divided in subsamples, consisted of sterilized soil artificially infested with suspensions of *R. solanacearum* at six different concentrations (10^2 to 10^7 CFU/g).

The methods of extraction established by Zhou *et al.* (26) and Kuske *et al.* (10) were modified and optimized in order to hasten the extraction process and to allow specific detection by PCR. This procedure was performed with the naturally or artificially infested soil samples.

The principal difficulty in designing a method to detect *R. solanacearum* by PCR in soil samples is the formulation of a DNA extraction method that is at once practical, rapid and able to prevent the action of inhibitors in order to guarantee the typical sensitivity of PCR without a previous pathogen culture step. During extraction, DNA can be lost by adsorption of nucleic acids to the surface of plastic containers or by degradation. In extracting DNA from soil, humic acids are the major contaminants that interfere with the quantification of DNA and its amplification. Contaminants in DNA extracts can inhibit the PCR Taq polymerase, interfere with the restriction enzyme digestion, and reduce the efficiency of bacterial transformation, and the specificity of DNA hybridization (26). During PCR, these substances hinder the cellular lysis necessary for DNA extraction, promote degradation of nucleic acid and inhibit polymerase activity (23). In this work, these problems were addressed by a two-step procedure. First, DNA was extracted from soil using the detergents CTAB and SDS together with proteinase K, but omitting mechanical disintegration, as *R. solanacearum* does not form spores. Afterwards, DNA in the extract was separated from humic acids by its higher molecular weight on a column of Sephadex G-100, mixed with PVP to adsorb phenolic material. This protocol allowed preparation of DNA from soil samples infested naturally (Fig. 1A) and artificially (Fig.1C) in a quality good enough to perform PCR with a high volume of sample in the reaction mixture. At the same time, this procedure was sufficiently rapid that a set of about six samples could be done in less than four hours.

R. solanacearum was also detected in the early stages of rhizome infection from *H. bihai* and *H. psittacorum* (Fig. 1B). Discolored areas near new shoots were perfused with 0.5 ml of TE buffer, using a 1 ml insulin-syringe with fine needle. Bacteria were flushed out of small rhizome pieces and afterwards lysed by heating in a water bath at 100°C for 10 min or digesting

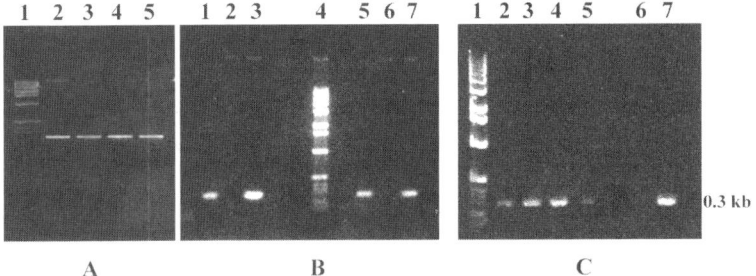

Fig. 1. A: PCR of DNA from soil naturally infested with *R. solanacearum*. Lanes: 1. 1kb ladder; 2. Soil cultivated with *H. bihai*; 3. Soil cultivated with *H. psittacorum*; 4 and 5. Soil cultivated with *Zea mays*. B: Detection of *R. solanacearum* in rhizomes infected with *Heliconia* spp. Lanes: 1. Rhizome of *H. bihai*; 2. Negative control, 3. Positive control; 4.1kb ladder; 5. Rhizome of *H. psittacorum*; 6 and 7. Negative and positive controls, respectively. C: Determining limit of detection of *R. solanacearum* in soil artificially infested with different concentrations of the bacterial suspension. Lanes: 1. 1kb ladder; 2. 10^7 CFU/ml; 3.10^6 CFU/ml; 4.10^5 CFU/ml; 5. 10^4 CFU/ml; 6.Negative control; 7.Positive control.

with lysozyme and proteinase K (24). The DNA extracts thus obtained were purified by gel filtration as above to remove phenolic compounds and other contaminants. As only a small quantity of tissue is required for this procedure, the diagnosis of infection can be performed even on precious or unique rhizome samples without compromising their viability and commercial value.

Thus *R. solanacearum* can be detected in many samples of soil and rhizomes of *Heliconia* spp. by a rapid PCR method that takes one day. In order to study the limit of detection of *R. solanacearum* in soil samples using this PCR protocol, sterilized soil was infested with different bacterial concentrations. In this experiment, the sensitivity of the method for soil samples approached 1 x 10^4 CFU/g of soil (Fig. 1C), a concentration below the critical limit of infection for tomato seedlings. This result corroborates the data of Lee and Wang (11) who found 1 x 10^4 CFU/g using different primers, also specific for *R. solanacearum*. Pradhanang (12) even obtained a sensitivity of 5 x 10^1 CFU/g of soil by a method where he processed for DNA extraction 20 g of a composite sample including 2g from 10 points in an area of 100 m^2. Priou *et al.*(13) detected 2-14.4 x 10^1 CFU/g soil using DAS-ELISA in samples incubated for 48 h at 28°C in an enrichment medium. This modified technique increased the sensitivity of the method but also elevated the cost and the diagnosis time with reduced practicality. Van der Wolf *et al.* (21), using the technique of immunofluorescence colony-staining (IFC) obtained a detection limit of 1×10^2 CFU/g soil, considerably better than the 1×10^4 to 1×10^6 CFU/g, found for the bioassay with tomato plants. However, their IFC was tarnished by cross-reactions with other bacteria taxonomically related to *R. solanacearum*.

Weller *et al.* (22) used fluorogenic probes in PCR for the detection of *R. solanacearum* in pure cultures, reaching a sensitivity of 1×10^2 cells/ml. However, sensitivity was much diminished when PCR was carried out with DNA extracted from inoculated potato tissues. Even so, the authors recommended this method to detect bacteria in potato seed. In the present work, the detection of *R. solanacearum* in soil samples collected from an area without living host plants demonstrates the ability of this bacterium to survive in these conditions. According to Shamsuddin *et al.* (17), even in the absence of plant tissue and with antagonistic microorganisms present, this pathogen stays alive in soil up to 2 years. The data in Fig. 1A indicate that the population density of *R. solanacearum* in the soils tested is equal or greater than the sensitivity limit of the test in artificially infested soil (1×10^4 CFU/g). Bacterial wilt of *Heliconia* in Brazil deserves additional studies involving host range, variability, survival, epidemiology and disease control.

Literature Cited

1. Assis, S.M.P., Rosa, R.C.T., and Mariano, R.L.R. 2000. Ocorrência de *Ralstonia solanacearum* e *Fusarium oxysporum* f. sp. *cubense* em *Heliconia* no Estado de Pernambuco, Brasil. Fitopatol. Bras. 25:319.

2. Buddenhagen, I.W., and Kelman, A. 1964. Biological and physiological aspects of bacterial wilt caused by *Pseudomonas solanacearum*. Annu. Rev. Phytopathol. 2:203-230.

3. Ferreira, S. 1990. Bacterial wilt on heliconia: Hawaii's experience. Heliconia Society International Bulletin 5: 9-11.

4. Ferreira, S., Pitz, K., and Alvarez, A. 1991. *Heliconia* wilt in Hawaii. Phytopathology 81:1159.

5. French, E.R., and Sequeira, L. 1970. Strains of *Pseudomonas solanacearum* from Central and South America. A comparative study. Phytopathology 60:506-512.

6. Hayward, A.C. 1995. Phenotypic methods for the differentiation of *Pseudomonas solanacearum*: biovars and supplementary observations. Pages 27-34 in: Techniques for Diagnosis of *Pseudomonas solanacearum* and for Resistance Screening Against Groundnut Bacterial Wilt. V.K. Mehan and D. McDonald, eds. ICRISAT Technical Manual n.1., India.

7. Hyde, K.D., McCulloch, B., Akiew, E., Peterson, R.A., and Diatloff, A. 1994. Strategies used to eradicate bacterial wilt of *Heliconia* (race 2) in Cairns, Australia, following introduction of the disease from Hawaii. Heliconia Society International Bulletin 6:7-9.

8. Jabuonski, R.E., and Hidalgo, A.O. 1987. Doenças bacterianas. Pages 85-93 in: Produção de Batata. F.J.B. Reifschneider, ccord. Linha Gráfica, Brasília.

9. Kelman, A., Hartman, G.L., and Hayward, A.C. 1994. Introduction. Pages 1-7 in: Bacterial Wilt - The Disease and Its Causative Agent, *Pseudomonas solanacearum*. A.C. Hayward and G.L. Hartman, eds. CAB International, Wallingford.

10. Kuske, C.R., Banton, K.L., Adorada, D.L., Stark, P.C., Hill, K.K., and Jackson, P.J. 1998. Small-scale DNA sample preparation method for PCR detection of microbial cells and spores in soil. Appl. Environ. Microbiol. 64:2463-2472.

11. Lee, Y-A., and Wang, C-C. 2000. The design of specific primers for the detection of *Ralstonia solanacearum* in soil samples by polymerase chain reaction. Botanical Bulletin of Academia Sinica 41:121-128.

12. Pradhanang, P.M. 1999. Optimization of sampling method for accurate detection of *Ralstonia solancearum* in naturally infested soil. ACIAR Bacterial Wilt Newsletter 16:2-5.

13. Priou, S., Aley, P., Fernandéz, H., and Gutarra, L. 1999. Sensitive detection of *Ralstonia solanacearum* (race 3) in soil by post-enrichment DAS-ELISA. ACIAR Bacterial Wilt Newsletter 16:10-13.

14. Seal, S.E., Jackson, L.A., Young, J.P.W., and Daniels, M.J. 1993. Differentiation of *Pseudomonas solanacearum*, *P. syzygii*, *P. pickettii* and the blood disease bacterium by partial 16S rRNA sequencing: construction of oligonucleotide primers for sensitive detection by polymerase chain reaction. J. Gen. Microbiol. 139:1587-1594.

15. Sequeira, L., and Averre, C.W. 1961. Distribution and pathogenicity of strains of *Pseudomonas solanacearum* from virgin soils in Costa Rica. Plant Dis. Rep. 45: 435-440.

16. Sewake, K.T., and Uchida, J.Y. 1995. Diseases of Heliconia in Hawaii. Hawaii Institute of Tropical Agriculture and Human Resources, Honolulu, Research Extension Series 159-4.

17. Shamsuddin, N., Lloyd, A.B., and Graham, J. 1978. Survival of potato strain of *Pseudomonas solanacearum* in soil. J. Austral. Inst. Agric. Sci. 44:212-215.

18. Silva, J.R. 1997. Coletânea de Informações Sobre o "Moko" da Bananeira. MARA, Brasília, (versão preliminar).

19. Stansbury, C., McKirdy, S., and Power, G. 2000. Moko Disease *Ralstonia solanacearum* Exotic Threat to Western Australia. Agriculture Western Australian 17. Available at:

<http:www.agric.wa.gov.au/programs/app/Industry/Hortguard/ananafa cts/Moko.pdf>

20. Takatsu, A. 2001. Moko da Bananeira no Brasil. Pages 439-452 in: Anais do Simpósio Brasileiro de Bananicultura. FUNEP, Jaboticabal.

21. Van der Wolf, J.M., Vriend, S.G.C., Kastelein, P., Nijhuis, E.H., Van Bekkum, P.J., and Van Vuurde, J.W.L. 1999. Immunofluorescence colony-staining (IFC) for detection and quantification of *Ralstonia* (*Pseudomonas*) *solanacearum* biovar 2 (race 3) in soil and verification of positive results by PCR and dilution plating. Eur. J. Plant Pathol. 106:123-133.

22. Weller, A.S., Elphinstone, J.G., Smith, N.C., Boonham, N., and Stead, D.E. 2000. Detection of *Ralstonia solanacearum* strains with a quantitative, multiplex, real-time, fluorogenic PCR (TaqMan) assay. Appl. Environ. Microbiol. 66:2853-2858.

23. Wilson, I.G. 1997. Inhibition and facilitation of nucleic acid amplification. Appl. Environ. Microbiol. 63:3741-3751.

24. Woo, T.H.S., Cheng, A.F., and Ling, J.M. 1992. An application of a simple method for the preparation of bacterial DNA. BioTechniques 13:696-698.

25. Yabuuchi, E., Kosako, Y., Yano, I., Hotta, H., and Nishiuchi, Y. 1995. Transfer of two *Burkholderia* and an *Alcaligenes* species to *Ralstonia* gen. nov.: proposal of *Ralstonia picketii* (Ralston, Palleroni & Doudoroff 1973) comb. nov. *Ralstonia solanacearum* (Smith, 1896) comb. nov. and *Ralstonia eutropha* (Davis, 1969) comb. nov. Microbiol. Immunol. 39:897-904.

26. Zhou, J., Bruns, M.A., and Tiedje, J.M. 1996. DNA recovery from soils of diverse composition. Appl. Environ. Microbiol. 62:316-333.

Use of GPS and GIS Technologies to Map the Prevalence of Moko Disease of Banana in the Amazonas Region of Brazil

R.A. Coelho Netto[1] and F.W. Nutter, Jr. [2]

[1]Instituto National de Pesquisa da Amazonia, Manaus, Brazil;
[2]Iowa State University, Ames, Iowa 50011 USA

Moko disease of banana, caused by *Ralstonia solanacearum*, causes a lethal disease of banana in many parts of the world, and is especially devastating to banana growers in the Amazon region of Brazil (4,5). In this region, Moko disease is the major production constraint limiting banana yields and explains why the Amazon region imports, rather than exports bananas. *R. solanacearum* survives in the soil, in the rhizosphere and in plant roots, and can be disseminated over long distances on vegetative propagation material (2). Although infested insects and farm implements have been implicated in the dissemination of the pathogen (1,5,7,15), there is little quantitative information on the prevalence and incidence of Moko in the Amazonas region. Moreover, little is actually known about how the bacterium is disseminated between banana plantations (5).

One of the basic tenets of integrated disease management is that the presence, distribution and intensity of any yield-reducing factor must be known (10,11). The coupling of global positioning systems (GPS) and geographic information systems (GIS) technologies with data on the prevalence and incidence of disease has tremendous potential to derive new information and hypotheses concerning factors contributing to disease risk (12). Quantifying the temporal and spatial spread of plant pathogens within and among host populations should lead to a better understanding of pathosystem dynamics as well as more effective disease management programs (9). Addressing the spatial aspect, we tried to determine if individual banana plantations infected with *R. solanacearum* affect the disease status of neighboring banana plantations.

The objectives of this study were to (i) quantify the prevalence and incidence of Moko disease of banana in 15 municipalities in the Amazonas region of Brazil; (ii) map the prevalence of Moko disease of banana in the Amazonas region; and (iii) determine if there is a greater risk for Moko disease in banana plantations subject to periodic flooding than in banana plantations not subject to periodic flooding.

Materials and Methods

SAMPLING AND ASSESSMENT METHODS

Fifteen municipalities in the Amazonas region were assessed for the prevalence (number of banana plantations with Moko disease/total number of plantations assessed X 100) and incidence (number of banana plants with Moko disease/total number of banana plants assessed) of Moko disease in 2001 (10). In this region, most banana plantations are owned by small land holders who grow approximately 50 to 300 banana plants. One hundred and seven banana plantations were arbitrarily selected for disease assessment. The number of banana plants assessed per plantation in our study ranged from 45 to 1,025. To determine if Moko disease was present within a plantation, banana plants exhibiting symptoms typical of those caused by *R. solanacearum* were cut near the base of a pseudostem and examined for vascular discoloration typical of Moko disease. If vascular discoloration was present, a 15-cm long section of the pseudostem was placed in a plastic bag and transported to the laboratory. The pathogen was isolated using a tetrazolium medium (4, 7) and isolated colonies were subjected to biochemical characterization (14), biovar determination (5), and pathogenicity tests to confirm that *R. solanacearum* was the causal organism.

GPS AND GIS TECHNOLOGIES

Geographic information systems provide a new set of tools to collect, store, retrieve, transform, and display spatial information for a specific population of sampling units (i.e., banana plantations with and apparently without Moko disease) (12). A global positioning system (GPS) instrument (Panasonic Model KX-G5500, Natsushita Electric Industrial Co., Osaka, Japan) was used to geospatially reference the position of each banana plantation. Universal Transverse Mercator (UTM) mapping units were then used to map the location of all banana plantations found to have Moko disease, as well as those with no evidence of Moko disease, using the geographic information systems (GIS) software program ArcView (ESRI, Redlands, CA) (12).

Chi-square analysis (16) was used to test the null hypothesis that the binomial parameter (Moko disease is present or not present) was homogeneous for all plantations (periodically flooded versus those not periodically flooded). Expected values were computed under the assumption that the null hypothesis was true (12).

Results and Discussion

DISEASE PREVALENCE

Moko disease was found in 5 of 15 municipalities in the Amazonas region in 2001 and disease prevalence within these municipalities ranged from 11 to 100% (Table 1). All isolates belonged to race 2, biovar 1. Disease prevalence averaged across all municipalities ($n = 107$) was quite high (29%).

DISEASE INCIDENCE

The incidence of Moko disease within the five municipalities found to have Moko disease ranged from 0.33 to 9.1% (Table 1). Because Moko results in plant death, this indicates that yield losses due to Moko disease within the five municipalities likewise ranged from 0.33 to 9.1%. These incidence values, however, are likely to underestimate the true impact of Moko disease on yield loss because dead plants in banana plantations (many probably killed by Moko disease) were not included in the incidence assessments. Understandably, Moko incidence within their own plantations was of greater concern to individual small plantation holders. Disease incidence (loss) within individual plantations found to have Moko disease ranged from 1 to 64%.

GIS MAPS

The locations of banana plantations subject to periodic flooding ($n = 52$) and those not subject to periodic flooding ($n = 55$) Were mapped using GIS technology. The locations of banana plantations found to have Moko disease versus plantations not found to have Moko disease were likewise mapped. When the two maps were superimposed, it was apparent that the presence of Moko disease is associated with banana plantations subject to periodic flooding by river water (data not shown). Moko disease occurred

Table 1. Prevalence and incidence of Moko disease of banana within and among municipalities in the Amazonas state in 2001.

Municipality	Prevalence (%)	Incidence (%)
Autazes	0	0
Careiro	0	0
Careiro da Varzea	0	0
Coadjas	20.00	2.03
Coari	65.38	5.53
Iranduba	0	0
Itacoatiara	11.11	0.33
Manacapuru	70.00	9.10
Manaus	0	0
Maues	0	0
Novo Airao	0	0
Presidente Figueiredo	0	0
Rio Preto da Eva	0	0
Silves	0	0
Urucurituba	100.00	7.28

in 30 of 52 (57.7%) plantations subject to periodic flooding, but in only 1 of 55 (1.8%) plantations not subject to periodic flooding.

CHI-SQUARE ANALYSIS

Chi-square analysis indicated that the null hypothesis that Moko disease would occur equally in both flooded and non-flooded banana plantations was strongly rejected ($\chi^2 = 40.55$, $P < 0.0001$), indicating that banana plantations subject to periodic flooding are at a much higher risk for Moko disease compared to banana plantations not subject to periodic flooding. Banana plantations within municipalities in the Amazon region can be considered as a system of either dependent or independent random varieties. It is quite probable that individual banana plantations subject to periodic flooding are having an impact on the disease status of neighboring banana plantations. Certainly, the dissemination of *R. solanacearum* is not limited to one dispersal mechanism and it is highly likely that several mechanisms for the dispersal of *R. solanacearum* are operating simultaneously. Thus, in addition to other known dispersal mechanisms such as the transport of infected vegetative planting material (5), root-to-root transmission (8), rain-splash (13), dispersal by farm implements (5, 15), and pathogen dispersal by insects (1, 4, 15, 17), the present study suggests that river water may also be contributing to the dispersal of *R. solanacearum*. Surface and irrigation (ditch) water is implicated in the epidemiology of potato brown rot disease,

Table 2. Chi-square analysis to test the hypothesis that there is a greater risk for Moko disease of banana in plantations periodically flooded versus plantations not subject to flooding.

	Moko present	Moko not present
Periodically flooded	30	22
Not flooded	1	54

which is caused by a phylogenetically and ecologically distinct group of *R. solanacearum* (3, 6, 18). Additional research utilizing green fluorescent protein (GFP) or antibiotic resistant-marked strains of *R. solanacearum* are needed to determine the relative importance and spatial scale (plant-to-plant; plantation-to-plantation) of each dispersal mechanism (9).

Literature Cited

1. Buddenhagen, I.W., and Elsasser, T.A. 1962. An insect-spread bacterial wilt epiphytotic of bluggoe banana. Nature 194: 164-165.
2. Buddenhagen, I.W., and Kelman, A. 1964. Biological and physiological aspects of bacterial wilt caused by *Pseudomonas solanacearum*. Annu. Rev. Phytopathol. 2: 203-230.
3. Elphinstone, J.G. 1996. Survival and possibilities for extinction of *Pseudomonas solanacearum* (Smith) Smith in cool climates. Potato Res. 39: 403-410.
4. French, E.R., and Sequeira, L. 1970. Strains of *Pseudomonas solanacearum* from Central and South America: A comparative study. Phyto-pathology 60: 506-512.
5. Hayward, A.C. 1991. Biology and epidemiology of bacterial wilt caused by *Pseudomonas solanacearum*. Annu. Rev. Phytopathol. 29: 65-87.
6. Janse, J.D., and Schans, J. 1998. Experience with the diagnosis and epidemiology of bacterial brown rot (*Ralstonia solanacearum*) in The Netherlands. OEPP Bulletin 28: 65-67.
7. Kelman, A. 1954. The relationship of pathogenicity in *Pseudomonas solanacearum* to colony appearance on a tetrazolium medium. Phyto-pathology 44: 693-695.
8. Kelman, A., and Sequeira, L. 1965. Root-to-root spread of *Pseudomonas solanacearum*. Phytopathology 55: 304-309.
9. Nutter, F.W., Jr., Schultz, P.M., and Hill, J.H. 1998. Quatification of within-field spread of soybean mosaic virus in soybean using strain-specific monoclonal antibodies. Phytopathology 88: 895-901.

10. Nutter, F.W., Jr. 2001. Disease assessment terms and concepts. Pages 312-323 in: Encyclopedia of Plant Pathology, O.C. Maloy and T.D. Murray, eds. John Wiley and Sons, Inc., New York.

11. Nutter, F.W., Jr., and Guan, J. 2001. Disease losses. Pages 340-351 in: Encyclopedia of Plant Pathology, O.C. Maloy and T.D. Murray, eds. John Wiley and Sons, Inc., New York.

12. Nutter, F.W., Jr., Rubsam, R.R., Taylor, S.E., Harri, J.A., and Esker, P.D. 2002. Geospatially-referenced disease and weather data to improve site-specific forecasts for Stewart's disease of corn in the U.S. corn belt. Computers and Electronics in Agriculture 37:7-14.

13. Ono, K. 1983. Ecological studies on the bacterial wilt of tobacco caused by *Pseudomonas solanacearum* E. F. Smith III. Distribution and spread of the pathogen in infected tobacco field under rainfall. Bull. Okayama Tob. Expt. Sta. 42: 149-153.

14. Sands, D.C. 1990. Physiological criteria – determinative tests. Pages 133-143 in: Methods in Phytobacteriology, Z. Klement, K. Rudolph, and D.C. Sands, eds. Akademiai Kiado, Budapest.

15. Sequeira, L. 1958. Bacterial wilt of bananas: dissemination of the pathogen and control of the disease. Phytopathology 48: 64-69.

16. Steel, R.G.D., Torrie, J.H., and Dickey, D.A. 1997. Principles and Procedures of Statistics, a Biometrical Approach, 3rd ed. McGraw-Hill Publishing Co., New York.

17. Vakili, N.G., Baldwin, Jr., C.H. 1966. Insect dissemination of the tomato race of *Pseudomonas solanacearum*, the cause of bacterial wilt of certain Musa species. Phytopathology 56: 355-356.

18. Wenneker, M., van Beuningen, A.R., Nieuwenhuijze, A.E.M., and Janse, J.D. 1998. Survival of brown rot and disinfection of surface water. Gewasbescherming 29: 7-11.

Diversity and Diagnosis of *Ralstonia solanacearum*

A.M. Alvarez

Department of Plant and Environmental Protection Sciences
3190 Maile Way, University of Hawaii, Honolulu, HI 96822 USA

A comprehensive analysis of pathogen diversity is essential for development of diagnostic tests of universal value. *Ralstonia solanacearum* is a heterogenous species with exceptional diversity among strains from different hosts and geographical origins. It is thus remarkable that despite the taxonomic complexity of this species, meaningful detection assays have been developed for ecological and environmental studies. This review will cover advances in assessing pathogen diversity and the resultant methodologies for pathogen detection and identification.

Early classifications of *R. solanacearum* divided the species into three races and at least seven subgroups of strains distinguished by pathogenicity on various hosts, colony morphology, biochemical type, lysotype, serotype and bacteriocin production (4, 5). Oxidation of six key carbon sources (maltose, lactose, cellobiose, mannitol, sorbitol and dulcitol) separated the species into four major biochemical types (biovars) that have been used to characterize strains worldwide (16). Utilization of trehalose and production of gas from nitrate were added to the above biochemical tests for further characterization, and strains were grouped into five biovars and five races (17, 18). A tropical variant of biovar 2 (2T or N2) has also been considered a sixth biovar (19; but see Fegan, this volume). Biovar classifications did not consistently correspond with race or pathotype classifications, except that race 3 (somewhat specific to potato) oxidized maltose, lactose and cellobiose but not mannitol, sorbitol or dulcitol, and was thus classified as biovar 2.

It is noteworthy that "races" of *R. solanacearum* are not analogous to "races" in other bacterial pathosystems, as for example, the races of *Xanthomonas oryzae* pv. *oryzae* affecting rice or *Pseudomonas syringae* pv. *glycinea* affecting soybean. In the latter cases, races are defined by differential reactions with cultivars of a single host species, whereas with *R. solanacearum* "races" consist of broader host range groupings, more consistent with the terms "pathotype" or "pathovar". Although assessments of race and biovar have been useful for describing strains worldwide, classification systems based on phenotypic characterization are inherently inconsistent. The new taxonomic scheme for the *R. solanacearum* species complex proposed by Fegan and Prior (this volume), addresses these inconsistencies by constructing a framework based on genetic classification.

Pathogen Diversity and Classification

THE SPECIES COMPLEX

A phylogenetic classification of *R. solanacearum* would be unimaginable without a series of detailed genetic analyses and increasingly refined methodologies used for strain comparison. Among the first studies on genetic diversity was a comprehensive analysis of a worldwide collection of strains using restriction fragment length polymorphism (RFLP) analysis, which divided the species into two major divisions and various subclusters or RFLP groups (7). Division 1 encompassed biovars 3, 4 and 5, while Division 2 contained biovars 1, 2 and N2 (= 2T) (7, 8,12). The existence of two major genetic clusters was confirmed by 16S rDNA sequence analysis (22, 31, 33). Gillings *et al.* (1993) showed a correspondence between RFLP groups of Cook and Sequeira (1991) and RFLP groups defined by *Hae* III digestion of an amplified endo-polygalacturonase gene fragment from *pehA*. Genetic analysis further demonstrated the close relationships between *R. solanacearum, P. syzygii* (Sumatra disease of cloves) and the blood disease bacterium (BDB) that affects some Musaceae in Indonesia (10, 11, 14, 27, 31). The latter two groups of strains are included in the *R. solanacearum* species complex (14).

Genomic fingerprinting methods, including fingerprinting by random amplified polymorphic DNA (RAPD) analysis, repetitive sequence based polymerase chain reaction (rep-PCR), PCR-restriction fragment length polymorphism analysis of the *hrp* gene region (PCR-RFLP), and amplified fragment length polymorphism (AFLP) have been used to analyze the diversity of *R. solanacearum* strains (20, 21, 26, 34). Relationships between biovar and phylogenetic groupings were seen, and certain genetic clusters revealed close relationships between strains with high levels of host specificity, but strains were mostly clustered by their geographical origins (20, 21, 26).

As more and more data have been assembled from genetic analysis of strains in the *R. solanacearum* complex, the inadequacy of classification based on phenotypic properties became increasingly apparent. In the new taxonomic framework proposed by Fegan and Prior (this volume), a hierarchal classification at taxonomic levels 1, 2, 3 and 4 (equivalent to species, subspecies, infrasubspecific groups and clonal lines) is based on genetic properties. "Phylotype" is used to designate major groupings at the proposed subspecies level, and "sequevar" is used for infrasubspecific groups. Phylotypes are identified by multiplex PCR based upon the ITS region. Sequevars are identified by endoglucanase (*egl*) gene sequence analysis (11). Sequevar-specific PCR tests for *Musa* (race 2) strains revealed a close correspondence between sequevars and multilocus groups (MLGs) described by Cook and Sequeira (1994). For example, MLGs 24, 25, and 28 containing ecotypes H/B, SFR/A and atypical race 2 banana strains, respectively, were equivalent to sequevars 3, 4, and 6 (Prior and Fegan, this volume). Relationships between races, biovars and the newly proposed phylotypes and sequevars also are clarified in the new proposal.

DNA fingerprinting methods, already widely used for analysis of the the overall diversity in the *R. solanacearum* species complex, would, according to the new proposal, be most appropriate for genetic analysis of clonal populations of strains (taxonomic level 4) rather than higher levels. Diversity analysis of local populations of strains from various hosts using AFLP, rep-PCR, and RAPDs have already been used for genetic fingerprinting of tomato strains in Thailand, pepper strains in Indonesia, pepper and tomato strains in Portugal, ginger strains in Japan, Hawaii and India, and potato strains in the Philippines (Alvarez *et al.*, Cruz *et al.*, Dittapongpitch *et al.*, Jover *et al.*, Mathew *et al.*, Natural, Thammakijjawat *et al.*, Tsuchiya *et al.*, pers. comm. and this volume). These diversity studies identified clonal lines that often were related to geographic origin and sometimes biovar classification, but they did not appear to lead to identification of specific sequences that could be used for DNA-based detection methods.

Detection and Diagnosis

A number of DNA-based and immunodiagnostic methods have been described for detection and identification of *R. solanacearum*. Detailed reviews are available that also cover comparative advantages of ELISA and DNA-based methods relative to their suitability for laboratories in less-developed countries (28, 29). Traditional test evaluation criteria, including sensitivity, specificity, reproducibility, feasibility, availability of reagents, facilities, operator experience, intended application and cost, determine whether the method is appropriate for a given field or laboratory situation. Recently, twenty official diagnostic laboratories in the European Union evaluated selected protocols, including selective isolation and enrichment, tomato bioassay, immunofluorescence, ELISA, fluorescent *in situ* hybridization (FISH), and PCR (Elphinstone, this volume). Some of these are described along with other methods below.

Molecular Diagnostics

Detection and identification by PCR. A number of primer sets have been developed for identification of R. solanacearum strains (13, 23, 30, 31). Multiplex PCR with internal PCR control and division-specific primers can be used for rapid strain identification (Fegan and Prior, and Prior and Fegan, this volume). A multiplex fluorogenic PCR (TaqMan) was developed using a species-specific probe-primer set and a second biovar specific probe-primer set to detect MLG26 and MLG 27 strains (race 3, biovar 2A) in potato extracts (38). A third probe-primer set was used as an internal PCR control to detect potato DNA. Pure cultures of R. solanacearum were detected at low concentrations (100 CFU/ml), but inhibitors in potato extracts raised the detection limits to 104 to 105 CFU/ml. Once the inhibition problem is resolved, the TaqMan assay will have advantages in routine indexing of potato tubers because of the increased specificity, speed, reliability, and possibility for automation (38).

The presence of inhibitory compounds in crude extracts of plant tissues or soil is a major drawback of PCR detection protocols. Poussier *et al.* (this volume) overcame the PCR inhibition either by capturing the DNA on magnetic microbeads prior to the amplification step or by DNA extraction from crude samples using a commercial kit. Both methods removed PCR inhibitors sufficiently to improve assay sensitivity.

Generation of microarrays. Microarray technology has opened the way to studies of functional genomics of R. solanacearum. Differences in gene expression among bacterial strains can be defined, providing insights on regulation of host specificity, hence races. Eventually, such studies should provide refined sequence-based diagnostic markers for detection and identification. Development of a DNA chip designed to detect R. solanacearum as well as other major quarantine pathogens of potato is underway (Elphinstone, pers. comm.).

IMMUNODIAGNOSTIC METHODS

A rapid, laboratory based, 40-minute test using ELISA format and a monoclonal antibody that detects most strains of *R. solanacearum* is available (Agdia, Inc., Elkhart, Indiana, USA). For field use, a lateral flow device, also based on a *R. solanacearum*-specific monoclonal antibody, has been developed by Central Science Laboratory, Sand Hutton, York, UK. In this test three drops of plant extract are placed into a sample well, and the liquid flows laterally from a release pad through an immunostrip across two detection sites into an absorbant filter pad. Antibody-coated latex particles attach to the target cells, which are then bound by a *R. solanacearum*-specific MAb at the first detection test line. Unbound antibody-coated latex beads are bound by an anti-mouse specific antibody at the second test line, which serves as a control. Postive and negative results are read within three minutes. This test kit enables direct sampling from plant tissues as well as from colonies growing on culture plates. An agglutination test for rapid identification of *R. solanacearum* colonies is also available (Adgen, Ltd., Auchincruive, Scotland).

Flow cytometry. Several cellular parameters can be simultaneously measured and quantified using a fluorescence-activated cell sorter, which electronically differentiates particles based on light scatter, absorption and fluorescence emission (32). Fluorescent probes can be used for a number of measurements, including DNA and RNA content, cell viability, membrane potential, intracellular pH, intracellular calcium flux, and enzymatic activity. For immunodetection, fluorescently labeled antibodies conjugated to fluorophores, such as phycoerythrin or fluorescein isothiocyanate, are used to target cell surface antigens. Samples containing bacterial mixtures react with appropriate antibodies. After incubation, samples are diluted in buffer, and cells are passed in a liquid stream, one cell per droplet, through a detection point. Light from a laser beam focused on the detection point is scattered and subsequently detected by electronic sensors that enumerate and size the particles, measure fluorescence and differentiate the fluorescing bacterial cells from nonfluorescing background cells and other particles (2,3).

Flow cytometry has several unique advantages over other immunodiagnostic methods for detection of bacterial plant pathogens in seed, soil, and environmental samples (1, 6). These include the ability to determine cell viability using green (SYTO 9) and red (propidium iodide) fluorescent dyes that distinguish between live and dead cells, respectively (37). Targeted cells also can be sorted from background populations permitting subsequent culture. The sensitivity of flow cytometry is not exceptionally high with detection thresholds between 10^3 to 10^4 CFU/ml. However, the ability to identify and characterize several bacterial populations simultaneously using different fluorescent dyes will permit new insights into dynamic interactions between various microbes in ecological studies. Flow cytometry promises to be a particularly useful tool for differentiating live from dead cells and for understanding the role of cells that fail to grow in culture (van der Wolf, this volume).

Large quantities of soil or plant material cannot be effectively assayed using detection methods that require exceptionally small sample sizes ranging from 2 to 50 µl as commonly prescribed for DNA-based or immunodiagnostic assays. Although the methods themselves may have adequate sensitivity, direct assay of field samples is statistically meaningless for predicting the presence of the pathogen in field soil or latently infected planting stock. In field situations, use of highly susceptible indicator plants is more effective. Susceptible Buffelspoort potatoes were used to trap and concentrate the pathogen from soil extracts prior to isolation (W. Van Broekhuizen, pers. comm.).

Various enrichment methods prior to ELISA or PCR also help to increase assay sensitivity. When soil suspensions were enriched with a semi-selective broth for 60 h prior to PCR, positive results were obtained with soil samples originally containing as few as 10^2 CFU per gram soil (24). A post-enrichment ELISA on a nitrocellulose membrane (NCM-ELISA) has been developed to detect latent infections in symptomless potato tubers (25). Pathogen populations are increased by adding 500 µl of tuber extract to an equal volume of a semi-selective broth and incubating for 48 h at 30 C with constant agitation. Aliquots of the enriched sample are then spotted onto a nitrocellulose membrane and reacted with a *R. solanacearum*-specific polyclonal antibody followed by goat anti-rabbit antibodies conjugated to alkaline phosphatase. Addition of substrate produces a purple color that indicates the presence of the pathogen. Assay sensitivity (2 to 20 cells per ml of tuber extract) was increased by six orders of magnitude following enrichment and was equivalent to the detection threshold of a nucleic acid spot hybridization procedure. Recently, using NCM-ELISA, detection probabilities of 95 to 99% were reported for sample sizes of 250 to 350 tubers, respectively (Priou *et al.*, pers. comm.). These and other efforts to evaluate *R. solanacearum* populations in agriculturally meaningful samples by enrichment and subsequent detection may eventually bridge the logistical gap between laboratory assays and field assessments.

Assays that depend on an enrichment step to achieve increased sensitivity face a different set of problems when the pathogen is not readily cultured. It was recently demonstrated that *R. solanacearum* can enter a dormant-like viable but nonculturable (VBNC) state in soil and plant tissues, and may be resuscitated in the presence of susceptible plant root exudates (15, 35, Van Elsas, this volume). The epidemiological significance of such cells has not yet been established, but the observation that *R. solanacearum* survives in the VBNC state indicates a need for inclusion of a resuscitation step in enrichment assays.

Polyphasic approaches to detection and identification have been important in determining survival rates of *R. solanacearum* race 3 populations in soil and the potato rhizosphere (35). Culturing methods coupled with immunofluorescence colony staining (IFC) and molecular methods, including fluorescent *in situ* hybridization (FISH), reporter gene technology (using *gfp*-expressing strains), PCR with *R. solanacearum* specific primers and PCR-DGGE were all used in a single study to evaluate the interactions between *R. solanacearum* and potential control agents in the tomato phytosphere (36). Such combinations of methods are essential for distinguishing culturable from nonculturable cells and for assessing the role of VNBC in soil and plant tissues.

Summary and Future Perspectives

Extensive studies on pathogen diversity have now permitted development of improved identification methods at the proposed species, subspecies and infrasubspecific taxonomic levels, but work is still needed to clarify the relationships between different groups of strains in the *R. solanacearum* species complex. For example, ginger strains, BDB strains, and other strains with restricted host specificities still have uncertain relationships within the larger taxonomic framework.

Rapid kits for species identification are presently available for field testing, and this permits subsequent removal of infected materials from planting stocks. Multiplex PCR using group-specific primers based on sequence information from the 16S-23S intergenic spacer region permits rapid identification of the four major phylotypes of *R. solanacearum*. Further, microarray technology is being developed for the study of gene function and host specificity.

A polyphasic approach to identification is most appropriate for studies of population ecology and epidemiology. The use of both immunodiagnostic and DNA-based detection techniques for locating and identifying bacterial populations should provide many new insights on the survival and infection process in soil studies. Finally, flow cytometry is among the promising immunodiagnostic tools that can be used to measure several populations simultaneously and to understand the epidemiological impact of VNBC cells in the rhizosphere and bulk soil.

Literature Cited

1. Alvarez, A.M. 2001. Differentiation of bacterial populations in seed extracts by flow cytometry. Pages 393-396 in: Plant Pathogenic

Bacteria. S. de Boer, ed. Kluwer Academic Publishers. Dordrecht, the Netherlands.

2. Boyce, E., and Steen, H.B. 1994. The physical and biological basis for flow cytometry of *Escherichia coli*. Pages 11-25 in: Flow Cytometry in Microbiology. D. Lloyd, ed. Springer-Verlag, Berlin.

3. Brailsford, M., and Gatley, M. 1994. Rapid analysis of microorganisms using flow cytometry. Pages 171-180 in: Flow Cytometry in Microbiology. D. Lloyd, ed. Springer-Verlag, Berlin.

4. Buddenhagen, I., Sequeira, L., and Kelman, A. 1962. Designation of races in *Pseudomonas solanacearum*. Phytopathology 52:726.

5. Buddenhagen, I.W., and Kelman, A. 1964. Biological and physiological aspects of bacterial wilt caused by *Pseudomonas solanacearum*. Annu. Rev. Phytopathol. 2:203-230.

6. Chitarra, L.G., Langerak, C.J., Bergervoet, J.H.W., and Van den Bulk, R.W. 2002. Detection of the plant pathogenic bacterium *Xanthomonas campestris* pv. *campestris* in seed extracts of *Brassica* sp. applying fluorescent antibodies and flow cytometry. Cytometry 47: 118-126.

7. Cook, D., Barlow, E., and Sequeira, L. 1989. Genetic diversity of *Pseudomonas solanacearum*: detection of restriction fragment polymorphisms with DNA probes that specify virulence and the hypersensitive response. Mol. Plant-Microbe Interact. 2:113-121.

8. Cook, D., and Sequeira, L. 1991. The use of subtractive hybridization to obtain a DNA probe specific for *Pseudomonas solanacearum* race 3. Mol. Gen. Genet. 227:401-410.

9. Cook, D., and Sequeira, L. 1994. Strain differentiation of *Pseudomonas solanacearum* by molecular genetic methods. Pages 77-93 in: Bacterial Wilt. The disease and its causative agent, *Pseudomonas solanacearum*. A.C. Hayward and G.L. Hartman, eds. CAB International. Wallingford, UK.

10. Eden-Green, S.J., and Sastraatmadja, H. 1990. Blood disease of banana present in Java. FAO Plant Prot. Bull. 38: 49-50.

11. Fegan, M., Taghavi, M., Sly, L.I., and Hayward, A. C. 1998. Phylogeny, diversity and molecular diagnostics of *Ralstonia solanacearum*. Pages 19-33 in: Bacterial Wilt Disease: Molecular and Ecological Aspects. P. Prior, C. Allen, and J. Elphinstone, eds. Springer, Berlin.

12. French, E.R., Aley, P., Torres, E., and Nydegger, U. 1993. Diversity of *Pseudomonas solanacearum* in Peru anad Brazil. Pages 70-77 in: Bacterial Wilt: Proc. Int. Conf. October 28-31, 1992. Kaohsiung, Taiwan. G.L Hartman and A.C. Hayward, eds. ACIAR Proc. No. 45.

13. Gillings, M.R., Fahy, P., and Davies, C. 1993. Restriction analysis of an amplified polygalacturonase gene fragment differentiates strains of

the phytopathogenic bacterium, *Pseudomonas solanacearum*. Lett. in Appl. Microbiol. 17:44-48.

14. Gillings, M.R., and Fahy P. 1994. Genomic fingerprinting: Towards a unified view of the *Pseudomonas solanacearum* species complex. Pages 95-112 in: Bacterial Wilt: The disease and its causative agent, *Pseudomonas solanacearum*. A.C. Hayward and G.L. Hartman, eds. CAB International. Wallingford, Oxon, UK.

15. Grey, B.E., and Steck, T.R. 2001. The viable but nonculturable state of *R. solanacearum* may be involved in long-term survival and plant infection. Appl. Environ. Microbiol. 67:3866-3872.

16. Hayward, A.C. 1964. Characteristics of *Pseudomonas solanacearum*. J. Appl. Bacteriol. 27:265-277.

17. Hayward, A.C. 1991. Biology and epidemiology of bacterial wilt caused by *Pseudomonas solanacearum*. Annu. Rev. Phytopathol. 29:67-87

18. Hayward, A.C. 1994. Systematics and phylogeny of *Pseudomonas solanacearum* and related bacteria. Pages 123-135 in: Bacterial Wilt. The disease and its causative agent, *Pseudomonas solanacearum*. A. C. Hayward and G. L. Hartman, eds. CAB International. Wallingford, UK.

19. Hayward, A.C, Sequeira, L., French, E.R., El-Nashaar, H.M., and Nydegger, U. 1992. Tropical variant of biovar 2 of *Pseudomonas solanacearum*. Phytopathology 82:608.

20. Horita, M., and Tsuchiya, K. 1999. Phenotypic characteristics and cluster analysis of Japanese and reference strains of *Ralstonia solanacearum*. Ann. Phytopathol. Jpn. 65: 604-611.

21. Horita, M., and Tsuchiya, K. 2001. Genetic diversity of Japanese strains of *Ralstonia solanacearum*. Phytopathology 91:399-407.

22. Li, X., Dorsch, M., Del Dot T., Sly, L. I., Stackebrandt, E., and Hayward, A. C. 1993. Phylogenetic studies of the rRNA group II pseudomonads based on 16S rRNA gene sequences. J. Appl. Bacteriol. 74:324-329.

23. Pastrik, K.H., and Maiss, E. 2000. Detection of *R. solanacearum* in potato tubers by polymerase chain reaction. Phytopathologische Zeitschrift 148: 619-626.

24. Pradhanang, P.M., Elphinstone, J. G., and Fox, R.T.V. 2000. Sensitive detection of *Ralstonia solanacearum* in soil: a comparison of different detection techniques. Plant Pathol. 49:414-422.

25. Priou, S., Gutarra, L., and Aley, P. 1999. Highly sensitive detection of *Ralstonia solanacearum* in latently infected potato tubers by post-enrichment ELISA on nitrocellulose membrane. EPPO/OEEP Bull. 29:117-125.

26. Poussier, S., Trigalet-Demery, D., Vandewalle, P., Goffinet, B., Luisetti, J., and Trigalet, A. 2000. Genetic diversity of *Ralstonia solanacearum* as assessed by PCR-RFLP of the *hrp* gene region, AFLP and 16S rRNA sequence analysis, and identification of African subdivision. Microbiology 146:1679-1692.

27. Roberts, S.J., Eden-Green, S.J., Jones, P., and Ambler, D.J. 1990. *Pseudomonas syzygii,* sp. nov., the cause of Sumatra disease of cloves. Syst. and Appl. Microbiol. 13: 34-43.

28. Seal, S. 1998. Molecular methods for detection and discrimination of *Ralstonia solanacearum*. Pages 103-115 in: Bacterial Wilt Disease: Molecular and Ecological Aspects. P. Prior, C. Allen, and J. Elphinstone, eds. Springer, Berlin.

29. Seal, S., and Elphinstone, J. 1994. Advances in identification and detection of *Pseudomonas solanacearum*. Pages 35-57 in: Bacterial Wilt: The disease and its causative agent, *Pseudomonas solanacearum*. A.C. Hayward and G.L. Hartman, eds. CAB International. Wallingford, Oxon, UK.

30. Seal, S.E., Jackson, L.A., and Daniels, M.J. 1992. Use of tRNA consensus primers to indicate subgroups of *Pseudomonas solanacearum* by polymerase chain reaction amplification. Appl. Environ. Microbiol. 58:3759-3761.

31. Seal, S.E., Jackson, L.A., Young, J.P.W., and Daniels, M.J. 1993. Differentiation of *Pseudomonas solanacearum, Pseudomonas syzygii, Pseudomonas pickettii* and the blood disease bacterium by partial 16S rRNA sequencing: construction of oligonucleotide primers for sensitive detection by polymerase chain reaction. J. Gen. Microbiol. 139:1587-1594.

32. Slavik, J. 1993. Fluorescent Probes in Cellular and Molecular Biology. CRC Press, Boca Raton, FL.

33. Taghavi, M., Hayward, C., Sly, L.I., and Fegan, M. 1996. Analysis of the phylogenetic relationships of strains of *Burkholderia solanacearum, Pseudomonas syzgii*, and the blood disease bacterium of banana based on 16S rRNA gene sequences. Int. J. Syst. Bacteriol. 46:10-15.

34. Thwaites, R., Mansfield, J., Eden-Green, S., and Seal, S. 1999. RAPD and rep PCR-based fingerprinting of vascular bacterial pathogens of *Musa* spp. Plant Pathol. 48:121-128.

35. Van Elsas, J.D., Kastelein, P., van Bekkum, P., van der Wolf, J.M., de Vries, P.M., and van Overbeek, L.S. 2000. Survival of *Ralstonia solanacearum* biovar 2, the causative agent of potato brown rot, in field and microcosm soils in temperate climates. Phytopathology 90:1358-1366.

36. Van Overbeek, L.S., Cassidy, M., Kozdroj, J., Trevors, J. T., and van Elsas, J.D. 2002. A polyphasic approach for studying the interaction between *Ralstonia solanacearum* and potential control agents in the tomato phytosphere. J. Microbiol. Methods 69-86.

37. Van der Wolf, J.M., Bonants, P.J.M., Smith, J.J., Hagenaar, M., Nijhuis, E., van Beckhoven, J.R.C.M., Saddler, G.S., Trigalet, A., and Feuillade, R. 1998. Genetic diversity of *Ralstonia solanacearum* race 3 in Western Europe determined by AFLP, RC-PFGE and Rep-PCR. Pages 44-49 in: Bacterial Wilt Disease: Molecular and Ecological Aspects. P. Prior, C. Allen, and J. Elphinstone, eds. Springer, Berlin.

38. Weller, S.A., Elphinstone, J.G., Smith, N.C., Boonham, N., and Stead, D.E. 2000. Detection of *Ralstonia. solanacearum* strains with a quantitative, multiplex, real-time fluorogenic PCR (TaqMan) assay. Appl. Environ. Microbiol. 66:2853-2858.

How Complex is the "*Ralstonia solanacearum* Species Complex"?

M. Fegan[1] and P. Prior[2]

[1] Cooperative Research Centre for Tropical Plant Protection, Department of Microbiology and Parasitology, The University of Queensland, St. Lucia, Queensland, Australia. [2] INRA, Unité de Pathologie Végétale, Domaine St Maurice, BP 94, 84143, Montfavet Cedex

R. solanacearum is a heterogeneous species; as Buddenhagen (2) pointed out, "there are many bacterial wilts and there are many '*Pseudomonas solanacearums*'", but is *R. solanacearum* a species complex? A species complex is defined as a cluster of closely related isolates whose individual members may represent more than one species. The term "species complex" was first applied to *R. solanacearum* by Gillings and Fahy (7) to reflect the phenotypic and genotypic variation within the species. Taghavi *et al.* (22) then expanded the concept of the *R. solanacearum* species complex to include two closely related organisms, the blood disease bacterium (BDB) and *Pseudomonas syzygii* as both of these organisms were found to fall within the diversity of *R. solanacearum* as defined by 16S rDNA sequence analysis. Studies of DNA-DNA homology of *R. solanacearum* strains have revealed that the relatedness between isolates of this species is often less than the 70% threshold level commonly expected within a species (15,20). Therefore we define *R. solanacearum* as a species complex.

A stable and meaningful taxonomy and nomenclature which accurately defines subspecific groups of *R. solanacearum* has to be the aim of taxonomists working on the *R. solanacearum* species complex. Such a taxonomic system will aid plant breeders, plant pathologists and quarantine officials who require a system of classification where strains can be grouped into clusters of isolates that relate to epidemiology, pathogenicity, host range and/or geographic origin. The taxonomic framework and methodology proposed below allows identification of subspecific groups within the *R. solanacearum* species complex and will improve our ability to predict the properties of *R. solanacearum* strains.

Diversity of *R. solanacearum*

Traditionally *R. solanacearum* has been classified into five races on the basis of differences in host range (1,12,16) and six biovars on the basis of biochemical properties (9,10,11). The work of Cook *et al.* (4) and Cook and Sequeira (3) employing restriction fragment length polymorphism (RFLP) analysis showed that *R. solanacearum* can be divided into two divisions: division 1 comprising strains belonging to biovars 3, 4 and 5, primarily isolated in Asia and division 2 comprising strains belonging to biovars 1, 2 and N2, primarily isolated in the Americas. Several other investigations employing molecular methods have confirmed this dichotomy within *R. solanacearum* (6,21,22). Taghavi *et al.* (22), using 16S rDNA sequence analysis, also revealed the existence of a subdivision within division 2 comprising isolates of *R. solanacearum* from Indonesia including the closely related organisms the blood disease bacterium (BDB) and *P. syzygii*. Further sequencing of the 16S-23S rRNA gene intergenic spacer region (ITS), the polygalacturonase gene and the endoglucanase gene (5) has supported the existence of the two divisions and the existence of the group of strains originating in Indonesia.

A recent PCR-RFLP analysis of the *hrp* gene region (17) demonstrated that certain African biovar 1 strains did not cluster with other biovar 1 isolates as was expected. An extended PCR-RFLP analysis of the *hrp* gene region complemented by amplified fragment length polymorphism (AFLP) and sequencing of the 16S rRNA gene (19) has provided further support for the existence of this group of strains. Phylogenetic analysis of the endoglucanase and *hrpB* genes has confirmed the presence of a group of strains originating in Africa (18).

Hence the picture has emerged that the *R. solanacearum* species complex is comprised of four broad genetic groups corresponding with geographic origin.

The Phylotyping Scheme: A New Scheme for Classifying *R. solanacearum*

A hierarchical classification scheme is proposed to reflect the known diversity within the *R. solanacearum* species complex. The scheme is outlined in Table 1. Under this classification system members of the *R. solanacearum* species complex can be subdivided into four phylotypes

Table 1. Hierarchical classification scheme for *R. solanacearum*.

Taxonomic level	Taxonomic equivalent	Nomenclature	Method of identification
Species	Species	*Ralstonia solanacearum* species complex	PCR Primers (eg 759/760) (14)
Phylotype	Subspecies	Phylotypes I, II, III and IV	Phylotype specific multiplex PCR based upon the ITS region
Sequevar	Infrasubspecific groups	Sequevars 1-23	Endoglucanase gene sequencing
Clone	Clonal Lines		Genome fingerprinting methods e.g. rep-PCR, RAPD, AFLP, PFGE, etc.

corresponding to the four genetic groups identified via sequence analysis (Figure 1). A phylotype is defined as a monophyletic cluster of strains revealed by phylogenetic analysis of sequence data, in this case the ITS region, the *hrpB* gene and the endoglucanase gene. Phylotype I is equivalent to division 1 defined by Cook *et al.* (3). This phylotype includes all strains belonging to biovars 3, 4, and 5; strains are isolated primarily from Asia. Phylotype II is equivalent to division 2 (1989), and includes strains belonging to biovars 1, 2 and 2T isolated primarily from America. Phylotype II contains the *R. solanacearum* race 3 potato pathogen, which has a world wide distribution, and the race 2 banana pathogens. Phylotype III contains strains primarily isolated from Africa and surrounding islands, strains belong to biovars 1 and 2T. Phylotype IV contains strains isolated primarily from Indonesia belonging to biovars 1, 2 and 2T. *R. solanacearum* strains in Phylotype IV have also been found in Australia and Japan. This phylotype also contains the two close relatives of *R. solanacearum*, *P. syzygii* and the BDB.

   The phylotype to which a strain belongs can be rapidly identified using a multiplex PCR based upon sequence information from the ITS region. This phylotype-specific multiplex-PCR employs four forward primers - one specific for each phylotype and a single reverse primer that is specific for the species (Table 2, Figure 1 and Appendix) and also includes the 759/760 primer pair described by Opina *et al.* (14). All *R. solanacearum*, BDB and *P. syzygii* strains generate the 280bp *R. solanacearum* species complex-specific fragment produced by amplification of template DNA by the 759/760 primer pair. All *R. solanacearum*, BDB and *P. syzygii* strains tested with the multiplex PCR produce a phylotype specific amplicon with the exception of strain ACH0732. Strain ACH0732 is the only *R. solan-*

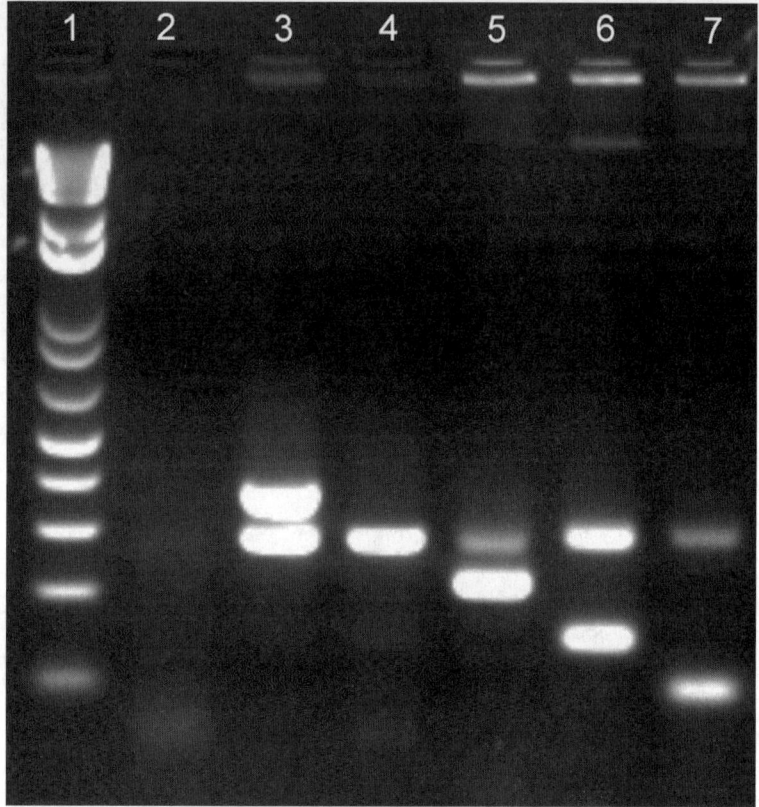

Fig. 1. Example of a multiplex PCR gel. Lane 1 molecular weight marker (1kb plus DNA ladder; Life Technologies); Lane 2 negative control; Lane 3 a representative phylotype II strain; Lane 4 ACH0732; Lane 5 a representative phylotype IV strain; Lane 6 a representative phylotype I strain; Lane 7 is a representative phylotype III strain.

acearum strain that varies in its phylogenetic position depending on the genomic region sequenced. Therefore using the phylotype specific multiplex PCR ACH0732 only produces the 280bp *R. solanacearum* species complex-specific fragment (Lane 4 in Figure 1).

Each phylotype is composed of a number of sequevars. A sequevar, or sequence variant, is defined as a group of strains with a highly conserved sequence within the area sequenced. Only if two or more strains sequenced have similar sequences has a sequevar been defined. Therefore single sequence clusters have not been given sequevar status (for example CIP10 in Figure 2). Sequevars are primarily defined upon partial endoglucanase gene sequences as a large number of strains have been sequenced in this region.

Table 2. Primers designed from the ITS region used in the phylotype specific multiplex PCR

Primer	Sequence (5' to 3')	Specificity	Amplicon size when paired with Nmult:22:RR
Nmult21:1F	CGTTGATGAGGCGCGCAATTT	Phylotype I	144bp
Nmult21:2F	AAGTTATGGACGGTGGAAGTC	Phylotype II	372bp
Nmult23:AF	ATTACSAGAGCAATCGAAAGATT	Phylotype III	91bp
Nmult22:InF	ATTGCCAAGACGAGAGAAGTA	PhylotypeIV	213bp
Nmult22:RR	TCGCTTGACCCTATAACGAGTA	All phylotypes	NA[1]

[1] Not applicable.

In the future it is hoped that sequence information from more strains from other areas of the genome, such as the *hrpB* gene, will be generated to confirm these sequevars. The endoglucanase gene of greater than 140 *R. solanacearum* isolates has been sequenced and over 20 sequevars have been identified (Figure 2).

Each sequevar may be composed of a number of clonal lines that may be identified using genomic fingerprinting methods such as PFGE, AFLP's or rep-PCR. In our experience rep-PCR is a fast and reproducible method for identification of clonal lineages within a sequevar.

The phylotyping scheme is highly discriminatory, flexible and additive allowing identification of further sequevars or even phylotypes. This phylotyping scheme is based upon genetic variation that accumulates relatively slowly in the genome of organisms at the level of the phylotypes and sequevars thus giving a long term global epidemiological perspective. However, the scheme also incorporates the finer resolving power of the genomic fingerprinting techniques to identify clonal lines below the level of the sequevar.

Because PCR facilities are not yet routinely applicable worldwide, an attempt has also been made to identify phenotypes associated with phylotypes or sequevars. This will allow phenotypic identification of these genetic groups. This approach is fundamentally different from the biovar scheme as it is attempting to identify a phenotype associated with an already identified genetic cluster of isolates. This work is ongoing but it is hoped that we will be able to use biochemical tests to identify the major genetic groups and thus allow laboratories that do not have ready access to sequencing technologies to accurately identify and place unknown isolates into this new typing scheme.

The biotyping scheme described here is based upon the work of Harris (8) and Hayward (9). Our results have confirmed the great degree of pheno-

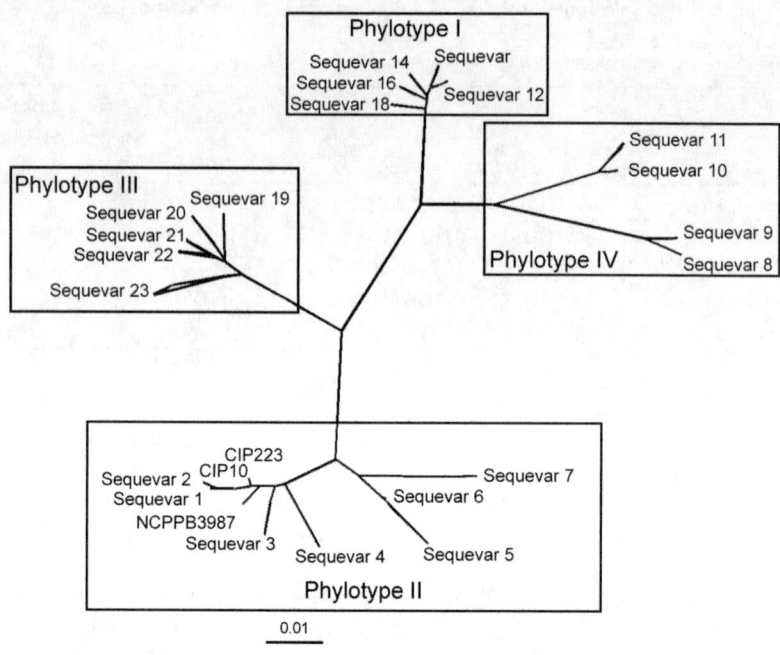

Fig. 2. Phylogenetic tree generated from partial endoglucanase gene sequence data showing the phylogenetic relationships of sequevars and phylotypes. The bar indicates 1 nucleotide change per 100 nucleotide positions.

typic diversity within biovar 1 isolates identified by Harris (8). This diversity is not surprising as this biovar is based on negative criteria for both disaccharides and hexose alcohols. The biotype scheme generates a unique metabolic profile for many sequevars based on a set of six substrates, namely maltose, manitol, malonate, trehalose inositol and hippurate (Table 2). Of the 56 strains tested in our collection, only the strain UW170 did not provide a biotyping profile consistent with the sequevar to which the strain belongs. Genetically this strain falls in phylotype II/sequevar 4 and it was expected that it would be of biotype 4. However, UW170 produced a biotype 3 profile which is characteristic of phylotype II/sequevar 3. The biotyping system needs to be fully validated on many other strains. Nevertheless, the scheme has already been useful in typing unknown strains of *R. solanacearum* isolated from pothos and from anthurium. The biotype of the isolates from these hosts was used to predict the phylotype and sequevar to which they belonged. The predicted phylogenetic positions were confirmed later by sequence analysis.

Table 2. Relationship of biotyping profiles and phylotype(s)

Biotype	Substrate[1]						Phylo-type(s)
	Maltose	Mannitol	Malonate	Trehalose	Inositol	Hippurate	
1	+	-	+	-	- *	+	II/1&2
2	+	-	+	+	+	+	II/ND
3	-	-	-	-	+	+++	II/3
4	-	-	-	-	-	+	II/4
5	-	-	+	- *	+	+	II/5
6	-	-	-	-	-	-	II/6
7	-	-	-	-	+	+	II/7
8	+/-	+	-	-	+	-	I/12-18
9	+	-	-	+	-	-	III/22
10	-	-	-	+	+	-	III/ND
11	+	-	-	+/-	+	+	III/8&9

[1] Substrates were filter sterilized and tested at a final concentration of 1% w/v in Ayers minimal medium with pH indicator. Tests were read after 14 days incubation at 28°C; NA, not applicable; *, alkalinisation; -, no acidification; +, acidification; +++, strains were considered positive for Hippurate if the media turned a deep black colour.

Comparison of the Phylotyping Classification Scheme to Previous Schemes

In comparison to race and biovar classification schemes we feel the phylotyping scheme proposed here more accurately reflects the diversity that we now know to be present in the *R. solanacearum* species complex.

Race 1, defined as strains “affecting tobacco, tomato, many solanaceous and other weeds, and certain diploid bananas” (1) is a very broad definition. Strains belonging to race 1 are found in phylotypes I and II and probably in phylotypes III and IV if host of origin can be used as a guide to which race a strain belongs. In contrast to race 1, races 2 and 3 have narrow host ranges and this is reflected in the narrow genetic diversity included within races. Race 3 strains belong to phylotype II, sequevars 1 and 2. Strains belonging to race 2 belong to phylotype II, sequevars 3, 4 and 6.

Strains representing biovars 1 and 2T are present in three of the four phylotypes and it is clear that simply identifying a strain as biovar 1 or 2T does not tell you much about the strain. The large degree of variation within strains of biovar 1 has previously been recognised phenotypically (8) and this is mirrored in the genetic variation found in biovar 1 strains. Most strains belonging to biovar 2 are equivalent to race 3 and therefore belong to phylotype II sequevars 1 and 2. However, some biovar 2 strains do not belong to race 3 and are found in phylotype IV sequevars 8 and 9.

This new scheme largely confirms the RFLP typing scheme (4). Phylotypes I and II are equivalent to the divisions 1 and 2 defined by Cook *et al.* (3). Phylotypes III and IV were not recognised by Cook *et al.* (4) as they did not study strains belonging to these two phylotypes. It would be expected that if strains belonging to these two phylotypes had been analysed using RFLP's then these two groups would have been identified earlier. Below the level of the phylotype at the sequevar level the RFLP and phylotyping schemes are also congruent with strains that belong to different MLG's also belonging to distinct sequevars. For example strains belonging to MLG's 24, 25, and 28, which contain moko disease causing strains of *R. solanacearum* are equivalent to sequevars 3, 4 and 6 respectively.

How Useful is the Phylotyping Scheme?

The DNA-DNA hybridisation values of certain strains of *R. solanacearum* are lower than would be expected of organisms belonging to the same species (15). Palleroni and Doudoroff (15) used strains representing biovars 1-4; the puzzling result from their analysis was the low DNA-DNA hybridisation values between strains representing biovar 1. The biovar 1 strains used by these authors originated from the USA, South America, Zimbabwe, and Reunion Island. When the same strains were analysed using the phylotyping scheme the strains from the USA and South America were found to belong to Phylotype II, whereas the strains from Zimbabwe and Reunion Island belonged to Phylotype III. This probably explains the low hybridization values. However, it does raise the question as to the taxonomic relationship of strains belonging to each phylotype. Are strains representing each phylotype related at the species or subspecies level? To adequately answer this question we require further information on the genotypic and phenotypic differences/similarities of representative strains of these two genetic groups.

The phylotyping scheme has also been used to help elucidate the unexplained results of Marín and El-Nashaar (13). These authors isolated biovar 1 strains from potato in Peru that apart from the biochemical tests used to differentiate the biovars were phenotypically and in pathogenicity the same as biovar 2/race 3 strains. When these strains were placed in the phylotyping scheme they were found to belong to Phylotpe II, sequevar 1 which contains only *R. solanacearum* biovar 2/race 3 pathogens of potato. When the strains were compared to other strains belonging to sequevar 1 using rep-PCR they produced a fingerprint the same as other strains within sequevar 1.

Table 3. List of strains with their PCR and biotype characteristics

Strain No	Origin	Host	Other No	Biovar[1]	Phylotype[2]	MLG	Biotype
UW20	Honduras	Banana		1	II/6	28	6
UW21	Honduras	Banana	R371, CIP21	1	II/6	28	6
UW181	Venezuela	Plantain	JT649, K261	1	II/6	28	6
DAR64836	Australia	*Musa* sp.		1	II/6	28	6
A3907	Hawaii	Heliconia		1	II/6	ND	6
A3909	Hawaii	Heliconia		1	II/6	ND	6
A3911	Hawaii	Heliconia		1	II/6	ND	6
UW 127	Peru	Plantain	CIP4	1	II/4	25	4
UW129	Peru	Plantain		1	II/4	25	4
UW131	Peru	Plantain		1	II/4	ND	4
UW160	Peru	Plantain	R282	1	II/4	25	4
UW162	Peru	Plantain	JT 648	1	II/4	25	4
UW163	Peru	Plantain		1	II/4	ND	4
CFBP1419	Costa Rica	*Musa* sp.	K163, JS847	1	II/4	ND	4
CIP20	Peru	Plantain	UW156, S249	1	II/4	25	4
UW70	Colombia	Plantain	CIP70	1	II/4	25	4
UW179	Colombia	Plantain	R368, CIP30	1	II/4	ND	4
UW175	Colombia	Plantain		1	II/4	25	4
CFBP2144	Colombia	Plantain	IW1509	1	II/4	ND	4
CFBP1412	Colombia	Plantain	NCPPB2314	1	II/4	ND	4
R368	Colombia	Plantain		1	II/4	ND	4
P515	USA	Pothos		1	II/4	ND	4
P548	USA	Pothos		1	II/4	ND	4
ANT307	FWI	Anthurium		1	II/4	ND	4
ANT11212	FWI	Anthurium		1	II/4	ND	4
UW170	Colombia	Heliconia	PD1453	1	II/4	ND	3
UW09	Costa Rica	Heliconia	JT644	1	II/3	24	3
UW11	Costa Rica	Heliconia		1	II/3	ND	3
UW135	Honduras	Banana	CIP7, S228	1	II/3	24	3
UW138	Costa Rica	Plantain		1	II/3	24	3
UW166	Costa Rica	Plantain	CIP27	1	II/3	ND	3
UW167	Costa Rica	Banana	R283, CIP125	1	II/3	24	3
CFBP1183	Costa Rica	Heliconia	JS793	1	II/3	ND	3
CFBP1409	Honduras	*Musa* sp	K135, JS77	1	II/3	ND	3
CFBP1482	Panama	*Musa* sp	K168, JS730	1	II/3	ND	3
CIP418	Indonesia	Peanut	MOH6	1	II/3	ND	3
CFBP2957	FWI	Tomato	MT5	1	II/5	ND	5
CFBP2958	FWI	Tomato	GT4	1	II/5	ND	5
CFBP3057	Burkina Faso	Tomato	JS912	1	II/5	ND	5
CIP301 [D1]	Peru	Potato	R311	1	II/5	3	5

Strain No	Origin	Host	Other No	Biovar[1]	Phylotype[2]	MLG	Biotype
CIP239	Brazil	Potato	R306	1	II/5	38	5
CFBP3858	Netherlands	Potato	JS907	2	II/1	ND	1
CIP 117	Nigeria	Potato	UW453	2	II/1	34	1
CIP309	Colombia	Potato	UW80, S206	2	II/2	27	1
CIP10	Peru	Potato	UW477, R569	N2	II/ND	29	2
ICMP7969	Kenya	Potato		1	II/7	ND	7
K60	USA	Tomato	UW25	1	II/7	1	7
JT528	Reunion Is.	Potato		1	III/19	ND	10
CFBP3059	Burkina Faso	Eggplant	JCG.AU28	1	III/23	ND	10
J25	Kenya	Potato		N2	III/22	ND	9
GMI1000	F-Guyana	Tomato		3	I/12	ND	8
CFBP765	Japan	Tomato	JS771	4	I/ND	ND	8
R288	China	*Morus alba*	JT659	5	I/18	ND	8
PSI07	Indonesia	Tomato		2	IV/8	ND	11
ACH0732	Australia	Tomato	UW433	2	IV/7	ND	11
R24	Indonesia	Clove	*P. syzygii*	NA	IV/10	ND	NA

[1.] Biovar and ecotypes of *Musa* sp strains of *R. solanacearum*; [2] Phylotype/Sequevar; known or not determinate (ND) RFLP-multi locus groups (3); 3. PCR primers (see Table 1) and products generated (+) or not (-); 4. Biotype NA, not applicable, see Table 2 for details of biotypes; UW; University of Wisconsin USA; R, Rothamsted Experimental Station UK; CFBP, Collection Française des Bactéries Phytopathogènes, France; CIP, International Potato Center, Peru; ACH, C. Hayward, University of Queensland, Australia

Conclusions, Predictions, and Speculations

The *R. solanacearum* species complex is composed of at least four genetic groups or phylotypes. Within these phylotypes there are subgroupings, sequevars, which correspond to clusters of isolates with similar pathogenicity or isolates of common geographic origin. By employing the phylotyping scheme outlined in this paper a view of the evolutionary relationships of the *R. solanacearum* species complex is gained. The additive nature of the scheme gives it great flexibility and allows addition of more genotypes as they are discovered. It is hoped that this scheme will be of use to plant breeders, plant pathologists and quarantine officials as it is able to distinguish epidemiological and ecological groupings of *R. solanacearum* strains and will thus help predict the biological properties of unknown strains. The vast majority of the *R. solanacearum* strains used in this study were collected from other strain collections and all were isolated from diseased crop plants. As more strains are isolated from environmental sources and other natural hosts of *R. solanacearum* it is expected that greater genetic diversity will be uncovered. Although it is possible that this new genetic diversity may lead to the description of new phylotypes it is, in our opinion, unlikely. However, it is almost certain that as more strains are sequenced more sequevars will be described.

Collecting and cataloguing strains of *R. solanacearum*, although very important, are relatively simple endeavours. However, it is more difficult to gather information on the biological, ecological and epidemiological properties of strains. Without both pieces of the puzzle it is impossible to use any taxonomic scheme to predict pathogenicity of strains or to aid in control of the disease. We suggest that research into the biological and eco-logical properties of strains should have high priority. It is our hope that the taxonomic framework based upon the evolutionary history of *R. solan-acearum* outlined in this paper will be used to better predict the properties of strains and aid in the successful control of the many bacterial wilts caused by *R. solanacearum*.

Literature Cited

1. Buddenhagen, I., Sequeira, L., and Kelman, A., 1962. Designation of races in *Pseudomonas solanacearum*. Phytopathology 52:726.
2. Buddenhagen, I.W. 1986. Bacterial wilt revisited. Pages 126-143 in: Bacterial wilt disease in Asia and the South Pacific: proceedings of an international workshop held at PCARRD, Los Banos, Philippines, 8-10 October 1985, edited by G. Persley. Canberra: ACIAR.
3. Cook, D., and Sequeira, L., 1994. Strain differentiation of *Pseudomonas solanacearum* by molecular genetic methods. Pages 77-93 in: Bacterial wilt: the disease and its causative agent, *Pseudomonas solanacearum*. A.C. Hayward and G.L. Hartman, eds. Wallingford, UK: CAB International.
4. Cook, D., Barlow, E., and Sequeira, L. 1989. Genetic diversity of *Pseudomonas solanacearum*: detection of restriction fragment polymorphisms with DNA probes that specify virulence and hypersensitive response. Mol. Plant-Microbe Interact. 2:113-121.
5. Fegan, M., Taghavi, M., Sly, L.I., and Hayward, A.C. 1998. Phylogeny, diversity and molecular diagnostics of *Ralstonia solanacearum*. Pages 19-33 in: Bacterial Wilt Disease: Molecular and Ecological Aspects. P. Prior, C. Allen, and J. Elphinstone, eds. Springer, Berlin.
6. Gillings, M., Fahy, P., and Davies, C. 1993. Restriction analysis of an amplified polygalacturonase gene fragment differentiates strains of the phytopathogenic bacterium *Pseudomonas solanacearum*. Lett. Appl. Microbiol. 17:44-48.

7. Gillings, M.R., and Fahy, P. 1994. Genomic Fingerprinting: towards a unified view of the *Pseudomonas solanacarum* species complex. Pages 95-112 in: Bacterial wilt: the disease and its causative agent, *Pseudomonas solanacearum*. A.C. Hayward and G.L. Hartman, eds. Wallingford: CAB International.

8. Harris, D.C. 1972. Intra-specific variation in *Pseudomonas solanacearum*. Pages 289-292 in: Proceedings of the Third International Conference on Plant Pathogenic Bacteria Wageningen 14 - 21 April 1971. H. P. Mass Geesteranus, ed. Wageningen: Centre for Agricultural Publishing and Documentation.

9. Hayward, A.C. 1964. Characteristics of *Pseudomonas solanacearum*. J. Appl. Bacteriol. 27:265-277.

10. Hayward, A.C. 1991. Biology and epidemiology of bacterial wilt caused by *Pseudomonas solanacearum*. Annu. Rev. Phytopathol. 29:67-87.

11. Hayward, A.C. 1994. Systematics and phylogeny of *Pseudomonas solanacearum* and related bacteria. Pages 123-136 in: Bacterial wilt: the disease and its causative agent, *Pseudomonas solanacearum*. A.C. Hayward and G.L. Hartman, eds. Wallingford: CAB International.

12. He, L.Y., Sequeira, L., and Kelman, A. 1983. Characteristics of strains of *Pseudomonas solanacearum*. Plant Dis. 67:1357-1361.

13. Marín, J.E., and El-Nashaar, H.M. 1993. Pathogenicity of the new phenotypes of *Pseudomonas solanacearum* from Peru. Pages 78-84 in: Bacterial wilt. ACIAR proceedings No. 45. G.L. Hartman and A.C. Hayward., eds. Canberra: ACIAR.

14. Opina, N., Tavner, F., Hollway, G., Wang, J.-F., Li, T.-H., Maghirang, R., Fegan, M., Hayward, A.C., Krishnapillai, V., Hong, W.F., Holloway, B.W., and Timmis, J. 1997. A novel method for development of species and strain-specific DNA probes and PCR primers for identifying *Burkholderia solanacearum* (formerly *Pseudomonas solanacearum*). Asia Pacific J. Mol. Biol. Biotech. 5:19-30.

15. Palleroni, N. J., and Doudoroff, M. 1971. Phenotypic characterization and deoxyribonucleic acid homologies of *Pseudomonas solanaceaum*. J. Bacteriol. 107:690-696.

16. Pegg, K.G., and Moffet, M. 1971. Host range of the ginger strain of *Pseudomonas solanacearum* in Queensland. Austr. J. Exper. Agric. Animal Husband. 11:696-698.

17. Poussier, S., Vandewalle, P., and Luisetti, J. 1999. Genetic diversity of African and worldwide strains of *Ralstonia solanacearum* as determined by PCR-restriction fragment length polymorphism analysis of the hrp gene region. Appl. Environ. Microbiol. 65: 2184-2194.

18. Poussier, S., Prior, P., Luisetti, J., Hayward, C., and Fegan, M. 2000. Partial sequencing of the hrpB and endoglucanase genes confirms and expands the known diversity within the *Ralstonia solanacearum* species complex. Syst. Appl. Microbiol. 23:479-486.
19. Poussier, S., Trigalet-Demery, D., Vandewalle, P., Goffinet, B., Luisetti, J., and Trigalet, A. 2000. Genetic diversity of *Ralstonia solanacearum* as assessed by PCR- RFLP of the hrp gene region, AFLP and 16S rRNA sequence analysis, and identification of an African subdivision. Microbiol. 146:1679-1692.
20. Roberts, S.J., Eden-Green, S.J., Jones, P., and Ambler, D.J. 1990. *Pseudomonas syzygii*, sp. nov., the cause of Sumatra disease of cloves. Syst. Appl. Microbiol. 13:34-43.
21. Seal, S.E., Jackson, L.A., and Daniels, M.J. 1992. Use of tRNA consensus primers to indicate subgroups of *Pseudomonas solanacearum* by polymerase chain reaction amplification. Appl. Environ. Microbiol. 58:3759-3761.
22. Taghavi, M., Hayward, C., Sly, L.I., and Fegan, M. 1996. Analysis of the phylogenetic relationships of strains of *Burkholderia solanacearum*, *Pseudomonas syzygii*, and the blood disease bacterium of banana based on 16S rRNA gene sequences. Int. J. Syst. Bacteriol. 46:10-15.

Appendix

MULTIPLEX PCR METHOD

Reactions were carried out in a total volume of 25 µl containing 1 x PCR buffer (supplied by the manufacturer of the polymerase) 1.5 mM $MgCl_2$, 0.2 mM of each dNTP, 2U of *Taq* Polymerase (Biotech International, Perth WA, Australia), 6 pmoles of the primers Nmult:21:1F, Nmult:21:2F, Nmult:22:InF, 18 pmoles of the primer Nmult:23:AF and 4 pmoles of the primers 759 and 760 (14). Reactions were heated to 96°C for 5 min and then cycled through 30 cycles of 94°C for 15s, 59°C for 30s and 72°C for 30s, followed by a final extension period of 10 min at 72°C. Samples (5 µl) of reaction mixtures were examined by electrophoresis through 2% agarose gels and bands were revealed by staining in 0.5 µg mL-1 ethidium bromide.

Occurrence and Epidemic Adaptation of New Strains of *Ralstonia solanacearum* Associated with *Zingiberaceae* Plants Under Agro-Ecosystem in Japan

K. Tsuchiya,[1] K. Yano[2], M. Horita[3], Y. Morita[2],
Y. Kawada[2], and C.M. d'Ursel[1]

[1] National Institute for Agro-Environmental Sciences (NIAES), Kannondai, Tsukuba, Ibaraki 305-8604, Japan;[2] Kochi Agricultural Research Center, Nankoku, Kochi, Japan; [3] National Institute of Agrobiological Sciences, Tsukuba, Ibaraki, Japan

Ginger (*Zingiber officinale*) and mioga (*Z. mioga*), perennial herbs belonging to *Zingiberaceae* family and which have long been cultivated in Japan, are important sources of spices, medicinal materials as well as food materials, all of which are obtained from rhizomes. On the other hand, *Curcuma* spp., an ornamental plant also belonging to the same family, was introduced from Thailand to Japan during the International Exhibition in 1989, and since then, it has been used as a planting material for cut-flower. In 1995, a bacterial wilt disease of *C. alismatifolia* caused by *Ralstonia solanacearum* occurred for the first time in the cultivated fields of a few localities in Kochi Prefecture, a southern district in Shikoku island, the leading production center of ginger which produces half of the total edible ginger production in the country (7). Subsequently, the outbreak of this disease spread to ginger fields in 1997, and since 1999 it has expanded successively to mioga plantations in the neighboring cities within the same Prefecture.

In Japan, prior to 1995 bacterial wilt had been recorded on 29 species in 14 families plants and not on any zingiberaceous plants. By the year 2001 the host range had expanded to 38 species in 20 families of plants.

Bacterial wilt of *Zingiberaceae* plants caused by *R. solanacearum* has been reported in several countries, such as U.S.A (Hawaii), Australia and Africa (2). In Asian countries, the occurrence of the disease has also been reported in the Philippines, Thailand, Indonesia, Malaysia, India, Sri Lanka and China (2). Strains of *R. solanacearum* attacking ginger and other zingiberaceous plants are shown to vary in their pathogenic specialization as well as serological and physiological properties.

Table 1. Biovar of zingiberaceous plant strains obtained from different origins

	Curcuma			Ginger					Mioga
	$J^a(11)^b$	T(6)	I(12)	J(11)	T(10)	I(14)	A(1)	C(2)	J(12)
Maltose	-	2+/4-	8+/4-	-	4+/6-	+	-	-	-
Lactose	-	2+/4-	8+/4-	-	4+/6-	+	-	-	-
Cellobiose	-	2+/4-	8+/4-	-	4+/6-	+	-	-	-
Mannitol	+	+	+	+	+	6+/8-	+	+	+
Sorbitol	+	+	+	+	+	6+/8-	+	+	+
Dulcitol	+	+	+	+	+	6+/8-	+	+	+
	bv4	bv3/4	bv3/4	bv4	bv3/4	bv3/4	bv4	bv4	bv4

[a] J: Japan, T: Thailand, I: Indonesia, A: Australia, C: China.
[b] ( ): number of strains tested. +: acid production; -: no acid production.

The objectives of the study were to characterize the strains causing wilting of ginger and two other zingiberaceous plants in Japan from pathological and physiological points of view and compare them with *R. solanacearum* strains that commonly cause wilting of tomato and other crops in Japan. Rep-PCR analysis was also conducted to compare genetic relatedness of these strains with those obtained from geographically different countries.

DISEASE SYMPTOMS

The development of disease symptoms in the three kinds of zingiberaceous plants used was similar. In the case of *C. alismatifolia,* the first symptom was curling of the leaves outwards, followed by yellowing of stems and leaves. In the cases of ginger and mioga, yellowing and wilting started from lower leaves, which quickly spread upwards until the whole plant became entirely golden brown and wilted. In advanced stages of the disease, the base of the pseudostems became watersoaked and rotten, readily breaking away from the rhizomes. The vascular tissues were discolored to dark brown or black. When the pseudostems and rhizomes were cut transversely, a white milky exudate oozed out from the cut edges.

BIOVAR DETERMINATION

All isolates tested in this study were identified as *R. solanacearum* and consisted of two biovars according to the classification by Hayward (1). All strains isolated from infected plants of curcuma, ginger and mioga in Japan were identical and have proved to be biovar 4, whereas those from Thailand and Indonesia consisted of both biovar 3 and 4, and those from Australia and China were biovar 4 (Table 1).

PATHOGENICITY

Pathogenicity of strains was tested in various hosts, including tomato, eggplant, sweet pepper, potato, tobacco and others as well as ginger and mioga in pots containing a horticultural soil-vermiculite mixture, following the methods of Winstead and Kelman (9). The hypersensitive reaction (HR) test on tobacco leaves was done as described by Lozano and Sequeira (6). Inoculated plants were incubated in greenhouse at 25 to 30° C under natural light. Severity of wilting was observed at 4 day-intervals and was rated based on the following scale: 1= no symptom, 2= leaf above inoculation site wilted, 3= two or three leaves wilted, 4= four or more leaves wilted, and 5= plant dead.

Following inoculation of ginger plants with the biovar 4 strains mentioned above, wilting occurred within 21 days after stem-inoculation and root-inoculation. The results of host range tests showed that the rate at which the plants became infected varied (Table 2). Both ginger and curcuma isolates infected and caused wilting of potato, zinnia and marigold and tomato (cv. Ponderosa did not wilt severely). The effect of mioga strains was similar to that of curcuma strains. In eggplant and sweet pepper, wilting was moderate and was accompanied with vascular browning or stunting. Tobacco, peanut, and sunflower did not wilt but developed vascular discoloration. On the other hand, the strains isolated from eggplant and tomato did not wilt ginger (Table 2), although they were more virulent to solanaceous plants and to other host plants such as turnip, kidney bean and soybean (data not shown) than the isolates from zingiberaceous plants.

REP-PCR

Genetic diversity of Japanese strains from three zingiberaceous plants was analyzed by PCR amplification based on repetitive DNA sequences (rep-PCR). The method described by Louws et al.(5) was employed using two primer sets, BOX and REP. PCR amplification was done following previously reported protocols (4). REP and BOX-PCR analysis was carried out using selected curcuma, ginger and mioga strains from Japan, Thailand, Indonesia, Australia and China. In addition, representative Japanese race 1 and 3, biovar 2, 3 and 4 strains isolated from various host plants including tomato, eggplant, sweet pepper and statice in Kochi Prefecture were also examined.

Table 2. Pathogenicity of *R. solanacearum* strains from zingiberaceous plants in Japan.

Plant tested (cultivar)	Pathogenicity [a]				
	Cur(8)[b]	Gin(11)	Mio(12)	Egg(5)	Tom(5)
Tomato (Ponderosa)	0-L	L-M	0-L	M-H	M-H
Tomato (Houkin No.2)	L-M	L-H	L-M	M-H	M-H
Eggplant (Senryo No.2)	L-M	M-H	L-M	M-H	M-H
Sweet pepper (Tosahime)	L-M	nt[d]	nt	L-H	M-H
Tobacco (Bright Yellow No.4)	0, HR[c]	0, HR	0, HR	L-M	0, HR
Potato (Danshaku)	L-M	M-H	L-M	M-H	M-H
Peanut (Han-waisei)	L-M	nt	nt	L-M	nt
Ginger (Tosa-ichi)	M-H	M-H	M-H	0-L	nt
Ginger (Sanshu)	M-H	M-H	M-H	0-L	0-L
Mioga (Natsu mioga)	M-H	M-H	M-H	0-L	0-L
Statice (Early Blue)	0-L	nt	nt	0-L	nt
Marigold (Bonanza Orange)	M-H	nt	nt	M-H	nt
Zinnia (Wollygig)	M-H	nt	nt	M-H	nt
Radish (Taibyo Sofutori)	0-L	nt	nt	M-H	nt
Strawberry (Toyonoka)	0-L	nt	nt	0-L	nt
Sunflower (Sunrich Lemon)	0-L	nt	nt	0-L	nt

[a] Results based on average disease indices of two to 10 plants. Disease severity was observed 21 days after inoculation and was rated using a scale of 0-5. H = high (4.1 to 5.0); M = moderate (2.6 to 4.0); L = low (1.1 to 2.5); and 0 = no symptom (1.0).

[b] Cur: cucurma, Gin: ginger, Mio: mioga, Egg: eggplant

[c] HR = hypersensitive response within 24 h.

[d] nt = not tested.

The DNA-profiles obtained with BOX-PCR were highly reproducible. Two distinct types of DNA fingerprints based on the presence or absence of a few bands were observed among Japanese strains from zingiberaceous plants. Type 1 consisted of all *Curcuma* strains isolated in 1995 and later dates, some ginger strains isolated in August, 1997 and all mioga strains (data not shown) isolated after 1999. On the other hand, Type 2 contained mostly ginger strains isolated in May, 1997 and later dates. However, neither the DNA patterns of indigenous *R. solanacearum* strains isolated from tomato, eggplant, sweet pepper and statice in Kochi Prefecture nor those of representative Japanese race 1 and 3, biovar 2, 3 and 4 were identical to any of the two types (Fig. 1).

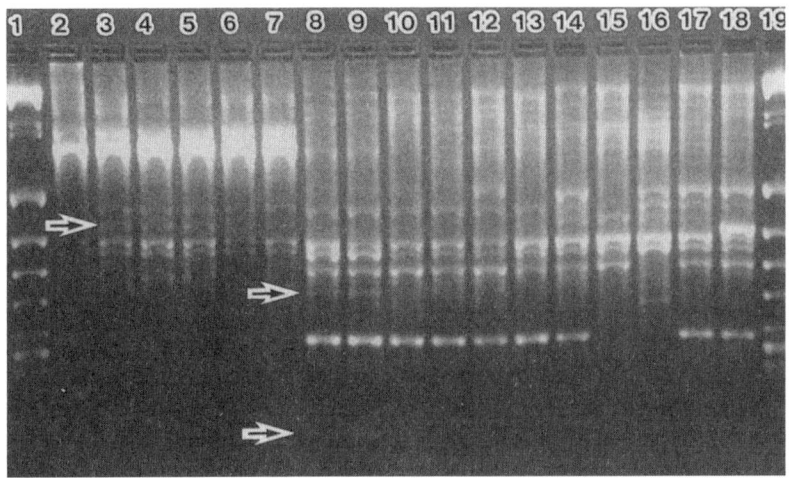

Fig. 1. BOX-PCR analysis of *R. solanacearum* strains isolated from ginger, curcuma and indigenous solanaceous host plants in Japan. Lanes 2-5: curcuma isolate; 6-9: ginger isolate; 10,11: eggplant isolate; 12: tomato isolate; 13,14: sweet pepper isolate; 15,16: tobacco isolate; 17,18: statice isolate; 1,19: markers: phiX174/*Hin*dIII+phiX174/*Hin*cII.

The DNA pattern of Type 1 strains was identical to that of several ginger and *Curcuma* spp. strains from Thailand, and that of Type 2 was identical to three ginger strains, one Australian (R277=Hayward 007a) and two Chinese (28a and 28b) (Fig. 2).

Discussion

Among the relatively few monocotyledonous plants severely attacked by *R. solanacearum* in Japan are those belonging to *Zingiberaceae*. The occurrence of bacterial wilt of ginger and two other zingiberaceous plants grown in the ginger production region has become an economically important problem. High degrees of similarity in both physiological and biochemical properties among the pathogens of the three zingiberaceous plants indicated that they were similar. Furthermore, all isolates from these plants have proved to be biovar 4. On the other hand, the reference strains from Thailand, Indonesia, China and Australia were either biovar 3 and/or 4 as previously reported (2).

The results of cross-inoculation tests to determine host range indicated that the zingiberaceous plant strains caused wilting of several host plants other than ginger and mioga, such as tomato (Houkin No.2), potato,

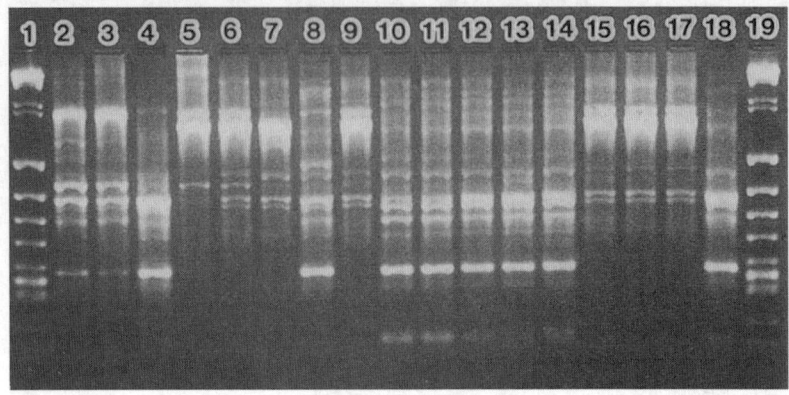

Fig. 2. BOX-PCR analysis of ginger strains obtained from geographically different origins. Lanes 2-4: Indonesian isolate; 5-9: Thai isolate; 10 and 11: Chinese isolate; 12-17: Japanese isolate; 18: Australian isolate; 1,19: markers: phiX174/*Hin*dIII+phiX174/*Hin*cII.

marigold, and zinnia, but failed to wilt tomato (cv. Ponderosa), tobacco, eggplant, and others.

Based on the results obtained from rep-PCR analysis, it was considered a possibility that Type 1 and Type 2 pathogenic strains from either curcuma or ginger were introduced independently through contaminated seed materials imported around 1995, and remained undetected until the first outbreak in *Curcuma* sp. in 1995 and subsequently in ginger in 1997. Furthermore, Type 1 strains were found in mioga after 1999. It was therefore concluded that the disease caused by these two exotic *R. solanacearum* strains started from different origins and has been spreading in epidemic proportions through separate routes.

It is not clear whether these strains attack only zingiberaceous plants in nature or not. To clarify this, field survey studies should be conducted using more effective diagnostic methods such as immunoassay and PCR using specific primers for the detection of pathogens in the fields as well as in the seed materials.

Literature Cited

1. Hayward, A.C. 1964. Characteristics of *Pseudomonas solanacearum*. J. Appl. Bacteriol. 27:265-277.
2. Hayward, A.C. 1994. The host of *Pseudomonas solanacearum*. Pages 9-24 in: Bacterial Wilt: The Disease and Its Causative Agent,

Pseudomonas solanacearum. A.C. Hayward and G.L. Hartman, eds. CAB International, Wallingford, U.K.

3. Hayward, A.C., Moffett, M.L., and Pegg, K.G. 1967. Bacterial wilt of ginger in Queensland. Queensland J. Agric. Anim. Sci. 24:1-5.

4. Horita, M., and Tsuchiya, K. 2001. Genetic diversity of Japanese strains of *Ralstonia solanacearum.* Phytopathology 91:399-407.

5. Louws, F.J., Fulbright, D.W., Stephens, C.T., and de Brujin, F.J. 1994. Specific genomic fingerprint of phytopathogenic *Xanthomonas* and *Pseudomonas* pathovars and strains generated with repetitive sequences and PCR. Appl. Environ. Microbiol. 60:2286-2295.

6. Lozano, J., and Sequeira, L. 1970. Differentiation of races of *Pseudomonas solanacearum* by a leaf infiltration technique. Phytopathology 60:833-838.

7. Morita, Y., Yano, K., Tsuchiya, K., and Kawada, Y. 1996. Bacterial wilt *Curcuma alismatifolia* caused by *Pseudomonas solanacearum.* Pro. Assoc. Pl. Protec. Shikoku. 31:1-6 (in Japanese).

8. Pegg, K.G., and Moffett, M.L. 1971. Host range of the ginger strain of *Pseudomonas solanacearum* in Queensland. Aust. J. Exp. Agric. Anim. Husb. 11: 696-698.

9. Winstead, N.N., and Kelman, A. 1952. Inoculation techniques for evaluating resistance to *Pseudomonas solanacearum.* Phytopathology 42: 628-634.

Characterization and Detection of *Ralstonia solanacearum* Strains Causing Bacterial Wilt of Ginger in Hawaii

A.M. Alvarez, K.J. Trotter, M.B. Swafford, J.M. Berestecky, Q.Yu, R. Ming, P.R. Hepperly, and F. Zee

Department of Plant and Environmental Protection Sciences, 3190 Maile Way, University of Hawaii, Honolulu, HI 96822 USA

Immunodiagnostic and DNA-based detection assays are needed for screening ginger rhizomes for *Ralstonia solanacearum* prior to planting in production fields. To determine the general applicability of potentially useful detection assays, representative *R. solanacearum* strains from a worldwide collection were characterized by polyphasic testing using bacteriological tests, metabolic profiles, reactivities to a panel of monoclonal antibodies (MAbs), RFLP and AFLP analyses. Ginger strains from Hawaii were serologically indistinguishable from strains representing races 1 and 2, but differed from some race 3 strains from potato. Genetic comparisons using RFLP and AFLP analyses indicated that ginger strains from Hawaii formed unique clusters (similarity indices above 0.90) and showed less similarity with strains from tomato, pepper, heliconia, banana, potato, and geranium. The relatively high degree of phenotypic and genotypic uniformity among ginger strains in Hawaii permitted development of a simple detection assay using two species-specific antibodies, Ps1 and Ps1a, which reacted with all ginger strains in the collection. MAb reactivity with virulent fluidal colonies as well as heated extracts containing EPS permitted use of a rapid ELISA to distinguish between *R. solanacearum* and bacterial contaminants (*Bacillus* sp., *Agrobacterium radiobacter*, *Comamonas acidovorus*, *Pseudomonas putida*, *Stenotrophomonas maltophilia* and *Enterobacter cloaceae*), which are frequently isolated from ginger rhizomes and overgrow *R. solanacearum* in culture. A capillary-based trapping technique combined with an immunodiagnostic assay was developed to detect *R. solanacearum* in mixed microbial populations. The assay is suitable for detecting the pathogen in wash water from ginger rhizomes and is intended for use in soil assays.

Bacterial wilt of ginger (*Zingiber officinale* Roscoe), caused by *Ralstonia solanacearum,* is a serious problem for ginger production in Hawaii, the Philippines, China, Japan, Thailand, Indonesia, Malaysia, India and Mauritius. The disease was very destructive on five farms in Australia from 1965 to 1970 but has not been recorded since then (A.C. Hayward, pers. comm.). Wilt disease has been the main cause of yield declines since 1993 in Hawaii, where losses up to 45% of the annual crop and complete destruction of individual fields have been recorded. In the absence of resistant cultivars, disease control is focused on screening and certification of pathogen-free propagative materials. No test has yet been adopted by growers for screening propagative materials. In addition, there is no soil test to determine the infestation levels of prospective production fields. Immunotrapping detection assays and DNA-based identification methods were investigated for screening ginger rhizomes prior to planting in production fields.

Characterization of Strains

To determine the general applicability of potential detection assays we first characterized 102 strains of *R. solanacearum* representing races 1, 2, and 3, from Central and South America, Asia, Hawaii and the Pacific using reactivities to a panel of MAbs, bacteriological tests, and metabolic profiles. The genetic diversity of the local population was determined by comparing strains with restriction fragment length polymorphism (RFLP) and amplified fragment length polymorphism (AFLP) analyses (2, 9).

PHENOTYPIC COMPARISONS

All ginger strains formed irregular, white fluidal or small pinpoint circular colonies on peptone-yeast extract and ginger extract agars. A characteristic diffusible brown pigment was evident after four days. Phenotypic variants (small red round colonies) were commonly observed during early stages of isolation, depending on strains and media, but both forms were positive in ELISA tests and both forms were virulent. All strains showed similar metabolic utilization patterns by API 20NE and Microlog™ (Biolog, Inc., Hayward, CA). The majority of strains were in Biovar 4, metabolizing sugar alcohols but not specific disaccharides (4, 5).

SEROLOGICAL COMPARISONS

All ginger strains tested were serologically identical, showing strong reactions with MAbs 1, 1a, and 10 but no reaction with MAb 2 (Fig. 1). Several race 1 strains from tomato and race 2 strains from banana and heliconia had the same reactivity patterns. Race 3 potato strains (A3445, A3447 and A3455) were distinct from the ginger strains as well as each other. A3447 reacted with all four MAbs, A3445 reacted only to MAb 10, and A3455 was negative for all the MAbs (data not shown).

MAbs Ps1 and Ps1a originally generated to antigens from peanut and heliconia strains, respectively (2), react with an extracellular polysaccharide (EPS) antigen produced by most virulent strains of *R. solanacearum* (7). The phenotypic switch associated with a loss of EPS production and a gain of motility in *R. solanacearum* (1) was detected by a loss of reactivity with both MAbs using heliconia strain, A3908 (3). Motile bacteria spread from colony margins in "fans" on motility agar, and when successively cultured on TZC medium, they frequently reverted to the small red colony type associated with avirulence. Several subcultures restreaked from the original colony failed to react with MAbs Ps1 and Ps1a, but all subcultures (both ELISA positive and ELISA negative) were positive by the OLI1-Y2 PCR test, confirming species identity (8). In contrast, ginger strains rarely lost reactivity with the MAbs following successive culture. Although small red colonies frequently appeared, the cultures reverted to the fluidal colony type, particularly when cultured on ginger agar. Reactivity of MAbs Ps1 and Ps1a with both colony types, as well as heated extracts containing EPS, permitted use of a rapid ELISA to distinguish between *R. solanacearum* and other bacteria (*Enterobacter cloaceae, Bacillus* sp, *Agrobacterium radiobacter, Pseudomonas putida, Comamonas acidovorus, and Stenotrophomonas maltophilia*), which are frequently isolated from ginger rhizomes and usually overgrow *R. solanacearum* in culture.

GENETIC COMPARISONS

Genetic comparisons of seven ginger strains by RFLP using twenty probes followed by restriction with *Eco*R1 or *Bam*H1 clustered the ginger strains (similarity indices above 0.92). The genetic diversity of the ginger strains and strains from other hosts was then examined using 451 AFLP markers (Fig. 1). Cluster analysis indicated that ginger strains from Hawaii formed a closely related group (similarity indices above 0.90), but they showed less similarity with strains from tomato, pepper, heliconia, banana, potato and geranium with an average genetic similarity of 0.855. The relatively high degree of phenotypic and genotypic uniformity among these ginger strains permitted development of a simple detection assay. Meanwhile, further analysis of the genetic diversity of a larger collection (now consisting of approximately 63 strains from ginger) is underway.

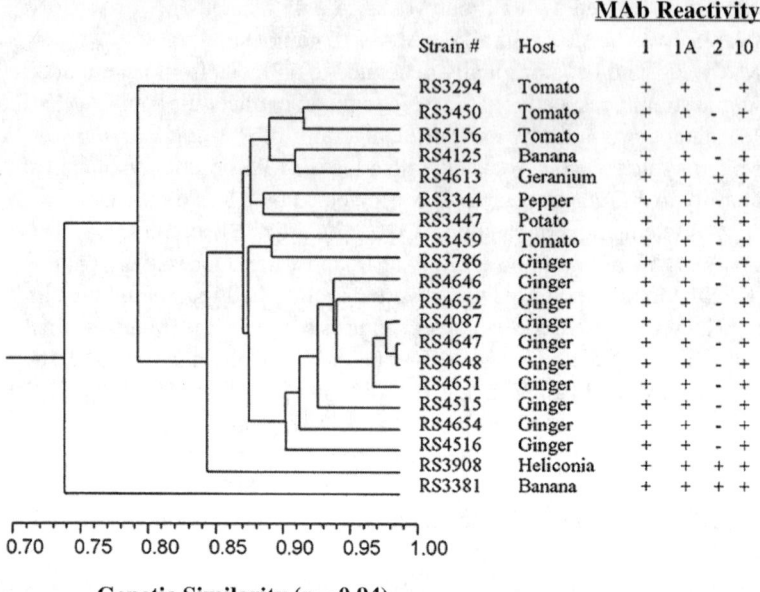

		MAb Reactivity			
Strain #	Host	1	1A	2	10
RS3294	Tomato	+	+	-	+
RS3450	Tomato	+	+	-	+
RS5156	Tomato	+	+	-	-
RS4125	Banana	+	+	-	+
RS4613	Geranium	+	+	+	+
RS3344	Pepper	+	+	-	+
RS3447	Potato	+	+	+	+
RS3459	Tomato	+	+	-	+
RS3786	Ginger	+	+	-	+
RS4646	Ginger	+	+	-	+
RS4652	Ginger	+	+	-	+
RS4087	Ginger	+	+	-	+
RS4647	Ginger	+	+	-	+
RS4648	Ginger	+	+	-	+
RS4651	Ginger	+	+	-	+
RS4515	Ginger	+	+	-	+
RS4654	Ginger	+	+	-	+
RS4516	Ginger	+	+	-	+
RS3908	Heliconia	+	+	+	+
RS3381	Banana	+	+	+	+

```
0.70   0.75   0.80   0.85   0.90   0.95   1.00
```

Genetic Similarity (r = 0.94)

Fig. 1. Phenogram based on simple matching coefficient of similarity among 20 *Ralstonia solanacearum* strains isolated from different host plants and analyzed by AFLP. Reaction of strains with anti-*R. solanacearum* monoclonal antibodies 1, 1A, 2, and 10 is shown on the right.

Immunotrapping Assay

The detection assay used the two species-specific antibodies (Ps1 and Ps1a), which reacted with all ginger strains in our collection. The assay was based on the assumption that motile variants of *R. solanacearum* show positive chemotaxis to a diffusion gradient of ginger extract.

PREPARATION OF CAPILLARY TRAPS

Ginger extract was obtained from fresh ginger root, ground and pressed through cheesecloth, then filtered to remove all solids. The extract was autoclaved and stored at 4 C. Liquified motility agar (Difco) was diluted with extract (4:1) in a microcentrifuge tube. A capillary (non-heparinized micro-hematocrit) was filled by capillary action and maintained in a horizontal position while the agar solidified. The periphery was sterilized by wiping with 70% ethanol. The capillaries were used immediately or refrigerated in a sterile Petri dish.

Capillary tubes containing motility agar and ginger extract were placed horizontally into suspensions containing 14 ml of the test sample (pure cultures or mixed bacterial populations). The motility agar became cloudy within 48 hours. The trap was then lifted from the sample with sterile forceps, the outside surface was sterilized with ethanol, and the agar plugs were removed by pushing a sterile needle through the tube. Contents were streaked onto TZC medium (6) and observed for colony development. A duplicate sample was mixed immediately with 150 µl carbonate-bicarbonate buffer (pH 9.6) and coated onto a 96-well microtiter plate (Falcon). ELISA was performed as described using MAb Ps-1, 1a, 2 and 10 (2). Negative controls included wells containing only CBC buffer, motility agar alone, ginger root extract alone, or a pure culture of *E. cloaceae* (strain B193). Positive controls were known *R. solanacearum* strains (A3908 from heliconia and A4651 from ginger).

R. solanacearum was detected by strongly positive ELISA reactions with contents of capillary tubes incubated in samples of mixed bacterial populations from leaf and soil extracts. When the contents of capillary traps were plated onto TZC medium rather than tested directly by ELISA, *R. solanacearum* was recovered from only two of nine samples (22%). The identity of the presumptive colonies was confirmed by ELISA after the first culturing cycle, but the positive reactions were lost following a second restreak because *R. solanacearum* was overgrown by acid producing, nonmucoid colonies. Not all fluidal colonies cultured from mixed suspensions were *R. solanacearum.* Several colonies resembling the ginger strains were negative for MAbs Ps1 and 1a on the first cycle but positive for MAb 10. On restreaking, they were overgrown by acid and EPS-producing colonies and were negative for all antibodies.

All negative controls reacted as expected. There was little background interference from the CBC buffer or the motility agar. Unidentified components of the ginger extract reacted with MAb Ps10, but the values were less than half of the readings obtained with positive controls.

Discussion

Ginger strains from Hawaii formed tight clusters both with RFLP and AFLP analyses, indicative of a clonal population with ca. 92% similarity. Low genetic variability may indicate that ginger wilt in Hawaii originated from a single introduction. A ginger strain (A3786) from the Philippines showed only 88% similarity with the Hawaiian ginger strains but 90% similarity with a race 1-tomato strain (A3459) from Peru.

In earlier work with a *R. solanacearum* strain from heliconia (A3908), we noted that subcultures taken from fans at edges of fluidal colonies failed to react with MAbs. Further subculturing resulted in development of small, red, avirulent, ELISA-negative colonies that produced no EPS (Alvarez *et al.*, 2000). The concern was that MAbs Ps1 and 1a would fail to react with motile cells attracted to the ginger extract and captured inside capillary tubes. However, when tubes became cloudy, the captured cells had already produced sufficient quantities of EPS for detection by ELISA. Furthermore, it appears that virulence or avirulence of ginger strains is not consistently related to colony type. Small red colonies reverted to fluidal colony morphology in the presence of ginger extract, and small red colonies were not consistently negative by ELISA. The capillary traps may thus be used to attract and concentrate motile cells of *R. solanacearum* present in extracts of plant tissues harboring mixed microbial populations. The assay can be used to detect ginger strains of *R. solanacearum* in wash water from ginger rhizomes that also contain *E. cloaceae*, and eventually it will be adapted to soil assays.

Literature Cited

1. Allen, C., Gay, J., Guan, Y., Huang, Q., and Tans-Kersten, J. 1998. Function and regulation of pectin-degrading enzymes in bacterial wilt disease. Pages 171-177 in: Bacterial Wilt Disease: Molecular and Ecological Aspects. P. Prior, C. Allen, and J. Elphinstone, eds. Springer, Berlin.

2. Alvarez, A.M., Berestecky, J., Stiles, J.I., Ferreira, S.J., and Benedict, A.A. 1992. Serological and molecular approaches to identification of *Pseudomonas solanacearum* strains from Heliconia. Pages 62-69 in: Bacterial Wilt. Int. Conf. Kaohsiung, Taiwan, ACIAR Proc. No. 45.

3. Alvarez, A.M., Swafford, M., and Berestecky, J. 2000. Differentiation of virulent and avirulent *Ralstonia solanacearum* strains with species-specific monoclonal antibodies. Phytopathology 90:S3.

4. Fegan, M., Taghavi, M., Sly, L.I., and Hayward, A.C. 1998. Phylogeny, diversity and molecular diagnostics of *Ralstonia solanacearum*. Pages 19-33 in: Bacterial Wilt Disease: Molecular and Ecological Aspects. P. Prior, C. Allen, and J. Elphinstone, eds. Springer, Berlin.

5. Hayward, A.C. 1964. Characteristics of *Pseudomonas solanacearum*. J. Appl. Bacteriol. 27:265-277.

6. Kelman, A. 1954. The relationship of pathogenicity of *Pseudomonas solanacearum* to colony appearance in a tetrazolium medium. Phytopathology 44:693-695.
7. McGarvey, J.A., Bell, C.J., Denny, T.P., and Schell, M.A. 1998. Analysis of extracellular polysaccharide I in culture and in planta using immunological methods: new insights and implications. Pages 157-163 in: Bacterial Wilt Disease: Molecular and Ecological Aspects. P. Prior, C. Allen, and J. Elphinstone, eds. Springer, Berlin.
8. Seal, S. 1998. Molecular methods for detection and discrimination of *Ralstonia solanacearum*. Pages 103-115 in: Bacterial Wilt Disease: Molecular and Ecological Aspects. P. Prior, C. Allen, and J. Elphinstone, eds. Springer, Berlin.
9. Vos, P., Hogers, R., Bleeker, M., Reijans, M., van de Lee T., Hornes, M., Frijters, A., Pot, J., Peleman, J., Kuiper, M., and Zabeau, M. 1995. AFLP: a new technique for DNA fingerprinting. Nucl. Acids Res. 23:4407-4414.

Flow Cytometry to Detect *Ralstonia solanacearum* and to Assess Viability

J.M. van der Wolf[1], V. Sledz[2], J.D. van Elsas[1],
L. van Overbeek[1], and J.H.W. Bergervoet[1]

[1] Plant Research International, Wageningen, The Netherlands
[2] University of Gdansk, Gdansk, Poland

Flow cytometry (FCM) is a technique in which rapid measurements on individual cells can be made as they flow in a fluid stream through a sensing point (1). Using a laser beam, multiple cellular parameters can be determined on the basis of light scattering and fluorescence. FCM has been shown to be a rapid and quantitative method for specific detection of plant pathogenic bacteria in crude extracts without the need of laborious sample extraction procedures (2). FCM, in combination with immunofluorescence antibody-staining of bacteria, provides an excellent alternative to the labour-consuming and tedious visual observations of stained cells in microscopy, a technique that is still widely used in Europe for tests on *Ralstonia solanacearum* in seed potatoes.

FCM will also be a valuable tool in epidemiological studies on plant pathogenic bacteria. Several fluorescent markers have been described, which can be used to distinguish live from dead cells on the basis of enzyme activity or membrane integrity of cells (3). Using these markers, the fate of the pathogen in ecosystems can be determined, in particular in combination with immunofluorescence antibody-staining.

FCM can also be used for sorting of subpopulations of cells with specific cellular parameters. Sorting will considerably enhance isolation of bacteria for full identification, in particular when samples contain high microbial backgrounds. In theory, up to 1 in 100,000 cells can be isolated with modern sorting equipment (1).

In this paper several applications of FCM for detection of (viable) cells of *R. solanacearum* are outlined.

Materials and Methods

IMMUNOFLUORESCENCE STAINING

Peelings taken over potato tuber heel ends were homogenised with a Pollähne press. After starch was settled, the supernatant was filtered through a Whatman 1 filter. Serial dilutions of *R. solanacearum* Biovar 2 strain in peel extracts and in 0.85% NaCl were prepared. Samples were incubated for 30 min with a FITC-labelled polyclonal rabbit antiserum diluted 200 times. Bacterial suspensions and peel extracts (100 μl) were pour plated in 300 μl Trypticase Soy Agar and incubated for 72 h at 27 °C to determine cell densities. Microscopical observations of cells stained with antibodies (IF) and fixed on microscope slides was done using an Orthoplan Leitz UV-microscope at a magnification of 625x.

VIABILITY STAINING

Pure cultures of *R. solanacearum* were incubated in the dark with Molecular Probes LIVE/DEAD stain containing SYTO9 and propidium iodide (PI) according to the manufacturers instructions. The green fluorescent dye SYTO9 penetrates live and dead cells and intercalates DNA, whereas the red fluorescent dye propidium iodide only penetrates dead cells. Cells were analysed by FCM, but were also microscopically examined to visually identify SYTO9 and PI positive cells.

FLOW CYTOMETRIC ANALYSIS

Flow cytometric analysis was performed on an EPICS XL (Beckman Coulter, Miami, FL) using EXPO32. The green fluorescence of FITC-labelled antibodies and SYTO9 was detected at FL1 (525nm) and the red fluorescence of PI was detected at FL3 (610nm). The flow cytometer was calibrated using Flow Count (XL (Beckman Coulter, Miami, FL). Approximately 10 μl of sample was analysed during 60 s. Live and heat-killed cells and mixtures of both were used for setting up colour compensation.

FLOW SORTING

Flow sorting was performed on an ALTRA HyPerSort equipped with MultiComp for colour compensation (Beckman Coulter Miami, FL). Green fluorescence of FITC or SYTO9 was detected at FL2 (525nm) and red fluorescence was detected at FL4 (610nm). Cells were sorted using a

Table 1. Flow cytometry for detection of *R. solanacearum* stained with FITC-labeled antibodies in (ten-fold) diluted potato peel extracts and in physiological saline

Concentration of *R. solanacearum* (CFU ml⁻¹)	Undiluted peel extract	Ten-times diluted peel extract	Physiological saline
0 (no antibodies)	605[1]	112	75
0	3001	759	440
2×10^2	n.d.	502	383
2×10^3	1861	1124	589
2×10^4	3715	3077	1576
2×10^5	4403	17242	10754
2×10^6	15202	96000	79693
2×10^7	83841	n.d.[2]	n.d.

[1] Number of fluorescent counts recorded by the flow cytometer in 60 s.
[2] n.d. = not determined.

70 µM HyPerSort tip at a sheath pressure of 45.0 psi, sample pressure of 44.5 psi and at 54.000 droplets per second. The sorting speed was approximately 12,000 sorting events per second. The tubing was sterilised using a 5% (v/v) NaOCl solution whereas the rest of the sorting chamber was sterilized using 70% (v/v) ethanol. To the waste container NaOCl tablets were added. After sorting, the sterilisation was repeated and the waste tubing was sterilised as well with a 5% (v/v) NaOCl solution.

Results

FCM analysis of antibody-stained cells added to potato peel extracts allowed detection of 2×10^3 to 2×10^4 CFU in the extracts if diluted ten-fold in physiological saline, but the detection limit increased to 2×10^5 CFU in undiluted extracts due to the high number of total events (Table 1). Suspensions of live and heat-killed cells of *R. solanacearum* and mixtures with 20%, 50% ,and 80% heat killed cells were incubated with SYTO9 and propidium iodide (PI). Within 10 min, the staining procedure was completed; no further increase in fluorescence signal was found anymore (results not shown).

FCM was used to determine the percentage of SYTO9 and PI stained cells of the total cells. A linear correlation was found between ratios of live and heat-killed cells and the percentage of Syto9 and PI stained cells (Fig. 1).

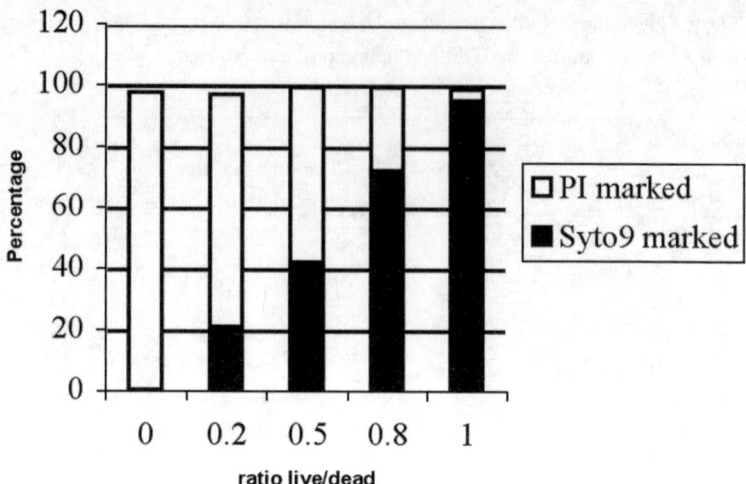

Fig. 1. Relation between ratio of live and dead cells and the percentage of PI and SYTO9 marked cells as determined by FCM.

The staining procedure is slightly bactericidal, as the percentage of PI-stained cells was higher after a 24 h incubation than after 1 h incubation period (Table 2). Peel extracts containing 3×10^6 CFU/ml of saprophytes were spiked with 10^7 cells per ml of *R. solanacearum* and stained with FITC-labelled antibodies. Green fluorescent cells were sorted and the number of target and non-target bacteria was determined in crude extracts and after sorting by plating on trypticase soy agar. The ratio target to non-target bacteria increased with a factor 55 from 0.6% *R.solanacearum* to 33.3%. SYTO9 or PI positive cells were also sorted and grown on media or used to infect tomato plants. The isolated SYTO9 -positive cells were able to form colonies whereas the PI-positive cells never formed colonies. When used to infect plants the PI-positive cells never caused symptoms but SYTO9-positive cells caused severe symptoms on the tomato test plants used.

A carbon-starved culture of *R. solanacearum,* incubated for 7 days at 27°C in demineralized water in the dark, and stained with SYTO9 and PI revealed two distinct SYTO9 peaks, but no PI positive peaks (Fig. 2). The SYTO9 positive- and negative cells were isolated using the ALTRA HyPerSort and grown on media or used to infect tomato plants. The SYTO9 positive fraction revealed colonies at a level of Log 2.52 CFU/ml, but in IF cell densities were Log 5.71 cells/ml. CFU numbers from the SYTO9 negative fraction were below the limit of detection whereas in IF, cell densities

Table 2. Effect of incubation period with SYTO9 and propidium iodide on flow cytometry measurements

% Dead Cells	1 h		24 h	
	SYTO9	PI	SYTO9	PI
100	0.2[a]	99.2	0.2	99.8
50	52.1	47.5	26.9	70.5
0	96.0	3.3	46.7	47.4

[a] Percentage of fluorescent cells compared with total cells recorded by FCM in 60 s.

were Log 6.05 cells/ ml. When tomato plants were inoculated with the SYTO9 positive cells (group A) severe wilting symptoms were found and the majority of the plants died within one week after inoculation. The lower leaves of test plants infected with the SYTO9 negative cells (group B) showed one week after inoculation a severe chlorosis when compared to water inoculated plants, but no wilting symptoms. Analysis of the plants treated with SYTO9 negative cells revealed the presence of both CFU and IF-stained cells one week after inoculation, indicating latent infections. Test plants inoculated with SYTO9 and PI only developed no symptoms.

Conclusions

Combination of FCM and cell staining with fluorescent labelled antibodies will allow rapid and quantitative detection of *R. solanacearum* in tenfold diluted peel extracts at a level between 10^3 and 10^4 cells per ml. After homogenisation of the plant material, sample preparation consists only of a simple filtration. FCM therefore provides an excellent alternative for the current immunofluorescence cell staining procedure, for which a laborious sample extraction procedure is requested to avoid interference from sample components, in particular autofluorescent particles, with visual observations.

Flow cytometric analysis of cultures of *R. solanacearum* using the membrane permeable DNA-binding dye SYTO9 together with the membrane impermeable DNA-binding dye PI allowed discrimination of live and dead cells. This staining procedure will be a helpful tool in studies of the fate of pure cultures of *R. solanacearum*. Staining of cells with FITC-labelled antibodies and propidium iodide may enable discrimination of dead and live cells also in a background of other micro-organisms. Cells stained with PI and SYTO9 retained viability for at least 1 h, enabling isolation of cells to confirm viability and identity.

Initial experiments with sorting of FITC-labelled cells showed a shift in the ratio of target to non-target bacteria by a factor of 55. It is expected that the method can be optimised, for example by adding a detergent, which will decrease clumping of cells. FCM and cell sorting will also be a helpful tool in studies on cells entering a viable but nonculturable (VBNC) state. It was reported already, that starvation of cells of *R. solanacearum* can result in formation of VBNC cells (3). In our study, FCM analysis of starved cells showed a division in clusters stained with SYTO9 at different levels of intensity. Hardly any cells were stained with PI and it was assumed that only a low percentage of the cells had really died. In contrast to the SYTO9 positive cells, the negative cells initiated only mild symptoms in tomato plants. It is speculated that a systemic acquired response has been induced by the SYTO9 negative cells thus reducing symptom expression in tomato plants, before cell multiplication can occur.

Literature Cited

1. Radbruch, A. 1999. Flow cytometry and cell sorting. 2nd edition. Springer-Verlag, Heidelberg.
2. Chitarra, L.G., Langerak, C.J., Bergervoet, J.H.W., and Van den Bulk, R.W. 2002. Detection of the plant pathogenic bacterium *Xanthomonas campestris* pv. *campestris* in seed extracts of *Brassica* sp. applying fluorescent antibodies and flow cytometry. Cytometry 47: 118-126.
3. Van Elsas, J.D., Kastelein, P., De Vries, P.M., and Van Overbeek, L.S. 2001. Effects of ecological factors on the survival and physiology of *Ralstonia solanacearum* bv.2 in irrigation water. Can. J. Microbiol. 47: 842 – 854.

Methods to Ensure the Detection by PCR of *Ralstonia solanacearum* in the Environment Using DNA Capture and a Commercial DNA Extraction Mini Kit

S. Poussier[1,2], J.J. Chéron[1], A. Couteau[1], and J. Luisetti[1]

[1] Pôle de Protection des Plantes, CIRAD, 7 chemin de l'IRAT, 97455 Saint-Pierre, La Réunion, France. [2] Laboratoire de Biologie Moléculaire des Relations Plantes-Microorganismes, INRA/CNRS, UMR 215, BP 27, 31326 Castanet Tolosan, France

Adapted prophylactic measures combined with the use of resistant cultivars is, up to now, the most effective way to reduce the incidence of *Ralstonia solanacearum*, the causal agent of bacterial wilt. In order to optimize the efficiency of prophylactic measures, powerful identification and detection tools of the bacterium in any potential inoculum source (plant, seed, water, soil) are required. However, the commonly used methods such as isolation on semi-selective medium (2, 7, 10), serological methods such as ELISA or immunofluorescence (6, 14), or pathogenicity tests on host plants (4, 9) for the diagnosis of bacterial wilt are often inadequate in terms of specificity, sensitivity or response time, especially for detecting the bacterium in soil.

DNA amplification offers many advantages over the above-mentioned techniques such as increased specificity, sensitivity and response time. Nevertheless, the PCR method has not yet become the diagnostic tool of choice for laboratories, mainly because of the inhibition of the amplification reaction by compounds contained in crude bacterial extracts which give false negative results or low detection sensitivity. Although a wide range of inhibiting substances have been reported, the identity and mode of action of most of them remain unclear (17).

The aim of this study was to compare several procedures to overcome PCR inhibition problems and to propose protocols ensuring a reliable PCR detection of low levels of *R. solanacearum* populations in natural settings.

Materials and Methods

Two *R. solanacearum* strains originating from Reunion island were used: JT516 isolated from potato and identified as a biovar 2, and JT519 from geranium rosat (*Pelargonium asperum*) and belonging to biovar 3. These strains were cultivated on a modified Granada and Sequeira (GS) medium, as described previously (12), supplemented by two antibiotics: nalidixic acid (50 mg/liter) and streptomycin (65 mg/liter) for strain JT516, rifamycin (120 mg/liter) and streptomycin (65 mg/liter) for strain JT519.

PREPARATION OF SAMPLES

Plants. Samples from plants (tomato, sweet pepper, eggplant, tobacco, geranium rosat, and pepper), cultivated in a field naturally contaminated by *R. solanacearum*, were collected. Stem fragments of a 3 cm-length were superficially disinfected with ethanol, sliced and ground into 5 ml of TENPP buffer [50 mM Tris, 20 mM EDTA pH 8.0, 100 mM NaCl, 5 % polyvinylpolypyrrolidone, (PVPP)], and allowed to sit for 30 min at room temperature.

Seeds. 500 tomato and eggplant seeds were artificially contaminated by soaking for 3 h at 4°C in 20 ml of bacterial suspensions (10^8 to 10^2 CFU/ml) prepared from 1-day-old cultures (strains JT516 or JT519), and then dried under air flow at room temperature. Bacterial populations associated with seeds were estimated by maceration of 45 seeds in 4.5 ml of Tris buffer (10 mM Tris-base, pH 7.2) overnight at 4°C.

Water. Samples (500 ml) of irrigation water were artificially contaminated by serial dilutions of strain JT519, giving a final concentration of 10^7 to 10 CFU/ml.

Soils. Four different natural soils identified as brown soil, ferrallitic soil, andosol and vertisol, were used. *R. solanacearum* was not detected in these soils as assessed by plating onto modified GS medium followed by PCR amplification (13). Samples (500 g) were artificially contaminated by known amounts of bacterial suspensions giving a final concentration of $2x10^7$, $2x10^5$ or $2x10^3$ CFU/g of soil. Twenty grams of soil were suspended in 100 ml of Tris buffer, and ground using Ultra-Turrax apparatus for 30 s. Then, from the collected supernatant, a bacterial fraction was separated from other soil components by centrifugation at 1000 X *g* for 5 min.

DNA capture and DNA extraction methods. Aliquots (1 ml) from all of the samples, prepared according to the above protocols, were simply boiled for 5 min and then cooled on ice to release DNA from cells before performing PCR amplification. Two rapid and simple methods were also assayed.

The first method is based on DNA capture through binding of a biotinylated specific probe to streptavidin-coated magnetic micro-beads (M-280, Dynal®). DNA capture was achieved according to the protocol described by Jacobsen (1995); the *R. solanacearum*-specific primers RS30 and RS31 (13) were biotinylated. The second method is based on DNA extraction by using mini spin columns from the QIAamp® DNA mini kit (Qiagen®). In both cases, the protocols were modified by the addition of 5 % of PVPP to the recommended lysis buffer.

All samples were also plated onto modified GS medium (12) for estimation of bacterial populations and comparison with PCR results. All assays were repeated at least three times.

PCR amplification. PCRs were performed using either primers OLI1-Y2 according to amplification conditions described by Seal *et al.* (1993), or primer pairs (RS30-RS31 followed by RS30a-RS31a and RS30b-RS31b) according to the nested-PCR procedure detailed by Poussier and Luisetti (2000). In all experiments, 1 µl aliquot of template DNA and water as a negative control were used for PCR.

Moreover, 500 ng/µl of bovine serum albumin (BSA) or protein 32 of T4 phage (P_{32}) were added to PCR mixtures to prevent any inhibition effect on PCR. PCR products were analyzed by electrophoresis on 1 % agarose gels at 5V/cm and visualized with UV light after ethidium bromide staining.

Results

PLANT SAMPLES

Plating onto modified GS medium and nested-PCR, using PVPP and BSA as additives to maceration buffer and PCR mixture respectively (13), allowed the presence of R. solanacearum to be detected in 86 samples while 27 samples were negative. Fourteen other samples were positive only by nested-PCR and 10 (mainly samples from geranium rosat) were positive only after plating. For the latter samples, the QIAamp® kit allowed the PCR detection of the bacterium whereas DNA capture led to variable response according to the sample.

SEED SAMPLES

Without performing DNA capture or DNA extraction using the QIAamp® kit, PCR products were observed from macerated seeds but only when they were highly contaminated (> 106 CFU/seed). Both DNA capture and the QIAamp® kit were found to be efficient procedures, and the sensitivity was excellent since the detection was still positive for seeds previously contaminated with bacterial suspension calibrated at 10^2 CFU/ml. Moreover, addition of BSA or P_{32} to the PCR reaction mixture enhanced the intensity of bands, however this effect was only observed for tomato seeds.

WATER SAMPLES (TABLE 1)

Without using DNA capture or the QIAamp® kit, the detection of *R. solanacearum* by nested-PCR was possible only in highly contaminated irrigation water (10^7 CFU/ml). DNA capture and the QIAamp® kit demonstrated a high sensitivity since detection was possible in irrigation water contaminated with 10 and 10^2 CFU/ml, respectively.

SOIL SAMPLES (TABLE 2)

Without performing DNA capture or the QIAamp® kit, PCR detection of *R. solanacearum* in soil was not possible. Without using PCR additives, DNA capture led to variable results: PCR detection of *R. solanacearum* in

Table 1. Influence of DNA capture and DNA extraction using QIAamp kit on the PCR detection of *Ralstonia solanacearum* in irrigation water.

	Inoculum concentration (CFU/ml)						
	10^7	10^6	10^5	10^4	10^3	10^2	10^1
Boiling	+	-	-	-	-	-	-
DNA capture	+	+	+	+	+	+	+/- *
QIAamp kit	+	+	+	+	+	+/- *	-

* : variable result according to the replication.

Table 2. Efficiency of procedures for detecting *Ralstonia solanacearum* by PCR according to the soil type and the inoculum concentration (CFU/g of soil).

	Brown soil	Ferrallitic soil	Andosol	Vertisol
Boiling	-	-	-	-
+/- BSA or P_{32}				
DNA capture	$2x10^3$	$2x10^7$*	$2x10^3$*	-
+ BSA or P_{32}	$2x10^3$	$2x10^3$	$2x10^3$	$2x10^3$
QIAamp kit	$2x10^7$	$2x10^3$	$2x10^3$	$2x10^3$
+ BSA or P_{32}	$2x10^3$	$2x10^3$	$2x10^3$	$2x10^3$

* : variable result according to the replication

brown soil and andosol whatever the inoculum concentration, in ferrallitic soil but only for highly contaminated samples, and no PCR detection in vertisol. Use of the QIAamp® kit led to PCR amplification whatever the soil type and the inoculum concentration, but for brown soil results were reproducible only for highly inoculated samples.

When BSA or P_{32} was added to the PCR reaction mixture, DNA capture or the QIAamp® kit enabled PCR detection of the bacterium whatever the soil type or the inoculum concentration.

Discussion and Conclusions

Our results showed that DNA capture and the commercial DNA extraction mini kit QIAamp® are powerful methods to overcome the PCR inhibition phenomenon. Both methods appeared very attractive compared to usual DNA extraction methods. Indeed, both methods require only few steps and simple handling without using hazardous chemicals such as phenol and chloroform. Moreover, we demonstrated that DNA capture using specific DNA probes associated with magnetic micro-beads permitted the effective separation of target DNA from non target DNA and from PCR inhibitors. DNA capture is an original method and is probably more specific than a similar and more usual technique called immunocapture (1, 3, 16) which uses antibodies instead of DNA probes. However, for some plant samples, the experimental procedure has to be improved to guarantee highly reproducible results. We showed that the QIAamp® kit is the most effective and reliable method to separate DNA from potential inhibitors and thus to allow the detection of *R. solanacearum* in all environmental samples so far tested. In addition, as a confirmation of the efficiency of the QIAamp® kit, we successfully detected the bacterium in the soil of a naturally contaminated field (results not shown), where up to now, the most effective means to detect the pathogen was the use of bait plants. This result demonstrates that this kit, which is already used for clinical samples, can also be recommended for the accurate detection of *R. solanacearum* and probably of many other plant pathogenic bacteria.

Furthermore, we showed that additives to buffer such as PVPP, or to PCR reaction mixture such as BSA or P32, are also useful in preventing inhibitory effects. These additives appeared very effective in improving the molecular detection of *R. solanacearum* in crude samples as already reported (8, 11).

The accurate and reliable PCR detection of *R. solanacearum* in soil samples is a major result of our work since, up to now, the commonly used methods for the detection of the pathogen are often inefficient mainly due to interactions with the abundant microbial flora in soil. Our next objective is the development and application of a PCR-based assay to quantify *R. solanacearum* populations in environmental samples, and more particularly in soil samples.

In conclusion, our study demonstrates that, using an appropriate procedure, PCR amplification can be considered as a useful and powerful alternative method for the detection of low levels of *R. solanacearum* populations in natural settings where the commonly used detection tools are often inefficient.

Literature Cited

1. Bukhari, Z., McCuin, R.M., Fricker, C.R., and Clancy, J.L. 1998. Immunomagnetic separation of *Cryptosporidium parvum* from source water samples of various turbidities. Appl. Environ. Microbiol. 64: 4495-4499.
2. Engelbrecht, M.C. 1994. Modification of a semi-selective medium for the isolation and quantification of *Pseudomonas solanacearum*. Bacterial Wilt Newsletter 10: 3-5.
3. Gelsthorpe, A.R., Gelsthorpe, K., and Sokol, R.J. 1996. Extraction of DNA using monoclonal anti-DNA and magnetic beads. BioTechniques 22: 1081-1082.
4. Graham, J., and Lloyd, A.B. 1978. An improved indicator plant method for the detection of *Pseudomonas solanacearum* race 3 in soil. Plant Dis. Rep. 62: 35-37.
5. Jacobsen, C.S. 1995. Microscale detection of specific bacterial DNA in soil with a magnetic capture-hybridization and PCR amplification assay. Appl. Environ. Microbiol. 61: 3347-3352.
6. Janse, J.D. 1988. A detection method for *Pseudomonas solanacearum* in symptomless potato tubers and some data on its sensitivity and specificity. Bull. OEPP/EPPO Bull. 18: 343-351.
7. Kelman, A. 1954. The relationship of pathogenicity in *Pseudomonas solanacearum* to colony appearance on a tetrazolium medium. Phytopathology 44: 693-695.
8. Kreader, C.A. 1996. Relief of amplification inhibition in PCR with bovine serum albumin or T4 gene 32 protein. Appl. Environ. Microbiol. 62: 1102-1106.
9. McCarter, S.M., Dukes, P.D., and Jaworski, C.A. 1969. Vertical distribution of *Pseudomonas solanacearum* in several soils. Phytopathology 59: 1675-1677.

10. Nesmith, W.C., and Jenkins, S.F. 1979. A selective medium for the isolation and quantification of *Pseudomonas solanacearum* from soil. Phytopathology 69: 182-185.

11. Picard, C., Ponsonnet, C., Paget, E., Nesme, X., and Simonet, P. 1992. Detection and enumeration of bacteria in soil by direct DNA extraction and polymerase chain reaction. Appl. Environ. Microbiol. 58: 2717-2722.

12. Poussier, S., Vandewalle, P., and Luisetti, J. 1999. Genetic diversity of African and worldwide strains of *Ralstonia solanacearum* as determined by PCR-Restriction Fragment Length Polymorphism analysis of the *hrp* gene region. Appl. Environ. Microbiol. 65: 2184-2194.

13. Poussier, S., and Luisetti, J. 2000. Specific detection of biovars of *Ralstonia solanacearum* in plant tissues by Nested-PCR-RFLP. Eur. J. Plant Pathol. 106: 255-265.

14. Robinson-Smith, A., Jones, P., Elphinstone, J.G., and Forde, S.M.D., 1995. Production of antibodies to *Pseudomonas solanacearum*, the causative agent of bacterial wilt. Food Agric. Immunol. 7, 67-79.

15. Seal, S.E., Jackson, L.A., Young, J.P.W., and Daniels, M.J. 1993. Differentiation of *Pseudomonas solanacearum*, *Pseudomonas syzygii*, *Pseudomonas pickettii* and the Blood Disease Bacterium by partial 16S rRNA sequencing: construction of oligonucleotides primers for sensitive detection by polymerase chain reaction. J. Gen. Microbiol. 139: 1587-1594.

16. Widjojoatmodjo, M.N., Fluit, A.C., Torensma, R., Verdonk, G.P.H.T., and Verhoef, J. 1992. The magnetic immuno polymerase chain reaction assay for direct detection of salmonellae in fecal samples. J. Clin. Microbiol. 30: 3195-3199.

17. Wilson, I. G. 1997. Inhibition and facilitation of nucleic acid amplification. Appl. Environ. Microbiol. 63: 3741-3751.

Variability of the Potato Bacterial Wilt Pathogen, *Ralstonia solanacearum* (E. F. Smith)Yabuuchi *et al.*, in the Philippines

Marina P. Natural[1], Lily Ann D. Lando[2] and Edna M. Jover[3]

[1]Professor, Dept. of Plant Pathology, University of the Philippines Los Baños, College, Laguna; [2]Associate Professor, Benguet State University, La Trinidad, Benguet and [3]Associate Professor, University of Southern Mindanao, Kabacan, Cotabato, Philippines

In the potato growing areas of Benguet and Mountain Province of the Cordillera Region and Bukidnon, Philippines, bacterial wilt has become very severe. Virgin forests have been denuded as farmers have cleared new areas for farming as a consequence of bacterial wilt on existing potato production areas. Baniqued (1998, pers. comm.) reported that in potato growing areas of the Cordillera Region, bacterial wilt has become so severe that some farmers have resorted to soil drenching with formaldehyde and bleach solutions or incorporating cement believing that they would gain temporary relief from the damage caused by the disease. Over 200 plant species have been recorded as hosts of the bacterium, and new host-pathogen combinations are continually being described. For example, Natural and Daquiaog (10) isolated *R. solanacearum* from wilting Indian trees, *Polyalthia longifolia* L. Individual plant species, such as potato, can be hosts to a number of distinct strains. Tomato was observed as the most susceptible host. Fresh isolates of the banana strains or from other hosts like peanut, ginger, or winged bean are highly virulent on tomatoes. Based on personal experience and results of undergraduate thesis, many banana isolates in our collection do not infect tomatoes anymore but remain virulent to bananas after months of storage in sterile distilled water.

This paper will focus on the variability of isolates from potato, based on the traditional but useful characterization like biovar classification, pathogenicity tests, and genetic analysis by polymerase chain reaction using REP-primers. Isolates were collected from Northern and Southern Philippines. Variability studies are important in breeding for host resistance, epidemiology, disease management, ecological competence, and phylogenetic and evolutionary relationships.

Variability of *Ralstonia solanacearum* Based on Host Range

The host range of the potato isolates from Benguet and a few areas in the Mountain Province, Cordillera Region, was very limited. More than 50% were pathogenic to potato only, 19% were pathogenic to potato and tomato and 26% were pathogenic to potato, tomato, and pepper. No potato isolate was able to cause wilt in ginger and banana. Combining the biovar data with the host range, it would seem that the race 3 true potato isolates comprise only 31%. These isolates belong to biovar 2 and are pathogenic to potato, or potato and tomato. Three isolates belong to biovar 2 but were pathogenic also to pepper and are therefore considered as race 1 or the solanaceous strain.

Of the 50 Bukidnon isolates collected, four were pathogenic to potato only and were biovar 2. Most (18 isolates or 54%) were pathogenic to potato, tomato, eggplant, and sweet pepper. Six isolates were pathogenic to the four crops mentioned plus ginger. This study showed that the potato strains from Bukidnon had a wider host range than the isolates from Benguet and Mountain Province. Except for the isolates that were pathogenic to potato only, the other isolates could have originally been isolates of tomato, eggplant, sweet pepper or ginger. Widespread potato production in Bukidnon started only about 5 years ago. The areas planted to potato could have previously been planted to the various crops susceptible to biovar 3 strains. The potato isolates from the Cordillera Region could have no contact with the other crops and did not have the capacity to infect them. Sweet pepper is one of the major crops in the highlands of Benguet and Mountain Province, accounting for 26% of the isolates being pathogenic to potato, tomato and pepper.

Understanding of the potential host range of strains of *R. solanacearum* endemic in any area, and recognition of the existence of strains specialized to particular hosts, is necessary in the effort to devise rational control strategies based on crop rotation.

Biovars

Many potato strains collected in Europe, southern South Africa, and other countries in temperate or mediterranean regions and at high elevations in the tropics are biovar 2, race 3 (1,3,5). The Philippine potato isolates have been found to be mostly biovar 3. Villa (12) who revived isolates maintained by Dr. N.L. Opina's group at the Institute of Plant Breeding (IPB), UP Los Baños and some recent isolates from Davao and Batangas provinces (elevation ~250-450 m asl) reported that 84.4% are biovar 3

Table 1. Biovar distribution of potato isolates of *Ralstonia solanacearum* in the Philippines

Scientist	Year	Number of Isolates	Percentage of biovars			
			I	II	III	IV
Valdez, R.B.	1985	111	0	5.4	70.3	24.3
Villa, J.E.	1997	64	0	16.6	84.4	0.0
Lando, L.A.D.	2002	74	0	30.1	69.3	0.01
Jover, E.M.	2001	50	0	8.0	88.0	4.0

while only 16.6 % are biovar 2. No biovar 1, 4, or 5 strains were isolated. A close look at the isolates indicates that a mixture of biovars 2 and 3 can be isolated in an area. It was noted that the old isolates maintained at IPB were all biovar 3 (25 out of 26 isolates) except for one biovar 2 that was isolated in Piat, Cagayan. A more recent collection of Lando (8) from Benguet, Northern Philippines, which is about 300 to 600m above sea level revealed that biovar 3 predominated (69.3%) followed by biovar 2 (30.1%). Biovars 2 and 3 often times occurred in the same field. There was only one municipality (Paoay, Atok) where all the six isolates were biovar 2. Jover (7) collected 50 isolates from Bukidnon, Southern Philippines (elevation ~300 to 450 m asl) and found that only four of the isolates were biovar 2 and were pathogenic only to potatoes (Table 1).

Genetic Variability of Potato Isolates as Determined by PCR

The combined analysis of ERIC and BOX primers revealed greater variability among the potato isolates. The isolates were clustered based in the area where they were collected (Figure 1). The southern Benguet cluster collected from Baguio, La Trinidad and the Sto. Tomas Experiment Stations were clustered together. Isolates from Bugias also grouped together based on the municipality from which they were collected. The northern Benguet isolates were grouped with isolates from Mankayan, Mt. Province. Mankayan is very near the northern Benguet border. A closer examination of the dendrogram revealed that isolates from adjacent towns were 75–80% similar. Clustering of isolates was not correlated with biovar classification. Biovar 3 isolates were distributed in different towns, either from southern Benguet or from northern Benguet and Mt. Province. The clustering of isolates was not correlated with pathogenicity to various crops.

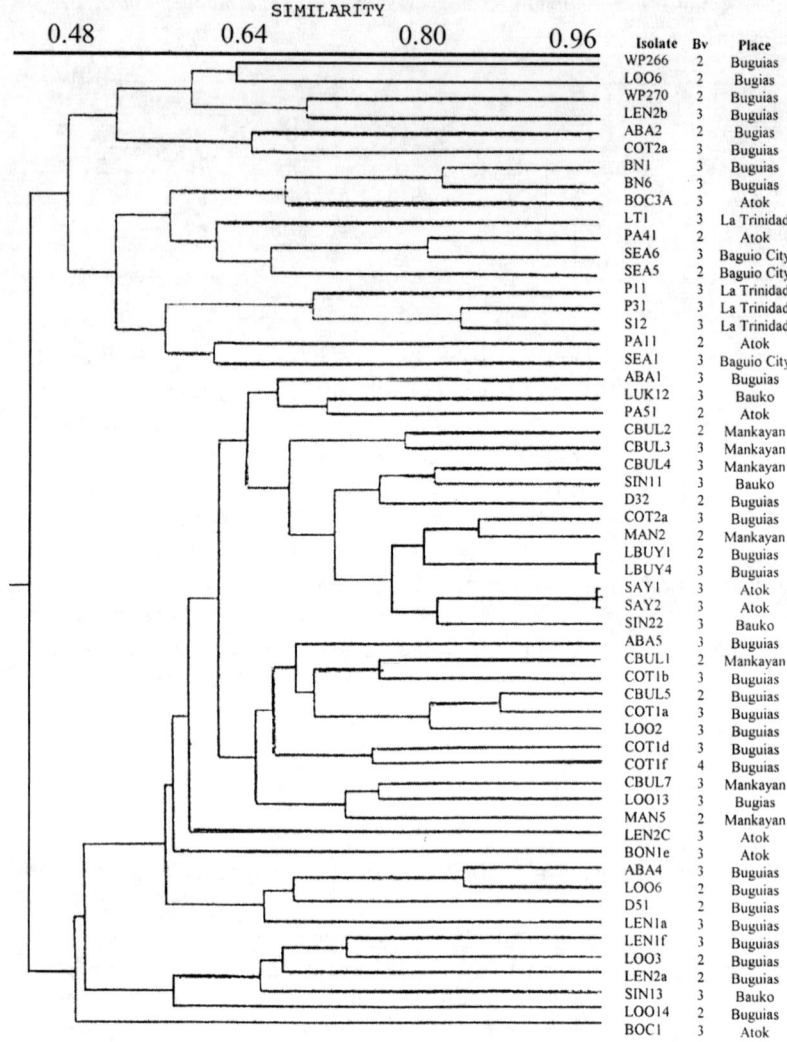

SIMILARITY

				Isolate	Bv	Place
0.48	0.64	0.80	0.96	WP266	2	Buguias
				LOO6	2	Bugias
				WP270	2	Buguias
				LEN2b	3	Buguias
				ABA2	2	Bugias
				COT2a	3	Buguias
				BN1	3	Buguias
				BN6	3	Buguias
				BOC3A	3	Atok
				LT1	3	La Trinidad
				PA41	2	Atok
				SEA6	3	Baguio City
				SEA5	2	Baguio City
				P11	3	La Trinidad
				P31	3	La Trinidad
				S12	3	La Trinidad
				PA11	2	Atok
				SEA1	3	Baguio City
				ABA1	3	Buguias
				LUK12	3	Bauko
				PA51	2	Atok
				CBUL2	2	Mankayan
				CBUL3	3	Mankayan
				CBUL4	3	Mankayan
				SIN11	3	Bauko
				D32	2	Buguias
				COT2a	3	Buguias
				MAN2	2	Mankayan
				LBUY1	2	Buguias
				LBUY4	3	Buguias
				SAY1	3	Atok
				SAY2	3	Atok
				SIN22	3	Bauko
				ABA5	3	Buguias
				CBUL1	2	Mankayan
				COT1b	3	Buguias
				CBUL5	2	Buguias
				COT1a	3	Buguias
				LOO2	3	Buguias
				COT1d	3	Buguias
				COT1f	4	Buguias
				CBUL7	3	Mankayan
				LOO13	3	Bugias
				MAN5	2	Mankayan
				LEN2C	3	Atok
				BON1e	3	Atok
				ABA4	3	Buguias
				LOO6	2	Buguias
				D51	2	Buguias
				LEN1a	3	Buguias
				LEN1f	3	Buguias
				LOO3	2	Buguias
				LEN2a	2	Buguias
				SIN13	3	Bauko
				LOO14	2	Buguias
				BOC1	3	Atok

Fig. 1. Cordillera Isolates. Dendrogram derived by unweighted pair group method, arithmetic mean based on amplified DNA band data obtained using combined ERIC and BOX primers, depicting similarities of potato *Ralstonia solanacearum* isolates collected in Cordillera Region, Northern Luzon.

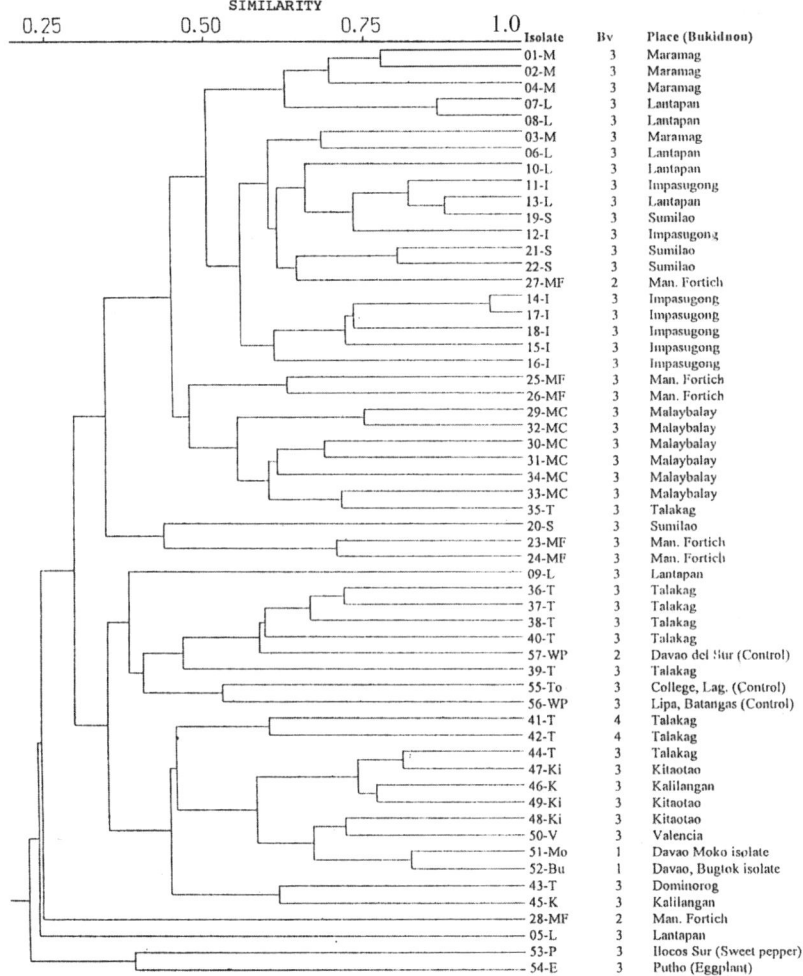

Isolate	Bv	Place (Bukidnon)
01-M	3	Maramag
02-M	3	Maramag
04-M	3	Maramag
07-L	3	Lantapan
08-L	3	Lantapan
03-M	3	Maramag
06-L	3	Lantapan
10-L	3	Lantapan
11-I	3	Impasugong
13-L	3	Lantapan
19-S	3	Sumilao
12-I	3	Impasugong
21-S	3	Sumilao
22-S	3	Sumilao
27-MF	2	Man. Fortich
14-I	3	Impasugong
17-I	3	Impasugong
18-I	3	Impasugong
15-I	3	Impasugong
16-I	3	Impasugong
25-MF	3	Man. Fortich
26-MF	3	Man. Fortich
29-MC	3	Malaybalay
32-MC	3	Malaybalay
30-MC	3	Malaybalay
31-MC	3	Malaybalay
34-MC	3	Malaybalay
33-MC	3	Malaybalay
35-T	3	Talakag
20-S	3	Sumilao
23-MF	3	Man. Fortich
24-MF	3	Man. Fortich
09-L	3	Lantapan
36-T	3	Talakag
37-T	3	Talakag
38-T	3	Talakag
40-T	3	Talakag
57-WP	2	Davao del Sur (Control)
39-T	3	Talakag
55-To	3	College, Lag. (Control)
56-WP	3	Lipa, Batangas (Control)
41-T	4	Talakag
42-T	4	Talakag
44-T	3	Talakag
47-Ki	3	Kitaotao
46-K	3	Kalilangan
49-Ki	3	Kitaotao
48-Ki	3	Kitaotao
50-V	3	Valencia
51-Mo	1	Davao Moko isolate
52-Bu	1	Davao, Bugtok isolate
43-T	3	Dominorog
45-K	3	Kalilangan
28-MF	2	Man. Fortich
05-L	3	Lantapan
53-P	3	Ilocos Sur (Sweet pepper)
54-E	3	Putho (Eggplant)

Fig. 2. Bukidnon Isolates. Dendrogram derived by unweighted pair group method, arithmetic mean based on amplified DNA band data obtained using combined ERIC-BOX-OPD 18 PCR primers, depicting similarities of potato *Ralstonia solanacearum* isolates collected in Bukidnon, Central Mindanao.

The Bukidnon isolates were analyzed using the combined data generated by ERIC, BOX and OPD-18 (a Rapid primer from Operon Technologies). Clustering of isolates was also based on the municipality where the isolates were collected (Figure 2). It did not, however, show that isolates from adjacent towns were more similar. The first major cluster was composed of isolates from Maramag, Lantapan and Impasugong. The next cluster has isolates coming from Manolo Fortich, Malaybalay and Talakag. Impasugong is in between Manolo Fortich and Malaybalay. Two isolates from Manolo Fortich separated to another cluster. The Talakag isolates formed another cluster that was only about 30 % similar.

The use of ERIC and BOX as PCR primers and a rapid primer OPD 18 indicates the existence of a great diversity in the population of potato isolates in the potato growing areas of the Cordillera region and Bukidnon. The presence of out-grouping isolates may indicate the movement of other strains, perhaps through exchange of planting materials. There is also a possibility that genetic exchange between and among these isolates have occurred over time within a geographic area.

The DNA homology pattern of nearly 200 different *R. solanacearum* strains collected from diverse geographical areas representing all five races and biovars were studied by Cook et al (2), and Cook and Sequeira (3). The characteristic most strongly correlated with RFLP data was geographical origin of the strain. This was corroborated by our studies. Division I contained all members of race 1/biovars 3, 4, and 5, and division II contained all members of race 1/biovar 1, and races 2 and 3. This is where the Philippine potato strains belong. They further demonstrated that probably, early in its evolution, *R. solanacearum* divided into two groups, and strains representing RFLP division I evolved in Australasia and division II in America. Race 3 strains that are isolated from Asia, Africa, and Australia are probably introduced with plant materials. Investigation into the fatty acid composition, membrane protein pattern, restriction analysis of a polygalacturonase gene fragment by polymerase chain reaction (PCR) amplification (4,5), and the sequence analysis of 16S rRNA genes (10) supports the broad classification of *R. solanacearum* strains into two divisions.

Acknowledgements

The authors would like to acknowledge the financial assistance provided by ACIAR and UP Los Baños, and the expert advice of Dr. Nenita L. Opina and the technical assistance of Mr. Joey Villa.

Literature Cited

1. Buddenhagen, I.W., and Kelman, A. 1964. Biological and physiological aspects of bacterial wilt caused by *Pseudomonas solanacearum*. Annu. Rev. Phytopathol. 2:203-230.

2. Cook, D., Barlow, E., and Sequeira, L. 1989. Genetic diversity of *Pseudomonas solanacearum*: detection of restriction fragment length polymorphism with DNA probes that specify virulence and hypersensitive response. Mol. Plant Microbe Interact. 2: 113-121.

3. Cook, D., and Sequeira, L. 1994. Strain differentiation of *Pseudomonas solanacearum* by molecular genetic methods. Pages 77-93 in: Bacterial Wilt. The disease and its causative agent, *Pseudomonas solanacearum*. Proceedings of an international symposium, Kaohsiung, Taiwan, ROC, 28-30 October 1992. G.L. Hartman and A.C. Hayward, eds. CAB International, UK.

4. Gillings M.R. and Fahy, P. 1994. Genomic fingerprinting: Towards a unified view of the *Pseudomonas solanacearum* species complex. Pages 95-112 in: Bacterial Wilt. The disease and its causative agent, *Pseudomonas solanacearum*. Proceedings of an international symposium, Kaohsiung, Taiwan, ROC, 28-30 October 1992. G.L. Hartman and A.C. Hayward, eds.

5. Graham, J. and Lloyd, A.B. 1979. Survival of potato strain (race 3) of *Pseudomonas solanacearum* in deeper soil layers. Aust. J. Agric. Res. 30:489-496.

6. Hayward, A.C. 1991. Biology and epidemiology of bacterial wilt caused by *Pseudomonas solanacearum*. Annu. Rev. Phytopathol. 29:65-87.

7. Jover, E.M. 2001. Hypersensitivity and pathogenicity tests, biovar classification and genetic analysis of *Ralstonia solanacearum* (EF Smith) Yabuuchi et al potato isolates collected in the Bukidnon province. PhD Dissertation, Central Mindanao University, Musuan, Bukidnon, Philippines.

8. Lando, L.A.D. 2002. Biovar classification, pathogenicity to various crops and genetic analysis of *Ralstonia solanacearum* (E.F. Smith) Yabuuchi et al potato isolates collected in Benguet, Northern Luzon. PhD. Dissertation, University of the Philippines Los Baños Graduate School, College, Laguna, Philippines.

9. Li, X., Dorch, M., Del Dot, T., Sly, L.I., Stackebrandt, E., and Hayward, A.C. 1993. Phylogenetic studies of the rRNA group II. Pseudomonads based on 16S rRNA gene sequences. J. Appl. Bacteriol. 74: 324-329.

10. Natural, M.P., and Daquiaog, V.R. 1996. Bacterial wilt of Indian tree (*Polyalthia longifolia* Benth and Hook). Philippine Phytopath. 32:127.

11. Valdez, R.B. 1986. Bacterial wilt in the Philippines. Pages 49-56 in: Bacterial wilt diseases in Asia and the South Pacific. G.B. Persley, ed. ACIAR Proc. No. 13. Canberra, Australia.

12. Villa, J.E. 1997. Comparison of techniques to detect *Ralstonia solanacearum* (E.F.Smith) Yabuuchi et al in potato (*Solanum tuberosum* L.) tubers. MS thesis, Philippines Los Baños Graduate School, College, Laguna, Philippines.

Improved Detection of *Ralstonia solanacearum* in Culturable and VBNC State from Water Samples at Low Temperatures

E.G. Biosca[1], P. Caruso[1], E. Bertolini[1], B. Álvarez[1], J.L. Palomo[2], M.T. Gorris[1], and M.M. López[1]

[1]Instituto Valenciano de Investigaciones Agrarias, IVIA, Apartado Oficial 46113, Moncada, Valencia, Spain. [2]Centro Regional de Diagnóstico, Apartado 61, 37080, Salamanca, Spain

Reports about the presence of *Ralstonia solanacearum* biovar 2 in surface water have increased in the past few years in Europe, irrigation water being one of the most important ways of dissemination of this pathogen (4, 5, 8, 13). In fact, *R. solanacearum* is able to survive in water for long periods as a free-living form or associated with *Solanum dulcamara*, in the absence of susceptible cultivated hosts (4, 5). This bacterium can be cultured and detected from water samples during warm months, but during colder months its isolation is usually unsuccessful (4, 5, 8, 11). In addition, it has been recently reported that *R. solanacearum* biovar 2 cells enter the viable but nonculturable (VBNC) state at low temperatures (7, 12). Since the aquatic environment is a reservoir and a vehicle of transmission for this bacterium, specific and sensitive methods are needed to prevent its spread from naturally contaminated water to healthy plants. Thus, the objectives of this work are to improve the detection of *R. solanacearum* from water samples at low temperatures and to evaluate the efficiency of serological and molecular techniques to detect VBNC *R. solanacearum* cells. To improve the detection of *Ralstonia solanacearum* biovar 2 from water samples at low temperatures, we have set up an enrichment procedure that can be combined with DASI-ELISA using specific monoclonal antibodies or PCR. Its ability to detect VBNC *R. solanacearum* cells was also evaluated. With these techniques we were able to detect up to 1-10 CFU/ml of *R. solanacearum* in water of different origins after shaking incubation for 72 h in modified Wilbrink liquid medium at 35°C as well as VBNC *R. solanacearum* cells, induced in water microcosms maintained at 4°C.

Materials and Methods

BACTERIAL STRAINS

Five strains of *R. solanacearum*, one isolated from water (IVIA 2167), three strains from potato (FATE 1609, PD 2762, IVIA 1602.1) and K60 (type strain) were used to prepare spiked water samples in preliminary experiments and for microcosm studies.

DETECTION OF *R. SOLANACEARUM*
IN NATURALLY CONTAMINED WATER SAMPLES

To improve the detection of *R. solanacearum* from water samples, we enriched them in modified Wilbrink broth (MWB) (2). MWB contains sucrose 10g, proteose peptone 5g, K_2HPO_4 0.5g, $MgSO_4$ 0.25g, $NaNO_3$ 0.25g, distilled water 900ml. The MWB was prepared in two steps. After sterilization a second part was added containing the same antibiotics and inhibitors as in SMSA broth (3) at the same concentrations, but omitting tetrazolium salts. Samples were mixed with this enrichment medium at 1:10. After shaking enrichment for 72 h at 35°C, we performed DASI-ELISA using specific monoclonal antibodies (2) or PCR using a modified protocol with existing primers (1,3) after a simple DNA extraction (9). Direct isolation on modified SMSA (mSMSA) medium (4, 6) was used for comparative purposes. When water temperature was below 10°C, water samples were also analysed by the most probable number (MPN) method (10). This involves the mathematical inference of the viable count from the fraction of multiple cultures that fail to show growth in a series of dilution tubes containing a suitable medium. Eleven water samples taken from a river water naturally contaminated with the bacterial wilt pathogen were analyzed.

DETECTION OF VBNC *R. SOLANACEARUM* CELLS

We also evaluated the ability of the enrichment and the developed techniques to detect viable but nonculturable (VBNC) *R. solanacearum* cells. The loss of bacterial culturability was only determined in solid medium according to the definition of Xu *et al.* (14). The dormant state was induced in water microcosms (inoculated with 10^7 CFU/ml) maintained at 4°C as described by van Elsas *et al.*(12).

Results and Discussion

After preliminary studies of detection of *R. solanacearum* in spiked water samples, we selected DASI-ELISA and PCR for their specificity, reliability and in the case of DASI-ELISA, for its usefulness in processing a large number of samples. Tables 1, 2, and 3 show the detection of *R. solanacearum* in natural river water samples taken at different temperatures, before and after enrichment at 29 and 35°C.

Direct isolation of *R. solanacearum* in natural river water samples at 7-8°C was only possible in some samples after plating 1 ml on mSMSA plates (15 cm ∅). Due to the low populations of *R. solanacearum* in these water samples (60-1 CFU/ml), the pathogen was detected before enrichment only by PCR.

Table 1. Detection of *Ralstonia solanacearum* biovar 2 in natural river water samples before enrichment.

No. samples	Month sampled	Water temp.	mSMSA[a]	DASI-ELISA	PCR
3	September	18°C	60	- (3/3)	+ (2/3)
3	October	14°C	15	- (3/3)	+ (2/3)
5	November	7-8°C	1	- (5/5)	+ (5/5)

[a] Average number of *R. solanacearum* CFU/ml detected.

Table 2. Detection of *Ralstonia solanacearum* biovar 2 in natural river water samples after 72 h of enrichment (1:10) at 29° and 35°C in MWB.

No. samples	Month sampled	Enrichment temp.	mSMSA[a]	DASI-ELISA	PCR
3	September	29°C	+ (1/3)	+ (1/3)	+ (2/3)
		35°C	+ (2/3)	+ (2/3)	+ (2/3)
3	October	29°C	+ (3/3)	+ (3/3)	+ (3/3)
		35°C	+ (3/3)	+ (3/3)	+ (3/3)
5	November	29°C	- (5/5)	- (5/5)	+ (4/5)
		35°C	- (5/5)	- (5/5)	+ (4/5)

[a] Average number of *R. solanacearum* CFU/ml detected.

Detection by DASI-ELISA and PCR was improved after enrichment, showing better results at 35°C. When water samples were at 7-8°C isolation was only successful when 10 ml of water in three replicates were analysed by the MPN method, with enrichment at 35°C being more efficient than at 29°C. The number of culturable *R.solanacearum* cells on MWB ranged from 43 to 9 CFU/100ml of water with 95% confidence limits. These methodologies detected 1-10 CFU/ml of *R. solanacearum* in water of different origins after shaking incubation for 72 h in selective enrichment media at 35°C. Further, these results demonstrate that *R. solanacearum* can survive in river water during colder months.

Table 4 shows that with DASI-ELISA and PCR it was possible to detect 10^4 and 1 VBNC CFU/ml, respectively, before enrichment. After enrichment we detected by isolation and ELISA 10^4 *R. solanacearum* CFU that had been unculturable on solid medium for one month. These results

Table 3. MPN enrichment (series of 3 tubes) of *Ralstonia solanacearum* biovar 2 in five natural river water samples after 4 days in MWB medium at 29° and 35°C.

No. samples	Volume analyzed[a]	Enrichment temp.	MPN tubes where *R. solanacearum* was confirmed by		
			mSMSA	DASI-ELISA	PCR
5	10 ml	29° C	+(7/15)	+(9/15)	+(9/15)
		35° C	+(13/15)	+(13/15)	+(15/15)

[a]Sampling of lower volumes yield less efficient (1ml) or unsuccessful (0.1 ml) detection.

Table 4. Detection of *Ralstonia solanacearum* biovar 2 cells after being in the VBNC state, with and without previous enrichment.

Dilutions of *R. solanacearum* VBNC CFU/ml	Detection					
	Before enrichment			After enrichment		
	SMSA	DASI-ELISA	PCR	*R.s.* on SMSA	DASI-ELISA	PCR
10^7- 10^5	-	+	+	+	+	+
10^4	-	+/-	+	+/-	+/-	+
10^3- 1	-	-	+	-	-	+

demonstrate the efficiency of an optimized liquid enrichment medium for the recovery of culturable cells of *R. solanacearum* during a longer period than on solid standard media. Gentle shaking provides aeration and more uniform availability of nutrients than in an agar medium where inhibitors may also occur. These protocols are appropriate for detection of stressed *R. solanacearum* cells in water samples at low temperatures.

Conclusions

The methodologies developed successfully combine high sensitivity due to the selective enrichment medium and incubation conditions with high specificity of the monoclonal antibodies and primers used.

Our results demonstrated the survival of *R. solanacearum* in naturally contaminated water at the low temperatures occurring during colder months and provide tools that may help to design new control strategies.

For the detection of the wilt bacterial pathogen from water samples at low temperatures we propose to use the MPN method with Modified Wilbrink's Broth for 72h at 35°C.

The detection of VBNC cells of *R. solanacearum* in water microcosms at low temperatures confirms the pathogen's survival in winter time.

Acknowledgements

This work was partially supported by the FAIR project PL 97- 3632 funded by the European Union. P. Caruso and B. Álvarez have a grant from the Instituto Valenciano de Investigaciones Agrarias, Valencia, Spain. E. G. Biosca and P. Caruso contributed equally to this study.

Literature Cited

1. Boudazin, G., Le-Roux, A.C., Josi, K., Labarre, P., and Jouan, B. 1999. Design of division specific primers of *Ralstonia solanacearum* and application to the identification of European isolates. Eur. J. Plant Pathol. 105:373-380.
2. Caruso, P., Gorris, M.T., Cambra, M., Palomo, J.L., Collar, J., and López, M. M. 2002. Enrichment-DASI-ELISA for sensitive detection of *Ralstonia solanacearum* in asymptomatic potato tubers using a specific monoclonal antibody. Appl. Environ. Microbiol. 68:3634-3638.

3. Elphinstone, J.G., Hennessy, J., Wilson, J.K., and Stead, D.E. 1996. Sensitivity of different methods for the detection of *Ralstonia solanacearum* in potato tuber extracts. Bull. OEPP/EPPO Bull. 26:663-678.
4. Elphinstone, J.G., Standford, H., and Stead, D.E. 1998a. Detection of *Ralstonia solanacearum* in potato tubers, *Solanum dulcamara* and associated irrigated water. Pages 133-39 in: Bacterial Wilt Disease: Molecular and Ecological Aspects. P. Prior, C. Allen, and J. Elphinstone, eds. Springer, Berlin.
5. Elphinstone, J.G., Standford, H., and Stead, D.E. 1998b. Survival and transmission of *Ralstonia solanacearum* in aquatic plants of *Solanum dulcamara* and associated surface water in England Bull. OEPP/EPPO Bull. 28:93-94.
6. Englebrecht, M.C. 1994. Modification of a semi-selective medium for the isolation and quantification of *Pseudomonas solanacearum*. Pages 3-5 in: Bacterial Wilt Newsletter. A.C. Hayward, ed. Australian Centre for International Agricultural Research, Canberra, Australia.
7. Grey, B.E., and Steck, T.R. 2001. The viable but nonculturable state of *Ralstonia solanacearum* may be involved in long-term survival and plant infection. Appl. Environ. Microbiol. 67:3866-3872.
8. Janse, J.D., and Schans, J. 1998. Experiences with the diagnosis and epidemiology of bacterial brown rot (*Ralstonia solanacearum)* in The Netherlands. Bull. OEPP/EPPO Bull. 28:65-67.
9. Llop, P., Caruso, P., Cubero, J., Morente, C., and López, M.M. 1999. A simple extraction procedure for efficient routine detection of pathogenic bacteria in plant material by polymerase chain reaction. J. Microbiol. Methods 37:23-31.
10. McCrady, M.H. 1915. The numerical interpretation of fermentation tube results. J. Infec. Dis. 17:183.
11. Palomo, J.L., Caruso, P., Gorris, M.T., López, M.M., and Garcia-Benavides, P. 2000. Comparación de métodos de detección de *Ralstonia solanacearum* en aguas superficiales. X Congreso de la Sociedad Española de Fitopatología, p 120. Valencia.
12. van Elsas, J.D., Kastelein, P., de Vries, Ph.M., and van Overbeek, L.S. 2001. Effects of ecological factors on the survival and physiology of *Ralstonia solanacearum* bv. 2 in agricultural drainage water. Can. J. Microbiol. 47:842-854.
13. Wright, A J. 1998. Legislative measures to prevent the introduction and spread of *Ralstonia solanacearum* in the European Union. Bull. OEPP/EPPO Bull. 28:513-518.
14. Xu, H., Roberts, N., Singleton, F., Atwell, R., Grimes, D., and Colwell R. 1982. Survival and viability of nonculturable *Escherichia coli* and *Vibrio cholerae* in the estuarine and marine environment. FEMS Microbiol Ecol. 8:313-323.

Subject Index

507

Phenotype conversion, 112, 207, 323, 329, 351, 359
Phylotype, 14, 205, 406, 415, 439
Piper spp. *See* long pepper
Potato, 1, 9, 29, 61, 81, 97, 125, 139, 145, 159, 167, 197, 205, 471, 493
  latent infection, 30, 169, 199, 208, 263
  resistance in, 197, 215, 229, 253, 261
Pseudomonas
  celebensis, 396, 415
  fluorescens, 103, 215, 375
  syringae, 278, 325, 339, 362, 375, 437
  syzygii, 397, 411, 449
Quantitative trait loci (QTL), 231, 301
Quarantine, 21, 121, 126
Ralstonia solanacearum
  colony morphology, 86, 366
  genome sequence, 335
Resistance. *See* individual hosts
Rhizobium
  leguminosarum, 103
  meliloti, 103, 375
Rhizome, solarization of, 185

Soil treatments, 39, 123, 148, 161, 178
Solanum dulcamara, 1, 13, 31, 82, 210, 501
  latent infection, 210
Solanum melongena. See Eggplant
Solanum tuberosum. See Potato
Survival, 114, 205
  soil, 32, 40, 206, 425
  water, 31, 40, 206, 214, 501
Tobacco, 9, 51, 123, 159, 161, 328, 359, 362, 486
  resistance in, 121, 230, 253, 279, 362
Tomato, 2, 9, 31, 57, 81, 111, 159, 177, 328, 330, 353, 362, 368, 373, 407, 471, 486, 493
  gene mapping, 301
  resistance in, 73, 133, 178, 230, 257, 277, 285, 301, 387
Viable but non-culturable (VBNC), 32, 40, 103, 207, 356, 442, 484, 501
Weed hosts, 1, 31, 73, 123, 145, 197, 213
  latent infection, 81
Xanthomonas campestris, 103, 362, 375
Zingiber officinale. See Ginger

Author Index

510